Tuberculosis of the Skeletal System

Bones, Joints, Spine and Bursal Sheaths

SEVENTH EDITION

SM Tuli
MBBS MS PhD FAMS
Senior Consultant
Department of Spinal Diseases and Orthopedics
Moolchand Hospital
Lajpat Nagar, New Delhi, India

Formerly
Chairman
Department of Orthopedics
Banaras Hindu University
Varanasi, Uttar Pradesh, India
Professor and Head
Department of Orthopedics
University College of Medical Sciences
New Delhi, India

Forewords
M Shantharam Shetty
Apurv Mehra
Raj Bahadur

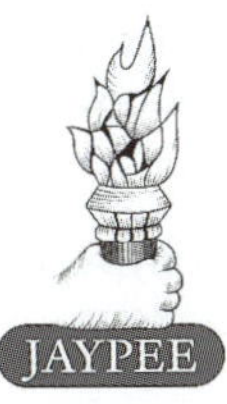

JAYPEE BROTHERS MEDICAL PUBLISHERS
The Health Sciences Publisher
New Delhi | London

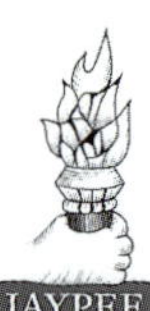

Jaypee Brothers Medical Publishers (P) Ltd

Headquarters
EMCA House, 23/23-B
Ansari Road, Daryaganj
New Delhi 110 002, India
Landline: +91-11-23272143, +91-11-23272703
+91-11-23282021, +91-11-23245672
e-mail: jaypee@jaypeebrothers.com

Corporate Office
4838/24, Ansari Road, Daryaganj
New Delhi 110 002, India
Phone: +91-11-43574357
Fax: +91-11-43574314
e-mail: jaypee@jaypeebrothers.com

Overseas Office
JP Medical Ltd.
83, Victoria Street, London
SW1H 0HW (UK)
Phone: +44-20 3170 8910
e-mail: info@jpmedpub.com

EU GPSR Authorised Representative
Logos Europe, 9 rue Nicolas Poussin
17000, La Rochelle, France
Phone: +33 (0) 6 67 93 73 78
e-mail: contact@logoseurope.eu

Website: www.jaypeebrothers.com

Website: www.jaypeedigital.com

Inquiries for bulk sales may be solicited at: jaypee@jaypeebrothers.com

***Tuberculosis of the Skeletal System* / SM Tuli**
First Edition: 1991
Seventh Edition: **2026**
ISBN: 978-93-7202-872-0
Printed at: Samrat Offset Pvt. Ltd.

Dedicated with Gratitudes to

Shanti Tuli and Ram Lal Tuli my Parents;
Prof KS Grewal, Prof PK Duraiswami and Prof Balu Sankaran my teachers;
and a large number of my stimulating students, and my ungrudging patients,
who provided me the opportunities to study and enjoy
the Science and Art of Medicine

Foreword to the Seventh Edition

It is indeed a privilege and an honor to be asked to pen the foreword for the *seventh edition* of this outstanding book, *"Tuberculosis of the Skeletal System"*, presented to the orthopedic fraternity of the world by a great teacher, clinician, surgeon, and researcher—*Professor Surendra Mohan Tuli.*

I had the unique opportunity to know Professor Tuli from my postgraduate days in Delhi in the late 1960s. His unparalleled quest for knowledge and his energy, even at this age, are God-given gifts bestowed on only a few.

Tuberculosis, as a disease, is as old as mankind. The transformation that has occurred—particularly in the management of *skeletal tuberculosis*—is remarkable. The journey from patients being crippled, deformed, and in chronic pain to achieving *normal functional ability and longevity of life* stands as a testament to persistent research and surgical innovation. Much of the credit for this achievement goes to *Dr Tuli,* who not only published this remarkable book in 1991 but has re-edited it *seven times*, each edition enriched with new insights and advancements for the betterment of patient's care and teaching.

From the concept of the *"middle path regimen"* to the various types of internal fixations, all are well illustrated across the *26 chapters* of this book. Truly, it is a *Bible of Skeletal Tuberculosis* for learning students, practicing clinicians, surgeons, and teachers across the globe. Professor Tuli has established a *legacy* for teachers and researchers to follow. Millions of patients around the world afflicted with skeletal tuberculosis owe a natural tribute to his great work.

We pray for his continued health. May his vision and mentorship keep guiding the orthopedic fraternity for generations to come.

I would like to conclude with these immortal lines:

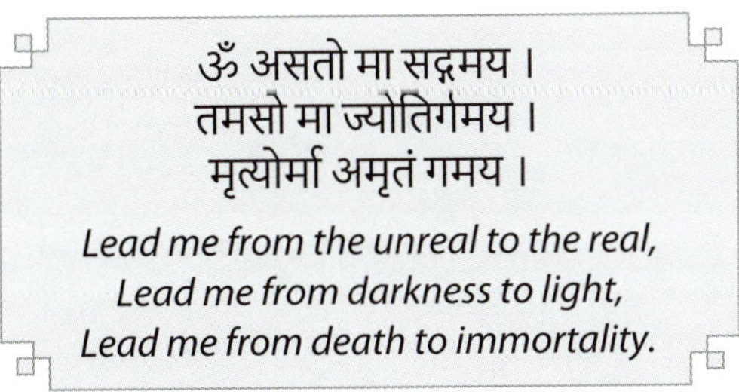

M Shantharam Shetty
MS(Orthopedics) FRCS(England) FACS FAMS
Pro-Chancellor, NITTE (Deemed to be University)
Chairman, Tejasvini Hospital Group of Institutions
AO Trustee 2006–2011 and Past Chairman AO Trauma India Council
Past President, Indian Orthopaedic Association
Mangaluru, Karnataka, India

Foreword to the Seventh Edition

"If" you are holding this book, I want you to know that here each chapter is a hand extended by the Legend himself Professor Dr SM Tuli and as if he himself whispers in each line "We will walk through this book together." The book's language connects with you right from the beginning, it embraces you with strong concepts, clear guidelines, and practical tips of not only understanding *Skeletal Tuberculosis* but also *Mastering* it. This line is very apt for this book, "Some stories are not written with ink they are carved into the heart."

"If" I have to pen down my favorite line from the book I loved this right from my residency days "*Mycobacterium* and humans have lived in symbiosis since the time humans arrived on Earth." This describes the in-depth analysis of not only the disease, the subject but also the life in broader perspective.

"If" you are holding this masterpiece edited seven times by Professor Tuli himself remember it is not for the bookshelf but it is for your table. The book goes beyond tuberculosis and it will enrich you with vast experience of Professor SM Tuli sir spanned over last seven decades. He thought of this book in 1975 worked relentlessly for 16 years to release its first edition in 1991 and subsequently edited it seven times with unparallel dedication. It is very aptly said that it is a gift from India to the world often described as *"With a touch of class and a stamp of authority"* lines Mr Harsha Bhogle would often use for cricketing shorts played by The great Mr Sachin Tendulkar.

"If" we only value that patience and calm mind can build great things and refer to shloka from *Bhagvad Geeta*.

"Shanay Shanay (शनैः शनैः)"

Which means "step by step".

It is absolutely true for the hardwork and dedication Professor Dr SM Tuli has shown in building this book, his devotion to patients, his teachings to his students, and love to his family members, each is built with human warmth which radiates from Professor Tuli's personality too. He always keeps saying to all of us *"The Learning Never Ends."*

"If—" was a poem written by Mr Rudyard Kipling in 1907 that got him the noble prize I would like to dedicate lines from it for Sir:

"If you can talk with crowds and keep your virtue,
Or walk with Kings nor lose the common touch,...
Yours is the Earth and everything that's in it
And—which is more—you will be a Man, my son!"

Dedicated to a "Man" whose life is an example for everyone and his work which will always stand in "History" as one of the greatest academic contributions.

Apurv Mehra
MBBS MS(Orthopedics) DNB(Orthopedics)
Author, Motivational Speaker
Founder, Conceptual Orthopedics
Vidya Jeevan Orthopedics Centre
and Vidya Jeevan Experience Centre
Director Orthopedics, Max Hospital, New Delhi, India

Foreword to the Seventh Edition

It is a distinct privilege to pen the foreword for the seventh edition of *"Tuberculosis of the Musculoskeletal System"*. I dreamt 50 years back to be student of Professor Tuli and God was kind enough to grace me with this lifelong opportunity at Banaras Hindu University, Varanasi. There can be no better recognition for me other than in my lifetime to write the foreword for the gospel on *"Musculoskeletal Tuberculosis"* written by none other than my own Guru—*Professor (Dr) Surender Mohan Tuli.*

For over six decades, Professor SM Tuli has stood as a colossus in the field of orthopedics, a "teacher of teachers" whose wisdom has shaped generations of surgeons. This textbook is not merely a compilation of facts; it is the repository of a philosophy—the "Middle Path"—that has brought sanity to surgical decision-making and relief to millions. This is a book which covers "A to Z of Tuberculosis" and recommended for clinicians, academicians and researchers dealing with musculoskeletal tuberculosis across all paths of career. It is beyond my comprehension to think that ever any student of orthopedics in my country can ever pass the exit examination of "Master of Orthopedics" or "Diplomat of National Board" without reading this compendium which I rate as equivalent to "Hutchinson's Clinical Methods in Medicine."

We stand today at a precarious juncture. "Biology is ever-evolving," and we face a post-pandemic landscape where the control of tuberculosis has regressed. We are witnessing a resurgence of neglected cases presenting with pathologies reminiscent of the prechemotherapeutic era-massive abscesses and severe deformities. Concurrently, the adaptive genius of *Mycobacterium tuberculosis* has birthed multi-drug-resistant (MDR) and extensively drug-resistant (DR) "superbugs" that threaten to render our standard pharmacopeia obsolete.

In this turbulent context, the seventh edition arrives not a moment too soon. It distinguishes itself by reaffirming the "Middle Path"—Professor Tuli's scientifically validated conviction that the "cold abscess" is a biologically active environment capable of resolution with chemotherapy. It reminds us that the goal of treatment is not radiographic perfection, but the restoration of the patient to a life of dignity and economic productivity.

This edition comprehensively modernizes that classic philosophy. It bridges past wisdom with the technological arsenal of the future, integrating molecular diagnostics like GeneXpert Ultra and next-generation sequencing. It incorporates the latest "BPAL" (bedaquiline, pretomanid, and linezolid) regimens. Reflecting the seismic shift toward shorter, all-oral cures for drug-resistant disease. Furthermore, it addresses "immune-potentiating techniques" and "neglected musculoskeletal injuries," reflecting a deep empathy for the suffering of the common man.

Professor Tuli remains an enigma-a clinician who can quote invictus and the latest WHO guidelines with equal fluency. This book is his "living" gift to the world. I am certain that this seventh edition will serve as a beacon of knowledge for orthopedic surgeons and neurosurgeons worldwide, guiding us through the "crossroads" of a changing disease spectrum.

I commend this volume to the medical fraternity with the highest enthusiasm and deepest reverence. Professor Tuli's life is the best lively expression and epitome of immortal words by Swami Vivekanand. *"It is a privilege to serve mankind, for this is the worship of God. God is here, in all these human souls".*

Raj Bahadur
BSc MSOrth FICA FIMSA FAMS FRCS FPASc FIIOPM
President, AIIMS Rishikesh, Uttarakhand, India
Director, Regional Spinal Injuries Centre
Former Vice Chancellor, Baba Farid University of Health Sciences, Punjab, India

Foreword to the First Edition

It is a pleasure to write this foreword to Dr SM Tuli's book *Tuberculosis of the Skeletal System*. It has a great deal of relevance to orthopedic surgeons in developing countries. Since many cases are missed in their early stages, particularly in adults when manifestations of the disease are masked by other problems of aging, it is important for all the physicians to be aware of the early clinicoradiological features.

With the spread of acquired immune deficiency syndrome to all the countries of the globe in some measure or other, there is every likelihood of the problem again cropping up in developed countries as well. This book is, therefore, timely. With the vast experience of the lifetime that Dr Tuli has had in the field, particularly in clinical diagnosis, operative and conservative management, it would be a reference book in the many libraries of the world. Dr Tuli has been an enthusiastic teacher and his talents as a writer have provided him with the tools required for clear message for the needs of busy residents and orthopedic surgeons. We also should remember that adult skeletal manifestations of tuberculous disease in affluent and developing countries quite frequently occur in patients with diabetes mellitus, an observation often forgotten by the young orthopedic surgeon. I wish the book and the author success in the endeavor to enlighten orthopedic surgeons and physicians all over the world.

Balu Sankaran
FRCS
Senior Consultant
Department of Orthopedics
St Stephen's Hospital
Tees Hazari, Delhi, India
Formerly, Director, General Health Services
Government of India
WHO Consultant in Orthopedics and Rehabilitation

Preface to the Seventh Edition

India has announced eliminating tuberculosis by the year 2025, much earlier than WHO target of global elimination by the year 2035. One can appreciate the concern and enthusiasm. However, chances of increase in the global burden of disease are not likely to decrease because of deprivations created by man-made tragedies or natural calamities. The data projected on World Refugee Day suggested that approximately 80 million people have been displaced worldwide due to war, persecution, and violence in 2018–2019. Pockets of deprivation create crowded living, undernourishment, smoking, alcohol and drug abuse, diabetes, and HIV infection, thus perpetuating and spreading mycobacterial infections and disease.

Of the 10 million new tuberculous infections reported globally (in 2018) 2.15 million are from India. According to WHO report, eight countries accounted for 66% of new patients: India, China, Indonesia, Philippines, Pakistan, Nigeria, Bangladesh, and South Africa. Disease notification, however, is still an area of concern.

In addition to high tuberculosis disease burden, these countries also account for maximum drug-resistant patients (nearly 130,000) to first-line multidrug resistance (MDR) antitubercular drugs. Most of the cases of drug resistance are due to lack of communication, compliance, and inadequate drugs.

World Health Organization has been warning the nations regarding antimicrobial resistance (AMR) when the "germs" do not respond to the drugs designated to kill them. AMR is increasing worldwide and can affect anyone, of any age, in any part of the world and relate to any germ, bacteria, and viruses.

Generally, there is no single way of managing orthopedic problems (infections), opinions of various scholars have been discussed. However, emphasis has been made on current, safe, effective, and cost-effective options. The present-day clinicians have the facilities to diagnose and treat the patients at a predestructive or early destructive phase. The outcome for most of such patients is nearly complete function and lasting healed status under the influence of effective antituberculous drugs. Surgical knife needs to be used as an adjunct for prevention and treatment of complications. Orthopedic clinicians today possess rich knowledge and skillful hands to make the most rational therapeutic options for the patients.

Pathological relations of *Homo sapiens* did get some global attention by the creation of international organizations, such as United Nations and World Health Organization after the World War II. Many enthusiastic members of the civil societies have also come forward to inform and educate the general population regarding various aspects of tuberculosis with sensitivity and concerns [Tuberculosis: India's Ticking Time Bomb—Chapal Mehra (Ed.)]. Resistant tuberculosis, such as other airborne diseases [coronavirus disease 2019 (COVID-19) included] has the potential for international spread. National TB Control Program of India is establishing MDR-TB centers attached to every medical college in the country.

The millennial generation observed the Global Havoc caused by COVID-19 (probably the first in their lifetime). This would hopefully induce introspection, redemption, and global empathy to care for each other rather than perpetuate man-made catastrophy. Civil societies all over the world must aim to make "Public Health Facilities" as a global requirement. All countries "rich" and "middle-income group" or "developing" have to join hands to mitigate human suffering and eliminate pockets of deprivation with availability of physical and digital communication. The earth at present is a global village and there is need for uniform and practical methodologies (the science has many) to control and eliminate at least the communicable diseases—if our neighbors are disease free, we will be disease free too. WHO sounds that nearly 4,100 people lose life due to tuberculosis daily in the world.

I pray the bright millennial generation is able to implement their efforts to eliminate (at least) tuberculosis and communicable diseases to make the Globe healthier place to enjoy life.

SM Tuli

Preface to the First Edition

Tuberculous disease in man predominantly affects the humanity in the eastern hemisphere of the world. Up to three quarters of the world's population lives in the eastern hemisphere and it is here that many live poorly nourished, overcrowded and in subnormal social conditions. Such pockets would keep on perpetuating human-cultures as media for the *Mycobacterium tuberculosis*. In an increasingly shrinking world, many persons from such pockets due to economic reasons would be interacting and dealing with the society in the affluent parts of the world. Thus, prevention and treatment of tuberculosis should not be a concern only of the East and poor but also of the West and affluent. For elimination of this disease from the face of mother earth, we must improve the social standards of life for all, and alleviate poverty.

Last three decades have seen such a tremendous improvement in the therapeutic armamentarium available in the biological control of tuberculosis that the present-day physician has picked up courage to challenge the long established norms for the treatment of skeletal tuberculosis. Removing or segregating such patients, to the sanatoria, aspiration of cold abscesses through the "antigravity points", dissemination of tuberculous infection as miliary tuberculosis or meningitis (especially after surgery), development of nonhealing postoperative ulcers and sinuses, amyloid disease due to chronic suppurations, treatment by enforced recumbency to patients in plaster-beds, plaster-jackets, and plaster-casts for 12 to 18 months should now form a part of history of medicine. With biological control of disease by the employment of modern antitubercular drugs, the present-day orthopedist and physician can give a better quality of life to the patient and better function to the involved joint. We have now broken the myth that, "antitubercular drugs do not penetrate the skeletal tuberculous lesions in sufficient concentrations", and "ankylosis of the joint is the only method to achieve no recurrence of disease". If diagnosed and managed effectively by "functional treatment" (i.e. by repetitive exercises of the joint rather than immobilization), early disease can resolve completely; in moderately advanced disease, many joints would heal with retention of functional arc of motion for many years; and in advanced disease of hip, elbow and other joints, surgical treatment can offer a mobile joint with healed status. Fusion may be confined predominantly for too painful and advanced a disease of the knee joint. One day in the burgeoning field of joint replacement (prosthetic or biological) more sophisticated mobilizing procedures may be available for the burnt-out disease. Though science and knowledge are universal, however, the art of its application to the people must naturally reflect the local concerns, priorities, resources, environments, social customs and the needs of the society. For this purpose, personal observations are discussed here with those of contemporary researchers reported in the easily accessible literature.

The first part of the book is devoted to the general principles, and therefore, is applicable to the disease of any part of the skeletal system. The second part is organized chapter-wise to each region of the body. Each chapter more or less follows a uniform pattern presenting pathogenesis, clinical features, radiological findings, differential diagnosis, methods of treatment, role of surgical treatment, surgical technique and relevant anatomy. Each chapter in the second part stands by itself, and both the novice and the relatively inexperienced would be able to follow the management with ease. Part three of the book deals with various aspects of tuberculosis of the spine which constitutes nearly 50 percent of all cases of osteoarticular tuberculosis. This part would be of special interest to physicians, neurologists and neurosurgeons in addition to orthopedic specialists. For convenience of consultation, the bibliography has been arranged separately for spinal tuberculosis and for extra-spinal tuberculosis. Some common references may be found in either part.

It is hoped that this book will be of great assistance to the trainees in orthopedics and infectious diseases, to the experienced surgeons working in the developing countries, to the specialists in the affluent societies (where the disease is misdiagnosed) who encounter this condition only infrequently, to the general medical practitioners on whom many patients would depend upon for follow-up treatment. Even the most experienced orthopedic surgeon would find enjoyment in perusing the illustrations and the text reflecting total change in the methodology of treatment.

This treatise is an expansion of the book *Tuberculosis of the Spine* written in 1975. I was encouraged to take up this project essentially because the younger generation of the enquiring orthopedic surgeons asked for it, whenever I interacted with them in the class, workshops and conferences. Whatever is presented here is based upon nearly 30 years of close observations on clinical behavior, radiological features, operative findings and laboratory studies. Most of the work referred to in this book was done in the Department of Orthopedics, Institute of Medical Sciences, Banaras Hindu University, Varanasi, Uttar Pradesh, India. It is but natural that cooperative effort of a large number of outstanding colleagues has been drawn upon. Over these years, wittingly or unwittingly, I provoked controversies and discussions on many areas of orthopedic tuberculosis. Many friends and colleagues were subjected to this harassment. I admire the tolerance shown towards me by Prof BP Varma (late), Prof TP Srivastava, Dr SV Sharma, Dr SC Goel, and Dr SK Saraf. I am indebted to them for the pleasure and profit of many stimulating exchanges of ideas during many years of fruitful association.

I would like to thank many of my technical staff and medical photoartists for their timely and continued assistance. Mr S Chaudhury, Mr OP Gupta, Mr GC Saxena, Mr AP Mathur, Mr K Raman, Mr Vipul Tuli helped in preparing the data, photographs, line illustrations, typescript and other associated jobs. Shri Jitendar P Vij (Group Chairman), Mr Ankit Vij (Managing Director) and Mr MS Mani (Group President) of M/s Jaypee Brothers Medical Publishers (P) Ltd, New Delhi, have been of tremendous help in the matters of editing, layout of text and illustrations, and printing. The get-up of this book speaks for itself.

Part of the material in this monograph appears in the articles in the Journal of Bone and Joint Surgery, Clinical Orthopedics and Related Research, Acta Orthopedica Scandinavia, and Tuberculosis of the Spine. JP Lippincott Company, Philadelphia, William and Wilkins Company, Baltimore, and Amerind Publishing Company, New Delhi, kindly permitted me to adopt and reproduce some of the illustrations which appeared in their respective publications: *Orthopedics Principles and their Application* by Sameul L Turek, and *Atlas of Orthopedic Exposures* by Toufick Nicola.

Acknowledgements would be incomplete without thanks to my loving wife Swarn whose conscientious assistance in preparation of the text, index, bibliography and correction of proofs, and affectionate understanding helped make this work possible. Dr Neena and Dr Varuna, our daughters, tolerated many of my eccentricities during the period of preparation of this book.

SM Tuli

Acknowledgments

No purposeful writing can be done without peace at home, and this was provided to me by my wife Swarn (literally meaning "gold"), and our daughters Dr Neena and Dr Varuna through different phases of life. All photographs were formatted for presentations by Mr Amit Kumar, the manuscript was typed-revised-retyped by Mr Kundan Kumar Thakur, all from VIMHANS Hospital, New Delhi, India. I am thankful to my associates Dr Varun Kapoor, Dr Mohapatra, and Dr Deepak Thakur who collected many illustrations and images for addition to seventh edition.

The preparation for the "next edition" in clinical subjects starts before the release of the current edition. The raw text material with many deletions, modifications, and additions reached the publishing house. Many new illustrations cut and pasted were sent for preparation for publication. The whole raw material was deposited in the publishing house as small bits over many months, where it was formatted as a beautiful book.

My sincere appreciation also goes to Shri Jitendar P Vij (Group Chairman), Mr Ankit Vij (Managing Director), and Mr MS Mani (Group President) of M/s Jaypee Brothers Medical Publishers (P) Ltd, New Delhi, India, for their support to this project.

The dedicated team coordinated by Ms Pooja Bhandari [Director—Production (Books and Journals)], Mr Ajay Kumar Sharma [DGM—Production (Books & Journals)], Ms Sunita Katla (Executive Assistant to Group Chairman and Publishing Manager), and all the Production Team Members at M/s Jaypee Brothers Medical Publishers (P) Ltd made the whole process of completion less stressful and more enjoyable.

I would also like to appreciate Ms Seema Dogra (Cover Visualizer), and Ms Lakshmi Popli (Proofreader), Mr Shubham Pundir (Typesetter), and Mr Varun Rajoria (Graphic Designer), Sabyasachi Hazra (Director—PG & PNR), Nikita Chauhan (Publishing Manager), Aarti Kushwah (Development Editor) of M/s Jaypee Brothers Medical Publishers (P) Ltd, New Delhi, for their hard work to complete this project.

I acknowledge them all and appreciate their contribution.

SM Tuli

Contents

Section 1: General Considerations

Section 3: Tuberculosis of the Spine

SECTION 1

General Considerations

CHAPTER 1

Epidemiology and Prevalence

Tuberculous bacilli have lived in symbiosis with mankind since time immemorial. In India, Rig Veda and Atharva Veda (3500–1800 BC approx.), Samhita of Charaka and Sushruta (1000 and 600 BC approx.), have mention of this disease by the name Yakshma in all its forms (Duraiswami and Tuli 1971). Greco-Roman civilization recognized it as phthisis or consumption (Formicola et al. 1987). Tuberculous lesions have been recorded in Egyptian mummies (3300 BC). In the Western World, the clinical features and communicability of tuberculosis were known before 1000 BC (Yeager 1963). Lichtor and Lichtor (1957) also reported paleopathological evidence of tuberculosis of bones, joints and spine in prehistoric humans.

Percival Pott first described tuberculosis of the spinal column in 1779, stating a classical description as destruction of the disc space and the adjacent vertebral bodies, collapse of spinal element and progressive kyphotic deformity. The physicians in the affluent countries do not have much experience in dealing with spinal tuberculosis and are, thus, unaccustomed to entertain the diagnosis of tuberculosis even for "appropriate clinical settings". Diagnostic delay in affluent societies is, thus not uncommon. Refugees, homeless, intravenous drug abusers, HIV patients, alcoholics, diabetics elderly, and people with poor nutrition are immunosuppressed and at the risk of infection. Therapeutically immunosuppressed, organ transplant recipients, patients on long-term prednisolone therapy, and patients on cancer chemotherapy are all at increased risk of tuberculous infection.

It was the celebrated French physician Laennec (1781–1826), inventor of the stethoscope, who discovered in the beginning of 19th century, the basic microscopic lesion, the "tubercle", the name by which the disease is universally known at present. It is an irony of fate that Laennec, himself at the early age of 45, fell prey to this dreaded disease.

The world at large has nearly 30 million people suffering from tuberculosis. Due to marked improvement in the socioeconomic status of affluent countries and the availability of therapeutically effective antitubercular drugs, up to early 1980s, there was great hope for complete elimination of the disease. Unfortunately, the optimism was shortlived because of the impact of acquired immunodeficiency syndrome (AIDS) pandemic. Tuberculosis has again become epidemic in many parts of the world (Barnes 1993, Patel 1995, Reichman 1997, Tuli 2013, Vielgut 2022, Panico 2023). After 1985, many affluent countries are recording an increase in the number of patients by 10–20% annually. According to current estimates of WHO, tuberculosis now kills 3 million people a year worldwide. There is paucity of authentic figures at the national level regarding the incidence of disease in India and other developing countries. However, it is estimated that India alone has got one-fifth of the total world population of tuberculous patients. Thus, there are nearly 6 million radiologically proven cases of tuberculosis in India, and perhaps a quarter of these are sputum positive (Editorial, Clinician 1968). Of all the patients suffering from tuberculosis, nearly 1–3% have involvement of the skeletal system.

Although osteoarticular tuberculosis was becoming a disappearing problem (prior to 1985) in many Western countries, however, in economically developing countries like Nigeria, India, Southeast Asia and Korea this continued to pose one of the major public health problems. A surgeon could gain experience in the management of tuberculosis of the bone and joints only if he chooses to work in economically less developed countries (Editorial, Br Med J 1968). The adjoining graph **(Fig. 1.1)** is a broad indicator of the incidence of tuberculosis in Europe. One can appreciate that marked reduction of the incidence occurred much before the discovery and availability of BCG vaccination or the effective antitubercular drugs. It is obvious that for a triumph over this disease the socioeconomic status of the society in general must be improved. Unfortunately, any major advances in the economic uplift of the people usually occur in small increments. Tuberculosis will exist in man so long as there are pockets of malnutrition, poor sanitation, living in crowded areas, exanthematous fevers, repeated pregnancies, immunodeficient states, alcohol and drug abuse, diabetes and advanced age present in the society. For the same reasons, and because of more frequent and convenient exchange of population (or migration) between various countries, even affluent countries can, however, not remain absolutely immune from this disease (Scott 1982, Hayes et al. 1996, Sandher 2007, Saudher 2007, Mallolas 1988, WHO 2012, Miller et al. 2013, Jutte et al. 2014, Dunn 2018, Vielgut 2022, Panico 2023, Rickent 2023). Nearly 82 million people were reported, displaced and enforced to migration due to man made tragedies (years 2021–2022).

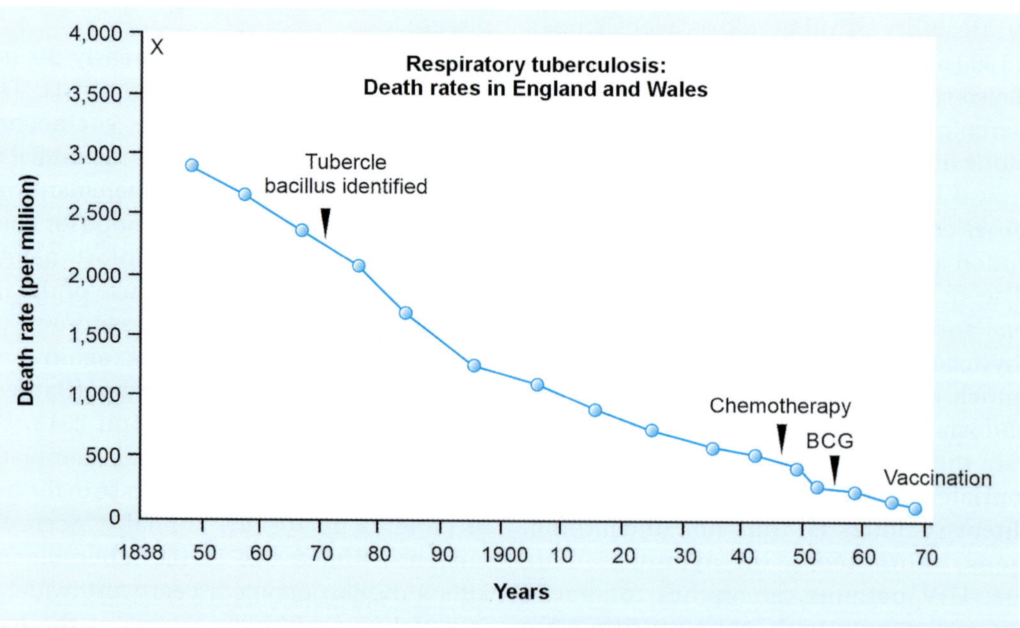

Fig. 1.1: It indirectly reflects the incidence of tuberculous disease in England. The incidence was markedly lowered not by chemotherapy or vaccination but by improvement in the socioeconomic and nutritional status of the society.

REGIONAL DISTRIBUTION

Like other skeletal structures, vertebral column may lodge any infectious process. The most common chronic vertebral infection, however, is tuberculosis. Even in a country like UK where tuberculosis was almost eradicated, Shaw and Thomas (1963) reported that out of 72 cases of surgically explored chronic infectious lesions of the spine, 52 (72%) were proved to be tuberculous, and 12 lesions (16.7%) were thought tuberculous on clinical and radiological grounds, though the isolation of the organism failed. Thus, nearly 88% of cases of chronic infections of the spine were of tuberculous origin. Similar observations were reported by Kemp et al. (1973) and Panico (2023) **(Fig. 1.2)**.

Vertebral tuberculosis is the most common form of skeletal tuberculosis and it constitutes about 50% of all cases of skeletal tuberculosis in

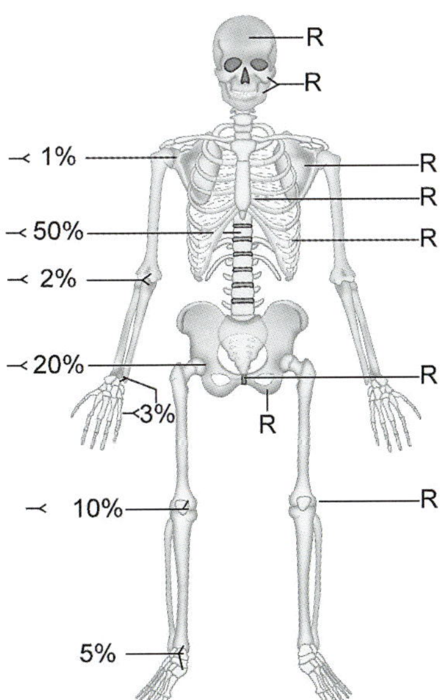

Fig. 1.2: Showing distribution of tuberculous lesions. Demographic data of patients visiting teaching hospitals in 20th century are different than the present data. A large number of patients now seek diagnosis and treatment in private sector. The data in this picture have been rounded-up to facilitate teaching and learning. Isolated lesions in skull, facial bones, mandible, scapula, sternum, rib, symphysis pubis, ischial tuberosity, patella do occur very rarely (R).

reported series (Sanchis-Olmos 1948, Wilkinson 1949, Girdlestone 1950, Sevastikoglou 1951, 1953, Mukopadhaya 1956, 1957, Falk 1958, Roaf 1958, Sinha 1958, Konstam 1963, Paus 1964, Grewal and Singh 1956, Tuli 1967, 2007, Martini 1988, Jain et al. 2007). The regional distribution of 1074 lesions of osteoarticular tuberculosis in 980 patients treated in the Department of Orthopedics, Banaras Hindu University, during the period 1965–1967 is shown in **Table 1.1**. In general, the regional distribution is in agreement with the figures from other centers of the world (Somerville and Wilkinson 1965, Sevastikoglou 1953, Sanchis Olmos 1948, Davies et al. 1984, Martini 1988, Pigrau-Serrallach et al. 2013). The work presented here is based upon personal observations, during the treatment of patients with tuberculosis of the skeletal system from 1965 to 2020. The number of cases which were available for various follow-up studies are mentioned in appropriate sections.

After 1987, sophisticated investigations like ultrasound, isotope bone scan, CT scan and MRI were available for most of the patients. The analysis of such investigations are mentioned in appropriate sections.

In a national survey of tuberculosis in England and Wales (Davies et al. 1984), the overall rates of tuberculosis were much higher in those of Indian subcontinental ethnic origin than in those of "white" descent. The Indian subcontinental patients were younger than the white patients, 55% were under 35 years as compared to 18% of the white group. The reasons for the differences are complex. The age of patients with orthopedic tuberculosis in developing countries tends to be even younger than in the Indian subcontinental patients in Britain.

INCIDENCE OF DISEASE AND INSTITUTIONAL DATA

With awareness of tuberculosis as a cause of osteoarticular infections and synovial diseases many patients would be treated by the neighboring family physicians. Not all patients

Table 1.1: Regional distribution of 1,074 lesions of osteoarticular tuberculosis (diagnosed clinically and by X-rays) amongst 980 patients in BHU Hospital (1965–1967).

Regions		***No. of cases***
Spine		440
Hip		81
Knee		89
Sacroiliac joint		69
Elbow		51
Ankle		43
Tarsal bones		39
Calcaneum		32
Metatarsals and phalanges		44
Greater trochanter and/or trochanteric bursa		21
Shoulder		17
Metacarpals and phalanges		28
Sternum		14
Clavicle and sternoclavicular joint		7
Wrist (carpal bones)		21
Ribs		19
Long bones of upper limb		14
Long bones of lower limb		19
Skull and facial bones		5
Pelvic bones		13
a. Pubic symphysis	6	
b. Iliac bone	5	
c. Ischial tuberosity	1	
d. Ischiopubic ramus	1	
Patella		1
Scapula		7
Total number of lesions		1,074

Note: There were 87 patients who had disseminated skeletal tuberculosis.

would need/seek the help of specialized hospitals. This would affect the observations of incidence of disease and the institutional data. The demographics data collected in a general teaching hospital between 1986 to 2019 would be different than those collected after 1965 because of the availability of better diagnostic facilities for clinical use.

The major areas of predilection are in the following order: Spine, hip, foot, knee, elbow, hand, shoulder, bursal sheaths and others. Mandible and tempromandibular joint appear to be the least common location where the tuberculous infection was observed by us in two cases from 1965 to 1994. There are, however, sporadic cases reported in the literature (Meng 1940, Sepheriadou-Mavropoulou 1986). One case of orbital tuberculosis was encountered by us recently.

PROPHYLAXIS AGAINST TUBERCULOSIS AND BCG VACCINATION

Selective immunization of groups at special risk is strongly recommended. These include household contacts of active cases, nurses, medical students, hospital workers and all those whose duties bring them in contact with patients or fomites. The protection afforded by BCG in the control of tuberculosis is estimated to be in the region of 80%.

It is customary to perform tuberculin test in each individual prior to BCG vaccination and to offer BCG only to those persons who do not react to tuberculin and are, thus, assumed to be uninfected previously. Normal reaction to BCG vaccination is a spontaneously regressive primary complex at the site of vaccination. The injection is made with a standard tuberculin syringe. For an adult 0.1 mL of the vaccine is injected intradermally proximal to the insertion of deltoid or lateral aspect of thigh. A satisfactory vaccination produces whitish wheal 5–7 mm in diameter. The wheal gets absorbed in 20–30 minutes. By 3–4 weeks an area of infiltration (induration) along with erythema develops at the site of vaccination. Between 4th and 5th week it develops into a papule (lump) 5–8 mm in diameter with a small nodule in its center. The papule increases in size to a maximum of

8–10 mm by about the 6th week. In many, a crust (scab) appears on the papule by about the 4th to 5th week. The crust may get detached leaving behind a superficial ulcer (5–6 mm diameter). The ulcer and the lesion heal slowly over 3–6 months leaving behind a scar. Rarely, there is delay in healing and regional lymph glands remain enlarged for a few months.

Even under the best conditions 10–20% of the vaccinated population may not get the protective immunity. About one case out of 10,000 vaccinated children in European countries may develop BCG osteitis, and extremely rarely a child may develop a generalized BCG infection. Fortunately, BCG osteitis runs a benign course (Shanmugasundaram 1982). The interval from BCG vaccination to onset of symptoms ranges from a few months to 5 years. The most common localizations are the epiphysis and metaphysis of long tubular bones, occasionally extending across the epiphyseal line. Nearly, 10% of the patients of BCG osteitis may have multiple lesions. Clinicoradiologically, the lesions resemble chronic osteomyelitis. Examination of the tissue removed would show histological picture resembling tuberculosis, culture may grow the same strain of BCG as was vaccinated, and guinea pig test is as a rule negative. Fortunately, these patients respond favorably to modern antitubercular drugs within about 6 months. BCG vaccination is being tried by us for immunopotentiation in desperate clinical cases of MDR and XMDR, and those reporting with recurrence of disease.

Helminthic infections have been suspected to predispose development of tuberculosis infection. Vitamin D may be another modulator for optimizing the normal human inmmune system.

Chemoprophylaxis

Chemoprophylaxis (a combination of isoniazid and rifampicin) may be considered in the infants and children staying in contact with an infected mother or attendants. Certain groups at special risk as mentioned above may be given chemoprophylaxis. Davidson and Le (1992) suggested rifampicin along with isoniazid for 3–6 months as prophylactic chemotherapy for:

- Close-contacts of an infectious tuberculous patient
- Persons with positive tuberculin test with abnormal chest X-ray without active disease but who have not received adequate antituberculous drugs
- Tuberculosis-infected persons without active disease when they develop high risk conditions such as diabetes, corticosteroid therapy, immunosuppressive therapy, HIV infection, hematological and reticuloendothelial malignancies, end-stage renal disease, silicosis, chronic undernutrition and weight loss
- Tuberculin skin test converters at any age
- Tuberculin skin test reactors younger than 35 years.
- We consider prophylactic medications mandatory as a perioperative umbrella, when a joint replacement procedure is being performed for a healed tuberculous arthritis.

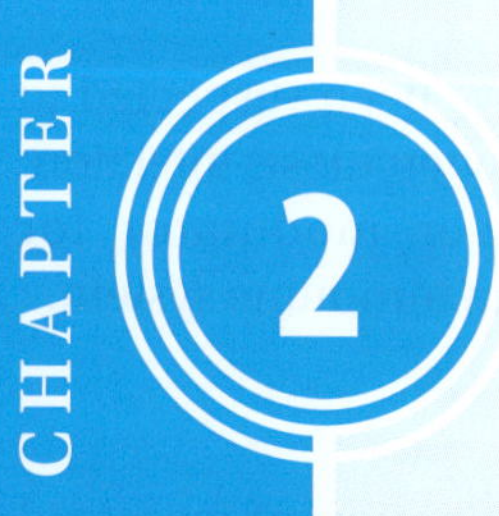

Pathology and Pathogenesis

Any osteoarticular tubercular lesion, is the result of a hematogenous dissemination from a primarily infected visceral focus. The primary focus may be active or quiescent, apparent or latent, either in the lungs or in the lymph glands of the mediastinum, mesentery or cervical region, or kidneys or other viscera. The infection reaches the skeletal system through vascular channels, generally the arteries as a result of bacillemia or rarely in axial skeleton through Batson's plexus of veins. Bone and joint tuberculosis is said to develop generally 2–3 years after the primary focus (Girling et al. 1988). Simultaneous involvement of paradiscal part of two contiguous vertebrae in a typical tuberculous lesion of the spine lends support to insemination of the bacilli through a common blood supply to this region. Simultaneous involvement of distant parts of the spine or the skeletal system, and associated visceral lesions suggest spread of infection through the arterial blood supply. Based upon radiological observations nearly 7% of cases of spinal tuberculosis had "skipped lesions" in the vertebral column and 12% had involvement of other bones and joints (excluding spine). About 20% of the cases on routine investigations had an evidence of tuberculous involvement of viscera and/or glands and/or other parts of the skeletal system. The incidence of concomitant involvement of more than one site or system is much higher, if assessment is made employing more recent sophisticated investigations. We have observed an additional subclinical (occult) active lesions in nearly 40% of cases who were investigated by whole body isotope bone scans or MRI.

EXPERIMENTAL TUBERCULOSIS

Hodgson et al. (1969) tried to produce spinal tuberculosis in monkeys, rabbits and guinea pigs by a variety of methods. The only technique which was found successful by them was injection of tubercular bacilli into the kidney, prostate and other abdominal and pelvic organs. This observation suggests that infection may spread directly from the visceral lesions to the vertebral column through the Batson's plexus of paravertebral veins.

Chronic tuberculous osseous lesions were induced consistently in 8–10 week old unvaccinated guinea pigs (Tuli et al. 1974) by the insertion of gelfoam impregnated with *Mycobacterium tuberculosis* into the metaphysial region through a drill hole in the distal part of the femur. Typical tuberculous lesions developed by 3 weeks. Of the animals that were killed 9 weeks or more after the inoculation, tuberculous lesions were observed in the lungs of all, in the liver in 33%, in the spleen in 9%, and in regional lymph nodes in all. In the same experimental studies (Tuli et al. 1974), local trauma by drilling the contralateral bone in the presence of tuberculous bacillemia failed to create a localized tuberculous osteomyelitis. Localized tissue necrosis and a prolonged contact between the bacilli and the damaged bone tissue markedly increased the possibility of development of osteomyelitis (Tuli et al. 1974, Norden 1970).

OSTEOARTICULAR DISEASE

Tubercular bacilli reach the joint space via the bloodstream through subsynovial vessels, or indirectly from the lesions in the epiphyseal bone that erode into the joint space. Articular cartilage destruction begins peripherally, in addition the tuberculous granulation tissue does not form proteolytic enzymes within the joint space, the central areas of the articular cartilage (weight bearing surfaces) are therefore, preserved for a long time (a few months) and provide the potential for good "functional recovery" with effective treatment. This is in contrast to the destruction of articular cartilage, in patients with pyogenic arthritis where proteolytic enzymes are produced.

The disease may start in the bone or in the synovial membrane, but in a short time in uncontrolled disease one infects the other. Typically, the initial focus starts in the metaphysis in the growing age, and at the end of the bone in adults. Radiologically, there is local destruction and marked demineralization. In bones with superficial cortical surfaces (such as metacarpals, metatarsals, phalanges, tibia, ulna), an osseous tuberculous lesion may produce thickening of bone (generally surrounding lytic areas) due to reactive subperiosteal new bone formation **(Figs. 17.1 and 17.6)**.

Cartilaginous tissue is resistant to tuberculous destruction. However, penetration of epiphyseal cartilage plate **(Figs. 9.2, 10.1 and 13.2)** predominantly occurs in tuberculous disease rather than in pyogenic infection. Metaphyseal tuberculous lesion may infect the neighboring joint through the subperiosteal space and through the capsule, or through the destruction of the epiphyseal plate. Once the tubercular process has reached the subchondral region (deep to the articular cartilage), the articular cartilage loses its nutrition and attachment to the bone, and may lie free in the joint cavity. Damage to the physis in childhood may result in shortening or angulation of the extremity.

In patients who have optimum or competent immunity, the disease generally starts as tuberculous synovitis and the course is usually slow. The synovial membrane becomes swollen and congested and there is synovial effusion. The granulation tissue from the synovium extends onto the bone at the synovial reflections eroding the bone. At the periphery of the articular cartilage, the granulation tissue forms a ring (pannus) which grows in the subchondral region and erodes the margins and surface of the articular cartilage. Flakes or loose sheets of necrosed articular cartilage, and accumulations of fibrinous material in the synovial fluid may produce "rice bodies" in synovial joints (and in tendon sheaths and bursae). Where articular surfaces are in contact, the cartilage is preserved for a long time because of the prevention of spread of the pannus. Necrosis of subchondral bone by the ingrowth of tuberculous granulation tissue (pannus) on each side of the joint line develops "kissing lesion" **(Fig. 9.3)** and/or "kissing sequestrae". The sequestrated articular cartilage and subchondral bone is usually contained in a small lytic area. Coke-like sequestrum contained in a cavity is characteristic of tuberculous infection **(Fig. 2.2)**.

ROLE OF TRAUMA

The relationship of trauma to osteoarticular tuberculosis has long been the subject of discussion and numerous publications. The present consensus, however, is that trauma probably draws the attention to a mild focus or it may activate a latent tubercular focus. Repeated mechanical strain in the mobile and weight bearing parts of the body (resulting in a minor hematoma or bone marrow edema) may determine the frequent localization of the disease in the lower part of dorsal and upper part of lumbar spine, and the weight bearing joints. Penetrating injuries on hand or feet may induce infection by non-typical mycobacteria.

THE TUBERCLE

Following the insemination of infection the initial response is in the reticuloendothelial depots of the skeletal tissues. This is characterized by accumulation of polymorphonuclear cells which are rapidly replaced by macrophages and monocytes (mononuclears), the highly phagocytic members of the reticuloendothelial system. The tubercle bacilli are phagocytosed and broken down, and their lipid is dispersed throughout the cytoplasm of the mononuclears, thus transforming them into epithelioid cells. Epithelioid cells are the characteristic feature of the tuberculous reaction. These are large pale cells with a large vesicular nucleus, abundant cytoplasm, indistinct margins, and processes which form an epithelioid reticulum. Langhans giant cells are probably formed by fusion of a number of epithelioid cells, these are formed only if caseation necrosis has occurred in the lesion, and often they contain tubercle bacilli. Their main function is to digest and remove necrosed tissue. After about a week, lymphocytes appear and form a ring around the peripheral part of the lesion. This mass formed by the reactive cells of the reticuloendothelial tissues constitutes a nodule popularly known as the tubercle. The tubercles grow by expansion and coalescence. During the second week, caseation occurs in the center of the tubercle by coagulation necrosis caused by the protein fraction of tubercle bacilli. The caseous material may soften and liquefy. Presence of caseation necrosis is almost diagnostic of tuberculous pathology (and of tuberculoid leprosy), such a tubercle is designated as "soft tubercle". A tubercle may, however, not show central caseation (hard tubercle) under the influence of treatment, or in the granulomatous inflammations caused by atypical (non-typical) mycobacteria, mycosis, brucellosis, sarcoidosis and foreign bodies (Williams 1983).

COLD ABSCESS

Marked exudative reaction is a common feature in tuberculous infection of the skeletal system. A cold abscess is formed by a collection of products of liquefaction and the reactive exudation. The cold abscess is mostly composed of serum, leukocytes, caseous material, bone debris and tubercle bacilli. The abscess, penetrates the ligaments in articular disease, bone and periosteum in osseous disease, and migrates in various directions following the facial planes and along the vessels and nerves. The "cold abscess" feels warm, though the temperature is not raised as high as in acute pyogenic infections. A superficial abscess may get secondarily infected, and clinically behave like pyogenic abscess; it may burst to form a sinus or an ulcer. The walls of an abscess, sinus or ulcer are covered with tuberculous granulations. The size of a cold abscess is not proportionate to the extent of destruction of the skeletal lesion. A huge abscess may be associated with radiological minimal destruction.

TUBERCULAR SEQUESTRA

Following the infection, marked hyperemia and severe osteoporosis takes place. Osseous destruction takes place by lysis of bone, which is thus softened and easily yields under the effect of gravity and muscle action, leading to compression, collapse or deformation of bones **(Fig. 2.1)**. Necrosis also takes place due to ischemic infarction of segments of bones. This change is secondary to arterial occlusion due to thromboembolic phenomenon, endarteritis and periarteritis. Ischemic necrosis has also been recognized as a contributing factor responsible for osseous and vertebral collapse (Cleveland and Bosworth 1942, Girdlestone 1950). As a result of ischemic changes sometimes sequestration takes place, usually appearing as "coarse sand" and rarely forming a definite radiologically visible coke-like sequestrum **(Fig. 2.2)**. Due to loss of nutrition the adjacent articular cartilage or the intervening disc get degenerated and may also become separated as sequestra **(Figs. 2.3 and 2.4A)**. Some of the radiologically visible smaller sequestra in tuberculous cavities (feathery sequestra) may be the outcome of calcification of the caseous matter **(Fig. 2.4B)**.

SPINAL TUBERCULOSIS

The intervertebral disc is not involved primarily **(Fig. 2.1)** because it is a relatively avascular structure. The early involvement of paradiscal

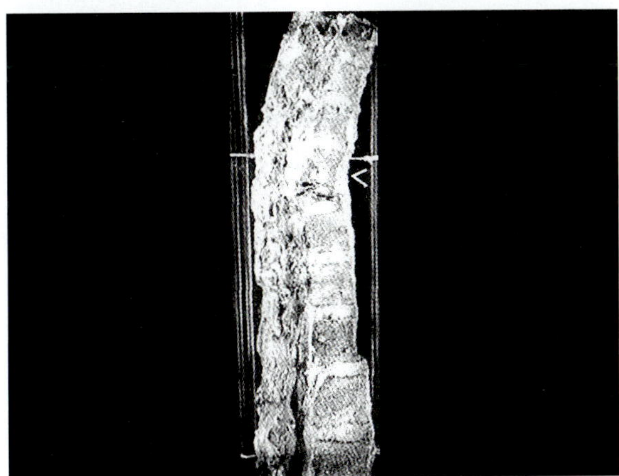

Fig. 2.1: A sagittal section of vertebral column showing the diseased area opposite to the arrow. Note complete obliteration of the intervening disc and destruction of the paradiscal vertebral bodies. The disc along the distal margin of the destroyed vertebra appears normal and shows bulging into the softened vertebral body above, softening of bones leads to collapse of vertebral bodies and kyphotic deformity.

Courtesy: Professor Gupta, IM, Department of Pathology, Banaras Hindu University (BHU).

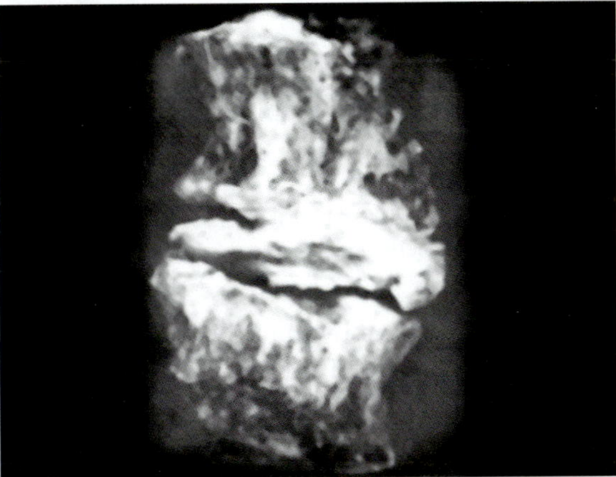

Fig. 2.3: An 18-year-old female presented with tuberculosis of the lumbar spine with persistent cauda equina type neural deficit. While doing decompression through the retroperitoneal sympathectomy approach the loose sequestrated bodies of lumbar 3 and 4 vertebrae just extruded out in the surgical field. Such an extensive sequestration is presumed to be due to thromboembolic phenomenon cutting off the major blood supply to the vertebral bodies.

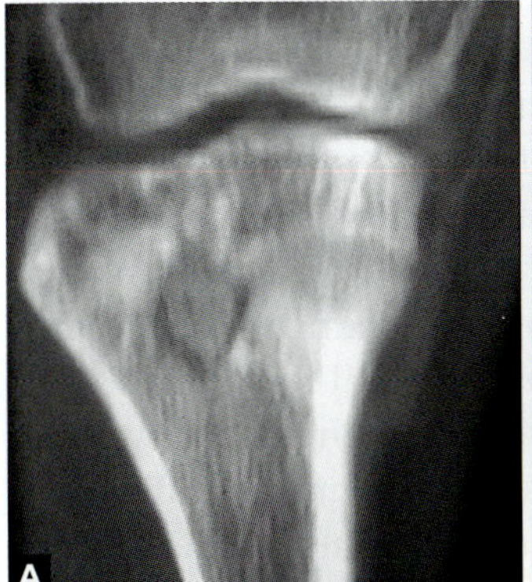

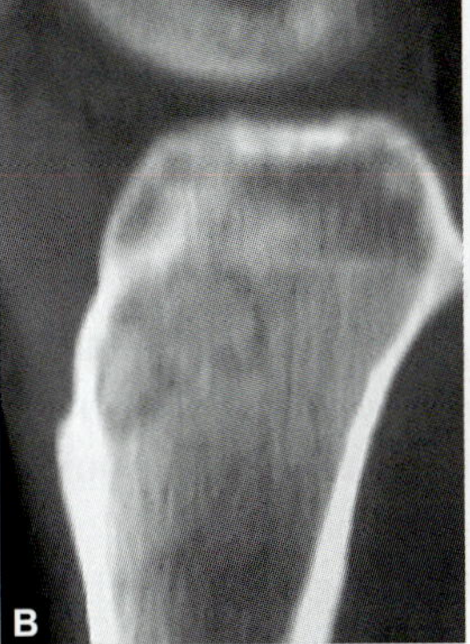

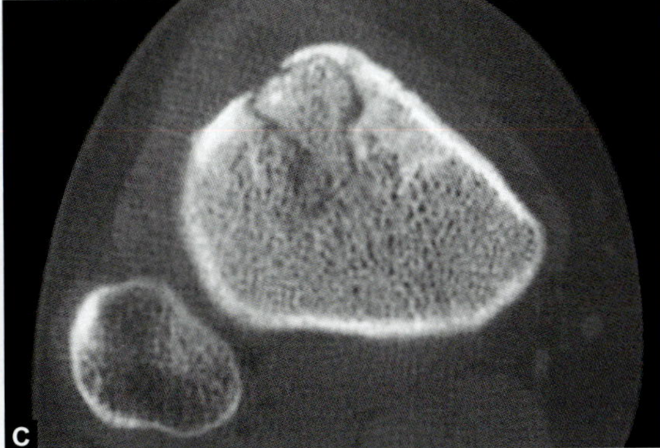

Figs. 2.2A to C: A soft feathery sequestrum (coke-like) contained in a cavity is almost characteristic of tuberculous infection of bone. CT scans of upper end of tibia showing the lesion in an early stage.

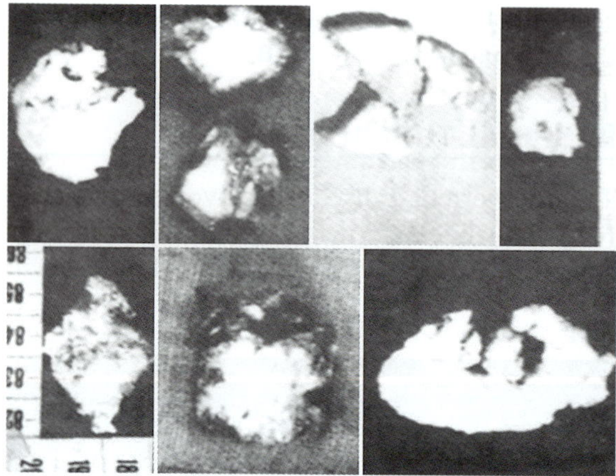

Fig. 2.4A: Big sequestra removed during operations for tuberculosis of the spine. The sequestrum in the right lower corner is from the disc, the rest are bony sequestra (the scales show centimeters).

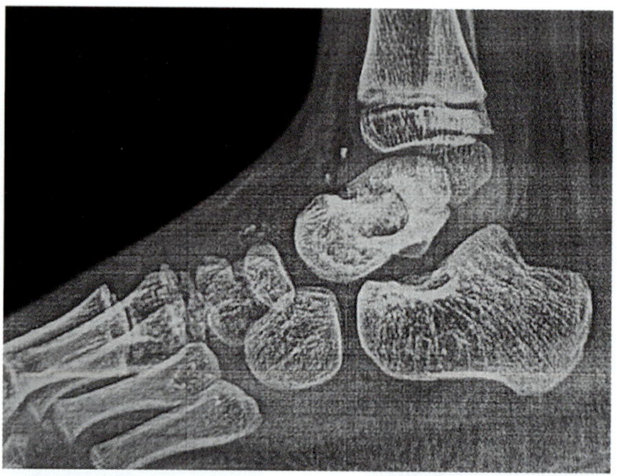

Fig. 2.4B: X-ray of Ankle shows a lytic lesion in talus containing soft sequestrum.

regions of vertebrae by the tuberculous process jeopardizes the nutrition of the disc. Such a necrosed or pathologically changed disc may also be invaded by the adjacent infectious process. The cartilaginous end plate is a sort of barrier, but once it has been invaded, destruction of disc progresses rapidly (Schmorl and Junghanns 1959). The radiological narrowing of the disc space may also be due to the disc breaking through the paradiscal margins of the diseased and softened vertebral bodies. This can be observed in many cases in MRI studies.

The tuberculous granulomatous debris and tuberculous abscess may be compressed between the sound vertebrae above and below and as a result lateral extension, propulsion (deep to the anterior longitudinal ligament) and retropulsion (in the extradural space deep to the posterior longitudinal ligament) of infected material may occur. The process may also spread and extend itself by osteoperiosteal infiltration, passing along deep to the anterior longitudinal ligament to involve and to destroy distant parts of vertebral column. Pressure on neural structures is more likely in the thoracic spine where the caliber of the vertebral canal is relatively small.

Initial involvement of more than two contiguous vertebrae does not seem to be common. When many adjacent vertebrae are affected, the disease may have extended from one to the other by contiguity. Involvement of several separated vertebrae was observed to occur in 1–4% of cases. Many small foci are not demonstrable radiologically. In our cases, 7% of patients had skipped lesions in the spine demonstrated by conventional radiography. The number of vertebrae involved and the extent of disease at each site is much more, if visualized by CT scan or MRI. Conventionally images of vertebral tuberculosis have been expressed as "paradiscal type" (most common), "central type"starting from the middle of vertebral bodies (creating vertebra plana), "anterior type" infected material spreading along the anterolateral surfaces of vertebrae deep to the anterior longitudinal ligament and periosteum, as "skipped lesions", multiple vertebrae involved in the spine with 2 or more uninvolved vertebrae between the obvious vertebral lesions, and as a clinically obvious visceral or generalized systemic tuberculosis. However in patients presenting with longstanding disease and the use of MRIs many lesions exhibit over lapping features.

TYPES OF THE DISEASE

For descriptive purposes two types of bone and joint tuberculosis are recognized. The "caseous exudative type" is characterized by more destruction, more exudation and abscess formation. The onset is less insidious, constitutional symptoms and local signs of inflammation and swelling are more marked, abscess and sinus formation occur commonly. The "granular type" is less destructive, has an insidious onset and course, and abscess formation is rare. Its classical example is that of caries sicca of shoulder **(Fig. 11.2)**. Generally, it is a dry lesion. In clinical practice, both types coexist, one predominating the other. The lesion in children is generally "caseous exudative type" while in adults it is more likely to be of "granular type" with minimal destruction.

FUTURE COURSE OF THE TUBERCLE

Before the availability of antitubercular drugs, the five-year follow-up mortality of patients of osteoarticular tuberculosis used to be about 30%. The modern antitubercular agents have greatly changed the outlook regarding the behavior of tuberculous lesions. Depending upon the sensitivity of tubercle bacilli, resistance and immune status of the patient, use of antitubercular drugs and the stage of the lesion at the inception of treatment, the tuberculous lesion may behave as follows: (i) It may resolve completely; (ii) The disease may heal completely with varying degrees of residual deformities and/or loss of function; (iii) The lesion may be completely walled-off and the caseous tissue may be calcified; (iv) A low grade chronic fibromatous granulating and caseating lesion may persist with grumbling activity; and (v) The infection may spread locally by contiguity, and systemically by bloodstream (disseminated disease) as seen in immunocompromised patients.

TUBERCULOSIS AS A LATE COMPLICATION OF "IMPLANT-SURGERY"

Occurrence of tuberculosis as a late complication of total hip replacement was reported by McCullough (1978) and Ueng et al. (1995). During the period 1990–2001, at GTB and Vimhans Hospitals, New Delhi, we had an opportunity to see 12 cases of osseous tuberculosis as a late complication (6–12 months postoperative) of surgery for closed fractures (two in hip joint, one each in femur and forearm) and hip joint arthroplasty. Extensive surgery and use of metal implants probably offered a very favorable nidus for localization of circulating mycobacteria in such cases. Operative intervention with instrumentations has resulted in many fold increase in unsuccessful outcome and persistence of infection (AndresCano 2018, Fehring 2019). Diabetic state, patients on corticosteroids, poor nutritional status and immune compromised state are predisposing factors in such a complication. A high suspicion index and laboratory examination of the diseased tissue would offer the diagnosis (Kumar et al. 2006).

The potential local and systemic toxicity of orthopedic implants is being debated and is under scrutiny (Keegan et al. 2007). There is always some inflammation in peri-implant tissues dominated by immunological and macrophagic reactions. Such inflamed areas offer a favorable nidus for circulating mycobacteria in susceptible humans. There are many potential hazards of nano-scale circulating metals and polyethylene particles on general immune system. Reigstad and Siewers (2008) reported a case of total hip replacement that developed tuberculosis after intravesicular BCG treatment of bladder cancer.

Implantation Tuberculosis

Present generation of orthopedic surgeons should be cognisant of tuberculous infection

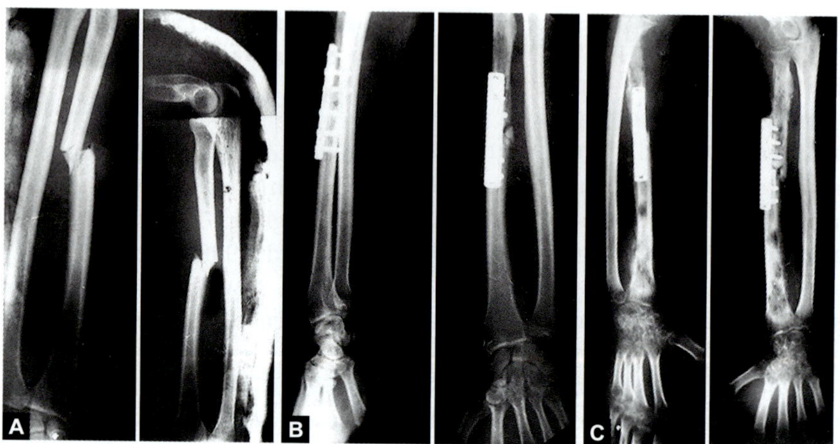

Figs. 2.5A to C: A 48-year-old man reported with a closed fracture of radius. (A) The fracture was treated by plating, the wound healed and stitches were removed 2 weeks after the surgery. (B) About one month later the forearm showed signs of low grade infection, there was dehiscence of the stitch line and there were multiple small undermined ulcers. "Implantation tuberculosis" was suspected as the X-rays showed multiple lytic areas throughout the radius. (C) Curettings from the lytic areas demonstrated caseating granulomas. There was complete resolution of infection and healing under the influence of antitubercular drugs during follow-up.

Courtesy: Dr Rajnish Gupta.

that may occur after any surgery in which bio-implants have been used or after treatment of compound fractures. The incidence of such an infection is not high, however unexplained dehiscence of wound, persistent seropurulent discharge, formation of ulcers with undermined edges, cavitations in the bones a few weeks or months after operation should arouse the suspicion of such an infection. Histological examination of the curettings from the sinuses, cavities and ulcers would establish the diagnosis. Acid fast bacilli may be demonstrated in a few cases by Ziehl–Neelsen staining or on culture. Atypical mycobacteria may be responsible for infection following compound fractures. The author has observed, analyzed and treated 12 cases **(Fig. 2.5)** collected during 1990 to 2001.

IMMUNOPATHOLOGY OF SKELETAL TUBERCULOSIS

Mycobacterium tuberculosis and *Homo sapiens* have lived in symbiosis since the ascent of man on earth. In addition to the innate immune response, mycobacterial specific adaptive cell mediated immunity (CMI) develops by interaction of mycobacteria with dendritic cells and macrophage. Human cell mediated immunity system can be regarded as having developed in response to mycobacterial infection and other infectious challenges. The immune response to infection by tubercular bacillus has been very effective due to which only about 5% of infected persons develop clinically evident primary (pulmonary) disease, and only a further 5% or so develop post-primary disease later in life (Stanford 1994). The very fact that a patient gets skeletal tuberculosis is a reflection of inherent poor protective response of his reticuloendothelial system at the time of infection (Tuli 1997). It is also possible that subtle changes may be brought about by mycobacterial infection itself, to weaken the immuno-regulatory system in man (Rook, Hernandez-Pando 1994).

The helper subset of T lymphocytes are central to cell-mediated immunity against tuberculous infection. These cells carry the CD4 antigen on their surface (CD4+ lymphocytes). In HIV disease, the virus enters and infects CD4 lymphocytes, kills these cells and progressively leads to a decline in the immunity of the host. In general, patients with CD4 cell counts greater than 500/mm^3 (total lymphocyte count greater than 2000/mm^3) should have normal immune response. However, CD4 lymphocyte count <200/mm^3 reflects a poor prognosis for any healing response. Reinfection of a previously infected individual (in childhood) who clinically remained disease free through life, can get the disease again when elderly because of waning immunity and comorbidities.

THERAPEUTICALLY REFRACTORY CASES

When a patient is not responding to effective multidrug therapy one should suspect the cause to be a resistant mycobacterium, nontypical mycobacteria, immune compromised host, or a patient on immunosuppressive therapy **(Figs. 2.6 to 2.8)**. One is impelled or tempted to do "excisional surgery" in such patients; however, postoperative outcome in such patients should be tempered or guarded. The patient would temporarily improve, however in many cases the disease continues to be active, sinuses and ulcers may reappear, or the operative wound may undergo dehiscence (Jain 2024).

Some of the therapeutically resistant patients may be cases infected by multidrug-resistant organisms (MDR). Despite excisional surgery with or without fusion the operative wounds in such cases break down with persistent discharging sinuses or ulcers. Immunomodulation as an adjunct to newer antitubercular drugs may be of great help in such a situation (Tuli 1999, Arora et al. 2006, Jain et al. 2012).

Cell mediated immunity is critical for protection against tubercular infection and also for healing of infection. What reduces cellular immunity: under or malnutrition, diabetes, prolonged use of steroids, Leflunomide, methotrexate, HIV, substance abuse, anti-onco drugs.

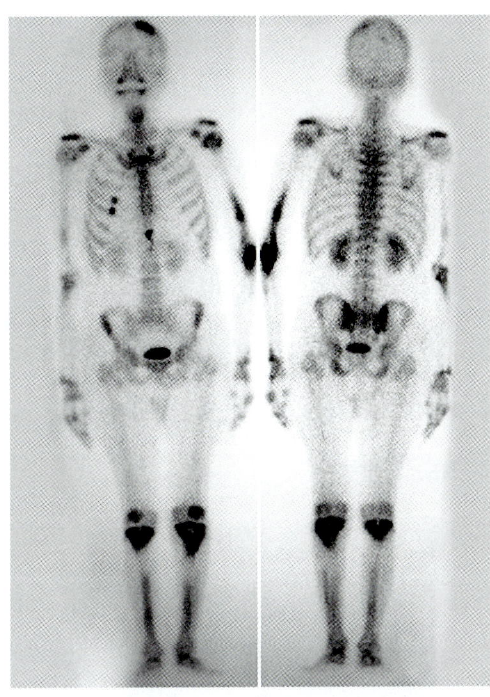

Fig. 2.6: Whole body isotope bone scan showing multiple hot areas in a patient who presented with clinically manifest active tuberculosis of both knees, left elbow and left skull bones. The patient was in an immune compromised state because of prolonged use of steroids for medical comorbidities. Other hot areas in right ribs, left humerus and spine had subclinical lesions.

IMMUNODEFICIENT STAGE AND LOOMING TUBERCULOSIS EPIDEMIC

In the Western countries up to 1915, nearly half of the surgical cases in the general hospitals were then suffering from "surgical tuberculosis". The incidence of tuberculous infection declined steadily in the affluent countries up to 1985 (Mitchison and Chalmers 1986), and it was considered to be a disappearing disease in those countries. In Asian and African countries, however, the disease continued in epidemic proportions. After 1985, due to emergence of AIDS pandemic there has been a dramatic reversal of trends in the affluent countries, the incidence of tubercular infection has started increasing at 10–20% per year. The most alarming features are

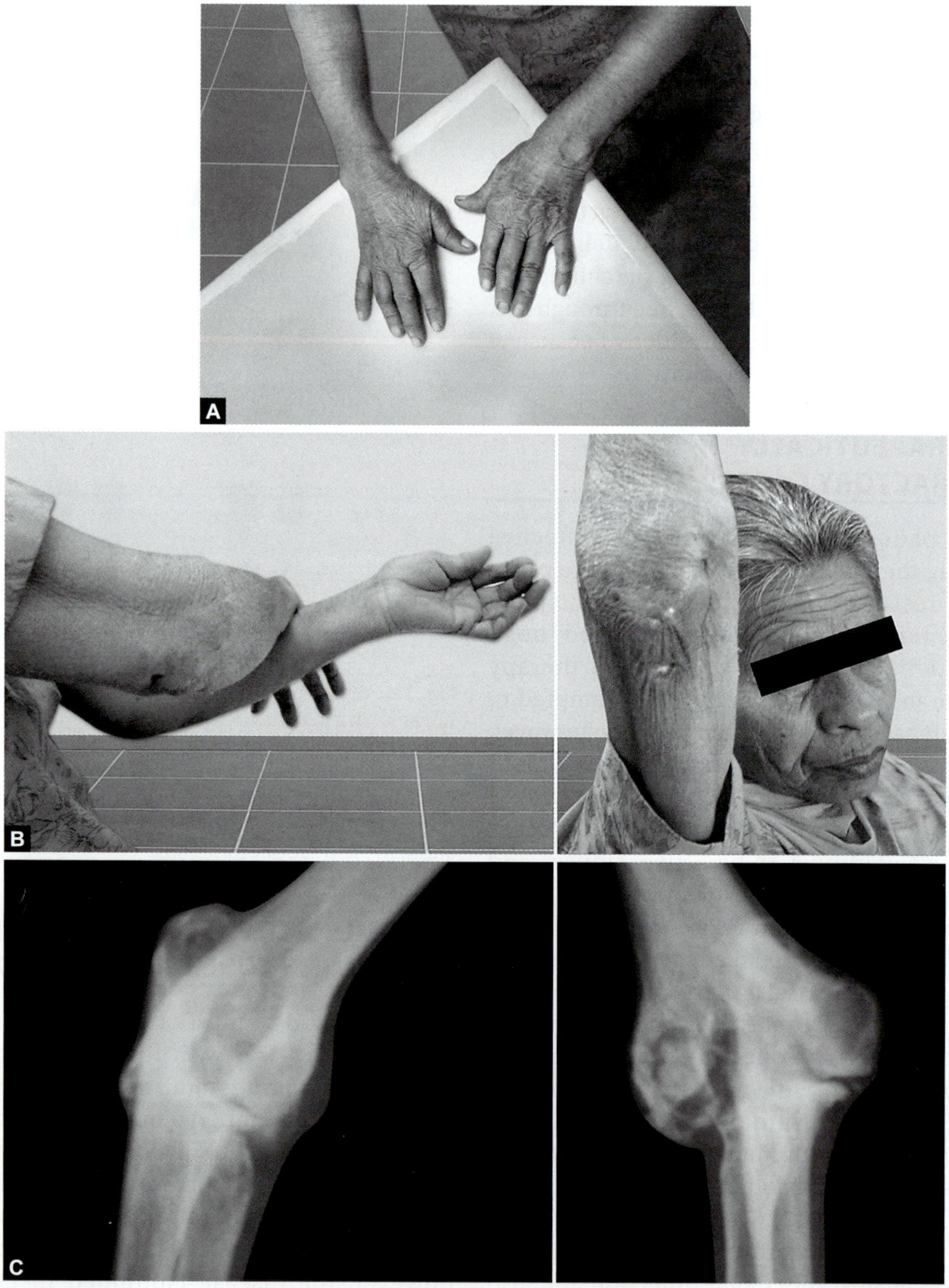

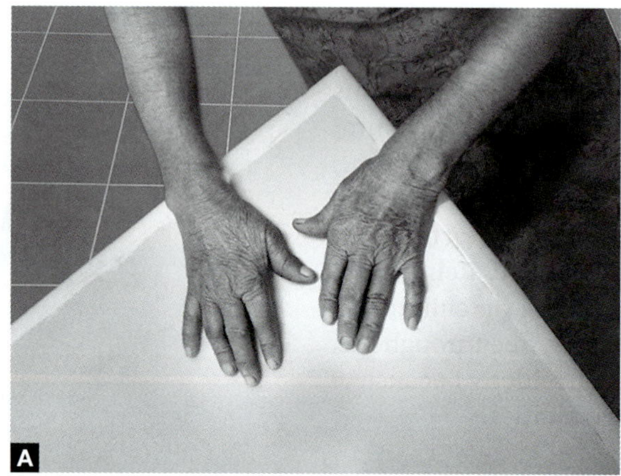

Figs. 2.7A to C: A physician's mother having generalized rheumatoid disorder. (A) hand showing arthropathy, was on methotrexate for >2 years. She then started showing ulcerations behind her right elbow (B). X-rays of the elbow (C) showed typical tuberculous lesion (soft sequestrum in cavities), histology proved the diagnosis of tuberculous infection.

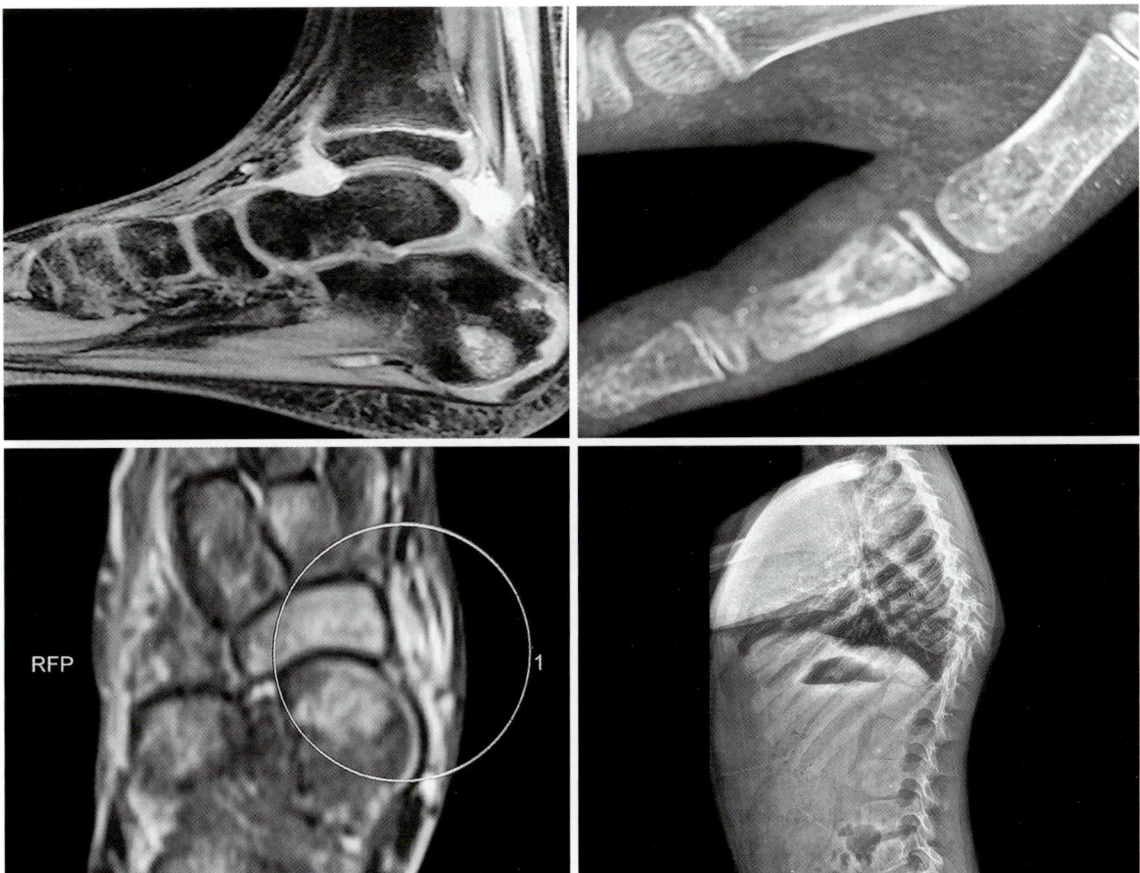

Fig. 2.8: Disseminated tuberculosis in a child: Observe lesions in spine D8–D9 proximal phalanx of thumb, calcaneum, and talar head.

that people with AIDS virus are getting infected with atypical tuberculous bacilli (which were earlier considered generally nonpathogenic), and many of these strains already show resistance to a large number of antitubercular drugs. HIV infected persons due to dysfunction of the host immune system have a very high incidence of getting primary tuberculosis, reactivation of the previous tuberculous lesion in the body and concomitant infection by another strain of tuberculous bacillus (different from that of initial disease—polymycobacterial) by exogenous route. HIV positive patients have been observed to have greater peridural abscess collection (Anley et al. 2012) as compared to other patients. The incidence of tuberculosis in patients with AIDS is almost 500 times the incidence in the general population (Barnes et al. 1991).

Patients with HIV and tuberculosis are a potential source for spread of drug resistant strains of tuberculous bacilli to other members of society. In countries where tuberculosis was no more endemic, the incidence of extra-pulmonary tuberculosis is considered a broad indicator of HIV infection in the society (Barnes et al. 1991).

HIV attacks the tissue macrophages and the thymic lymphocytes which are *Homo sapiens* defense against infection with *Mycobacterium tuberculosis*. *Tuberculosis* appears early during HIV infection before the appearance of other opportunistic infections. In addition to new tuberculous infections, dormant foci of tuberculosis are very likely to be reactivated after HIV infection (Jellis 2002, Liebert et al. 1996). In advanced HIV disease, any operative wound would heal poorly and provide a portal for secondary bacterial infection which may create a life-threatening situation. Patients with neurological complications would die of horrendous bedsores, uncontrolled urinary infection and septicemia. However, if osteoarticular tuberculosis is treated efficiently in patients with early HIV disease, there is no reason why the patient should not live for 5–10 years until the HIV disease advances to its final stage (Jellis 2002). The ultimate prognosis is not of tuberculosis but of HIV infection.

IMMUNOMODULATION

In multidrug resistant cases (MDR) and those who were considered therapeutically refractory, CD4 cell count were analyzed to be lowered (Arora 2002). Attempts were made by us in such cases for immunomodulation. The following outline is suggested: 150 mg of levamisol is given at night for 3 consecutive days at weekly intervals for a total of 45 tablets. Four injections are administered once a month. The first and second are 0.1 mL intradermal BCG injections, and the third and fourth are intramuscular DPT (diphtheria + pertussis + tetanus vaccine) injections. Clinically, a favorable response was observed in 85% of patients. The above-mentioned immunomodulation regime in conjunction with second-line drugs demonstrated upgradation of CD4 count after 4–6 months of therapy (Arora et al. 2006). Jain et al. 2012, Tuli 1999, 2014 also reported beneficial effects of immunomodulation in therapeutical refractory cases of spinal tuberculosis.

Antigens from *Mycobacterium vaccae* strain (NCTC 11659) were deriving special attention for immunotherapy of mycobacterial infections in general (Stanford and Stanford 1994). The efforts, however, have not been successful. BCG vaccination has been known to provide some degree of immune protection for various mycobacterial infections. Direct BCG vaccination without tuberculin testing is considered safe and acceptable to the persons being vaccinated. Though the mechanism of influence on immune response after mycobacterial vaccination remains speculative, however, it is considered that macrophages get activated to become more effective killer cells against mycobacteria, probably it switches off the tissue-necrotizing aspects of the Koch's phenomenon, and it replaces an inappropriate immune reaction by an appropriate one against mycobacterial infections (Stanford and Gange 1994). Many mycobacterial cell envelop bases vaccines are being investigated in animal models to evaluate the protective response against tuberculosis.

Clinically for immunopotentiation we found the following technique effective and therapeutically acceptable by the patients: Injection BCG 0.1 mL intradermal at one month interval for maximum three injections. After 1-month gap from the last injection (of BCG) start injection DPT (diphtheria, pertussis, tetanus) intramuscular, give three injections at one month interval.

CHAPTER 3

The Organism and its Sensitivity

MYCOBACTERIUM TUBERCULOSIS

Historically in the Western countries before generalized use of pasteurization, there were many reports which showed a fairly high incidence of bovine type of bacillus responsible for osteoarticular tuberculosis. Approximately, 85% of cases of skeletal tuberculosis under the age of 10 years were considered due to bovine bacilli (Girdlestone 1950). Investigations by many workers in this field have shown that most of the strains responsible for skeletal tuberculosis in Indian subcontinent were of the human type. Perhaps, in Indian subcontinent, the universal habit of taking milk after boiling may be responsible for the absence of bovine type of infection. Konstam (1962) wrote that as after weaning no fresh milk was consumed in Ibadan it was presumed that the causative organism was the human type. Generally, only typical *Mycobacterium tuberculosis* are considered to be pathogenic. Sweany et al. (1943) considered yellow colored colonies of acid fast bacilli to be avirulent. In our investigations during 1969–1971 at Banaras Hindu University (Lakhanpal et al. 1974, 1976), 92% of cultures had grown typical *Mycobacterium tuberculosis*, whereas 8% of the positive cultures showed the growth only of chromogenic acid fast bacilli. These were considered to be pathogenic by us as these were the only organisms cultured in these cases.

Mycobacterium tuberculosis is a slow growing aerobic organism with a growth doubling time of about 20 hours in conditions favorable to the bacillus. In unfavorable conditions, it will grow only intermittently or remain dormant for a prolonged period to regrow whenever the host defense system becomes deficient. Ideally speaking the diagnosis of tuberculous infection should be confirmed by the demonstration of tubercle bacilli in the skeletal tuberculous lesion. However, this has not been possible in all the cases in any series (Grange 1989, Martin et al. 1989, Moon et al. 2002), probably because skeletal tuberculosis is a paucibacillary disease. In general, the load of mycobacteria in pulmonary lesions is 10^7 to 10^9 whereas in osteoarticular disease the load is $<10^5$. Incidence of positive cultures for acid-fast bacilli in osteoarticular tuberculous lesions has been reported by various workers to be between 40 and 88% [Dahl 1951, Dobson 1951, Holmdahl 1951, Wilkinson 1953, Weinberg 1957, Hald (jr) 1964, Kemp et al. 1973, Masood 1992]. Direct smear examination of tuberculous material obtained during operation or obtained by aspiration of the infected synovium (from joints, bursae and tendon sheaths) or involved lymph nodes or the tuberculous osseous cavities, may yield a positive result for tubercle bacilli **(Fig. 5.5)** if the sample contains >10,000 bacilli per mL. The highest positivity was observed in our material from fresh cases of tendovaginitis (Arora 1994), and in cases of disseminated tuberculosis probably having an immune compromised state. In general, the number of mycobacteria present in skeletal tuberculosis is approximately 10^5/mL of the pathological material.

MYCOBACTERIUM CULTURES

In our efforts at Banaras Hindu University, positive results were obtained in 60.5% of cases of osteoarticular tuberculosis submitted for culture examination during 1965–1974. Proof of tuberculosis by submitting the material both for culture and guinea pig inoculation was available in 89% of cases (Lakhanpal et al. 1974). Tubercle bacilli were found less frequently, the longer the period of medications and the longer was the duration of clinical disease, before submitting the material for microbiological investigation. In our series, a number of positive cultures were obtained if the material was incubated for 20 weeks. *Mycobacterium* culture methods are slow and insensitive enough in bacillary pulmonary tuberculosis, these difficulties get greatly magnified in paucibacillary osteoarticular disease. The search for simpler, cheaper, and hopefully more reliable immunological and biochemical detection techniques have uptil now been fraught with disappointment (Grange 1989). Martin et al. (1989) suggested the use of a broth medium in addition to egg-based or agar-based culture media especially for paucibacillary disease. They reported encouraging result by cultures maintained for 8 weeks. Guinea pig inoculation is, at present, considered uneconomic.

The best material for microbiological assessment appears to be centrifuged residue material from a large quantity of abscess, curettings from the walls of a cold abscess prior to secondary infection, and curettings from the lining of sinus tracts as close to the base (source) as possible. Of the 22 cases, Karlson (1973) reported to be positive for bone and joint tuberculosis, the break up for the type of organism was *M. tuberculosis* 16, *M. avium* complex 2, *M. kansassi* 2 and *M. scrofulaceum* 2. All microbiological investigations in a clinically suspected case of tuberculosis should include studies for *Mycobacterium tuberculosis*, pyogenic organisms, atypical mycobacteria and fungi.

SENSITIVITY OF ORGANISM

There are only a few reports regarding culture and sensitivity of tubercle bacilli isolated from osteoarticular lesions. Resistance to streptomycin has been reported to be 7–10% (Orell 1951, Harris 1952). Hodgson and Yau (1968) reported one out of 32 cases of tuberculosis of the spine resistant to streptomycin, PAS and INH. Smith et al. (1950) found 10.7% cases of skeletal tuberculosis which responded unfavorably to streptomycin. Kemp et al. (1973) determined sensitivities in 57 cases of spinal tuberculosis and found drug resistance only in 3 instances.

Of the strains of *Mycobacterium tuberculosis* isolated from various tuberculous lesions, the resistance has been reported to be 9–22% for streptomycin, 4–14% for PAS, and 8–24% for INH from various centers of the world (Singh 1956, Ganguli 1960, Hillerdal et al. 1961, Gangadharan 1967, Pablos-Mendez 1998). Higher incidence of resistant strains has been reported from patients who had antitubercular drugs for >3 months before culture and sensitivity (Bickel-William 1948, Medlar 1951, Bell 1961, Gupta 1962, Goyal 1962, Gangadharan 1967). Resistance to thioacetazone has been reported in 5–15% of strains (East Africa BMRC 1963, Menon 1965).

In our study (1970–1974), out of typical strains, 16.7% were resistant only to streptomycin, 12.5% were resistant only to PAS, 20.8% were found to be resistant only to INH. Resistance against thioacetazone was observed in 8.3% cases. All the anonymous acid fast bacilli were resistant to commonly used antitubercular drugs, viz. streptomycin, PAS, INH and thioacetazone. No strain of typical *Mycobacterium tuberculosis* was found to be resistant to all the 3 first line

Table 3.1: Results of sensitivity tests of 52 cultures from skeletal tuberculous lesions (1969–1971 BHU study) positive for tubercle bacilli.

Drugs tested	*Total*	*Sensitive*	*Resistant**	*Resistant** to all 4 drugs*
Streptomycin	52	40	8	
PAS	52	42	6	4
INH	52	38	10	
Thiacetazone	52	44	4	

*Resistant only to one drug, these were typical mycobacteria.
**Resistant to all the 4 drugs tested, these were atypical mycobacteria.
Source: Lakhanpal VP, Singh H, Sen PC, Tuli SM. Bacteriological study in osteoarticular tuberculosis. Ind J Orthop. 1976;10:13-7.

antitubercular drugs. In fact, the typical bacilli, which were observed to be resistant to one first line antitubercular drug, were found sensitive to the rest of the drugs tested **(Table 3.1)**.

Incidence of drug resistance amongst USA war veterans was reported as 3.2% for streptomycin, 2.8% for INH, 4.4% for PAS, 9.7% for ethambutol, 0.8% for rifampicin during 1972–1973 (Hobby 1974, Hobby et al. 1974). The incidence of resistance in New York was 15.1% to INH, 13.9% to streptomycin, 6.3% to PAS and 1.2% for ethambutol (Steiner 1974). The resistance reported from Madras was 8.7% to INH, 8.7% to streptomycin and 3.8% to both (Tuberculosis Research Center, Madras 1981). Amongst the therapeutically refractory patients of spinal tuberculosis resistance was present to INH 92%, rifampicin 81% and streptomycin 69% (Mohan et al. 2013). Resistance to anti-TB drugs in a teaching hospital in delhi was detected in 8% of new patients and 25% of previously treated patients (Sural 2021).

DISEASE CAUSED BY ATYPICAL MYCOBACTERIA

The term atypical mycobacteria refers to mycobacteria other than *M. tuberculosis* and *M. bovis.* These mycobacteria are also addressed as nontuberculosis mycobacteria (NTM). Rarely these organisms may be responsible for infective lesions in the skeletal system. Synovial sheath infections are more common with atypical mycobacteria than infection of osseous tissues. Of the 77 positive cultures, the organisms (obtained in BHU Hospital between 1969–1971) were typical in 73, and photochromogen *Mycobacterium kansassi* in 4. The clinical and radiological picture of the lesions produced by atypical mycobacteria as a rule does not resemble the classical, typical osteoarticular lesions (Karlson 1973, Lakhanpal et al. 1980). Typical mycobacteria are as a rule not resistant to more than one main drug, whereas most of the atypical mycobacteria are found resistant to many commonly used drugs (Lakhanpal et al. 1976, Goyal 1962, Runnyon 1959).

With atypical mycobacterial infections human-to-human transmission does not generally occur. Often a history of trauma (possible direct inoculation) such as puncture wound, steroid injection, surgery, or exposure to contaminated marine life is found. Many patients may have concomitant diabetes, or immuno-suppression for organ transplantation, or may be infected with human immunodeficiency virus (HIV) (Sunderam et al. 1986). In culture reports, atypical mycobacteria were often disregarded as contaminants. However, in the presence of predisposing factors (vide supra), the atypical mycobacterial growth should be considered significant and pathogenic. Disease caused by atypical mycobacteria (Sutker et al. 1979, Tanaka et al. 1993), and emergence of multidrug-resistant strains is an alarming and common observation seen in tuberculous disease in HIV patients.

Extensive work is being done in many laboratories to understand the intermediary metabolism of mycobacteria. It may help us to appreciate subtle differences between virulent and avirulent strains, and between sensitive and resistant strains (Suryanarayana-Murthy 1966, Ramakrishnan et al. 1972, Dewan et al. 1987).

Atypical mycobacteria (NTM) which have been isolated from tuberculous lesions of skeletal system are *M. kansassi, M. marinum, M. avium* complex, *M. scrofulaceum, M. chelonae, M. intracellulare, M. fortuitum* (Lakhanpal 1980, Runnyon 1959, Sutker et al. 1979, Tanka et al. 1993, Satoskar 1999, Danaviah et al. 2007, Park et al. 2014, Sudrezl et al. 2019). There are more chances of atypical mycobacterial infections in HIV patients, Numerous etiologic species of Mycobacteria responsible for infection of stray animals like cows, dogs, cats have been described.

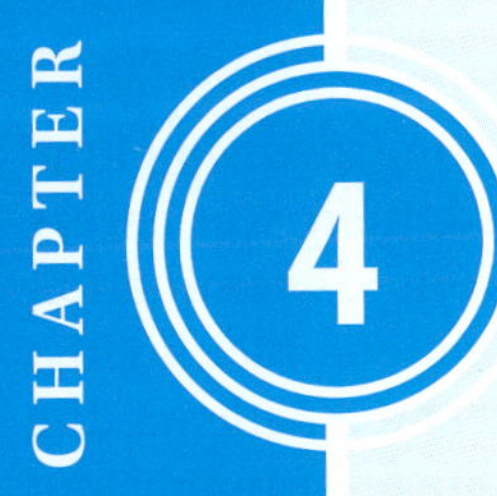

Evolution of Treatment of Skeletal Tuberculosis

The evolution of treatment of tuberculosis of bones, joints and spine has passed through different phases of development. The availability of antitubercular drugs (1948–1951), a significant milestone, divides the treatment of tuberculosis into two eras:

1. **Preantituberculor era**: When such patients were treated either by orthodox conservative regime or by various operative procedures.
2. **Postantitubercular era**: Two different lines of treatment developed over the years.
   a. Operative in all cases in conjunction with antitubercular drugs (Wilkinson 1950, 1969, Hodgson et al. 1956, 1960, Mukopadhaya 1956, 1957, Buchman 1961, Donaldson 1965, Stock 1962, Cameron 1962, Risko 1963, Fellander 1955, Orell 1951, Kondo and Yamada 1957, Silva 1980, Chahal 1980).
   b. Antitubercular drugs in all cases with operation for failures or complications (Tuli 1967–84, Roaf 1958, 1959, Seddon 1956, Friedman 1966, 1973, Kaplan 1959, Konstam and Blesovsky 1962, Stevenson and Manning 1962, Martini 1980–88, Versfeld 1982).

PREANTITUBERCULAR ERA

Preantitubercular Conservative Treatment

Orthodox Treatment (Bick 1976)

In ancient India, the Atharvans (1800–1000 BC) used to treat cases of skeletal tuberculosis with "Sipudru", a herbal preparation and sunshine (Duraiswami and Tuli 1971). Hippocrates (450 BC) and Galen (AD 131–201) tried to correct kyphotic deformity due to tuberculosis of the spine, by manual pressure, traction and mechanical appliances but failed **(Fig. 4.1)**. The orthodox conservative treatment was entirely constitutional in its character and strongly advocated recumbency, better nutrition, immobilization by means of body casts, plaster beds and braces. The value of heliotherapy and open air was extolled in specialized hospitals or sanatoria. Average time of hospitalization varied between one and 5 years. Rest as the fundamental of treatment was strongly advised and practised by John Hilton (1863) and Hugh Owen Thomas (1875). The unique combination of Sir Robert Jones (1923) and Dame Agnes Hunt enhanced these principles and placed the benefit of country hospitals at the disposal of such patients where they could receive fresh air,

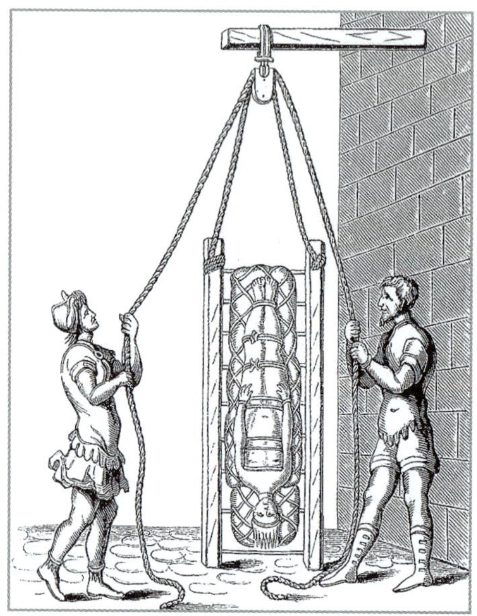

Fig. 4.1: Mechanical methods of correction of the obvious deformity in spinal tuberculosis, used by earlier workers; the results were usually futile and sometimes disastrous.

sunshine, adequate food and rest. These dictums still constitute part of the routine treatment of tuberculosis, especially in economically underdeveloped countries, because most of the patients suffering from tuberculous infection, due to their economic strata live in subnormal conditions.

Natural Course of Skeletal Tuberculosis without Chemotherapy

Before the availability of antitubercular chemotherapy, osteoarticular tuberculosis passed through three stages spanned over a period of 3–5 years. The stage of onset lasted from one month to one year (synovial disease) during which the localized disease developed into a warm tender swelling with marked localized osteoporosis and minimal destruction. In the second stage of destruction (lasting for 1–3 years), the disease progressed till there was gross destruction of joint with deformity, subluxation, contractures and abscess formation. The abscesses finally ruptured and drained as sinuses with frequent secondary pyogenic infection. With superimposed pyogenic infection, the general defense mechanism of the patient was markedly lowered, there was severe cachexia, frequent tuberculous dissemination (milliary tuberculosis, tuberculous meningitis) and death of nearly one-third of the patients. The survivors entered the third stage of repair and ankylosis, occurring after 2–3 years of onset of the disease. There was improvement in the patient's general condition. The abscesses resorbed, sinuses underwent healing, and the destroyed bones were remineralized. The diseased area generally healed with fusion in a deformed position. Bony fusion (generally the outcome with superimposed pyogenic infection) was preferred because absence of joint motion meant minimization of recurrence of infection and progress of deformation. When healing took place by fibrous ankylosis, the surgeons considered it unsatisfactory because such joints had pain on movement and weight bearing, reactivation of infection was frequent (with chances of amyloid disease) and deformation aggravated with the passage of time. The primary aim prior to the availability of chemotherapy was to achieve the "stage of repair and ankylosis" of the diseased joint or spine in the least disabling position by plaster cast immobilization for 2–3 years.

Results of Orthodox Conservative Treatment

Results on the whole were unsatisfactory. On the bases of total number of patients treated, only 30–44% of cases were found to have full working capacity (Alvik 1949, Dobson 1951, Fellander 1955, Fox 1962). The rest of the patients were either dead (30–50%) or severely crippled. In Dobson's (1951) series, out of 394 cases 31% developed paraplegia and 25% of paralyzed patients died. Girdlestone and Somerville (1965) also reported 28% mortality out of 130 nonparaplegic cases treated by orthodox method. LaFond (1958) reported 57% of mortality and 39% of relapse rate in adult skeletal tuberculosis. Kyphosis could develop or increased while the patient was being treated in a plaster bed (Paus 1964). Recovery from paraplegia was reported in about one-third of the cases (Alvik 1949, Griffiths, Seddon and Roaf 1956, Kaplan 1959). However, the failure of the conservative treatment in preventing the onset of paraplegia was also well recognized (Dobson 1951).

Prechemotherapy Operative Treatment and its Results

Disappointing results of orthodox conservative treatment in the pre-chemotherapy era induced the attending physicians to evolve more direct surgical excision of the diseased bones and joints. Most of the earlier operations were for drainage of abscesses or sinuses. Unfortunately, all such procedures resulted in persistent serious sinus and ulcer formations, and death of patients. The general outlook regarding surgery, therefore, was aptly summarized by Calot (1930) as, "Surgeon who, so far as tuberculosis is concerned, swears to remove the evil from the very root, will only find one result awaiting him—the death of his patient". Probably because of such a gloomy picture of the "direct operation on the diseased area" the surgeons tended to develop "distant operations" without opening the site of disease. Albee (1911, 1930) and Hibbs (1912, 1918, 1928) introduced and developed posterior spinal fusion, and extra-articular operations for fusion of hip and shoulder joints were developed by Britain (1952) **(Fig. 4.2)**.

The aim of these operations was to shorten the period of immobilization in bed and plaster casts, and provide a permanent internal stability (fusion) to the diseased parts (as no motion implied least chance of activation of disease). Such operations were carried out from 1911 onwards. Over the years, it became increasingly obvious that extra-articular fusions only reduced the pain and did not create postoperative nonhealing tuberculous ulcers and sinuses. Nothing dramatic happened to the diseased area where pus, debris and necrotic bone remained enmeshed in dense fibrous tissue, the disease persisted sometimes mildly active, in other cases dormant only to flare up at any provocation. Of the survivals in general nearly 50% were assessed "healthy and fit", about 30% were "improved", and 20% remained "not healed". The posterior spinal operations had nothing to offer to the paraplegic patients who failed to respond to the standard sanatoria treatment.

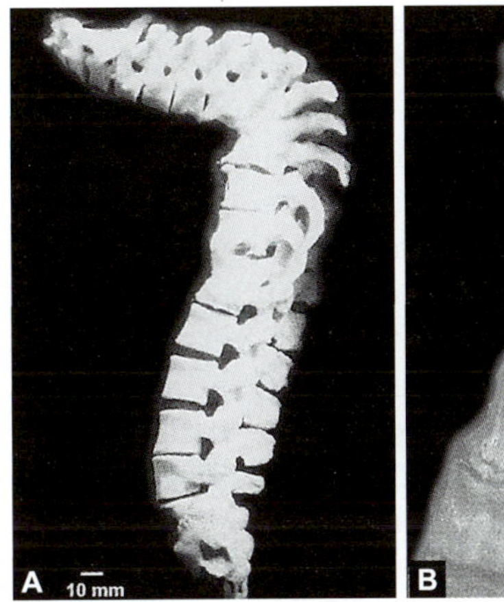

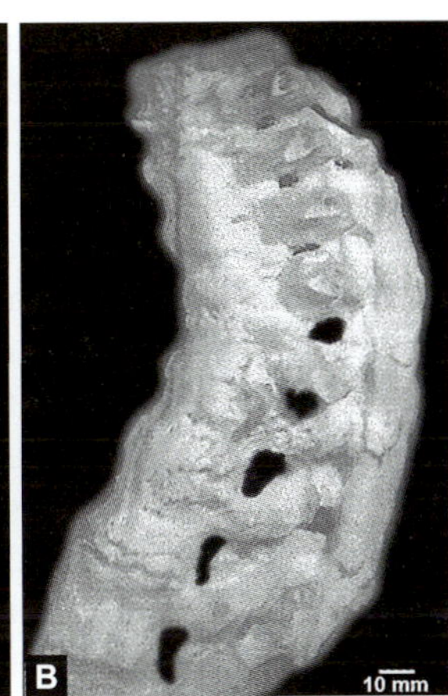

Figs. 4.2A and B: (A) Involvement of 14 vertebrae; and (B) Successful posterior fusion with arrested disease and deformity. Specimens of pre-anti TB drugs era.

Courtesy: Galler Collection Museum, Switzerland.

POSTANTITUBERCULAR ERA

Streptomycin became available for clinical use in 1947, PAS in 1949 and INH in 1952. The period for chemotherapeutic triumph was ushered in. However, in the wake of enthusiasm of surgical attack on skeletal tuberculosis the standard treatment practised and advocated during 1950 to 1960 was universal focal surgery in conjunction with antitubercular drugs (Bailey 1972, Wilkinson 1950, 1955, Kondo and Yamada 1957, Deroy 1952, Hodgson 1956, Compere 1952, Ostman 1951, Severance 1951, Smith 1950, Orell 1951, Mukopadhya 1956, Weinberg 1957, Roaf 1959).

Addition of streptomycin lowered the rate of relapse and the death rate due to tuberculosis; on the other hand it increased the return to productive activity of the patients. Average relapse rate with addition of streptomycin alone decreased by 30–35% (Falk 1958).

The most spectacular effect of the drugs was disappearance of sinuses, ulcers and abscesses despite extensive surgery, and the elimination of the danger of postoperative dissemination of tuberculous infection. Simultaneously, however, many surgeons (Kaplan 1959, Stevenson 1954, 1962, Konstam 1962, Friedman 1966, 1973, Tuli 1967–1985, Martini 1980–1988, Versfeld 1982) reported of excellent results by antitubercular drugs alone, confining surgery to failures or complications only. With the passage of time, indications for surgery have become universally more selective, less for the biological control of disease, but more for prevention and correction of deformities/complications, and for improving the quality of function of the diseased joints (Martini 1988, Tuli 1985, Moon et al. 2002, Hoffman et al. 2002, Rajasekaran et al. 1998, Jain 2007, Rajasekaran et al. 2013).

Most of the workers at present continue the chemotherapeutic regime for 12–18 months. For optimal results, the drugs must be used in combination, for a long time and uninterruptedly. Citron (1972) emphasized that major cause of poor results and discrepancy of results of various regimes is irregular drug administration. He suggested that supervised intermittent drug therapy (say twice a week) may be the answer for patients who are known to be irregular with self-administration of drugs. If for any reason the first combination of antitubercular drugs cannot be used, other combinations of newer drugs **(Table 6.1)**, as mentioned in the Chapter 6 on Antitubercular Drugs, can be confidently used.

The chief limitation of antitubercular drugs is development of resistant strains of tubercle bacilli. If only one drug is used there are very high chances of emergence of resistant strains, however, it is unusual for bacilli to be resistant to a combination of 2 or more drugs. As stated earlier, in our series none of the typical *Mycobacterium tuberculosis* cultured were observed to be resistant to more than one antitubercular drug *in vitro* (Lakhanpal et al. 1976).

Most of the clinical research work regarding the efficacy of antitubercular drugs has been carried out in the treatment of pulmonary tuberculosis. The results of the treatment of skeletal tuberculosis cannot be exactly similar because of different nature of tuberculous lesion in the two situations. At present, considerable discussion is taking place about the degree of healing which can take place without operative treatment. Many workers (Stevenson and Manning 1954, 1962, Konstam et al. 1958, 1962, 1963, Kaplan 1959, Friedman 1966, Medical Research Council 1973–1982, Martini 1980–1988, Tuli 1967–1985) have reported remarkable healing of osteoarticular tuberculosis with drugs alone. However, there are always some cases who require to be treated by surgery. Indications of continuation of drug treatment or of operation can be rationally controlled by serial radiography and imaging at about 3–4 months intervals. Progressive destruction or imperfect or slow healing in spite of antitubercular drugs (used for 4 months or more) are reasonable indications for surgery in early stages.

The knowledge about the exact effect of the modern antitubercular drugs on osteoarticular tuberculosis is still inadequate. However, certain facts are now quite clear (Somerville and Wilkinson 1965). Osseous tubercular lesions are relatively more resistant than synovial lesions. With prolonged antitubercular therapy histological appearances lose their characteristic forms. In a typical tubercle, the epithelioid cells become less compact. Tubercle becomes unrecognizable because the epithelioid cells and lymphocytes become widely scattered. The caseous area in the center of tubercle may become small or even undergo resorption. Fibrosis, however, still remains a significant feature in tuberculous joints treated by prolonged antitubercular therapy and immobilization. Early stage articular tuberculosis is now best treated by range of motion active exercises within the limits of pain while on multidrug therapy (functional treatment), most of these patients can achieve a healed status with functional arc of motions.

Sinuses and Ulcers

Before the advent of antitubercular chemotherapy, sinus formation was regarded as one of the most dreaded complications of skeletal tuberculosis, and surgery of tuberculosis was usually complicated by the formation of sinuses (Evans 1952, Harris 1952). Under the influence of antitubercular drugs most of the sinuses are observed to heal within 3–4 months without surgical intervention (Bosworth 1952, 1963, Hald 1954, Kaplan 1959, Konstam and Blesovsky 1962, Paus 1964, Tuli 1970, 1971). With triple drug therapy healing of sinuses is no more a problem. It is not associated even with extensive surgery done to remove the tubercular focus. Sinuses which fail to respond to drug therapy alone, would heal by change of drugs combined with or without curettage or excision of the sinus tracks. Failure of sinuses and ulcers to heal or their appearance while the patient is on drug therapy suggests infection by resistant organisms or immunosuppressed state of the patient.

Relapse of the Disease or Recurrence

Falk (1958) reported a relapse rate of 20% in cases of skeletal tuberculosis treated with streptomycin during the years 1946–1948. Kaplan (1959) reported 2% recurrence rate among 130 patients. In Konstam and Blesovsky's (1962) series, out of 207 patients only one had recurrence. The low rate of relapse is probably due to effective antitubercular drugs available these days. Yeager (1963) observed that prolonged use of "combined antimicrobial therapy has lowered the relapse rate to its lowest point in our history". Results of various series treated by "orthodox", "conservative ambulatory", "conservative nonambulatory" and "radical operative" procedures are summarized in **Tables 23.1 and 23.5**. The results of orthodox treatment obviously were poor because in those days antitubercular drugs were not available. The series treated by antitubercular drugs, conservatively or in conjunction with radical surgical extirpation on the whole gave good results. The incidence of healing by conservative antitubercular therapy in different series varies between 83 and 96.8%. In the series treated by excisional therapy, the incidence of healing has been between 80 and 96%. As skeletal tuberculosis runs an insidious and chronic course with occasional reactivation or relapse many years later, it is obvious that exact incidence of recurrence can never be calculated accurately. An average figure at present, for patients followed-up for 5–10 years after the completion of the drug therapy, would be 2–5% (Tuli 1985). Martin (1970) reported reappearance of cold abscesses in 35 cases after 2 years, and in 54 cases after 3 years or more, out of 359 cases treated by chemotherapy.

At present, treatment of skeletal tuberculosis is both systemic and local. Systemic therapy consists of relative rest, general supportive measures and prolonged chemotherapy. Modern antitubercular drugs are the most important therapeutic measures in skeletal tuberculosis. It has accelerated the rate and quality of recovery, and has minimized the incidence of mortality, complications and recrudescence **(Fig. 4.3)**.

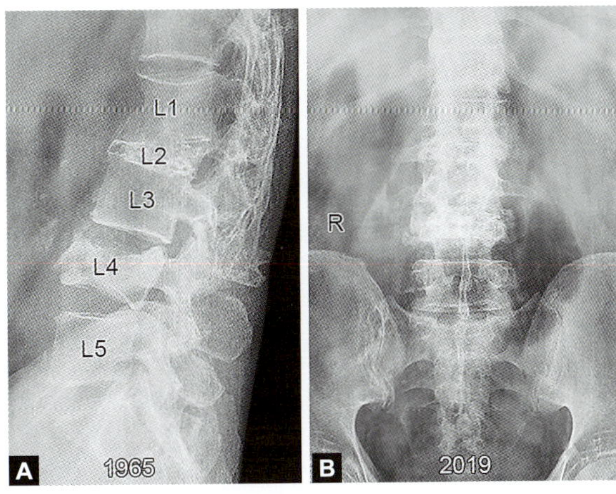

Figs. 4.3A and B: The classical posterior spinal fusion done 54 years ago (1965); Note excellent result. Patient now reported for a new tuberculous lesion at adjacent distal level (delayed recrudescence) at L4 in 2019.

Patients with early disease, sensitive organisms and favorable pathological lesion (i.e., absence of large cavitations, ischemic tissue and infarcted bone) can achieve full clinical healing with antitubercular chemotherapy without surgical intervention. Antitubercular drugs must be continued for about 18 months and must include isoniazid. Total elimination of mycobacteria from the body is impossible because some microbes will continue staying in the host intracellularly for many years. Immunity of the patient must be maintained at optimum level throughout the life-span to minimize reactivation of disease **(Fig 4.3)**.

Nene et al. (2018) observed patients who were treated by anti-TB drugs for 6 month, no reactivation was observed upto 24 month of follow-up. Many workers (as above), however, have reported recurrence of disease or reactivation at the "healed lesion" >10 years after completion of the drug therapy at the first visit **(Fig. 4.3)**. Common causes are diabetes, HIV infection, prolonged use of corticosteroids, disease modifying agents, substance abuse, alcoholism, oncological drugs, poor nutrition, morbid obesity and senior age any time during the life span of the patient. We prefer using "healed status" of disease rather than cure for tibercular infection.

CHAPTER 5

Diagnosis and Investigations

GENERAL CLINICAL PICTURE

Skeletal tuberculosis mostly occurs during first three decades of life; no age, however, is immune. In the affluent societies, the disease is being reported essentially in the elderly (Mann 1987, Autzen 1988, Mitchison and Chalmers 1986). The characteristics are insidious onset, monoarticular or mono-osseous involvement and the constitutional symptoms like low-grade fever and lassitude (especially in the afternoon), anorexia, loss of weight, night sweats, tachycardia, and anemia. Local symptoms and signs are pain, night cries, painful limitation of movements, muscle wasting, and regional lymph node enlargement. During acute stage, the protective muscle spasm is severe holding the diseased area immobilized. During sleep, the muscle spasm relaxes and permits movement between the inflamed surfaces resulting in pain causing the typical night cries (especially in children). In neglected cases or those with compromised immunity, the patient may present with tuberculous ulcers and sinuses. Tubercular ulcers are typically flat, irregularly shaped excavations of skin (5–15 mm), the margins are pigmented and the borders are undermined. The ulcers may show seropurulent discharge and pale granulations. Some of the ulcers may have continuity with the deeper sinus tracts.

DIAGNOSIS

In developing countries, in general, diagnosis of tuberculosis of bones and joints can be reliably made on clinical and radiological examination (Shanmugasundaram 1982, Hoffman et al. 1993, Sankaran 1993). However, such a situation is becoming increasingly difficult in affluent countries where tuberculosis has been reduced almost to the status of a rare disease, and the present generation of doctors are unfamiliar with it's skeletal manifestations. In such situations and whenever in doubt, a positive proof of the disease must be obtained employing semi-invasive or invasive investigations. In the affluent societies, corticosteroids, alcoholism, prolonged illness, diabetic state, HIV infection, anticancer chemotherapy, immunosuppressive drug therapy (for rheumatoid disorders and organ transplants), and old age are the probable predisposing factors. Since 1985, however, there is reappearance of tuberculosis in all forms in the developed countries as well.

The delay in diagnosing a case of tuberculous arthritis is quite common in the affluent industrialized world (Wray and Roy 1987, Halsey et al. 1982, Newton et al. 1986). Therefore, skeletal tuberculosis must be included in differential diagnosis of chronic/subacute monoarticular arthritis, chronic abscess, draining sinus, chronic

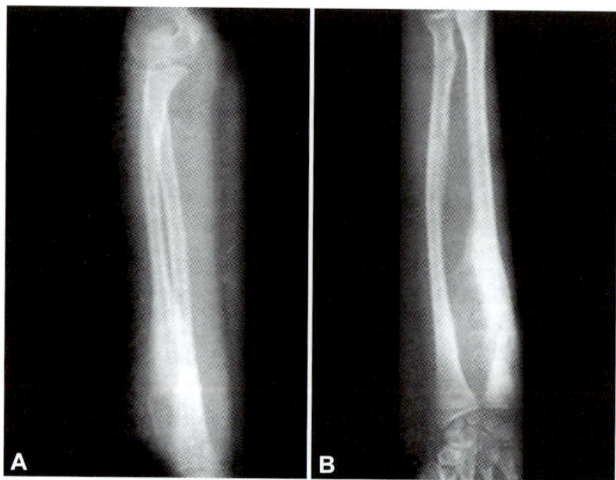

Figs. 5.1A and B: (A) "Tumor-like" appearance in the distal ulna of a young girl. Histology proved the diagnosis of tuberculous infection. The drugs completely resolved the lesion (B).

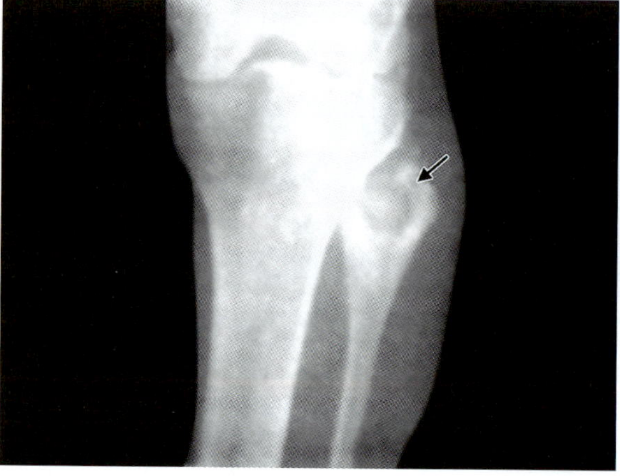

Fig. 5.2: Tuberculosis of upper end of fibula. Note a typical coke like sequestrum contained in a cavity.

swelling **(Fig. 5.1)** or osteomyelitis (Wolfgang 1978, Su et al. 1985, Martini 1986, Chatterjee et al. 2003).

The following investigations are useful in a routine case.

Roentgenogram

Anteroposterior and lateral views of the part, and an X-ray of the chest are mandatory. Localized osteoporosis is the first radiological sign of active disease. The articular margins and bony cortices become hazy, (giving a "washed out" appearance) there may be development of areas of trabecular or bony destruction and osteolysis. The synovial fluid, thickened synovium, capsule and pericapsular tissues may cause a soft-tissue swelling. With the involvement of articular cartilage, the joint space (articular cartilage space) shows diminution in the X-rays. As the destructive process advances there may be collapse of bone, subluxation/dislocation, migration and deformity of the joint. The epiphyseal growth plate may be destroyed to cause irregular growth or premature fusion. Rarely, hyperemia adjacent to the growth plate may, temporarily, stimulate the longitudinal growth. With healing of the disease process, there is remineralization and reappearance of bony trabeculae and sharpening of cortical and articular margins. Changes in the bone are discernable in the routine X-rays 2–4 months after the onset of disease. In early disease, it is wise to have identical X-rays with contralateral region (by the same exposure) wherever possible to discern the earliest abnormal signs. This is easily possible for elbow, wrist, hand, hips, knees, ankle, and feet.

In the center of a tuberculous cavity, there may be a sequestrum of cancellous bone or calcification of the caseous tissue, which gives an appearance of an irregular soft, feathery, coke like sequestrum ("image en Grelot") contained in the cavity **(Figs. 5.2 and 10.1)**. Sequestration of a segment of bone, particularly in cancellous region, may take place due to ischemic infarction **(Figs. 2.2, 5.3 and 5.4)**. If secondary infection supervenes or there is a sinus formation, subperiosteal new bone formation can be seen along the involved bones. The subperiosteal reaction occurs much earlier in pyogenic arthritis. Plaques of irregular calcification (dystrophic calcification) if present in the wall of a chronic abscess **(Fig. 5.5)** or sinus, in any **(Fig. 20.9)** case is almost diagnostic of tuberculous infection of long-standing (Sharma 1978, Griffith et al. 2002).

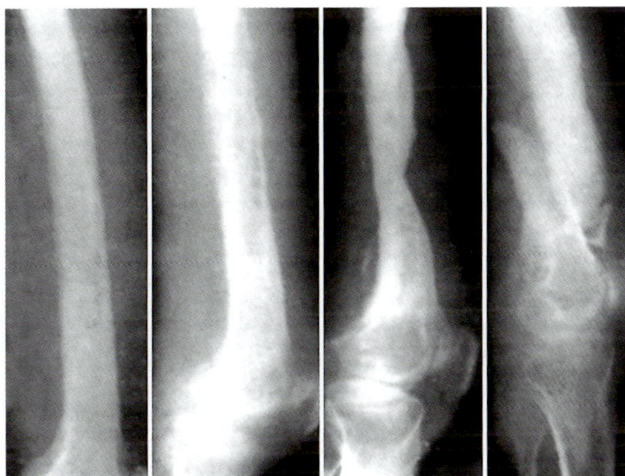

Fig. 5.3: X-rays of an adult from 1980 to 1996. The "atypical osteomyelitis" of femur had a deroofing operation done, however, unfortunately the tissue diagnosis was not available. The disease healed with minor recrudescence off and on. In 1996, the patient had a fracture as a result of minor trauma which resulted in reactivation of infection. Histological examination of the pathological tissue proved the diagnosis of tuberculosis.

Courtesy: Professor NK Aggarwal, CMC Ludhiana.

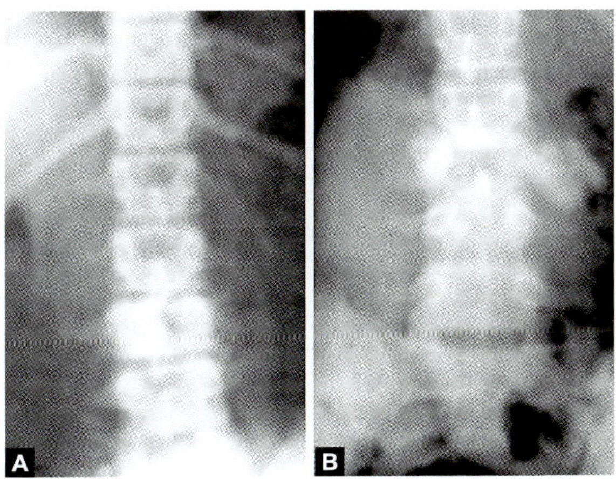

Figs. 5.4A and B: X-rays of an adult female show (A) Increased density of lumbar 3 vertebral body with a vertical break, (B) shows wide separation of the sequestrated fragments of the vertebral body 4 weeks later.

Tomography and computerized axial tomography demonstrate the localization and extent of bone and soft-tissue lesions, and immensely help in needle or core biopsy (Cropper et al. 1982).

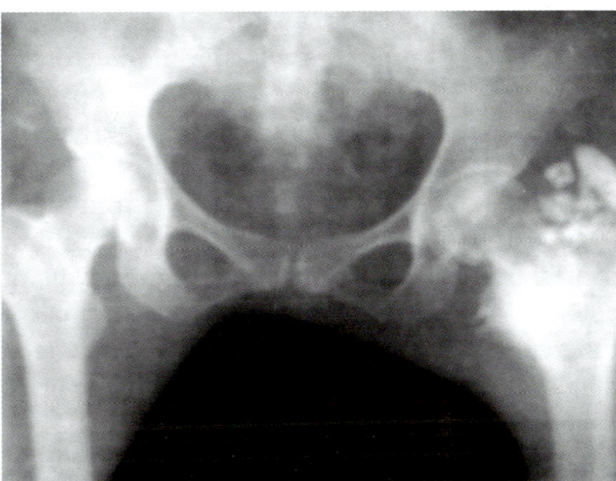

Fig. 5.5: Dystrophic calcification is visible around the left hip joint in a patient who had gluteal bursal tuberculosis of long-standing.

Blood

A relative lymphocytosis, low hemoglobin, and raised erythrocyte sedimentation rate are often found in the active stage of disease. Raised ESR, however, is not necessarily a proof of activity of the infection. Its repeated estimation at 3–6 months intervals gives a valuable index to the activity of the disease. There are, however, some patients who may not exhibit raised ESR despite the presence of clinically obvious active disease.

Mantoux (Heaf) Test

As a rule, a positive reaction is present in a patient with tuberculous disease of some standing (1–3 months). A negative test, in general, rules out the disease. Rarely, the tuberculin test may be negative although active tuberculosis is present, as in severe and disseminated tuberculosis, during high fever or certain exanthemata, after virus vaccination, recent viral infection or steroid therapy, or in immunocompetent state, or severe under-nutrition or extremes of age.

Biopsy

Whenever there is doubt (particularly in early stages) it is mandatory to prove the diagnosis by obtaining the diseased tissue (granulations and/

or synovium and/or bone and/or lymph nodes). Microscopic examination of aspiration cytology (Bailey 1985), core biopsy, needle biopsy or open biopsy would reveal typical tubercles in untreated cases of shorter duration of disease. Epitheliod cells surrounded by lymphocytes in the configuration of a tubercle (even without central necrosis or peripheral foreign-body giant cells) is an adequate histological evidence of tuberculous pathology in a patient who has been diagnosed so clinicoradiologically (Newton et al. 1986, Aggarwal et al. 2012, Kafla 2022). If one has decided to do a biopsy from the diseased joint and bone, one should also obtain the enlarged regional lymph nodes for examination. For the disease of knee and foot, it is essentially/only the deep inguinal lymph nodes that are diagnostic. At the time of open biopsy of a joint or an osseous lesion, a wise orthopedic surgeon would perform synovectomy or curettage/debridement as a part of therapeutic measures.

Histopathological features distinguish between infective lesions and malignant disease on one hand, and between a suppurative and a granulomatous condition on the other hand. The infections of bone and joints that present as granulomatous lesions in order of frequency are tuberculosis, mycotic infection, brucellosis, sarcoidosis, and tuberculoid leprosy.

Examination of synovial fluid in early cases of tuberculosis is marginally helpful; it shows a leukocytosis in which polymorphs predominate (10–20 thousand white blood cells/mL). The glucose content is markedly reduced, protein levels are elevated with a poor mucin clot. Synovial joint aspirate is an excellent material for polymerase chain reaction (PCR) for tuberculosis.

Guinea Pig Inoculation

The tuberculous pus, joint aspirate, liquefied granulation tissue, curettings from the depth of sinus or ulcers, or diseased material may be injected into the guinea pig intraperitoneally. Examination in positive cases discloses tubercles on the peritoneum 5–8 weeks later. This investigation is considered uneconomical, and clinically not practicable, however, it perhaps offers the most reliable proof of tuberculous pathology.

Smear and Culture

The material prepared for guinea pig inoculation may also be submitted for smear and culture examination for acid-fast bacilli (Chapter 3). Direct smear examination of the pathological material, in cases with the disease of short duration and who were not previously on antitubercular drugs, may reveal acid-fast bacilli in the synovial fluid aspirate in 10%, in the synovial tissue in 20%, in the regional lymph nodes in 30% **(Fig. 5.6)** and in the osseous cavities or destroyed areas in 10%. Cultures are likely to be positive in 30–60% of such material. Demonstration of acid-fast bacilli by direct smear facilitates a prompt diagnosis, the cultures generally take 8 weeks.

Despite the above-mentioned investigations, there are certain cases (20%), particularly those already treated or those with chronic disease of long-standing, in which it is not possible to confirm the exact diagnosis. Highest proof of

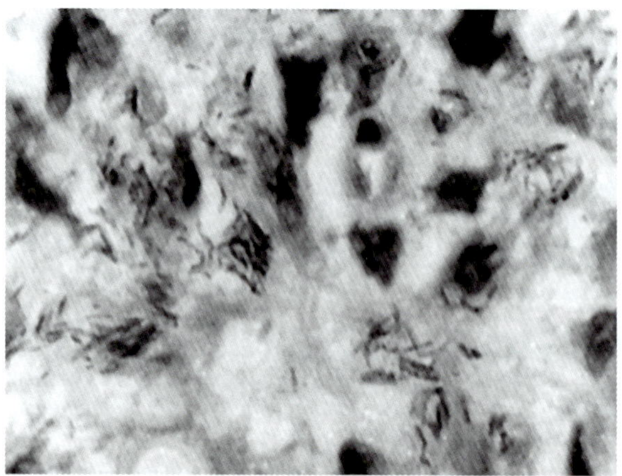

Fig. 5.6: Material obtained by fine-needle aspiration from the enlarged lymph nodes in the axilla of a patient suffering from tuberculosis of second metacarpal and elbow joint. One can see a large number of tuberculous bacilli as happens in immunocompromised states.

tuberculous disease would be obtained if the diseased material is submitted for direct smear, histology, culture, and guinea pig inoculation, simultaneously (Lakhanpal et al. 1974, Hald 1964). Microbiological examination of the washings of a dry lesion is as a rule of no avail. Aspirates of paravertebral abscess or diseased tissue from spinal tuberculosis seldom demonstrate mycobacteria (Moon 2002).

Isotope Scintigraphy

Most of the cases of skeletal tuberculosis are easily diagnosed on clinical and radiological findings, however, common and indiscriminate use of antibiotics has created an environment in which "low-grade" pyogenic infections can mimic any infection. Scintigraphy has become a common diagnostic technique in affluent countries. The three currently utilized isotopes in imaging patients with suspected/early skeletal tuberculosis are technetium-(^{99m}Tc), gallium-(^{67}Ga), and indium-(^{111}In). Of all these, technetium-99m scintigraphy is extremely sensitive and only misses a small percentage of infections. The major drawback is, however, lack of specificity. A technetium scan may show increased uptake in osteoporotic fractures, infections, stress fractures, healing traumatic fractures, inflammation due to degenerative osteoarthrosis or malignancies, and is not therefore diagnostic (Nocera et al. 1983, Goris 1986). A positive scan does localize the suspicious region for future observations, and for identifying an easily accessible site for obtaining material for tissue diagnosis (Bhatnagar et al. 2000).

Serological Investigations

Stroebel et al. (1982) reported that an enzyme-linked immunoabsorbent assay (ELISA) for antibody to mycobacterial antigen-6, demonstrated, at a cut-off 1:32, sensitivity of 94% and specificity of 100% in the serologic diagnosis of bone and joint tuberculosis. Consistency of these observations have not gained acceptance for routine use. Serological investigations are, however, useful in differential diagnosis of brucellosis, typhoid infection, and syphilitic infections.

In a study (1979–1999), Hoffman et al. (2002) reported their observations on polymerase chain reaction (PCR) for tuberculosis of knee joint. Of the 10 patients who had histological caseating granulomas or a positive AFB culture or both, only 4 had a positive result by the nested PCR method, giving 40% sensitivity for tuberculosis. He, however, observed no false positive test (100% specificity). Polymerase chain reaction (PCR) for tuberculosis is being critically analyzed in clinical situation. The best material for this test is clear fluid from cold abscesses, joints, pleural cavities or ascities. A negative test does not exclude tuberculosis. However, a positive report is of value if there is clinical evidence of active inflammation (Gollwitzer et al. 2004). Held et al. (2014) used "GenXpert" PCR on pathological tissues obtained from spinal tuberculosis in South Africa. They reported 95% of sensitivity and 96% specificity, and also detected MDR-Tb in 5.8% of specimens. Though PCR is considered highly specific for tuberculous bacillus, however, it may overlook other species of mycobacteria. PCR is of significance if the patient has clinically active inflammatory picture because the PCR may be positive even if the *Mycobacterium* is dead, formalin preserved (Jambekar et al. 2006) or the test material contains only a fragment of the bacterium. Monoarticular disease with non-specific histologic evaluation, a negative culture, and a negative PCR for tuberculosis is a diagnostic problem, to be differentiated from pauciarticular juvenile rheumatoid arthritis. If the characteristic histologic fibrinoid necrosis of rheumatoid disease is not detected in biopsy material, repeated clinical assessment would help in management of such cases.

Quanti FERON-TB Gold blood tests have been reported with sensitivities and specificities of 84% and 95% however, they are not useful in TB endemic areas due to the populations common exposure with asymptomatic latent (inactive) infection rather than active disease during growing years. Similarly, PCR may be falsely positive in tissues or body fluids in patients from TB endemic areas from specimens obtained from nontuberculous lesions (Broderick et al. 2018). Immune-based testing may indicate exposure to tuberculous infection but not clinical disease.

Osteoarticular involvement due to brucellosis must be considered in differential diagnosis of tuberculosis in any person from the endemic areas, having a contact with animals and consuming unpasteurized or unboiled milk. Any area of the skeletal system may be involved either as monoarthritis or as oligoarthritis; hip is the commonest joint affected (Mousa et al. 1987, Benjamin and Khan 1994). The diagnosis is best established by identification of the causative organism, agglutination tests or by tissue biopsy. Seventy-five cases of bone and joint tuberculosis from orthopedic department at BHU Hospital during 1970–1973, were submitted for serological investigations for brucellosis. None of them, however, showed a positive Smith and Wright test for brucella antibodies (Varma and Krishnamurthy 1973 unreported). Skeletal involvement by brucella is extremely rare below the age of 3 years.

In a patient with concomitant meningitis, cerebrospinal fluid examination may be of diagnostic help: sugar level is less than 2/3 of the blood level, protein level is >50 mg/mL (may form a web on standing), cell count is elevated with predominant lymphocytes, mycobacteria may be positive in about 25%, and PCR may be of help.

Modern Imaging Techniques

CT scans (essentially the X-rays in transverse sections) are helpful in demonstrating small destroyed areas (lytic cavities) in the bone and marginal erosions much before these can be seen in X-rays. Swelling in the soft tissues caused by tissue edema, granulations, exudations or abscess formation can also be demonstrated much earlier. All these changes are, however, not specific **(Fig. 5.7)**. Similar changes can be detected in trauma, nontuberculous infections and neoplasms. This investigation is a good choice for detecting disease in difficult areas like craniovertebral region, cervicodorsal region (C7 to D3), lumbosacral region, sacroiliac joints, sacrum, and posterior elements of vertebrae, ribs and sternum. Encroachment of the vertebral canal and dystrophic calcification in the soft tissue can be easily detected. CT guided/directed needle biopsy is an effective method of obtaining tissues for pathological and microbiological diagnosis (Azouz 1981) **(Fig. 5.8)**.

MRI would confirm whatever one can see in plain X-rays and CT scans. However, it also shows the predestructive lesions like demineralization, edema or inflammation of the bone in active disease which is more extensive than the areas of radiological destruction in the bone **(Figs. 5.9 and 5.10)**. Once the radiological changes have established, no great advantage is gained by radioisotope scanning or MRI. Encroachment of the vertebral canal, displacement of the dural

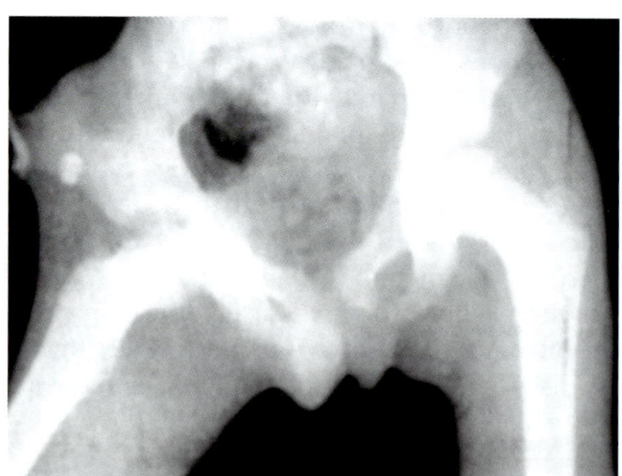

Fig. 5.7: Plain X-ray for pain, limping and deformity of right hip joint revealed an abduction-external rotation deformity, moderate degree of diminution of the right hip joint space, and soft-tissue swelling. CT scans of the right hip (diseased) compared with the normal hip do not show any features pathognomonic of tuberculous pathology. The changes observed in the CT scan of the same patient are shown in **Figure 5.8**. Unusual deformity of flexion, abduction and external rotation in this child was because external rotation rested the thigh on bed for relief of pain.

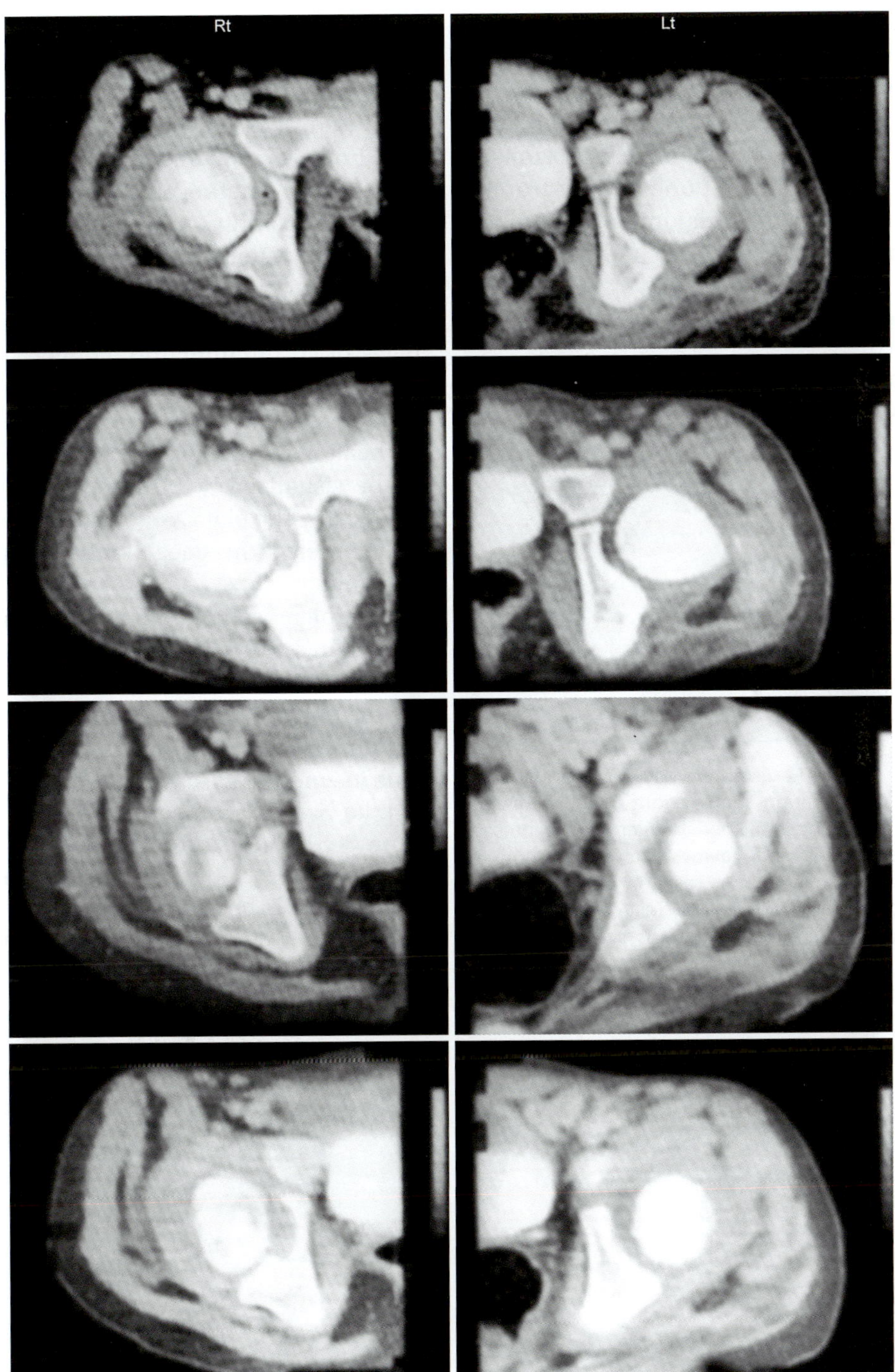

Fig. 5.8: CT scans of the patient shown in **Figure 5.7** show periarticular soft-tissue swelling in the right hip, irregular diminution of the joint space, presence of subchondral fracture of femoral head, irregularity in its shape, and areas of destruction in the femoral head and acetabulum. Tuberculous nature of pathology was confirmed by histology of the diseased tissue from right hip joint.

sheath, localized tuberculoma, generalized granuloma, shrinkage of the cord substance, myelitis (edema of cord), myelomalacia, syrinx formation of cord can be appreciated by the study of MRI T1- and T2-weighted images. Erosions of the surface or margins of bone and dystrophic calcification (calcified debris) in the soft tissues, however, cannot be appreciated in the MRI. MRI also does not show early involvement of posterior elements of vertebrae (pedicels, posterior facet joints, transverse processes, laminae and spinous processes) any better than CT scan. MRI, however, can suggest the nature of "soft-tissue mass" whether it is composed of fibrous tissue, granulations, thin exudate, thick pus or a mixed lesion (Bell et al. 1990, Deroos et al. 1986, Desai 1994, Griffith et al. 2002, Skoura 2015).

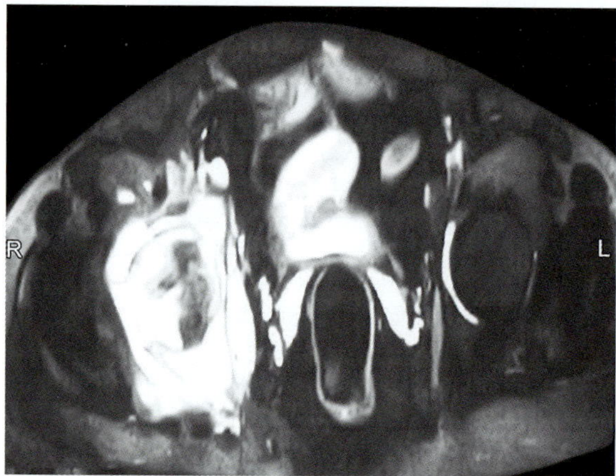

Fig. 5.9: The typical T2-weighted MRI picture of active "infection" or "inflammation" shows bright signal of effusion in the right hip joint and in the periarticular synovial bursae. The destroyed bones and cavities show collection of infective material or inflammatory reaction, essentially "non-specific changes" of bone edema and fluid collection. When in doubt arthrotomy and tissue diagnosis is mandatory.

Osseous tuberculosis passes through stages of (i) inflammatory edema and exudate (predestructive phase), (ii) necrosis and cavitation, (iii) destruction and deformation, and (iv) healing and repair. The predestructive stage can be visualized by MRI and probably also by bone scans. The plain X-rays and CT scans are not likely to detect the stage of inflammatory edema and exudate.

The role of gadolinium as a contrast medium in MRI has not yet been fully established in infective lesions; fibrous tissue is expected to give greater enhancement on T1-weighted images. Gadolinium enhancement is also considered of value in epidural abscess.

Like X-rays a repeat of CT scans and MRI about 3–5 months after the onset of treatment may show deterioration of the pathological process, this is because these images somewhat lag behind the pathophysiological changes

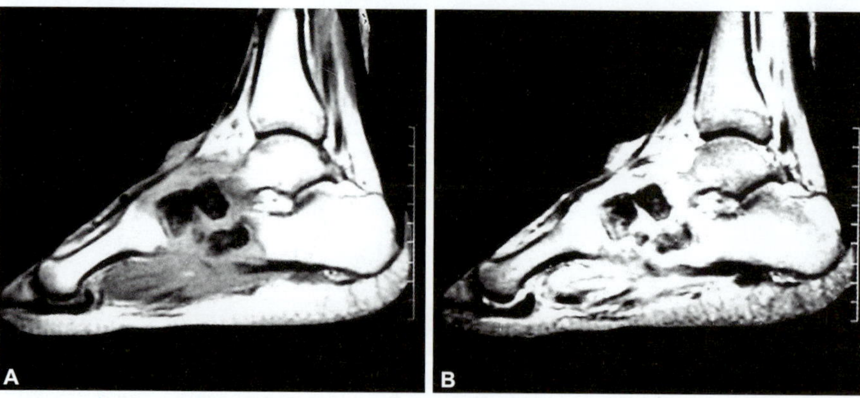

Figs. 5.10A and B: In MRI sequestrated bones show as signal voids. Note the typical signals of inflammatory reaction and collection of low signals in T1 (A), and high signals in T2 (B) images surrounding the sequestrated tarsal bones (showing signal voids).

that are taking place in the infected area, it should not cause unnecessary alarm. Repair of any infective lesion takes place by highly vascular granulation tissues. MRIs do not differentiate between the signals of reparative granulations and the granulations of active infection. The next follow-up by MRI 5–6 months after effective chemotherapy would show resolution or reduction in the extent of tissue edema, reduction in the size of paravertebral or paraosseous soft-tissue shadows, resolution or fibrosis of soft-tissue abscesses, reduction in the degree of encroachment of vertebral canal. X-rays and CT scans should show improvement like remineralization, reduction in the size of eroded areas and cavities, and sclerosis of osseous borders. If 6 months after the start of antituberculous chemotherapy there is deterioration of the clinical, laboratory and imaging features, a representative biopsy from the diseased area is mandatory to ascertain the underlying pathology. Distortion of the shape of the bone or spine, large areas of destruction and cavities and big sequestra do not undergo significant resolution.

Ultrasonography has been employed by various workers to estimate the presence of soft-tissue abscesses and its behavior under treatment. Sophisticated investigations are not warranted in clinically palpable and radiologically visible soft-tissue abscesses. However, small abscesses or soft-tissue masses can easily be appreciated in the CT scans and MRI.

Tuberculosis the Great MIMIC—Diagnostic Dilemma

Any tuberculous lesion may have overlapping features with almost any non-tuberculous pathology (vide supra). However, rarely one may come across another pathology coexiting with tuberculosis. It is sometime difficult to understand the "cause and effect" relationship or suspicion of coexistence. During a course of 60 years (1960–2020), we encountered skeletal tuberculosis coexisting with rheumatoid disorders, ankylosing spondylitis, hematological and visceral malignancies, lymphoproliferative disorders, transplant patients, immunosuppressive conditions, AIDS disorders. Coexistence of cancer and tuberculosis (Harikrishan 2012) and spondylolisthesis with tuberculosis (Chadha 2006) has been observed by other authors as well **(Figs. 5.11 and 5.12)**.

Despite the availability of ultrasonography (especially useful for tenosynovitis), CT scan and MRI, skeletal tuberculosis still maintains its reputation as a great mimic (Boutin 1998, Griffith et al. 2002). In early predestructive disease tuberculous infection, regardless of the site, may have overlapping features with nontuberculous infections, neoplastic disease, inflammatory conditions, sequele of metabolic disorders and trauma. Whenever in doubt, tissue diagnosis by aspiration and biopsy would help diagnosis before the onset of debilitating destructive disease. Gradient-echo MRI can demonstrate hemosiderin within the synovium which is characteristic of pigmented villonodular synovitis. Ultrasound may be an ideal first-line investigation for tenosynovitis to confirm the diagnosis and reveal the degree and extent of tendon and tendon-sheath involvement (Griffith et al. 2002). It can also reliably show large or medium sized psoas abscesses. Of all the patients who were subjected to generalized scanning (MRIs, isotope bone scan, PET-scan) >40% exhibited additional foci of subclinical active infection in the skeletal system or viscera or lymph nodes.

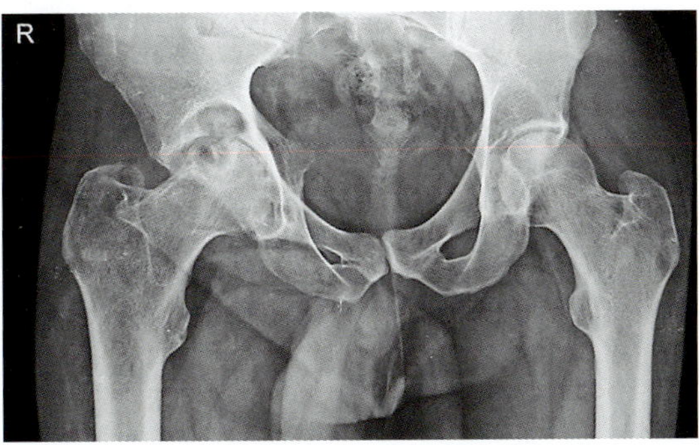

Fig. 5.11: X-ray of hip joint showing a "kissing lesion" (typical of tuberculous infections) astride the joint, suggesting infection through a common blood supply.

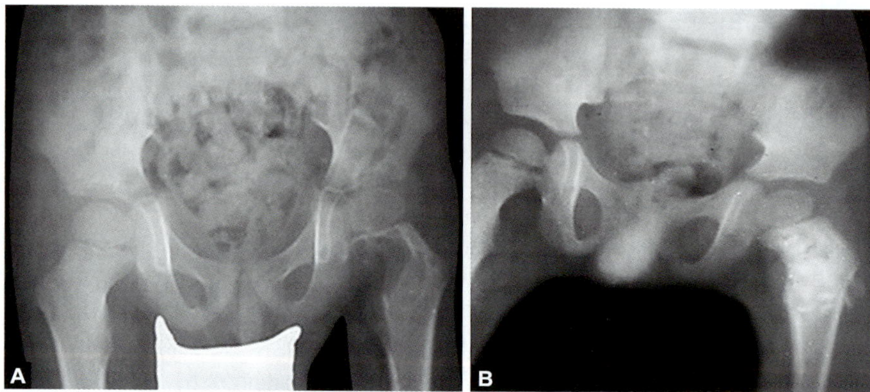

Figs. 5.12A and B: Tuberculosis can mimic any pathology and any pathology can mimic tuberculosis. If a patient does not respond favorably by 2–3 months, a possibility of an alternative pathology must be kept in mind. This child did not respond favorably (A). Curettage and bone grafting was done. The tissue diagnosis was eosinophilic granuloma (B).

Poncet's Disease or Tubercular Rheumatism

Poncet (1897) described cases of polyarthritis occurring in patients with tuberculosis. There is controversy over the existence of an association between polyarthritis and tuberculosis other than by chance. However, cases of polyarthralgia and polyarthritis associated with tuberculosis (usually extra-articular tuberculosis), continue to be described (Allen 1981, Southwood et al. 1988). Wilkinson and Roy (1984) reported a case of Poncet's disease in which one symptomatic joint was culture-positive (TB), however, as a rule the joint aspirate shows a watery or straw colored fluid which is negative on culture. During a period of 25 years, we observed 5 patients suspected to be tubercular rheumatism, majority were patients on antitubercular drugs, in a few the tuberculous disease had healed, ankle and knee were most commonly affected. The symptoms subsided in all the cases spontaneously by physiotherapeutic measures and the use of nonsteroidal anti-inflammatory drugs for a few weeks. With changing demographics many patients with long-term healed tuberculous infection may present with localized or generalized pains in bones and joints at senior age. Arthralgia can also be induced as a drug reaction to antitubercular chemotherapy (especially pyrazinamide). Generally, serum uric acid levels are raised and uricosuric drugs would relieve pains.

CHAPTER 6

Antitubercular Drugs

STREPTOMYCIN(S)

It was first discovered by Schatz, Bugie and Waksman in 1944 (Krantz and Carr 1958). Streptomycin exhibits both bacteriostatic and bactericidal activity toward sensitive organisms. The predominance of one activity over the other seems to depend on the concentration of streptomycin, the period of contact with the organism, the number, the rate of growth, and the sensitivity of the bacilli involved and the nature of medium. However, the main action appears to be bactericidal (Winder 1964). The bactericidal action of streptomycin is exerted only on growing and replicating organisms. In the case of multiplying and sensitive strains of tubercular bacilli, streptomycin probably damages the cell membrane by interfering with the synthesis of membrane protein, enters the cell and subsequently interferes with cytoplasmic protein synthesis (Winder 1964). This bactericidal action has been divided into two major phases: (i) initiation, which involves protein synthesis and which probably represents an effect of streptomycin on the membrane resulting in entry of streptomycin into the cell; (ii) the lethal phase which involves a further attack by streptomycin, possibly on a process other than protein synthesis. Under the influence of streptomycin, bacteria may become elongated and swollen and may stain irregularly (Winder 1964).

Eighth nerve damage is reported due to streptomycin toxicity. Streptomycin sulphate is more likely to affect the labyrinthine division leading to vertigo, and dihydrostreptomycin is more likely to damage the acoustic division, thus causing deafness. Crofton (1960) stated that the tendency to nerve complications are high by the presence of even a mild degree of renal insufficiency because then streptomycin is not excreted as fast as normally. Highest serum levels are generally reached in about 2 hours and the greater part is excreted in urine within 24 hours. Eighth nerve complication is reported to be minimized by simultaneous administration of 25 mg of calcium pantothenate daily (Somerville and Wilkinson 1965). Other rare complications are aplastic anemia, neutropenia, drug rashes, drug hypersensitivity, nausea and vomiting. All these require a careful detection and suitable treatment. In severe case, streptomycin may be completely withdrawn or a dosage schedule of alternate days or twice a week may be tried. In patients above the age of 45 years, streptomycin may enhance respiratory paralysis by interacting with neuromuscular blocking agents, especially while giving anesthesia.

PARA-AMINOSALICYLIC ACID (PAS)

It was discovered by Lehman in 1943 (Krantz and Carr 1958). The inhibitory effect is bacteriostatic, not bactericidal and the staining properties of the organism are not affected. PAS exerts its inhibitory action on the growth of mycobacteria by interfering with folic acid biosynthesis. PABA (para-amino benzoic acid) is used by microorganisms in the synthesis of folic acid, and PAS competes with PABA for the active site of an enzyme involved in the synthesis of folic acid (Winder 1964). This drug is not as effective as streptomycin and isoniazid. At best, it is a useful adjuvant to streptomycin or isoniazid to prevent development of resistant strains. By oral administration it is rapidly excreted; the highest blood level is reached within an hour. Its most important side effects, especially with higher doses, are symptoms of gastrointestinal irritation. The bulk of the drug markedly increases the chances of noncompliance, the recommended dose being 10–20 g per day.

ISONIAZID (INH-H)

It was discovered by Fox in 1951 (Krantz and Carr 1958), and became available for clinical use in late 1951. It is bactericidal and has two phase action on bacteria, one reversible and occurring even when cell growth is inhibited; the other irreversible, requiring growth. The enzyme peroxidase transfers isoniazid into the cell where it (INH) inhibits the synthesis of phospholipid fraction, insoluble carbohydrate containing fraction and nucleic acid, which are essential for the growth and viability of mycobacterium (Winder 1964).

Isonicotinic acid hydrazide (INH) is probably the most potent antitubercular drug. The potential effectiveness of INH alone or in various combinations was not well appreciated till the reports of its effectiveness appeared in the literature in the series mainly treated by domiciliary regime without strict bed rest and without universal surgical extirpation (Madras Experiments 1959, 1960, 1961, Konstam 1958, 1962, 1963, Friedman 1966, Dickson 1967, Watts 1996, Dhillon et al. 2001, 2002, Shembekar 2002). After oral or parenteral administration of INH the drug metabolizes to various inactive compounds. Only free INH has been found to have antimicrobial activity. Thus, it was speculated that the therapeutic usefulness of INH depends upon the metabolic pattern of the subject. On the basis of serum levels of biologically active INH the individuals have been segregated into "rapid inactivators", "intermediate inactivators" and "slow inactivators" (Harris 1963). Individual or racial variation in the response to drug therapy would, thus, depend upon the sensitivity of the mycobacterium and the metabolic pattern of the individual.

Isoniazid has the property of causing vasodilatation in the diseased area, thus permitting greater quantities of antibiotics to reach the lesion. Furthermore, the molecule of isoniazid is smaller than that of streptomycin and it is considered that isoniazid is able to reach the bacilli even within the macrophages.

The most important complications are the neurotoxic effects of isoniazid due to depletion of vitamin B factors. Neurotoxic complications may take the form of peripheral neuritis, muscular twitchings, paresthesiae, and psychological disturbances. These should be treated by administration of 50 mg of pyridoxine, 100 mg of nicotinamide and other B complex factors daily. Rarely skin rashes or gastrointestinal symptoms or hepatitis may develop.

Cases of skeletal tuberculosis as a rule require prolonged courses of large doses of antitubercular drugs, so it is essential to be aware of the possible toxic complications; their onset is often insidious and may continue for sometime even after the causative drug has been discontinued **(Table 6.1)**.

ETHAMBUTOL(E)

Average daily recommended dose of ethambutol is 25 mg/kg for first 60 days to be followed by 15 mg/kg, it may be continued for a period of about 1.5–2 years. Like other antitubercular drugs the daily requirement may be given as a single dose or in divided doses. Most important complication is retrobulbar neuritis and optic neuritis which fortunately recover on stopping the drug. Therefore, during ethambutol administration

Table 6.1: Commonly prescribed and useful antitubercular drugs and their toxicity.

Drugs	*Daily adult dose and administration*	*Minimum inhibitory concentration: μg/mL for human mycobacteria*	*Main drug toxicity*
Streptomycin (injection) (SM) C	20 mg/kg maximum 1 g (In children and elderly twice a week)	1–2	Vestibular damage, deafness, fever, rashes, contact dermatitis, nephrotoxicity
Isoniazid (INH)* C F	300–400 mg in single/ two divided doses	0.1–0.2	Peripheral neuropathy, behavior disorders, convulsions, hepatitis, hypersensitivity, osteomalacia like
Ethambutol (ETB) S F	15–25 mg/kg in single/ two divided doses	1–3	Retrobulbar neuritis with loss of vision, warned by diminution of visual field and acuity, and color blindness
Rifampicin (RCN) C F	450–600 mg in single/ two divided doses	0.25–1.0	Pinkish staining of urine, sweat and saliva, liver damage, bowel upset, rashes "flu-like" symptoms (purpura rarely)
Pyrazinamide C F	40 mg/kg in single or two divided doses	10–20	Hepatotoxicity, gouty arthritis (hyperuricemic arthralgia)
Fluoroquinolones C F	400–600 mg/day	1–2	GI upset, rashes, transient liver disturbances
Para-aminosalicylic acid (PAS)	12 g in single/two divided doses	1–4	GI disturbances, rashes, fever, lymphadenopathy, hepatotoxicity, drowsiness
Thioacetazone S	150 mg single dose	1	Anorexia, nausea, vomiting, liver damage, marrow depression
Ethionamide/ Prothionamide S	1 g single dose	10–20	GI upsets, abnormal liver tests, peripheral neuritis, convulsions
Cycloserine S	1 g single dose	5–10	Brain damage, mental disturbances, epilepsy
Capreomycin C (injection)	15 mg/kg single dose	2–3	Nephrotoxicity, others like streptomycin, 8th nerve damage
Kanamycin C (injection)	15 mg/kg single dose (maximum 1g/day)	8–16	Auditory toxicity, nephrotoxicity
Clofazimine C F	100–200 mg/day	1–5	GI upset, headache, red discoloration
Amikacin (injection) C	15 mg/kg/day	4–8	Ototoxicity, nephrotoxicity
Minocyclines S	100–200 mg/day		GI disturbances, rashes, vestibular and hearing disturbances
Rifabutin	150 mg–500 mg		Orange-brown staining of urine, saliva and cramps
Linezolid	600–1000 mg/day		GI upset, vision disturbance
Ciprofloxacin	500–1000 mg as two divided doses		GI upset, headache, insomnia
Clarithromycin	500 mg as two divided doses		GI upset, hepatotoxicity
Coamoxiclav	2 g twice a day		GI upset
Myser	250 mg twice a day		Hepatotoxicity, nephrotoxicity

*INH must form a part of any multidrug therapy.

Note: Thioacetazone is contraindicated in HIV positive patients because of risk of severe skin reactions.

C-bactericidal, F-first line drugs, S-bacteriostatic, GI-gastrointestinal.

Of all the Fluoroquinolones Levoflox (10 mg/kg twice a day), Ofloxacin (12–20 mg/kg), Moxifloxacin (7–10 mg/kg) have been found to be favorable for long-term clinical use.

visual acuity, red-green color vision and gross peripheral visual fields must be frequently examined. Special care must be taken if this drug is to be administered to a child. It is metabolized by oxidation in the liver. Hepatic and renal dysfunction may increase the risk of toxicity.

RIFAMPICIN(R)

It is a potent semisynthetic antibiotic, like pyrazinamide it has the ability to kill so-called "persisters"—mycobacteria that lie dormant, often within the cells. Absorption is complete and rapid after administration on an empty stomach. The presence of food causes marked variation in serum concentrations, though it does not seem to interfere with the efficacy of the drug. The distribution of rifampicin is extensive and the patient should be warned about red-brown coloration of body fluids like sweat, tears, urine, feces, etc. It is subject to hepatic metabolism and transferred to bile. The metabolism is principally by deacetylation. The deacetylated metabolite is active. The excretion of rifampicin is both biliary and renal, and modification in dosage are required in patients with hepatobiliary or hepatorenal insufficiency. Side effects include minor elevation of SGPT and serum bilirubin, erythematous reactions, fatigue, headache, ataxia, the influenza like syndrome, and rarely renal dysfunction. Clinically important reduction of effects of concurrent therapy, include the efficacy of oral contraceptives, antiepileptic drugs, anticoagulants and hypoglycemic agents. Daily recommended dosage is 450–600 mg for an adult (10–20 mg/kg).

PYRAZINAMIDE(Z)

This drug is especially bactericidal to mycobacteria multiplying intracellularly at low pH levels. Many studies have shown, especially in pulmonary disease, that inclusion of pyrazinamide in the first 3 months of the treatment program can reduce the later relapse rate, and allow a shorter duration of continuation therapy. It is well-absorbed after oral administration and is eliminated principally by hepatic metabolism. Only about 3% of an oral dose is excreted unchanged in the urine in the first 24 hours. Like isoniazid, pyrazinamide penetrates well into cerebrospinal fluid, and it may, therefore, be especially indicated in tuberculous meningitis, and paraplegia. When the drug is not well tolerated it commonly causes nausea, flushing, arthralgia, and hepatotoxic reactions. Daily requirement is 1.5–3 g for adults, given as divided doses or as a single dose (40 mg/kg).

THIOACETAZONE WITH OTHER DRUGS

It was found by the East African/British Medical Research Councils (1963) to be as effective a regimen as isoniazid with PAS and no more toxic. In India, too, it was observed to be of equal efficacy to INH-PAS combination, though a higher incidence of side effects with thioacetazone containing regimen were observed (Tuberculosis Chemotherapy Center, Madras, 1966). We used isoniazid (300 mg)-thioacetazone (150 mg) combination as a single daily dose at bedtime for treatment in place of INH and PAS combination only for economic reasons or in patients who developed reaction to PAS or were considered resistant to PAS. Most important complications of prolonged thioacetazone therapy are liver damage and skin rashes. At present, we do not consider thioacetazone to be a safe drug for outpatient treatment. It should be avoided in HIV patients because of severe exfoliative dermatitis it can induce.

ALTERNATIVE REGIMENS

Isoniazid, rifampicin, pyrazinamide, ethambutol and streptomycin are the most effective, fairly safe and not too costly drugs. Careful combination of these drugs can tackle majority of cases of tuberculosis. These drugs are distributed at effective concentrations in almost all organs and body fluids, especially if the bones, synovial membrane and meninges are inflamed. The effectiveness is, however, blunted by the development of resistant strains due to abuse of chemotherapy and noncompliance by patients, and when tuberculosis is caused by atypical and resistant organisms particularly in HIV infected patients.

Drug Resistance in Tuberculosis

Main cause of MDR-TB in the Indian subcontinent is mismanagement of infections, inadequate therapy, crowded living, poor nutrition, compromised immunity and personal hygiene (Agoramoorthy 2017). MDR-TB is a disease that does not respond to at least isoniazid and rifampicin. XMDR-TB is a form of MDR-TB having additional resistance to fluoroquinolones (Q) and one of the injectables like amikacin, capreomycin, or kanamycin (Km).

Where resistance to first group of antitubercular drugs is apparent (as may be interpreted from drug sensitivity tests and/or more reliably from the failure of response on clinical and radiological grounds after 3–6 months of drug treatment) it is necessary to switch on to newer drugs such as amikacin (injection), fluoroquinolones, rifabutin, clofazimine, clarithromycin, etc., in various combinations **(Table 6.1)** (Bastian 1999).

Newer drugs that have been suggested as alternatives for therapeutically refractory cases are morphazinamide (dynazide), ethionamide (Et), capreomycin, Km, viomycin, cycloserine. All these are more toxic and should be considered second line antituberculous drugs for the treatment of multiple drug resistant disease. At present, PAS bas been replaced by ethambutol or rifampicin. Streptomycin should be used essentially as a paraoperative drug.

Newer drugs like bedaquiline and delamanid are being tried for drug resistant cases, however such patients need more closer observations, regarding the side effects and more serious complications like cardiac arrhythmia and mortality.

CORTICOSTEROIDS AND NONSTEROIDAL ANTI-INFLAMMATORY DRUGS

Use of corticosteroids is not recommended routinely. It is dangerous to give cortisone as patient's disease may not be sensitive to the antitubercular drugs being administered. However, cortisone may help keep alive a moribund patient till the antitubercular drugs can take effect. In active tuberculosis cortisone may be given, if indicated, only with concomitant administration of effective antitubercular drugs. Preoperative corticosteroids may be justified in a patient with advancing paralysis where some delay is anticipated or entailed prior to an operative decompression. Moon et al. (2002) recommended the use of nonsteroidal anti-inflammatory drugs (NSAIDs) for the relief of the pain in early painful stage of disease. They felt destructive changes and bone resorption attributable to non-specific synovial membrane inflammation would be minimized by the use of NSAIDs. We have used cyproheptadine (antihistaminic) during early period of treatment. It helps improve loss of appetite, has a mild sedative effect and possibly minimizes allergic reaction. Steroids may have a useful role in patients with severe hypersensitivity reactions. A short course of anabolic hormones may help a debilitated patient to be prepared for surgery. A postoperative course of 7–15 days of corticosteroids may be employed in patients of paraplegia where decompression entailed some degree of handling of cord (e.g., anterior transposition of cord in cases of severe kyphosis).

THE ROLE OF ANTITUBERCULAR DRUGS

The addition of antitubercular drugs (1950–1960) brought improvements in the results of surgical procedures. Fuller value of the effect of antitubercular drugs, however, was not evaluated till about 1965 as it took many years before the effect of any regime could be definitely appreciated in skeletal tuberculosis. Konstam (1963) aptly wrote, "often it seems to me as if surgeons generally did not appreciate the full power of the new antituberculous drugs." Bosworth and Wright (1952) compared the results of their patients before the availability of antitubercular drugs, from 1941 to 1946, and the cases after their availability, from 1946 to 1951. In the first series, the mortality was 21.1% and in the latter 5.8%. Thus, mortality was reduced by 72.5% because of the effect of antitubercular drugs.

The great Madras Experiments (1959–1961) established the supremacy and efficacy of the antitubercular drugs beyond doubt. Here patients with lung disease were treated successfully under conditions far from sanatoria. The availability and employment of first line drugs changed the behavior of tuberculous disease in general. "Lesions can be much more readily controlled, the victims are fewer, infection is less feared, hospitalization is tremendously shortened and the disease is now under control. The younger men in the profession can have no conception of the dreadful situation previously existing, in which skeletal tuberculosis constituted almost as great a disaster as metastatic neoplastic disease," (Mercer 1964). At present, drugs are considered so effective that they have made time honored virtues of sanatorium treatment, rest, nutritious diet and good accommodation combined with isolation, remarkably unimportant (Fox 1962, 1964). Role of streptomycin, INH and PAS was fully evaluated in pulmonary tuberculosis in the great Madras Experiments, and it has been found that these drugs are very effective. A triple drug regime of streptomycin, INH and PAS was virtually 100% effective in pulmonary tuberculosis (Menon 1966, Pamra 1967) which can be treated adequately at home, even under conditions far from sanatoria (Fox 1962, 1964, Lauckner 1959, 1964). Lattimer et al. (1962) reported that excisional therapy had been successfully avoided because of the effectiveness of long-term, multiple drug therapy. In their 4-year follow-up of cases of advanced renal tuberculosis treated with streptomycin, isoniazid and para-aminosalicylic acid for 2 years, there was 100% successful conversion of urine cultures. In skeletal tuberculosis also, gradually the effective role of these drugs was realized. Many workers (Chofnas 1964, Dickson 1967, Friedman 1966, Konstam 1958, 1962, 1963, Friedman and Kapur 1973, Medical Research Council 1973, Tuli et al. 1967–1984, Martini et al. 1980–1988, Coventry 1994, Moon et al. 1997, 2002, Rajashekaran et al. 1998, 2013), reported the encouraging effects of these drugs in varying combinations in the treatment of tuberculosis of the skeletal system. The American Thoracic Society in 1963, also agreed on the curative power of the chemotherapy in skeletal tuberculosis and concluded, "effectiveness of chemotherapy has obviated the need for surgical therapy". Deep seated radiological abscesses get absorbed, or healed by calcification without surgical intervention (Kaplan 1959, American Thoracic Society 1963, Stevenson and Manning 1962, Tuli et al. 1967–75).

The availability of specific antituberculous drugs has revolutionized the outcome of treatment of spinal tuberculosis, however, chemotherapy cannot completely replace the surgical treatment. Their use has improved the results of conservative and radical restorative operative treatments (Arct 1968, Donaldson 1965, Goel 1964, Hodgson 1960, Stock 1962, Kondo 1957, Risko 1963, Vyaghreswarudu 1964, Wilkinson 1969, Martin 1970, Tuli 1975, 1984, Martini 1988).

In general (Shembekarr and Babhulkar, 2002), for the large population of mycobacteria actively multiplying in the decreased area, INH, RCIN, streptomycin and ethambutol are effective. Against the small population multiplying slowly inside the macrophagic cells, pyrazinamide is the most effective drug followed by INH and RCIN. Against intermittently multiplying bacilli in solid caseous lesions rifampicin is most effective.

Adverse drug reactions (ADRs) have been observed mostly during the intensive phase of treatment (Prasad et al. 2021), however if the patients are on regular clinical observation, most of ADRs are treatable.

PENETRATION OF ANTITUBERCULAR DRUGS

Surgery was generally considered necessary to aid recovery on the supposition that drugs are unable to gain access to tuberculous abscesses and necrotic bone (Hodgson 1956, Wilkinson 1955, 1969). Even if they reach the lesion they were considered "not as effective because caseous and necrotic tissue produce substances which are antagonistic to the action of antibiotics; bacilli are also considered less vulnerable to drugs in caseous necrotic tissue because they may be in a state of resting phase and they become more inert than normal because of oxygen deprivation (Somerville and Wilkinson 1965). Roaf (1958) suggested that the avascular scar tissue may serve as a barrier behind which the tubercle bacilli may live protected from the chemotherapeutic drugs". While it is true that *Mycobacterium tuberculosis* has been found in excised tissue after a year of chemotherapy, its presence does not necessarily result from the failure of chemotherapeutic agents to reach it. Many nonviable or nonreproducible acid fast bacilli are consistently found in surgical specimens after long periods of antitubercular drug therapy (Friedman 1966). However, the presence of the organisms in smears is of significance only if they can be cultured (Falk 1958). The viable bacteria found in excised tissue after prolonged chemotherapy are often drug resistant (Hall 1956) and their presence is not a reflection on the ability of the antitubercular drugs to reach them. Moreover, the studies of Barclay (1953) and Canetti (1955) revealed by the use of radioactive tagged isoniazid that this drug is freely diffusible into all tissues including bone, as well as into abscess cavities and even into dried caseous material, in sufficient concentration to destroy bacilli. As pointed out earlier, isoniazid has a property of causing vasodilatation at the area of disease, thus the drugs are brought to the lesion in greater quantities (Somerville and Wilkinson 1965). Mackaness (1952) demonstrated that INH enters macrophages and is as active against intracellular tubercle bacilli as against those growing in a liquid medium *in vitro*. Streptomycin also enters within caseous areas and even thick-walled abscesses (Fellander et al. 1952, Canetti 1955, Somerville 1965), and other antitubercular drugs are also presumed to reach the site of tubercular lesions. Lindberg (1967) demonstrated the presence of radioactive dihydrostreptomycin in necrotic region and the abscess of skeletal tubercular foci produced experimentally in the guinea pigs. Similar observations regarding dihydrostreptomycin in tubercular foci were made by Andre (1956) and Hanngren (1964). Hanngren (1959) also observed the diffusion of radioactive para-aminosalicylic acid in tuberculous abscesses. Tuli et al. (1974) demonstrated in experimentally produced chronic osseous tuberculous lesions that streptomycin penetrates readily into the osseous lesions. After a single intramuscular injection, streptomycin was observed in the tuberculous abscess in concentrations much higher than that considered sufficient to have inhibitory effect on human type of *Mycobacterium tuberculosis*. Further (Tuli et al. 1977, 1983) observations in our laboratories have also revealed appreciable concentrations of streptomycin, rifampicin and ethambutol in the tuberculous material obtained from patients of osteoarticular tuberculosis **(Table 6.2)**. Qi-qiu et al. (1987) made similar observations. Finally, the clinical response of skeletal disease under chemotherapeutic treatment, with bone healing that is more rapid and more consistent than was seen before the use of the chemotherapeutic agents, and marked diminution of the incidence of relapse or recurrence led many workers (Dickson 1967, Friedman 1966, Konstam 1958–1963, Tuli et al. 1967–1975) to infer that the antitubercular drugs are indeed reaching the site of infection and there is no osseous barrier or gradient for their penetration **(Fig. 6.1)**.

Table 6.2: Concentration of antitubercular drugs in clinical osteoarticular tuberculosis, 3 hours after systemic administration of the drug in a single therapeutic dose (Tuli 1977, 1983, BHU Study).

Drugs	Number of samples from			Average concentration mg/mL			
	Blood	Abscess	Joint	Serum	Abscess	Joint	MIC
Ethambutol	24	25	5	3.7	4.8	4	2
Rifampicin	20	16	8	11	4.8	4.8	1
Streptomycin	52	55	14	13	6	19	1
*Pyrazinamide	8	8	—	50	4.8	—	20

* In patients on drug for 2 weeks (Mahajan 1990—unreported).
(MIC: minimum inhibitory concentration as mg/mL for *Mycobacterium tuberculosis* in clinical material)

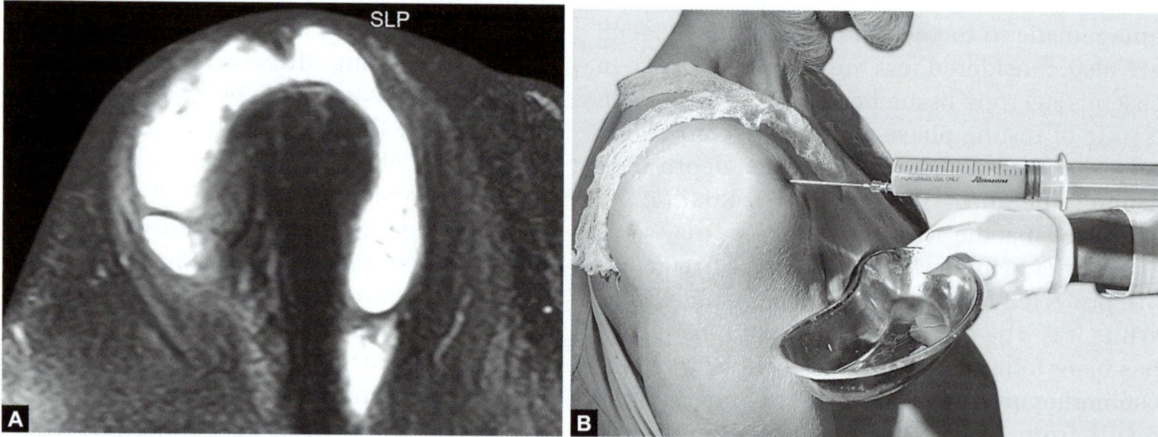

Figs. 6.1A and B: This senior citizen was on anti-cancer therapy for prostatic malignancy. He developed tuberculosis of his right shoulder probably the result of immunocompromise. (A) MRI showing the collection in shoulder. He was put an anti-TB drugs. The aspirate from the shoulder swelling shows the pinkish color of rifampicin (B) proving adequate penetration of drugs into skeletal tuberculous lesions.

Skeletal tuberculosis is only a localized manifestation of a systemic infection, and thus no local surgical procedure is a substitute for adequate and prolonged systemic anti-tuberculous therapy **(Fig. 6.1)**. Even Hodgson and Stock (1956–1960) and other workers advocated antituberculous drugs for 18 months to 2 years along with the radical excisional surgery. Dutt et al. (1986) reported that a short-course chemotherapy (9 months) with INH and rifampicin was as effective in newly diagnosed and drug-susceptible cases as the conventional therapy for 18–24 months in extrapulmonary tuberculosis. The consensus based upon the observations of a large number of workers is that in skeletal tuberculosis the multidrug therapy must be continued for 18–24 months.

CHAPTER 7

Principles of Management of Osteoarticular Tuberculosis

PROGNOSIS AND COURSE

As mentioned earlier, the use of modern antitubercular drugs has revolutionized the outcome of treatment of bone and joint tuberculosis. Death due to uncontrolled disease, meningitis, miliary tuberculosis, amyloidosis, paralysis and crippling seen frequently before the availability of antitubercular drugs is now rare (LaFond 1958, Girdlestone 1965, Meltzer 1985). If a patient is diagnosed early and treated vigorously, healing can be accomplished without residual ankylosis of the joint. Extensive surgery even in active disease is now possible without the fear of spread or formation of unhealing sinuses. The chances of reactivation are least if the healed status is achieved with remineralization and restoration of destroyed bones, or bone block formation in the vertebral disease, or healing of an articular disease with near complete function, or bony ankylosis of a grossly destroyed joint, or a stable painless fibrous ankylosis.

At the stage of tuberculous arthritis, if the disease remains closed the natural outcome is generally a fibrous ankylosis. If an abscess discharges and sinuses with secondary infection develop, the outcome may be a bony ankylosis. The position of ankylosis on healing is determined by the presence or absence of effective splintage. Prognosis regarding movements in tuberculosis of joints depends upon the stage/extent of the disease when the specific treatment was started **(Table 7.1)**.

CLASSIFICATION OF ARTICULAR TUBERCULOSIS

In untreated cases, tuberculous disease of a joint passes through the following stages **(Fig. 7.1)**. Each stage has fairly clear clinical and radiological picture, and the extent of anatomical involvement. These stages have specific implications for nonoperative or surgical management and the outcome of treatment **(Table 7.1)**. This classification permits more valid comparison of various series. Broadly speaking the classification of articular tuberculosis is as follows.

Stage I: Synovitis

Range of movements present is >75%. Limitation of movements is only in terminal degrees or in selective directions. Clinically, soft tissue swelling and synovial effusion is present **(Figs. 7.1 and 7.2)**. Radiologically, only soft tissue swelling and osteoporosis of the articular ends may be present, there is no evidence of destruction or erosion of bone, or diminution of the joint space.

Stage II: Early Arthritis

There is preservation of movements between 50 and 75%. Restriction of movements is in all directions. Radiologically, in addition to above (stage I), slight diminution of the vertical height of the joint space (articular cartilage space) and marginal erosions of the articular surfaces

Table 7.1: Staging of tuberculosis of the joints and its outcome in general.

Stages		*Clinical*	*Radiology*	*Usual effective treatment*	*Expectation*
I	Synovitis	Movements present >75%	Soft tissue swelling, osteoporosis	Chemotherapy and movements. Rarely synovectomy	Retention of near full mobility
II	Early arthritis	Movements present 50–75%	In addition to I, moderate diminution of joint space and marginal erosions	Chemotherapy and movements. Rarely synovectomy or debridement	Restoration of 50–75% of mobility
III	Advanced arthritis	Loss of movements of >75% in all directions	In addition to II marked diminution of joint space and destruction of joint surfaces	Chemotherapy and surgery. Generally arthrodesis in lower limbs	Ankylosis$
IV	Advanced arthritis with subluxation/ dislocation	Loss of movements of >75% in all directions	In addition to III, joint is disorganized with subluxation/dislocation	Chemotherapy and surgery, generally arthrodesis	Ankylosis*
V	Aftermath/ terminal of gross arthritis	Gross deformity and ankylosis	In addition to IV, grossly deformed articular margins ± degenerative osteoarthrosis	Chemotherapy and surgery, Arthrodesis/ corrective osteotomy	Ankylosis*

* After completion of growth of involved bones for elbow and hip, one may, if desired, obtain a fairly mobile joint by excision-arthroplasty, without fear of recrudescence.

$ Currently for major joints (hip, knee) arthroplasty is a rational option. After 2–3 years of healed status, under 3–5 months of anti-TB drugs umbrella.

is present. There is no gross destruction of the articular bone **(Fig. 7.1)**.

Stage III: Advanced Arthritis

There is nearly 75% loss of movements and the restriction is in all directions. Radiologically, in addition to above II, there is marked diminution of the joint space, and gross destruction of the articular margins and bone ends.

Stage IV: Advanced Arthritis with Subluxation or Dislocation

In addition to the above III, there is joint deformity caused by subluxation or dislocation. As an example wandering/migrating acetabulum or pathological dislocation of hip, triple deformity of knee, anterior subluxation/dislocation of wrist joint, anterior or posterior, subluxation of ankle, etc. (Figs. in Chapters 8, 9 and 13).

Stage V: Terminal or Aftermath of Arthritis

It is ankylosis of the joint. Articular margins may be adapted to the deformed position, there may be subchondral eburnation of bone (in case of fibrous ankylosis) and changes of degenerative arthritis, there may be bony ledge or buttress formation in case of long-standing. Gross appearance of the joint surface may be irregular, cobbled, deformed, pock-marked and devoid of articular cartilage (Figs. in Chapter 8).

PRINCIPLES OF MANAGEMENT

General

The general and systemic treatment is like that of tuberculosis in general. Any concomitant disease must be treated to build the general body resistance. Hospitalization is necessary only for

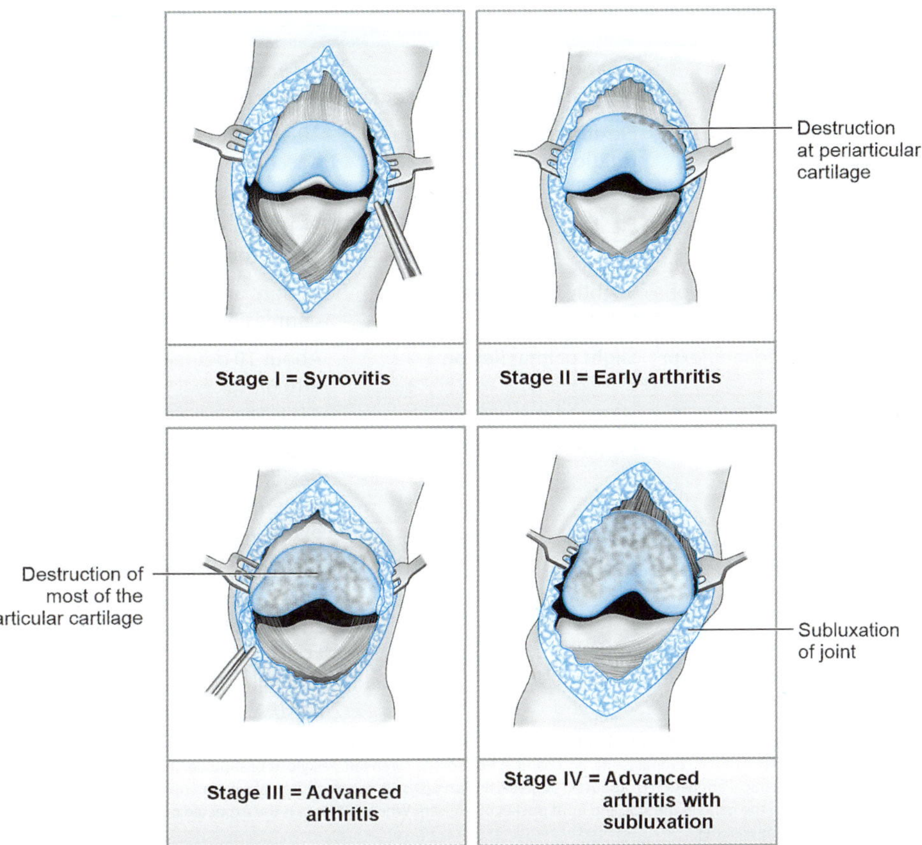

Fig. 7.1: Diagrammatic representation of various stages of articular tuberculosis.

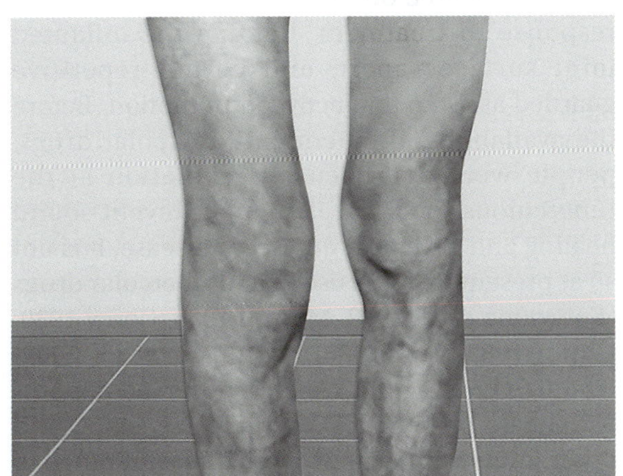

Fig. 7.2: Clinical picture of tubercular synovitis of right knee. There is fullness of parapatellar fossae, bulging of suprapatellar pouch and wasting of quadriceps muscle.

complications, and for those requiring traction to correct deformities under supervision.

Rest, Mobilization and Brace

All patients are advised to sleep on hard bed. A plaster bed is necessary only for a minority of children with neural complications. In the treatment of craniovertebral, cervical and cervicothoracic lesions, traction is used in the early stages to put the diseased part at rest. This is particularly done for cases with neural deficit and those with pathological subluxation/dislocations. The patients with neural deficit are hospitalized and treated in recumbent position till return of adequate motor power.

In active stage of disease, the joints are given rest in the position of function **(Table 7.2)**. In

Table 7.2: Positions of "ease" and "function" of diseased joints.

Joint	*Site of maximum swelling*	*Position of maximum capacity or "position of ease"*	*Desired position of ankylosis, and center of functional arc*
Hip	Proximal part of Scarpa's triangle	Flexion, abduction, external rotation	10–30 degrees of flexion directly related to age, neutral position regarding abduction, adduction and rotation
Knee	Suprapatellar bursa, either side of patellar tendon	Flexion	5–10 degrees of flexion to allow foot to clear ground on walking
Ankle	Anterior and either side of Achilles tendon	Slightly flexed and inverted	At right angle (Plantigrade neutral) ± 5 degrees of external rotation
Wrist	Deep to extensor and flexor tendons	Slight palmar flexion	About 10 degrees of dorsiflexion to allow a firm grasp
Elbow	On either side of triceps tendon	Flexion 90 degrees plus semi-pronation (mid-prone)	90 degrees of flexion and semi-pronation. In bilateral disease left at 45 degrees of flexion and right at 105 degrees of flexion to permit reach the upper and lower external orifices
*Shoulder	Deep to deltoid along the biceps brachii tendon and in axilla	Abducted	Absolute recommended angles are abduction 50 degrees between vertebral border of scapula and long axis of humerus. Forward flexion 30 degrees between vertical and the long axis of humerus, internal rotation 30 degrees

*In clinical practice, the "saluting position" of the upper limb offers a rough guide to the position for arthrodesis. The shoulder looks abducted 80 degrees, flexed 40 degrees, elbow slightly anterior to the coronal plane, and hand in front of the forehead. Ankylosis of shoulder in optimum position permits; the arm to fall to the side of the trunk, allow clinical abduction of about 90 degrees, flexion up to 80 degrees, internal rotation up to 90 degrees, permitting patient to reach any part of face/head and place the hand in the side and front pocket of trousers. When ankylosis is the expected outcome ensure 5 degrees of external rotation at the destroyed joint (hip/knee/ankle)

the presence of gross destruction, especially in the disease of hip, knee and ankle, continuation of the immobilization may lead to spontaneous sound ankylosis. Cases with early disease are put on one hourly intermittent guarded active and assisted exercises (functional treatment) under cover of antitubercular drugs with the aim of retaining a useful range of movements in the functional arc of the involved joint. In the presence of deformities, traction is used to correct the deformity and to put the diseased part at rest. Gradual mobilization is encouraged with the help of suitable braces/appliances soon after the start of treatment while the healing was progressing.

Traction is one of the best available method to correct a deformity, maintain the limb in the functional position throughout the treatment, offer unhindered observation regarding the local response to treatment, holding the inflamed joint surfaces apart, and permit repetitive guarded assisted and active joint motion. Before the availability of potent antitubercular drugs, people were apprehensive of motion at the tuberculous joint lest it should prevent sound healing and flare up a quiescent disease. It is not so at present with the use of antitubercular drugs (Katayama et al. 1962, Martini 1980, Chow 1980, Gupta 1982, Tuli 1985, Babhulkar et al. 2002, Hoffman et al. 2002). We have observed patients with healed tuberculosis of hip, knee, elbow and other joints with 50% or more of useful range of motion (in the functional arc) who did not accept arthrodesis. They did not develop recrudescence of the disease over a period of 10–15 years of follow-up.

Functional Treatment of Articular Tuberculosis

Maintenance of traction and intermittent active and assisted motion of the joint within the range of tolerable pain, during the process of healing, in all probabilities encourages development of healthy synovial membrane and well-lubricated useful fibrocartilage adapted to the function of the joint (Albrook and Kirkaldy-Willis 1958, Calandruccio and Glimer 1962, Wilkinson 1969). The repair with retention of joint mobility, occurring spontaneously on conservative lines or after operative procedures like synovectomy, debridement, excision arthroplasty, is dependent upon proliferating mesenchymal reparative cells. These cells under the influence of "repetitive motion" may be induced to metaplasia to synovial membrane and to fibrocartilage **(Fig. 8.23)**. This may permit return of reasonable function even in a joint damaged by infection, and maintain a lasting healed status of the disease (Sankaran 1993, Tuli 2002, Shanmugasundaram 2005).

Ambulation in the initial stages is without weight bearing. As the disease heals and pain subsides weight bearing is permitted accordingly. During all this period, the joint is continually observed. If symptoms or signs increase, the patient goes back a stage; if there is steady progress, he goes forward (Thomas' test of recovery). At no time the movements or degree of weight bearing is forced beyond tolerable discomfort. This is expressed as the "*functional treatment*" of articular tuberculosis.

Guarded weight bearing in the lower limbs is started 3–6 months after the subsidence of signs of activity. The braces/appliances are gradually discarded after its use for about 2 years.

Abscess, Effusion, Ulcers and Sinuses

Palpable abscesses and large joint effusions are aspirated and one gram of streptomycin alone or combined with injectable isoniazid is instilled at each aspiration. However, considering the sufficient local concentration of antibiotics achieved after parenteral administration the need for local instillation may be obviated. Open drainage of the abscesses may be performed if the pus is too thick or aspiration failed to clear them. Not all radiologically visible paravertebral abscesses require to be drained, drainage was incidental when decompression was performed for paraplegia or when debridement of the diseased vertebrae was performed for active tuberculosis. Prevertebral abscess in the cervical region is drained when complicated by difficulty in swallowing or breathing. Drainage of a large paravertebral abscess may also be considered when its radiological size increases markedly in spite of the treatment.

Sinuses in a large majority of cases would heal within 6–12 weeks under the influence of systemic antitubercular drugs. A small number (<1%) may require longer treatment and excision of the tract with or without debridement. It is important to remember that sinus ramification is always greater than can be appreciated, complete surgical excision is indeed impracticable, and fortunately unnecessary.

Antitubercular Drugs (Chapter 6)

No significant complications are encountered due to multidrug regime in patients with active disease. Where resistance or allergy to the most preferred drugs is apparent it is necessary to switch on to other drugs in various combinations. Rifampicin has nearly replaced streptomycin. Streptomycin at best may be employed as a paraoperative drug. In the ever changing scene of more potent, less toxic **(Table 6.1)**, and hopefully not too costly antitubercular drugs, it may be unrealistic to stick to one particular drug regime, however, at present it is important to stress to maintain the drugs for a minimum of one year, preferably 18 months and in some cases for 24 months. Our current general policy for an average adult is to start with "*intensive phase*" treatment, comprising of daily dosage of isoniazid 300–400 mg, rifampicin 450–600 mg and fluoroquinolones 400–600 mg for 5–6 months. All replicating sensitive mycobacteria are likely to be killed by this bactericidal regime. The *"continuation phase"* treatment should last for 9–10 months where the aim is to attack the persisters, slow growing or intermittently growing or dormant or intracellular mycobacteria. It comprises of isoniazid and pyrazinamide (1500 mg per day) for 4–5 months (pyrazinamide is considered to have maximum penetrability to kill intracellular mycobacteria) to be followed by isoniazid and rifampicin for another 4–5 months. The slow growing mycobacteria by this phase of treatment hopefully would be in their "state of replication", the combination of isoniazid and rifampicin is considered the safest and most effective treatment to eliminate such organisms. The *"prophylactic phase"* consists of isoniazid and ethambutol (1200 mg) for 3–4 months. This is the time when the treated patient is back to his normal working environments. The aim is to offer prophylaxis to the patient during the time his body is developing adequate protective immunity. The doses and drugs were modified and other drugs were used, according to the weight of the patient, existing comorbidities and any adverse drug reactions.

If an operative treatment is anticipated or planned, it is wise to avoid the administration of >2 hepatotoxic drugs (e.g., INH and rifampicin combination) for 3–4 weeks prior to surgery. Nearly 10% of patients who have been on >2 hepatotoxic drugs for 3 weeks or more may show evidence of significant hepatic dysfunction on investigations. The dysfunction may be higher in patients having poor nutritional status. Halothane like anesthetic agents should be avoided during surgery on these patients.

For a long time, many workers perpetuated the presumption that antitubercular drugs do not penetrate into the diseased area in effective concentrations (Chapter 6). Universal radical excisional surgery was then advocated by many workers (Silva 1980) to encourage effective penetration of drugs into the diseased region. There is, however, overwhelming evidence to prove that modern antitubercular drugs indeed readily reach the osteo-articular tubercular lesions in effective concentrations (Katayama et al. 1954, 1962, Tuli et al. 1974, 1977, Friedman 1973, Canetti 1955, Fellander et al. 1952, Barclay 1953, Lindberg 1967, Andre 1956, Hanngren 1959, 1964, Moon 1997, Rajasekaran et al. 1998, Moon et al. 2002). In clinical practice, if the activity of a tuberculous lesion does not come under control, the cause is not failure of the drugs to reach the lesion in sufficient concentrations. The cause lies in other factors such as acquired or genetic resistance of the infecting organisms to the drugs being administered, and the pathological nature of the skeletal lesion, e.g., gross destruction of bones and joints and presence of large sequestra.

Relapse of Osteoarticular Tuberculosis or Recurrence of Complications

Exact assessment of the incidence of relapse or recurrence of complication is not possible because these problems may occur at any period during the lifetime of a patient, whether the initial treatment included excisional surgery or not **(Figs. 7.3 and 7.4)**. Reactivation or development of complications has been observed even during the era of antitubercular drugs as late as 20 years or more after apparent healing (Martin 1970). The cause of reactivation of the disease in spite of apparently adequate treatment at the time of initial therapy, appears to be lowered nutritional status of the patient or acquisition of immune compromised state. The relapse rates reported by Paus (1964) and Kaplan (1959) were 11% and 2% respectively. In Konstam and Blesovsky's (1962) series, only one of 207 patients had recurrence.

After the availability of modern drugs, the incidence of relapse in our patients treated after 1972 seems to be 2% in those followed-up for 5–10 years. Nearly 50% of cases with recurrence of the disease at the first site, or development of tuberculosis in any other part of the skeletal system, on close questioning would reveal that they did not continue drugs for >12 months. This is a strong pointer against accepting "short duration regimes" while treating osteoarticular tuberculosis. Other precipitating factors may be prolonged use of systemic cortisone therapy,

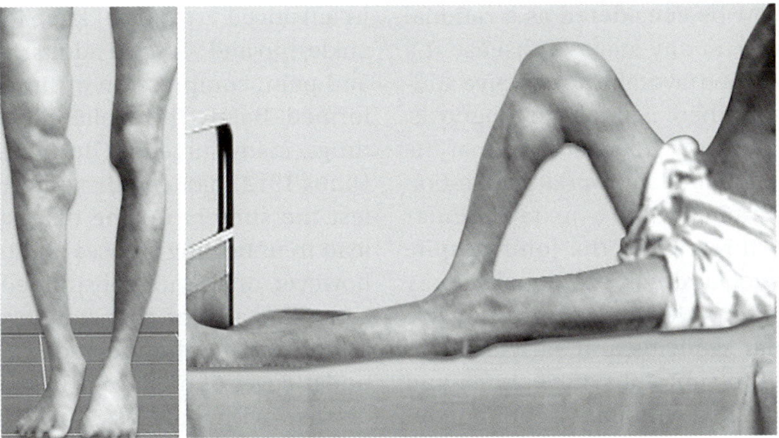

Fig. 7.3: Clinical photographs of a patient who was treated by antitubercular drugs and subtotal synovectomy (right knee) in 1969. The disease healed completely with retention of full range of movements. He reported with recurrence of disease in 1986 after a gap of 15 years. The disease healed again under the influence of newer drugs

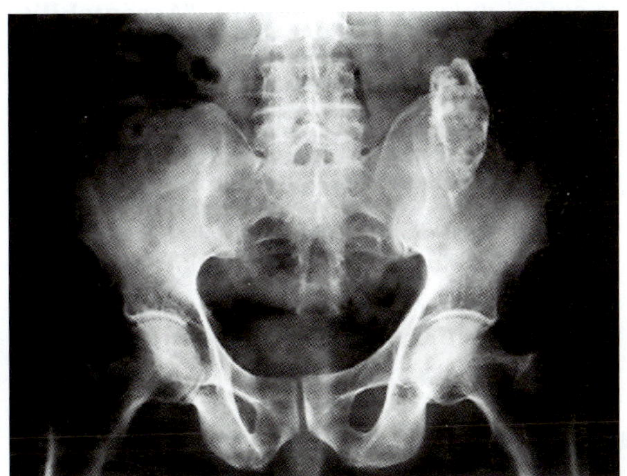

Fig. 7.4: X-ray of a patient treated for lumbar spine tuberculosis 20 years ago showing a calcified left psoas abscess. He has now developed diabetes and active tuberculosis of right sacroiliac joint

immunosuppressive drugs, malnutrition, development of diabetes, alcoholics or immune deficient state. Any surgical procedure or a significant injury to the once infected area may reactivate the disease, an adequate course including newer antitubercular drugs must be given to prevent it. Special health measures may be required in possible noncompliant patients (alcoholics, drug addicts, insane) to ensure suitable medications.

Surgery in Tuberculosis of Bones and Joints

Surgery is at best an adjunct to the systemic antitubercular therapy of the patient. No surgical resection is a substitute for a prolonged course of antitubercular drugs and supportive therapy. A trial of conservative treatment is justified in most of the cases before surgery is contemplated. Nonoperative treatment is usually adequate in pure synovial tuberculosis (without articular involvement), low grade or early arthritis of any joint, and even advanced (stage III, IV) arthritis, especially in the upper extremity.

If operative procedures are to be undertaken it should take place after the general condition of the patient is stabilized under the protective cover of drug therapy and before the development of drug resistance. In general a minimum of 1–3 weeks of drug therapy and general supportive treatment is advisable before any major surgical intervention.

Extent and Type of Surgery

Fusion of a major joint is now rarely indicated as a primary mode of treatment. Reconstruction or reposition of joints, juxta-articular osteotomies, soft tissue releases and arthroplasties to obtain, mobile, stable joints with biological control of disease should now be considered as a rational method. In general, at any stage of disease if a lesion is not responding favorably to effective antitubercular drugs, or there is doubt in diagnosis, or it is a case of refractory recrudescence of the infection, exploration and appropriate operation is considered mandatory. If a juxta-articular osseous focus is threatening the joint despite adequate antitubercular drugs, excisional surgery of the focus may be performed. Nonresponsive cases of tubercular synovitis and early arthritis may be subjected to subtotal synovectomy and synovectomy combined with joint debridement, respectively. Debridement should be limited to infected synovium, sequestra, pockets/cavities of pus and sinuses. In advanced tubercular arthritis of hip and elbow in adults (nonresponsive cases or cases who did not obtain acceptable range of movements), excisional arthroplasty is offered. Postoperatively, all these patients where the aim was mobility, are treated by frequent repetitive active and assisted movements of the operated joint with an aim to obtain a functional arc of movements. Low friction arthroplasty is being tried in patients with healed tubercular arthritis (Chapter 8). However, arthroplasty performed in patients with active tuberculous disease has proved disastrous (Mitchison and Chalmers 1986).

In advanced arthritis of knee joint (and rarely in ankle, hip and wrist) in adults, for gross deformity and pain, compression arthrodesis may be performed. Before the availability of antitubercular drugs, many surgeons (Brittain 1952, Albee 1911, Hibbs 1912) pioneered extra-articular operations lest the surgery on the diseased tissue should lead to unhealing sinuses and ulcers. At present, however, one is not constrained to remain extra-articular, any of the standard techniques of arthrodesis may be adopted in tubercular arthritis under cover of modern drugs. In cases of healed disease with painless ankylosis in deformed position, a juxta-articular corrective osteotomy may be performed (for hip, knee and ankle or any joint) to bring the joint to the best position of function. Whenever the aim of operative treatment is sound ankylosis of the joint, **"Acceptability Test"** prior to arthrodesis of any major joints like hip, knee, ankle-foot, elbow should be mandatory. Postarthrodesis operation, immobilization in plaster cast should be continued till solid fusion was obvious radiologically (3–6 months). Arthrodesis/fusion of hip and knee joints cause gross disturbance of kinematics of locomotion over the years. Arthroplasty operations are now considered a more rational choice for these joints, after the disease in the joint and any other system

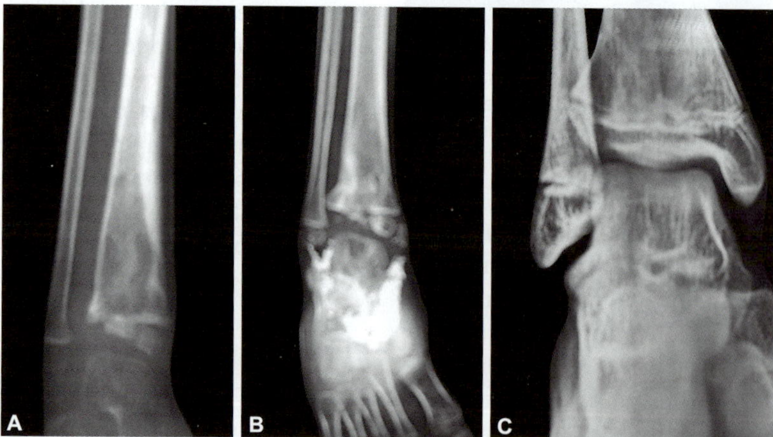

Figs. 7.5A to C: During growing years there is remarkable potential for repair and regeneration. X-rays of a child (A) at presentation (histologically proved tuberculosis) showing a cystic lesion in distal tibia; lateral half of growth plate is not visible (fragmentation). (B) One year after ATT and ROM exercises. (C) At 4-year's follow-up note the restoration of bone and the growth plate and near normal bone texture.

of body has remained healed for >2–3 years. Joint replacement arthroplasty procedures are best done under an umbrella of anti-TB drugs for 3–5 months.

Healing of Disease

With modern antitubercular drugs and a suitable treatment, osteoarticular tuberculosis can be observed to pass through the following stages; invasion and destruction (at onset), control and regression, and healed stage. A healed stage is identified by disappearance of all systemic features of activity, disappearance of local warmth, tenderness, spasm, abscess, sinuses, and return of painless motion (in early disease). Repeated erythrocyte sedimentation is normal or does not show a progressive increase in it's value. Radiologically, there is remineralization, and restoration of bony outlines and trabeculae and sharpening of cortical and articular margins. MRI would show/reveal resolution of edema of soft tissues and bones, and synovial fluid collection. The destroyed areas of bone may get reconstituted, sometimes the marrow of the diseased bone after healing gets replaced by fat. Restorative abilities of the osteoarticular system under the influence of present antitubercular drugs are amazing **(Fig. 7.5)**.

SECTION 2

Extra-spinal Regional Tuberculosis

CHAPTER 8

Tuberculosis of the Hip Joint

Tuberculous disease of the hip is very common, the frequency of involvement is next only to spinal tuberculosis. In any long series, hip disease constitutes nearly 15% of all cases of osteoarticular tuberculosis (Martini 1988, Babhulkar 2002). The initial focus of tuberculous lesion may start in the acetabular roof, epiphysis, metaphyseal region (Babcock's triangle), or in greater trochanter **(Fig. 8.1)**. Rarely the disease may start in the synovial membrane and may remain as synovitis for a few months. Tuberculosis of the greater trochanter may involve the overlying trochanteric bursa without involving the hip joint for a very long time. As the upper end of femur is entirely intracapsular the joint gets involved rapidly from any osseous lesion situated within the capsular attachments, the disease becomes "osteoarticular", and destruction of articular surfaces of femoral head and acetabulum takes place. When the initial focus starts in the acetabular roof, the joint involvement is late and severity of symptoms mild, therefore, by the time the patient first reports to the hospital extensive destruction of the bone is already present. A cold abscess usually forms within the joint, the inferior weaker part of capsule or rarely the acetabular floor may be perforated and the cold abscess may present anywhere around the hip joint such as femoral triangle, medial, lateral or posterior aspects of thigh, ischiorectal fossa, or pelvis. The abscess tracks away from the hip joint mostly along the neighboring vessels and nerves to reach the surface. The intrapelvic abscess above the attachments of the levator ani muscle tracks upwards to point in the inguinal region; whereas those below this muscle, track into the ischiorectal fossa.

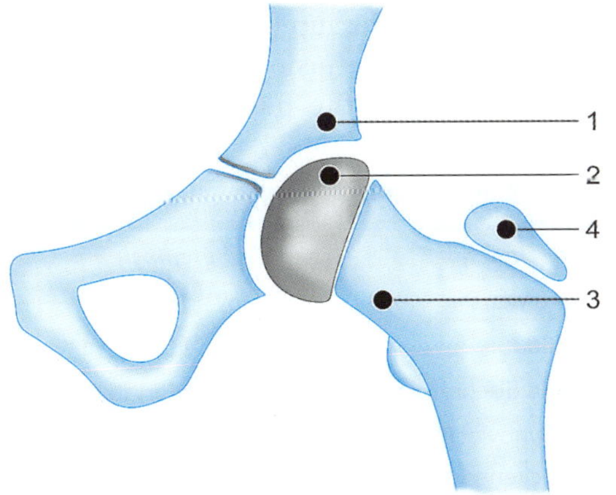

Fig. 8.1: Diagrammatic representation of the location and frequency of osseous origin of tuberculosis of the hip joint; (1) upper part of acetabulum (the commonest); (2) femoral head/epiphysis; (3) femoral neck/metaphysis; (4) greater trochanter (the least common).

CLINICAL FEATURES

Like osteoarticular tuberculosis in general commonest age of start of illness is during first 3 decades. Pain, limping, deformity and fullness around the hip are the presenting symptoms when the disease is active. Pain is often referred to the medial aspect of the knee and is maximum toward the end of the day. A child may wake from sleep due to night cries. In developing countries, nearly 8% of patients may have clinically palpable cold abscesses with or without sinuses, and nearly 10% of patients may present with varying degrees of pathological subluxation or dislocation of the hip.

The limp is the earliest and commonest symptom. The patient while walking puts as little pressure on the diseased hip joint (for a short time) as possible (i.e., has shortest possible stance phase of the affected side) giving rise to the typical antalgic gait. To get relief from the pain of an active hip disease while changing position in the bed, the patient may support or lift the involved limb with the contralateral normal limb, or the patient may "apply traction" on the painful hip by pushing down on the dorsum of foot with the opposite foot while recumbent. So long as the disease is active, physical examination will reveal tenderness by direct pressure on the hip in the femoral triangle, or medial to the greater trochanter posteriorly or indirectly, by bitrochanteric pressure or thumping. Muscle spasm can be appreciated in the lower abdominal muscles, and in the adductors of the thigh on attempting sudden abduction-external rotation at the hip joint. In untreated cases, the disease of the hip joint passes through different stages as follows (Chapter 7, **Table 8.1** adapted from Babhulkar and Pandey 2002, **Table 8.2**).

Tubercular Synovitis (Stage I)

In synovitis, or early disease of the hip joint due to a juxta-articular osseous lesion causing "irritable hip", the joint is held in the position of maximum capacity, that is flexion, external rotation and abduction, causing apparent lengthening. There is no true/real shortening. Only extremes of movements are limited and painful. X-rays may show only soft tissue swelling, with or without rarefaction of the hip bones **(Fig. 8.2)**.

The differential diagnosis at this stage is from traumatic synovitis, rheumatic/rheumatoid disease, nonspecific transient synovitis, low-grade pyogenic infection, Perthes' disease, juxta-articular disease causing irritation of the joint, spasm of the iliopsoas muscle due to an abscess in its sheath or overlying inflamed lymph nodes/viscera, slipped capital femoral epiphysis and avascular necrosis of femoral head. Careful clinico-radiological examination and noninvasive investigations repeated at 3–6 weeks intervals usually help establish the exact diagnosis. Ultrasonography has been shown to be a useful investigation to appreciate the swelling of the soft tissues of the hip joint. MRI at this stage may show synovial effusion and varying degree of bone edema. If the pathological nature is

Table 8.1: During growing years common hip conditions that require attempt at differentiation.

	Irritable hip	*Septic hip*	*Perthes' hip*	*Tuberculosis hip*
Age	3–9 years	1–6 years	4–8 years	Any age
Pain	Mild	Severe	Mild	Severe
Weight bearing	Comfortable	Uncomfortable	Mild discomfort	Uncomfortable
Images	↑ Synovial fluid Thickened synovium	↑ Synovial fluid Thickened synovium Subperiosteal erosion	↑ Synovial fluid Thickened synovium Hyperdense femoral head	↑ Synovial fluid Thickened synovium Eroded articular margins
Synovial fluid aspirate	Sterile	Pus cells ++	Sterile	Mycobacteria ±
NSAIDs response	Favorable	Symptomatic	Temporary	Temporary

Aspirate by inserting the needle (A) proximal to the greater trochanter directing toward the femoral head; or (B) insert the needle almost vertically from anterior aspect – 1.5 cm lateral to the palpable femoral artery and 1–2 cm distal to the mid-inguinal point.

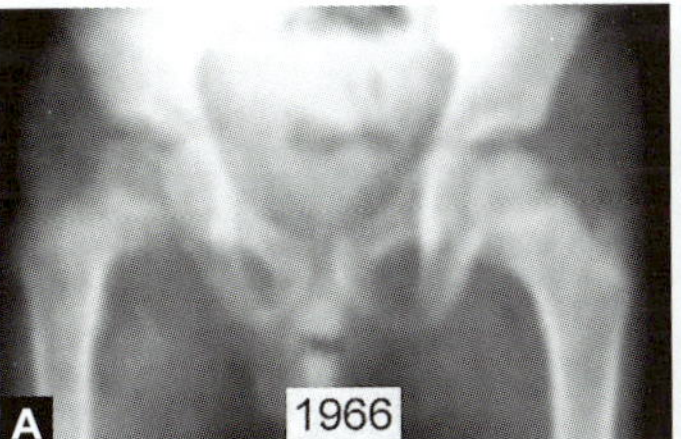

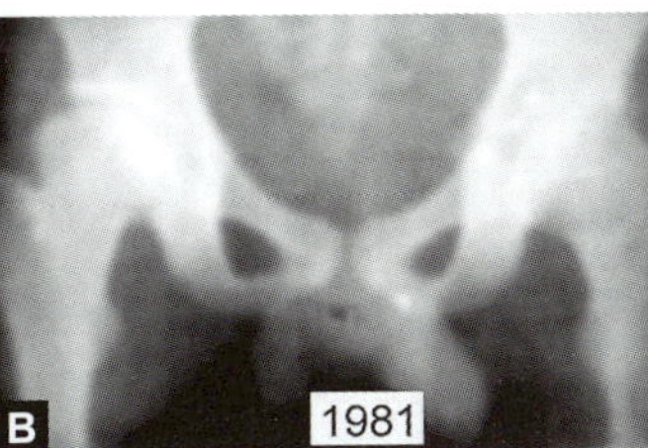

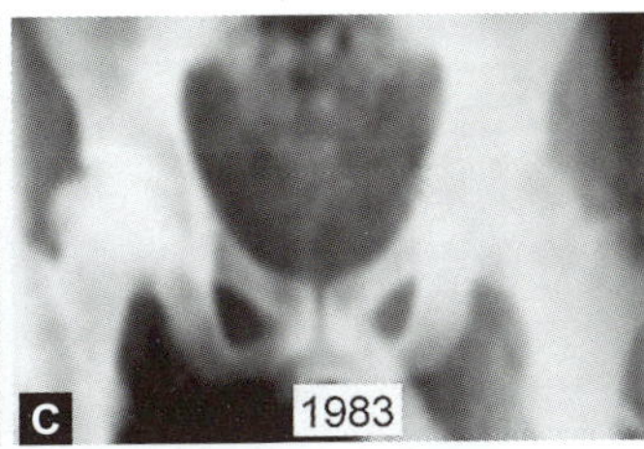

Figs. 8.2A to C: Successive X-rays of a patient of tuberculous synovitis of right hip, treated by antitubercular drugs, traction, repetitive exercises and guarded weight bearing (for 2 years). Except moderately uncovered large femoral head and mild **coxa-valga**, there was no functional disability on healing of disease and follow-up of 17 years.

Table 8.2: Clinicoradiologic classification of tuberculosis of the hip.

Stages	*Clinical findings*	*Radiologic features*
1. Synovitis	Flexion, abduction, external rotation, apparent lengthening	Soft tissue swelling, haziness of articular margins and rarefaction
2. Early arthritis	Flexion, adduction, internal rotation, apparent shortening	Rarefaction, osteopenia, marginal bony erosions in femoral head, acetabulum or both, No gross reduction in joint space
3. Advanced arthritis	Flexion, adduction, internal rotation, true shortening	All of the above and destruction of articular surface, reduction in joint space
4. Advanced arthritis with subluxation/dislocation	Flexion, adduction, internal rotation with gross shortening	Gross destruction and reduction of joint space, wandering acetabulum

There is progressive loss of motion in various stages; least in stage of synovitis and gross in arthritis with subluxation/dislocation. For comfort from pain during long decubitus some patients may continue the position of abduction and external rotation, keeping the thigh resting on the bed.

undiagnosable, biopsy must be obtained from the representative diseased tissue for bacteriological, PCR and histological investigations.

Early Arthritis (Stage II)

As the disease advances, actual destruction or damage to the articular cartilage sets in. The local signs become more prominent and due to the spasm of adductors and flexors the hip assumes a deformity of flexion, adduction (presenting as apparent shortening) and internal rotation. There is true/real shortening of not >1 cm, appreciable muscle wasting, and restriction of movements, due to pain and muscle spasm, in all directions. X-rays show localized osteoporosis, slight diminution of the joint space due to decrease in the vertical height of the articular cartilage and localized erosions at the articular margins **(Fig. 8.6)**. MRI at this stage may show synovial effusion, synovial thickening, minimal areas of bone destruction and osseous edema.

Advanced Arthritis (Stage III)

With further advancement of destruction, clinical signs of flexion-adduction-internal rotation deformities, restriction of movements, muscle wasting **(Figs. 8.3 to 8.5, and 8.7 to 8.16)**, true and apparent shortenings are exaggerated. The tendency of the patient to sleep on the side of the uninvolved hip further contributes to the flexion, adduction and internal rotation deformity. There is gross destruction of articular cartilage and bones of the femoral head and acetabulum **(Fig. 8.5)**. The capsule is further destroyed, thickened and contracted.

Advanced Arthritis with Subluxation or Dislocation (Stage IV)

With further destruction of acetabulum, femoral head, capsule and ligaments, the upper end of femur may displace upwards and dorsally in the wandering or migrating acetabulum, leaving

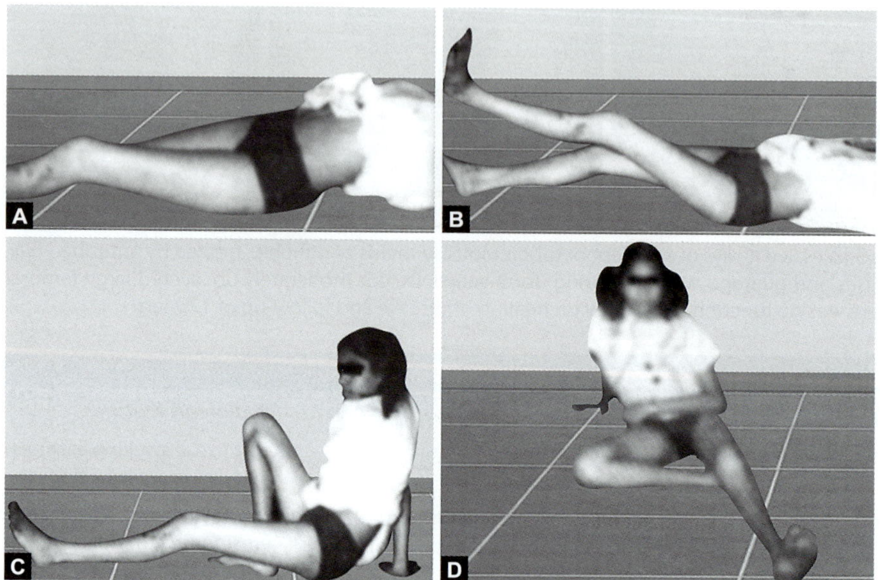

Figs. 8.3A to D: Clinical pictures of a young patient with advanced tuberculous arthritis of left hip joint. (A and B) Note fixed flexion deformity of 45 degrees; (C) Shows the position the patient adopts, to ease herself using an Indian-type of toilet; (D) Shows the posture while sitting on the floor. Being a young patient she manages these postures because of the compensatory movements at the lumbar spine; with advancing age such compensations become more difficult.

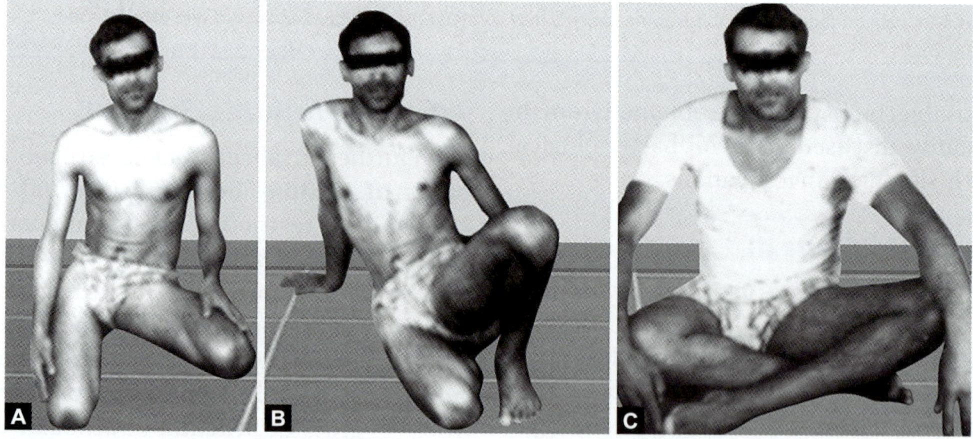

Figs. 8.4A to C: (A and B) show the method of attending to the social needs in a 35-year old man whose right hip was ankylosed at 40 degrees of flexion. (C) The same patient was able to squat and sit cross-legged after excisional arthroplasty of right hip joint.

its lower part empty and Shenton's arc broken **(Figs. 8.7, 8.8, 8.10 to 8.13, 8.19 to 8.25)**. Rarely the destruction of capsule and acetabulum may be so severe as to lead to frank pathological posterior dislocation of the femoral head **(Fig. 8.13)**. This severe variety of tuberculous infection can rarely be encountered in children.

Sometimes the hip may show protrusio acetabuli **(Figs. 8.7 and 8.8)**. In some cases, the femoral head and neck are grossly destroyed, collapsed and small in size (coxa breva) **(Fig. 8.10)** contained in an enlarged acetabulum producing a mortar–pestle appearance (Shanmugasundaram 1983).

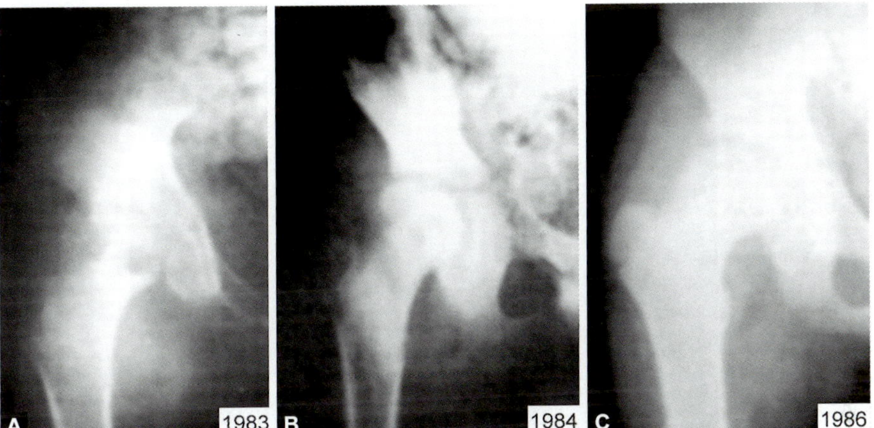

Figs. 8.5A to C: X-rays of a case of tuberculosis of the right hip joint at presentation (A) showing destructive changes in the acetabulum and the femoral head. There is wandering acetabulum, lower part of the acetabular cavity is empty and the femoral head is uncovered. The patient was treated by antitubercular drugs, skeletal traction and repetitive exercises for the right hip joint. X-rays (B) one year, (C) 3 years after the treatment show improvement of anatomy, reformation of joint margins and space, restitution of destroyed trabeculae, and coxa magna. Despite persistence of the wandering acetabulum the patient obtained a painless, 80% mobile and stable hip joint.

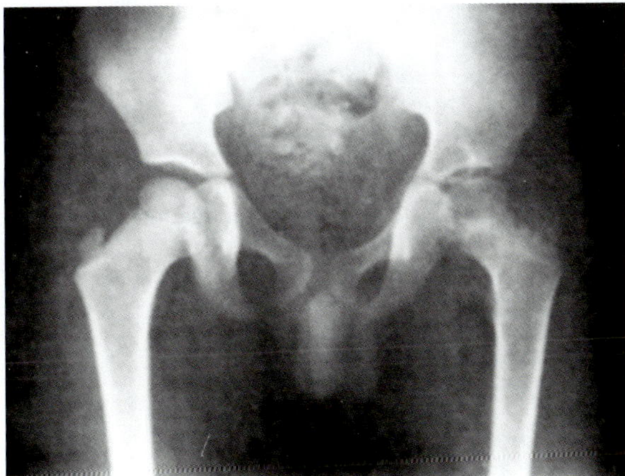

Fig. 8.6: A child with tuberculosis of the left hip joint, early arthritis (stage II) resembling the "normal hip" appearance. Note slight diminution of the joint space and a juxta-articular lytic lesion in the acetabular roof.

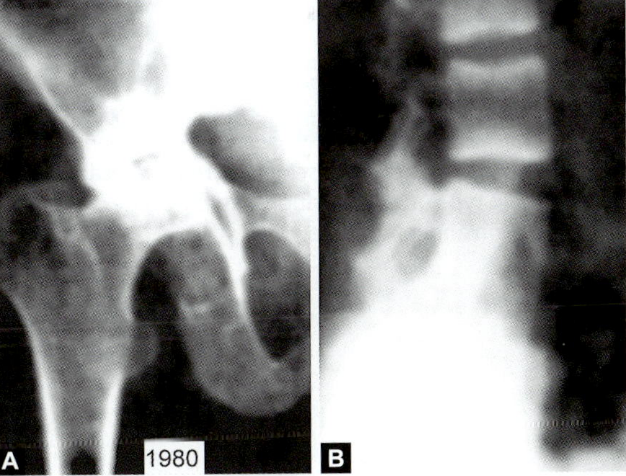

Figs. 8.7A and B: Advanced tuberculous arthritis (stage IV) of right hip joint: Note destruction and deformation of femoral head, wandering acetabulum, upward migration of femoral head, break in the Shenton's arc, empty lower part of the acetabulum, and protrusio acetabuli. The patient also had concomitant tuberculous spondylitis involving lumbar 4–5 vertebrae.

In general, the movements at this stage are grossly restricted, however, some cases with the radiological appearance of wandering acetabulum, protrusio-acetabuli, or mortar-pestle picture may retain fairly good range of movements for a long time **(Fig. 8.11)**. In some cases of aftermath of tuberculous arthritis with the disease healed in the displaced position, the femoral head may be supported by a buttress (false acetabulum) formed over its posterosuperior aspect **(Figs. 8.12 and 8.13)**.

In certain cases of tuberculous arthritis (Stages II, III and IV), the hip may not assume the classical triple deformity of flexion, adduction and internal

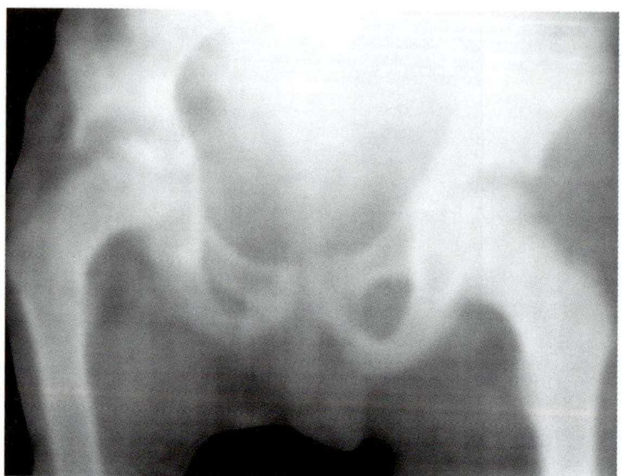

Fig. 8.8A: Active tubercular arthritis of right hip joint. Note localized osteoporosis, break in the Shenton's arc, widened acetabulum, **protrusio acetabuli**, avascular capital femoral epiphysis (Perthes type) and mild coxa vara.

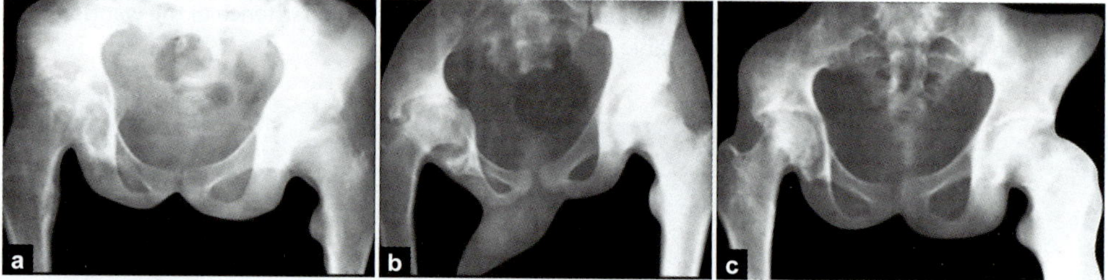

Figs. 8.8B(a to c): Another case of **protrusio acetabuli** showing the outcome of treatment with ATT and ROM exercises. TB-hip protrusio type (a) presentation = fuzzy borders, osteoporosis (b) one year after ATT (c) 3 years after treatment, improved mineralization and joint space.

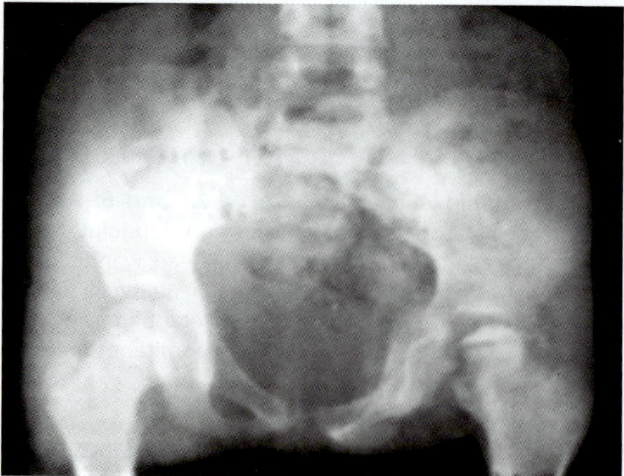

Fig. 8.9A: X-ray of a child with tuberculosis of left hip joint. One can appreciate diminished joint space, indistinct joint margins, subluxation of femoral head, avascular **(Perthes type)** capital femoral epiphysis and cavities in the femoral neck (Stage IV).

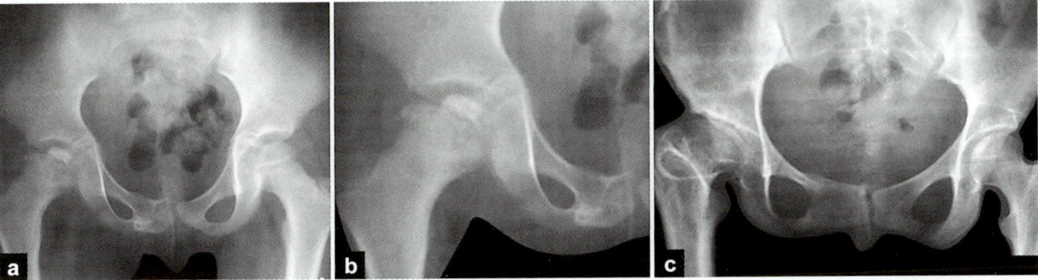

Figs. 8.9B(a to c): Another case of **Perthes-type** tuberculous infection showing the outcome of ATT and ROM exercises. (a and b) TB Hip Perthes' type: sclerotic physis, metaphyseal osteoporosis: Also note TB of right pubic bone. (c) Healed status resembles healed Perthes'–coxa-magna + short neck (coxa-breva), enlarged right pubic bone.

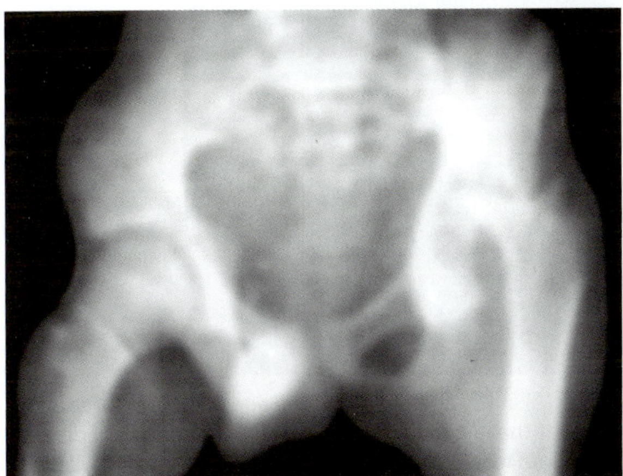

Fig. 8.10A: Tubercular arthritis of left hip joint (stage IV). Note break in the Shenton's arc, emptying of lower half of acetabulum, wandering acetabulum and grossly destroyed femoral head and neck **(mortar-pestle appearance)**.

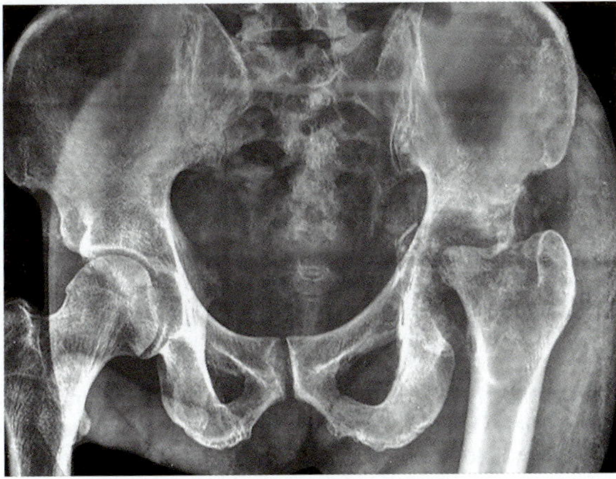

Fig. 8.10B: Another case showing **mortar-pestle appearance** in a healed status of infection. He managed his life up to 60 years of age when he sought medical care for pain in the left joint.

rotation, instead the deformity may be that of flexion, abduction and external rotation **(Figs. 8.14 and 8.16)** with the lateral aspect of thigh of the diseased hip resting on the bed. This may be due to continuous adoption of the latter posture for relief of pain, or due to the destruction of iliofemoral Y ligament by the tuberculous process. In some cases, there is lack of correlation between the radiographic appearance of the hip disease and the range of movements possible in the joint.

If the limb has been plastered for >12 months (as was the practice in first half of 20th century), the growth plates around the knee may undergo premature fusion producing marked shortening and limitation of movements (once called "frame knee"). During growing age in some patients, hyperemia and overgrowth of the femoral head and neck may lead to coxa magna which is often associated with moderate valgus deformity and anteversion of the femoral neck, and some degree of adaptive changes in the acetabulum resembling acetabular "dysplasia". Coxa vara may also occur rarely following a destructive lesion in the femoral head and neck (leading to arrested growth of capital physis) in the presence of normal growth of the greater trochanter.

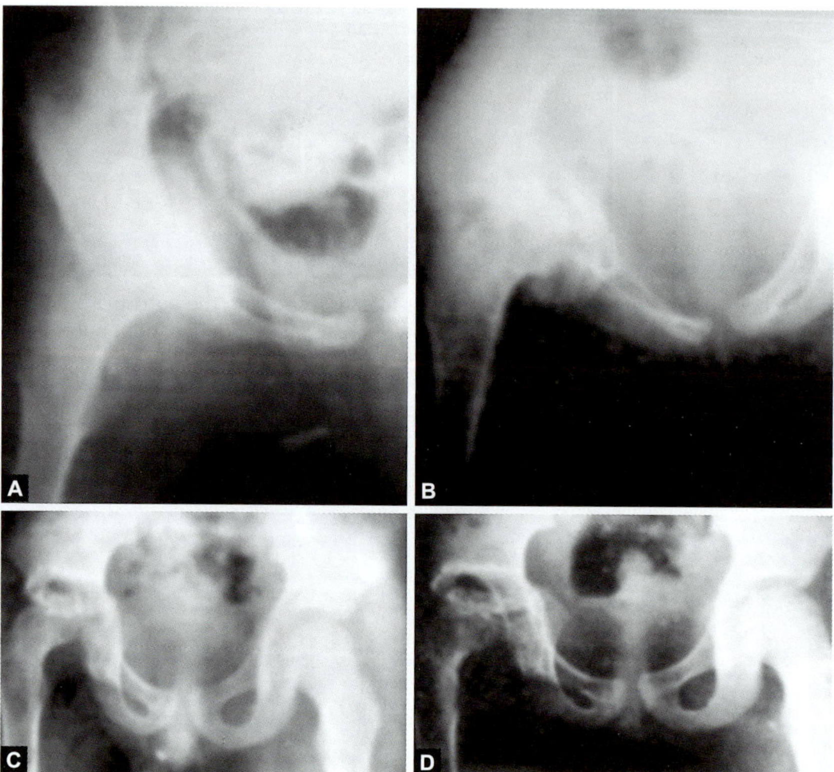

Figs. 8.11A to D: Serial X-rays of a child treated by functional method: (A) at the age of 5, (B) at the age of 6, (C) at 8 years and (D) at 9 years of age, 5 years after the onset of treatment. The patient at the last follow-up had complete healing of disease, though radiologically the femoral head was flattened and the acetabulum was irregular, and **wandering** the boy was able to squat, sit cross-legged and do normal physical activities.

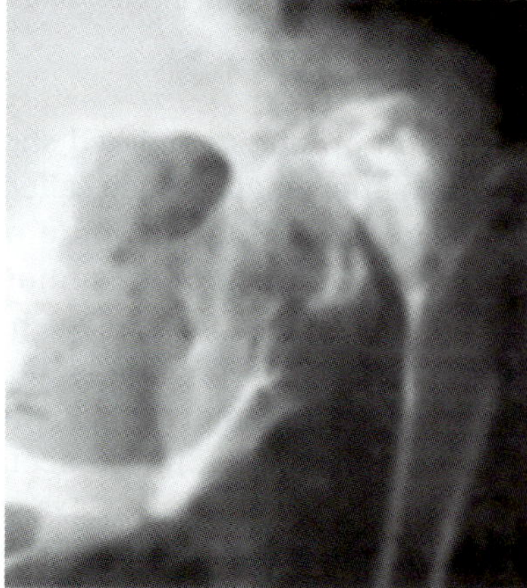

Fig. 8.12: Radiograph showing aftermath of tuberculous arthritis of left hip joint. Note empty acetabulum, coxa magna with dislocation and flattening of the femoral head, and formation of a **secondary false acetabulum** superior and dorsal to the original acetabulum.

Classification of the Radiological Appearance (Figs. 8.5 to 8.17)

Shanmugasundaram (1983) suggested a radiological classification for tuberculous disease of the hip applicable for the lesions in children (C) and adults (A). Following radiological types are suggested by him: "normal" appearance (C); travelling acetabulum (C, A); dislocated hip (C); Perthes' type (C); protrusion acetabuli (C, A); atrophic type (A); "mortar and pestle" type (C, A). There is a relationship between various radiological types and the functional outcome (Campbell and Hoffman 1995). If the disease occurs during childhood (growing period), chronic hyperemia would lead to enlargement of femoral head epiphysis and metaphysis (coxa magna), thromboembolic phenomenon of selective

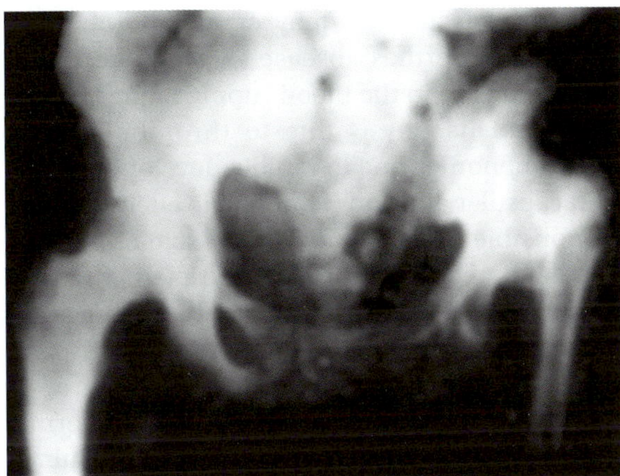

Fig. 8.13: A 26-year-old male suffered from tuberculous infection of left hip joint when he was 9-year-old. The disease healed by traction and antitubercular drugs. The patient had managed his routine activities with a shoe-raise of 6 cm. Now 17 years after the onset of disease, he has started complaining of pain in the left hip region probably due to degenerative changes in the **secondary hip joint**. Note on the left side empty acetabulum, pathological dislocation of hip joint, probable formation of a secondary acetabulum, and hypoplastic pelvis and femur.

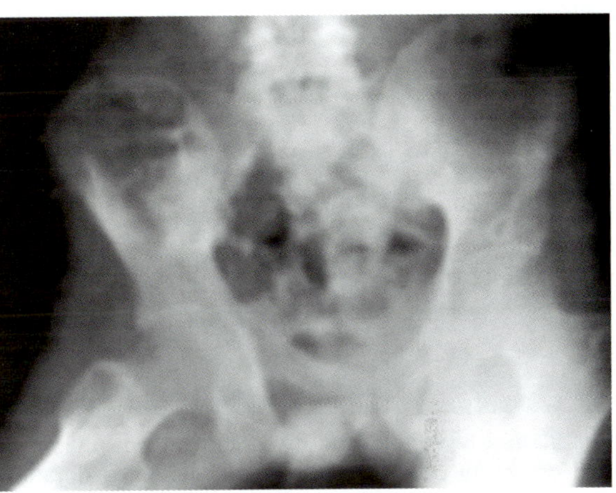

Fig. 8.14: X-ray of tubercular arthritis of right hip joint. The limb has attained the unusual deformity of flexion, abduction and external rotation (maximal capacity of intracapsular space).

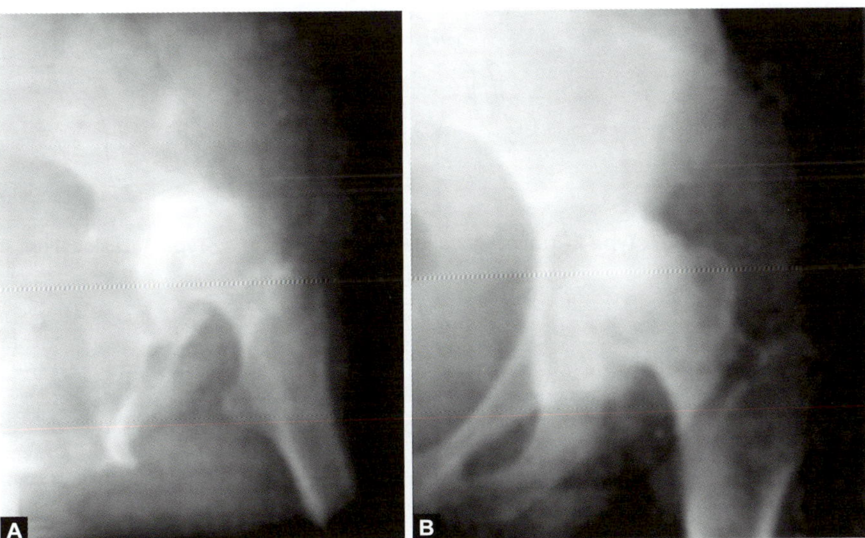

Figs. 8.15A and B: At the age of 18 years, this young lady was treated by traction, exercises, and antitubercular chemotherapy. The disease healed and she obtained a painless, stable and mobile hip joint. Having enjoyed the ability of sitting cross-legged and squatting for 22 years (A), she has now reported for pain in the hip joint due to secondary degenerative changes. The recent clinical examination revealed range of flexion of hip joint from 0 to 90 degrees, the X-rays revealed a wandering acetabulum, diminished joint space, spheroidal uncovered femoral head and **secondary degenerative** change in the left hip joint at 40 years of age (B).

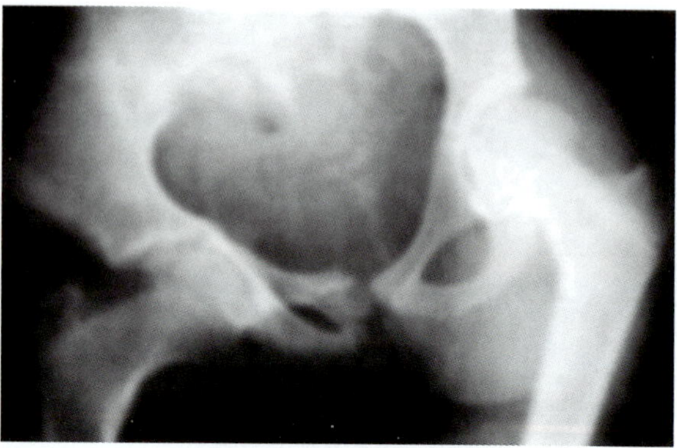

Fig. 8.16: A 6-year-old boy, presented with pain, limping and deformity of right hip joint for 2 months duration. Plain X-rays revealed an abduction deformity of right hip and moderate degree of diminution of the joint space. One can note the uncovering of the contralateral (left) femoral head due to marked fixed abduction deformity of the right hip. Tuberculous nature of pathology was confirmed from the tissue obtained while preforming arthrolysis and synovectomy on right hip joint.

terminal vasculature may create the changes resembling Perthes' disease **(Figs. 8.8 and 8.9)** gross decrease in the blood supply of the femoral head and its physis due to thromboembolic phenomenon or due to rapidly developing tense intracapsular effusion (tamponade effect) may be responsible for reduction in the size of femoral head and neck (coxa breva), restricted growth of capital femoral epiphyseal plate in the presence of normal growth of trochanteric growth-plate would lead to coxa vara, and restricted growth of trochanteric physis in the presence of normal growth of femoral head physis would result in coxa valga. Vascular changes can also occur due to destructive osseous cavities (affecting intraosseous circulation) in the upper end of femur, by a sudden pathological dislocation, or as a complication of operative intervention.

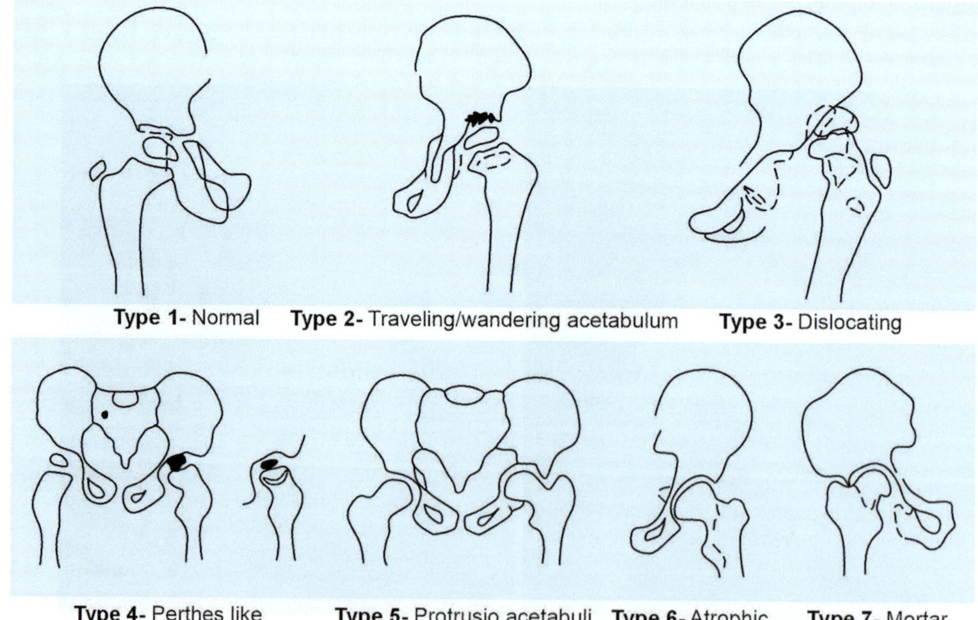

Fig. 8.17: Radiological types of tuberculosis of hip. Rarely a tuberculous hip joint may be healed with bony-ankylosis, more chances if there is concomitant pyogenic infection.

Courtesy: Shanmugasundram, 1983.

More than one factor may be responsible for the radiological appearance in a particular case.

Rarely, simultaneous damage to the trochanteric physis and femoral head physis would result in generalized hypoplasia of upper end of femur (coxa breva). Campbell and Hoffman (1995) while treating children with tuberculosis of hip joint observed a close relationship between the radiological type and the therapeutic outcome; "good-results" were obtained in 92% of "normal type", 80% of Perthes' type, 50% of dislocating type, 29% of travelling-acetabulum and mortar-pestle type. If the radiological joint space was reduced to 3 mm or less, the outcome could be predicted as poor.

PROGNOSIS

The outcome of prognosis with modern antitubercular drugs depends essentially on the stage of the disease when the treatment is initiated (Caparros 1999, Silber 2000, Babhulkar 2002, Saraf 2014). Early disease (synovitis or early arthritis) may heal leaving a normal or nearly normal hip joint **(Figs. 8.2 and 8.20 to 8.24)** (Moon et al. 2012). Healing in the state of advanced arthritis generally results in fibrous ankylosis. If correction of deformities was not achieved by timely and appropriate treatment (traction, splintage or operation), the ankylosis is likely to occur in a non-functional position of flexion and adduction. The diseased limb may show gross shortening a few years after the treatment. This is usually the result of gross destruction of hip bones, damage to proximal femoral physis, and occasionally premature fusion of distal femoral physis if the limb has been immobilized for >1 year.

Some of these cases may be associated with a tuberculous cavity situated in the femoral neck. The femoral head then passes through the typical phases such as metaphyseal osteoporosis, diminution of the vertical height of the capital femoral epiphysis, increased density, fragmentation, collapse of the proximal segment, and development of coxa-magna with healing. Such patients require to be treated like Perthes' disease with simultaneous coverage by effective antitubercular drugs.

MANAGEMENT

All patients during active stage are treated by multidrug therapy, and traction to correct the deformity **(Figs. 8.18 and 8.34)** if present and to give rest to the part. In the presence of abduction deformity, for better control of the pelvis, bilateral traction (well leg traction) is mandatory, otherwise traction to the deformed limb alone would increase the abduction deformity further. Traction relieves the muscle spasm, prevents or corrects deformity and subluxation, maintains the joint space, minimizes the chances of development of migrating acetabulum and permits close observation of the hip region. Any palpable cold abscess may be aspirated with instillation of streptomycin with or without isoniazid.

If there is favorable clinical response the same treatment should be continued. In cases which do not have gross ankylosis, active assisted movements of the hip are started as soon as the pain has subsided. The hip mobilization exercises are gradually increased to 5–10 minutes every hour during the period the patient is awake, and within the limits of tolerable pain. With the traction applied, the patient may be progressively encouraged to sit and touch his forehead to the knee, sitting in squatting position and putting the thigh in abduction and external rotation. Usually after 4–6 months of treatment the patient may be permitted ambulation with suitable orthosis and crutches. The ambulation should be non-weight bearing for first 12 weeks and partial weight bearing for the next 12 weeks. Nearly 12 months after the onset of treatment, crutches or orthosis may be discarded. Excellent results are obtained by the above non-operative regime in majority of cases of synovial disease, in many cases with early arthritis **(Figs. 8.19 to 8.26)** and in some cases of advanced arthritis **(Figs. 8.5, 8.11, 8.15, and 8.19 to 8.26)**.

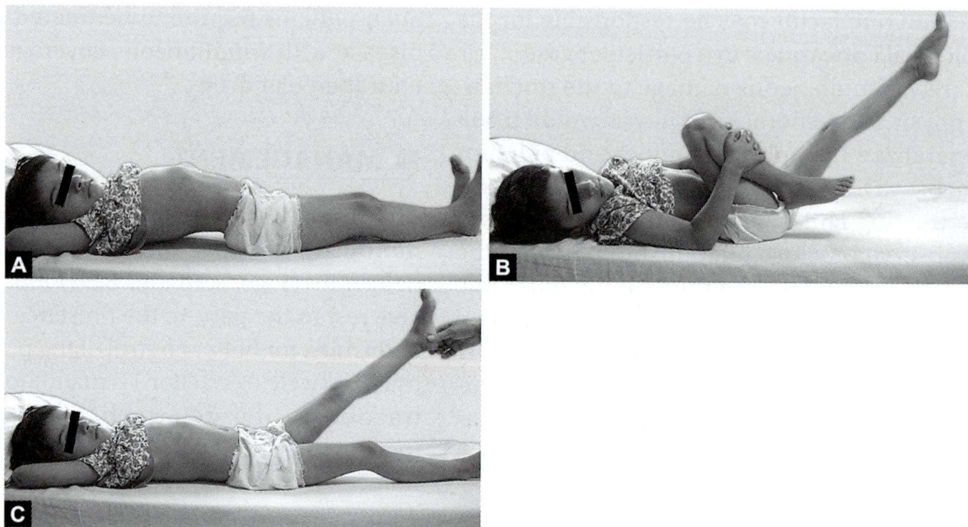

Figs. 8.18A to C: Fixed flexion deformity is the commonest deformity in an established hip infection. Flexion deformity (Left Hip) gets hidden by (A) exaggerated lumbar lordosis. Oblitrate the lordosis: flexion deformity becomes manifest; (B) by performing Thomas test or (C) by holding the hip in the deformed position.

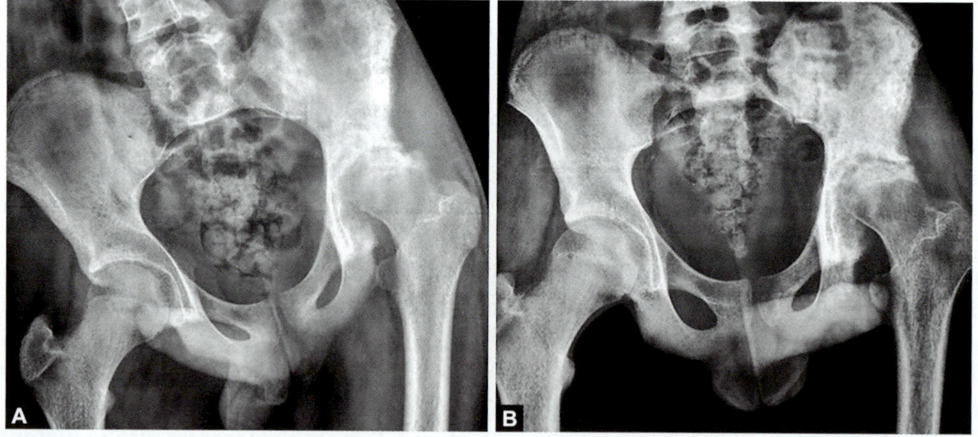

Figs. 8.19A and B: (A) X-ray of an advanced arthritis of left hip joint. Note **wandering acetabulum** and adduction deformity. (B) After 3 months of traction and the ATT-drugs, note improvement in texture of bone and deformity, and re-appearance of the joint space. Effective traction relieves spasm, pain, corrects deformities, displacements, improves joint space, permits ROM exercises.

With the employment of effective anti-tubercular drugs destruction of more than half of the articular surface is not always incompatible with a useful range of joint motion (Hodgson and Fang 1981), therefore, decision to perform excision or arthrodesis should not be made in a hurry **(Table 8.2)**. If the response to nonoperative treatment is unfavorable, one should perform synovectomy or debridement of the diseased joint as needed. Occasionally, on opening the hip joint the disease may be more advanced than anticipated. When the disease is well under control, protected ambulation is started 3–6 months after the operation.

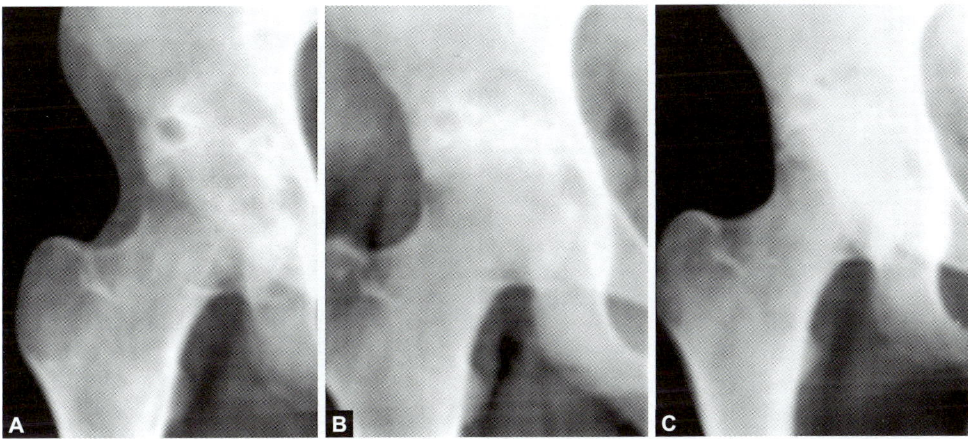

Figs. 8.20A to C: Follow-up X-rays of a young engineer who was treated by antitubercular drugs, traction and active assisted exercises, (A) for early tuberculous arthritis of right hip joint. Observe a supra-acetabular cavity at presentation (A) and its healing process (B). The patient maintained the healed status, with 70% function of the joint. The X-ray 8 years after completion of treatment (C), shows slight diminution of the articular cartilage space and almost normal texture of bones.

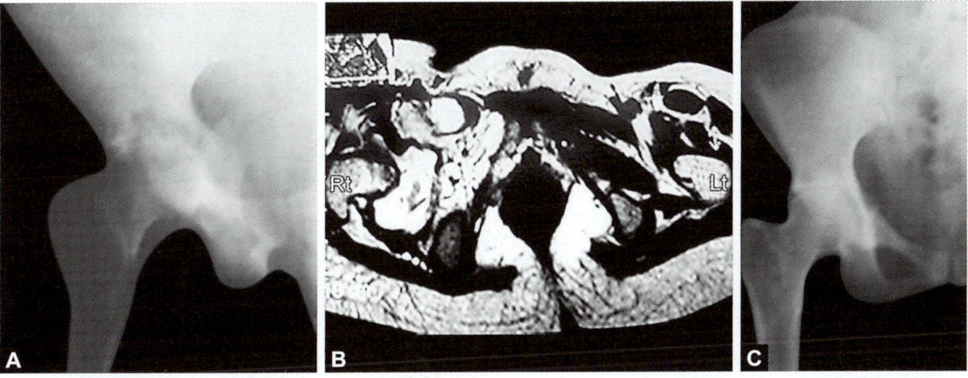

Figs. 8.21A to C: X-ray (A) and MRI (B) of right hip joint at presentation. X-ray shows eroded acetabulum, gross diminution of joint space (stage III). MRI shows collection of fluid within the joint, it also shows a suppurating lymph node anteriorly. She was treated at home by traction (for a few weeks), multidrug therapy and range of motion exercises; (C) shows the healed status by restoration of the bone architecture and the joint space one year after the start of treatment.

In *advanced arthritis,* the usual outcome is gross fibrous ankylosis. The traction regime and functional exercises in the initial stages help to overcome the deformities and permit assessment regarding the retention or return of any useful range of motion. Once gross ankylosis is anticipated and accepted, the limb should be immobilized with the help of a plaster hip spica for about 4–6 months. The **ideal position for ankylosis of hip joint** in adults is neutral between abduction and adduction, 5–10 degrees of external rotation, and flexion depending upon age (between 10 degrees in children and 30 degrees in adults). About 6 months after onset of the treatment or the application of hip spica, whichsoever is earlier, partial weight bearing should be started first in a single hip spica (for about 6 months), and later on with the help of an orthosis and crutches for nearly 2 years.

In an analysis of results of traction regime for tubercular arthritis, Sandhu (1983) reported healing of disease in 98% of cases. Of the 41 patients,

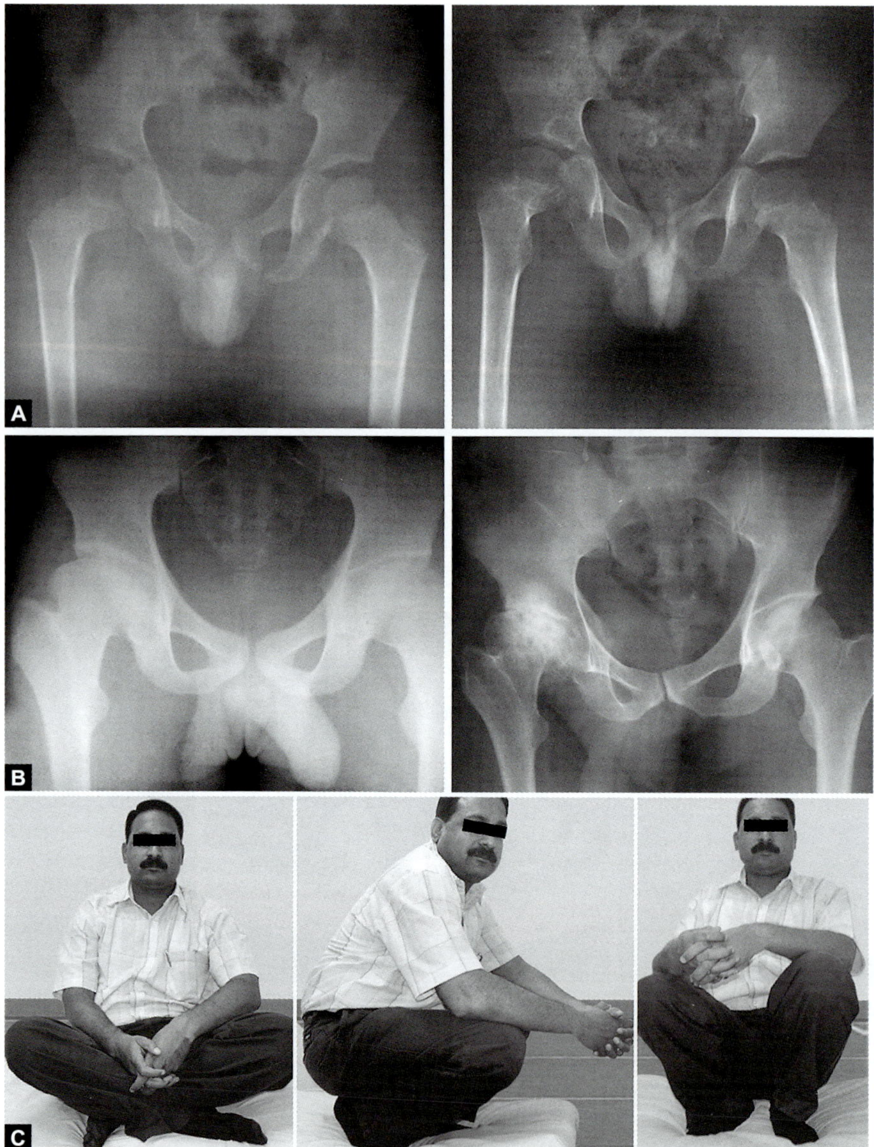

Figs. 8.22A to C: (A) Four years male presented in 1966 as TB right hip joint. Treatment was multidrug therapy, ROM exercises and traction at home. Patient followed up to 2006. (B) During growing age there is remarkable potential for recovery of disease and retention of joint movements despite coxa magna. (C) At 44 years age note the remarkable function of right hip joint. In due course he may be justifiably suitable for right hip replacement.

40 had healed with retention of appreciable range of movements; the average range was flexion 69 degrees, abduction 22 degrees, adduction 19 degrees, external rotation 22 degrees and internal rotation 24 degrees. One patient who had secondary infection ended up in bony ankylosis. In 5 patients, corrective osteotomy was indicated for unacceptable deformity.

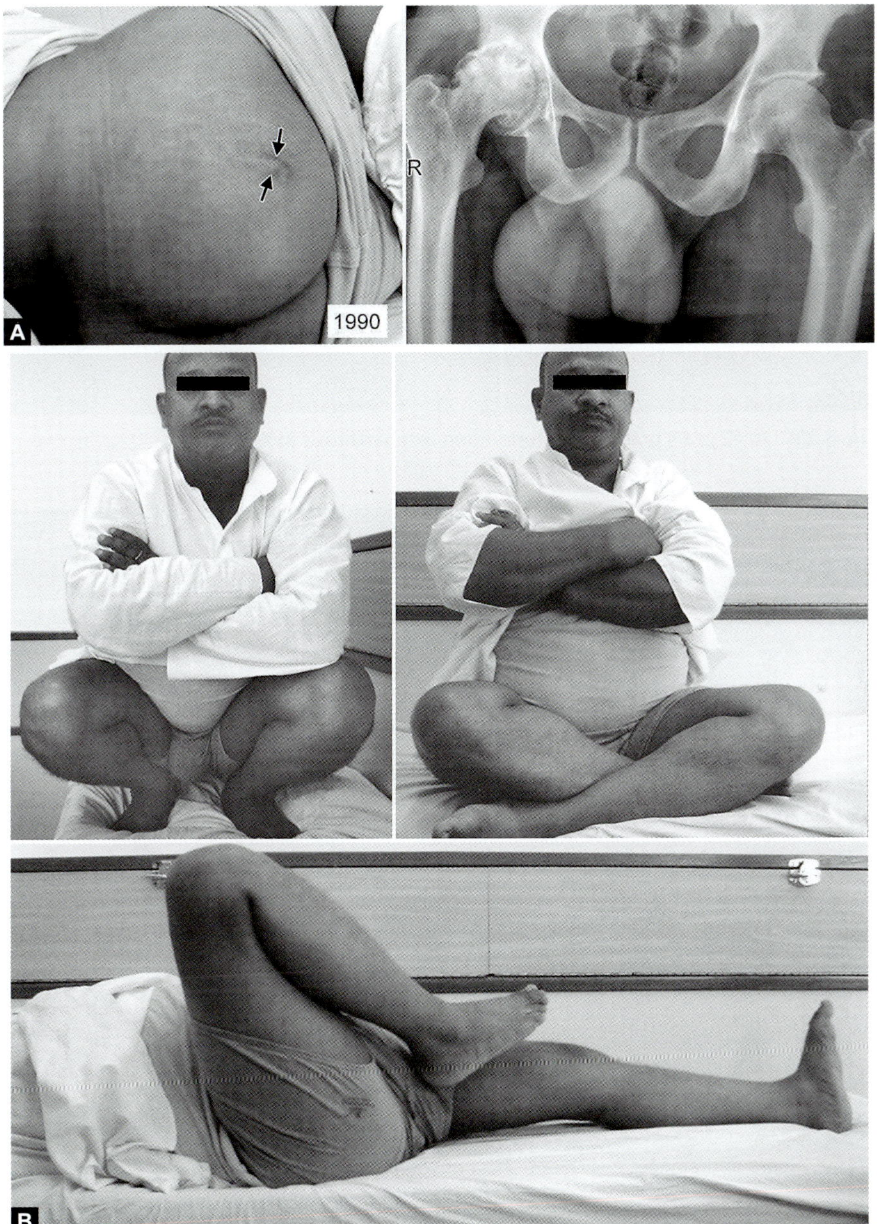

Figs. 8.23A and B: (A) A 20 years male developed right hip TB (stage II ±), treated by drugs, drainage of gluteal abscess right hip TB (Scar) and ROM exercises. At 22 years follow-up (now aged 42 years) he has very good function. X-rays show secondary osteoarthrosis. (B) At age 42 years clinical function despite osteoarthrosis in X-rays.

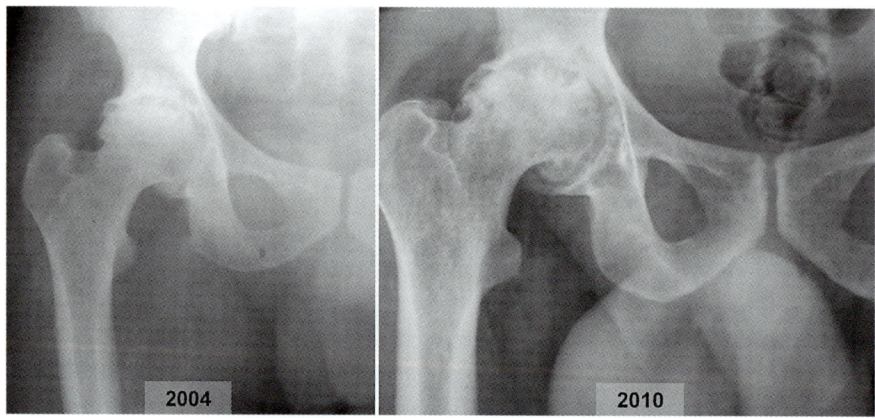

Fig. 8.23C: At 42 years gradually deteriorating osteoarthrosis in X-rays.

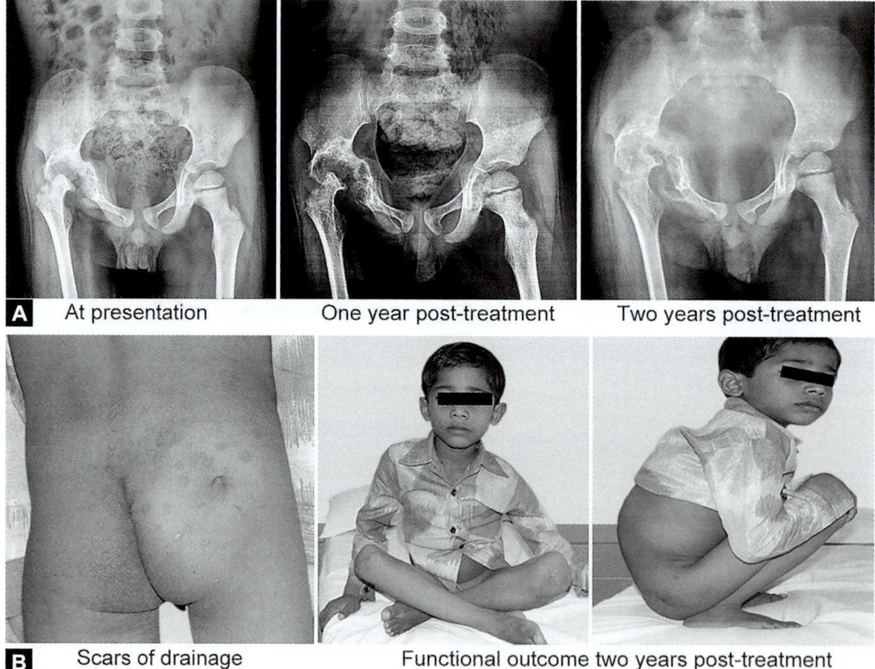

Figs. 8.24A and B: In children, expectant treatment is justified with multidrug therapy, and active/assisted ROM exercises. Despite gross destruction of femoral head and its growth plate, and gross destruction of acetabulum producing **"wandering" acetabulum** and **"protrusio" acetabulum** the infection healed with nearly complete range of motion.

Management in Children

In children with arthritis, the deformity and subluxation/dislocation is corrected or minimized by employing traction. Rarely, one may require correction of the deformity by applying plaster under general anesthesia with or without adductor tenotomy. Failure to achieve correction of gross deformities and minimization of subluxation/dislocation in children warrants open arthrotomy, synovectomy and debridement

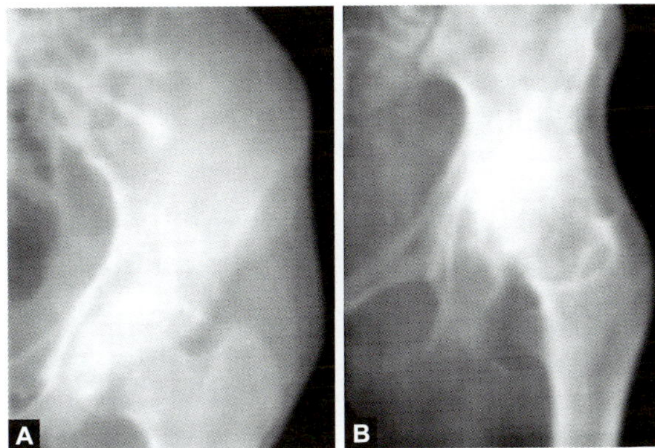

Figs. 8.25A and B: Tuberculosis of the left hip joint with destruction of the weight bearing part of the iliac bone (A). The patient did not receive specific treatment and in the next 3 years developed wandering acetabulum with gross ankylosis of the hip joint (B). Tuberculous pathology was proved from the tissues at the time of excisional arthroplasty—specimen in **Figure 8.27**.

of the diseased joint and improvement of displacement. Arthrodesis of the grossly destroyed hip joint or excisional arthroplasty in children is contraindicated till the completion of growth potential of the proximal femur. Children presenting with disease healed with gross deformity (flexion more than 30 degrees, adduction more than 10 degrees or abduction more than 10 degrees), require an extra-articular corrective osteotomy to enable them to walk better till they reach skeletal maturity. In some children, the disease may heal with gross fibrous ankylosis. If there is no gross distortion of anatomy of the hip joint subtotal excision of the contracted fibrous capsule (*arthrolysis*) followed by traction and repetitive exercises may restore a useful range of movement for a few years (Agarwal et al. 2014, Saraf 2015).

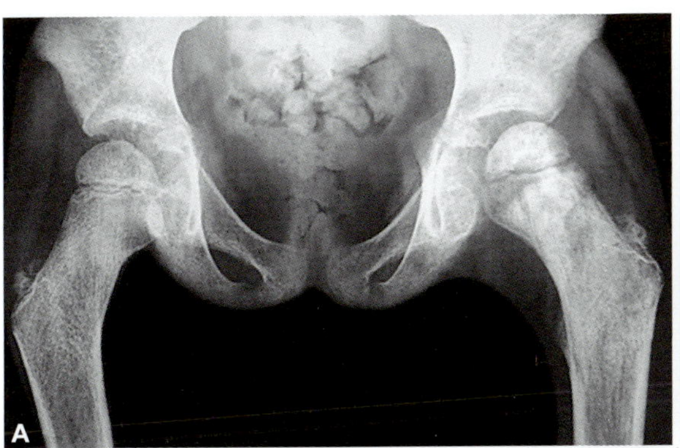

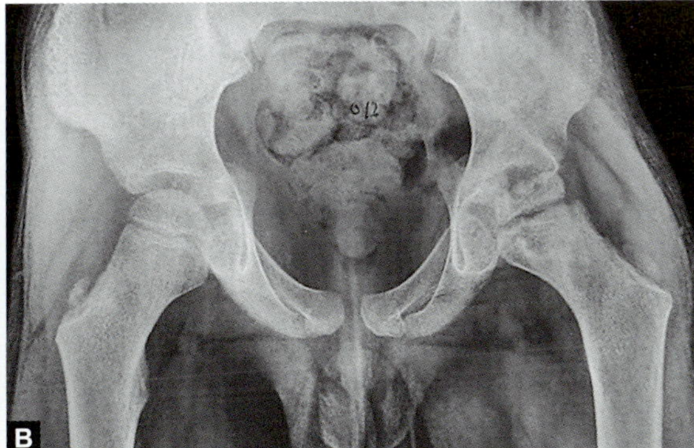

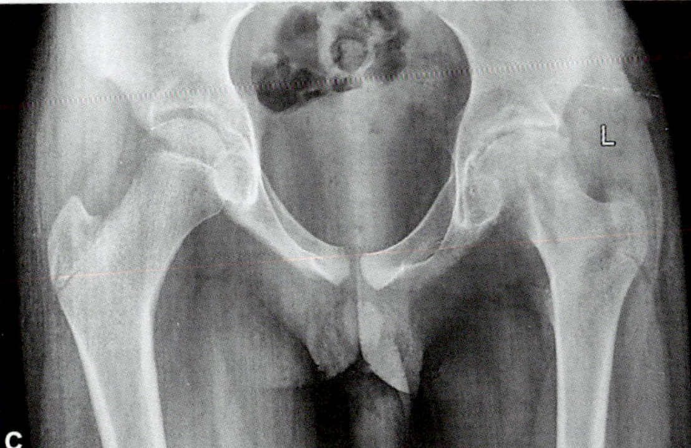

Figs. 8.26A to C: Potential of recovery for childhood tubercular lesions. Left hip shows irregular destruction of femoral head and neck (A). Patient was treated by anti-TB drugs and functional regime. During the healing process the X-ray showed Perthes like changes (B). Approximately 18 months after, the X-ray show near normal texture and shape of bones (C).

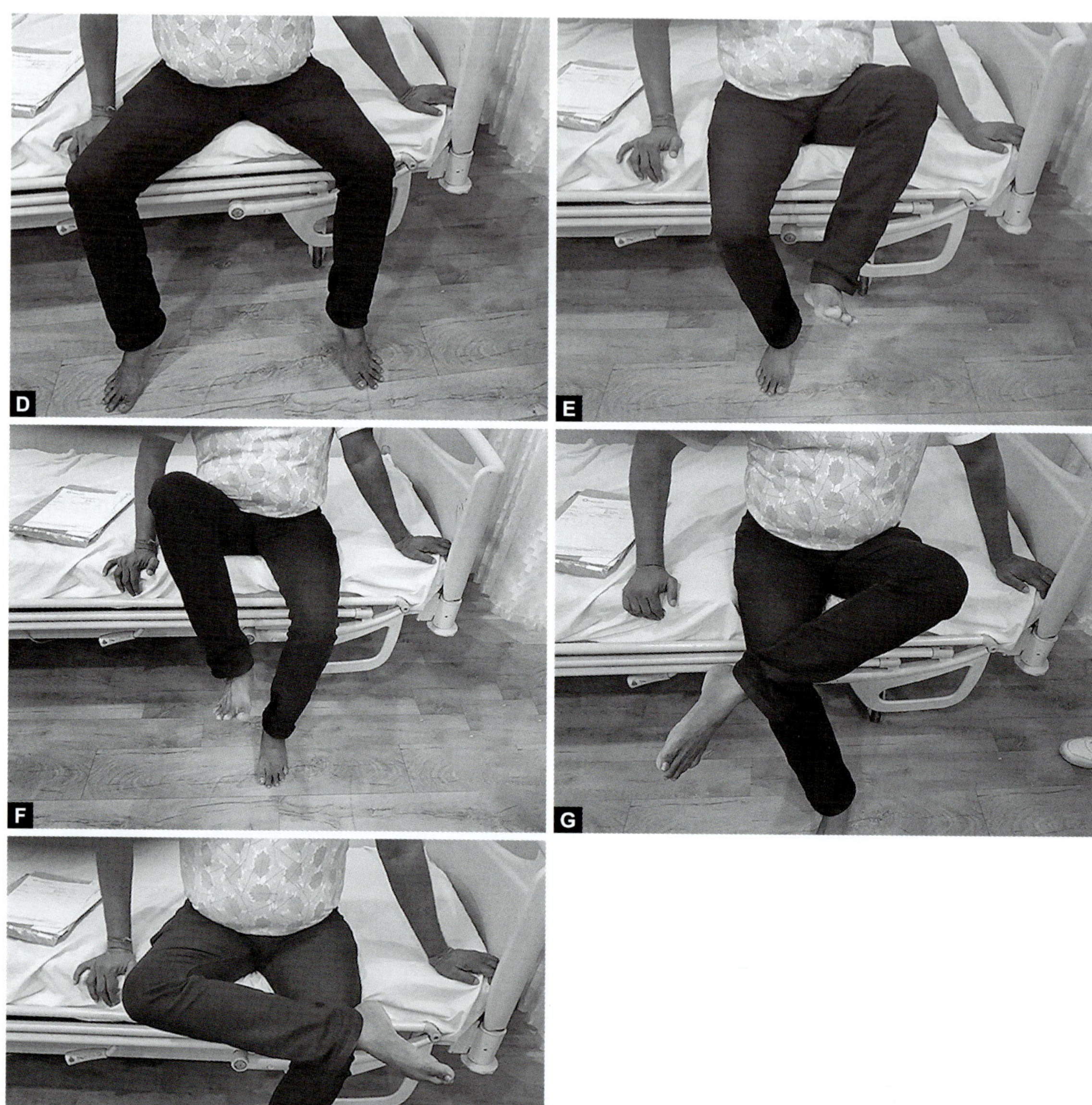

Figs. 8.26D to H: A 2012 at presentation with follow-up to 2024. Healed disease left joint is an adult patient, observe the functional outcome.

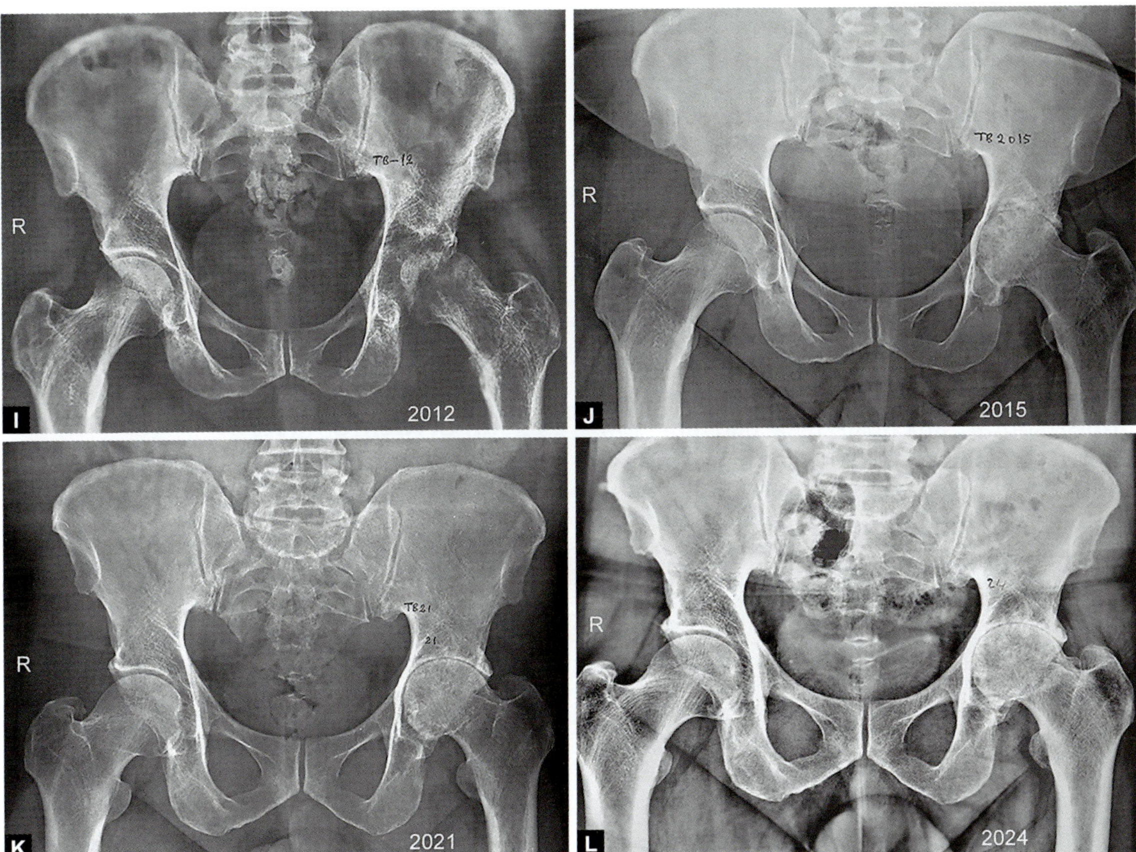

Figs. 8.26I to L: (I) Increased joint space in left hip joint, erosions in acetabular and in femoral head and osteoporosis. (J and K) One can appreciate the role of anti-TB drugs with "function" treatment in adult having tuberculosis of left hip joint and (L) early degenerative enthesophytes, observe the healed statins: reduced joint space restored bone density.

Table 8.2: Guidelines for treatment according to clinical presentations.

Guidelines for indications and operations in tuberculosis of hip	
Therapeutically refractory or doubtful diagnosis	Arthrotomy, synovectomy, debridement
Dislocation/subluxation during active stage of disease	Arthrotomy and repositioning of joint
Juxta-articular non-resolving lesion threatening the joint	Debridement of the lesion
Unacceptable gross ankylosis of hip in active stage of disease in adults	Excision arthroplasty
Partial ankylosis with healed disease with "useful range" of motion	Juxta-articular femoral osteotomy to bring the range of motion to the "functional arc" or arthrolysis
Bony ankylosis of hip in non-functioning position	Juxta-articular corrective femoral osteotomy to bring the fused joint to the best functioning position
Painful ankylosis of hip in adults	Excisional arthroplasty or replacement arthroplasty
Unacceptable ankylosis with healed disease (>3 years)	Replacement arthroplasty

INDICATIONS FOR SURGICAL TREATMENT

If the response to conservative treatment is not favorable or the outcome is unacceptable, the following selective operative procedures are useful and have stood the test of time **(Table 8.2)**.

Osteotomy

Patients presenting with sound ankylosis in non-functional position require upper femoral corrective osteotomy. Sometimes an unsound (fibrous-painful) ankylosis in a bad position becomes an osseous fusion (sound-painless) by a high femoral corrective osteotomy. This operation is a simple extracapsular procedure and can be done at any age. The ideal site for corrective osteotomy is as near the deformed joint as possible.

Arthrodesis

Before the availability of effective antitubercular drugs, one preferred to perform an **extra-articular fusion**. Bone grafts were used to bridge the gap between the ischium and femur (ischiofemoral arthrodesis, **Fig. 8.32**) or between the ilium and femur (iliofemoral arthrodesis, **Fig. 8.33**). With availability of modern drugs, however, direct intracapsular fusion is favored between the rawed surfaces of femoral head and the acetabulum. Classically, this operation is indicated in an adult presenting with unsound (painful fibrous ankylosis) ankylosis with active or healed disease. This procedure should be deferred so long as the bones of the hip joint have any growth potential. Young adults with sound bony ankylosis in functioning position learn to adopt themselves for active life **(Figs. 8.3 and 8.4)**. One has, however, to resort to chair and commode toilet system.

Excisional Arthroplasty

In the Indian subcontinent, Japan, China, South-east Asia and Middleeast, majority of people do not like to accept a stiff hip joint. In these countries, squatting, sitting cross-legged, and kneeling are essential socioeconomic activities. Girdlestone's excision arthroplasty can be safely carried out in healed or active disease after the completion of growth potential of bones of the hip joint. This procedure provides a mobile, painless hip joint with control of infection and correction of deformity **(Figs. 8.27 and 8.28)**. However, some degree of shortening (3.5–5 cm) and instability is unavoidable. On an average, there is an addition of 1.5 cm to the preoperative shortening. Application of postoperative traction

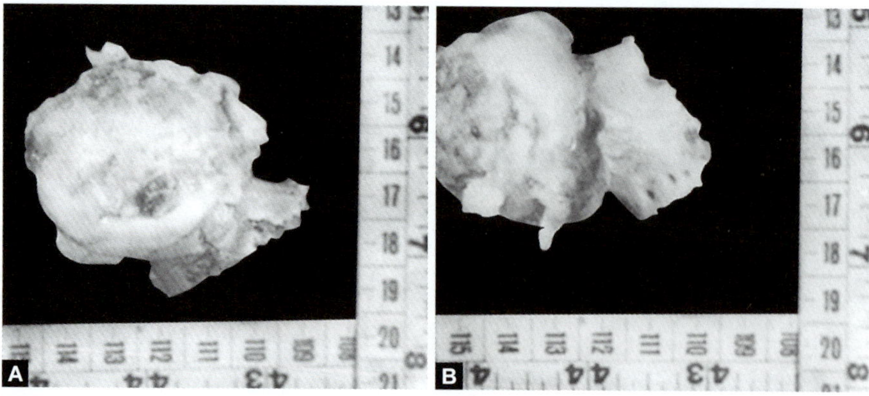

Figs. 8.27A and B: Gross appearance of the excised femoral head of the case of **Figure 8.25**. The articular cartilage is destroyed and eroded at many places, loose tags of the cartilage (A) are hanging (in the view on right), subchondral bone (B) shows cobbled appearance, the head is flattened and deformed.

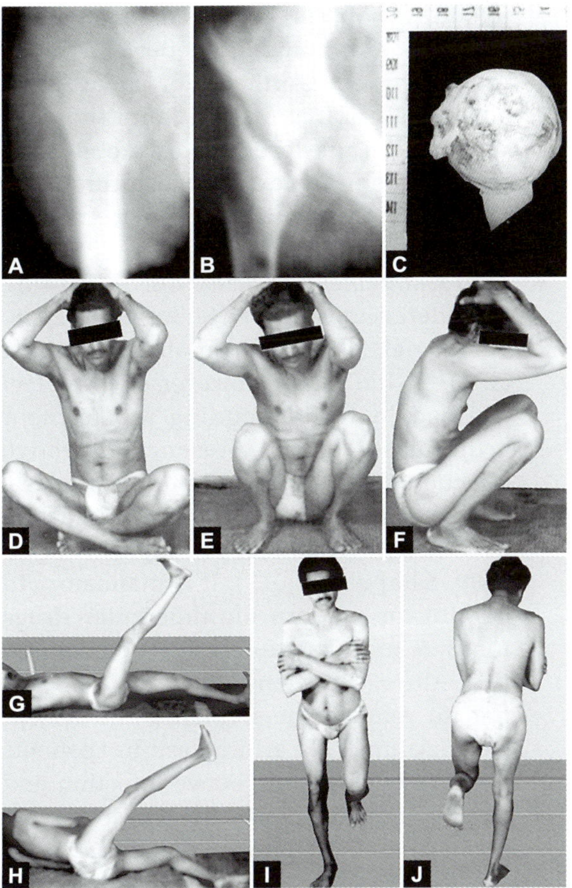

Figs. 8.28A to J: Composite picture of a patient of excision arthroplasty of right hip joint 5 years after the operation, showing the radiological appearance and functions of the joint. The excised femoral head (inset) shows the subchondral bone denuded of the articular cartilage. The remnant small patch of articular cartilage is showing the pock-marked appearance, (A) soon after surgery, (B) 5 years after surgery, (C) excised femoral head, (D to J) various activities performed by the patient at 5 years postoperative follow-up.

Courtesy: Tuli SM, Mukherjee SK. Excision arthroplasty for tuberculous and pyogenic arthritis of the hip. J Bone Joint Surg. 1981;63B:29-32.

for 3 months minimizes shortening and gross instability (Tuli and Mukherjee 1981, Saraf 2015).

We have observed 80 patients of tuberculous arthritis of hip joint treated by a mobilization procedure (by excision arthroplasty) for a period of 2–9 years. With the employment of effective antitubercular drugs the chances of recrudescence are no more in such patients than in those who obtained sound ankylosis. 90% of our patients, observed between 1965 to 1980, were able to squat and kneel **(Fig. 8.28)**, 85% were able to sit cross-legged, 60% were able to stand on the operated extremity unsupported, 90% were able to lift the limb straight against gravity, almost all were able to climb up the stairs using a walking-stick, 5% of patients required a change to newer drugs for control of their infection. With long follow-up radiologically, there was improvement in bone texture and remodeling of the bones of the false joint **(Fig. 8.28)**. 11% of patients did not feel satisfied with the result because of development of reankylosis of the joint. No patient was made worse. For a long time, it was considered that the most successful treatment for tuberculosis of the hip joint was to achieve a sound bony fusion, lest any mobility should cause reactivation (Girdlestone 1950, 1965, Mukopadhaya 1956) of the disease. There are, however, exponents (Adjrad and Martini 1987) who noted a favorable response to antitubercular chemotherapy in all their 40 patients treated by obtaining a sound ankylosis or by operative arthrodesis. We now safely recommend excision arthroplasty for active or healed tuberculous arthritis in adults without any apprehension of increased incidence of reactivation of the infection.

Stage of Disease and Operative Procedure (Table 8.2)

a. In *synovial stage*, if the disease is not responding favorably or the diagnosis is uncertain, arthrotomy and synovectomy should be carried out. In a similar clinical response in early arthritis, in addition to synovectomy removal of loose bodies/rice bodies, debris, pannus covering the articular cartilage, loose articular cartilage and careful curettage of osseous juxta-articular foci should be carried out (joint clearance or joint debridement). Postoperatively triple drug therapy, traction, intermittent active and assisted exercises should be continued for 4–6 weeks. Ambulation with suitable braces and orthosis should be started (according to the time-table as mentioned above) 3–4 months after the operation depending on the control of disease.

b. With *advanced arthritis* with or without dislocation/subluxation it is unlikely that the joint would attain a healed status with retention of good range of movements. However, with the modern effective antitubercular chemotherapy and employment of traction regime, it is surprising how some cases maintain good functional range of movements **(Figs. 8.5, 8.11, 8.15, 8.18 and 8.21 to 8.24)**, and therefore, ankylosis should not necessarily be the aim. If there is some "joint space" visible, *arthrolysis* and release of contracted capsule can minimize the deformity and improve the range of motion. Some of these patients may report back, with pain due to secondary osteoarthrosis after having enjoyed many years of useful mobility of the hip **(Figs. 8.15 and 8.20 to 8.24)**.
c. When *ankylosis is the aim* or the expected result in a patient with growth potential, the hip should be immobilized, during early stage of treatment in 10–15 degrees of abduction because with fibrosis during convalescence and healing there is a tendency toward adduction. A few degrees of flexion deformity of the hip joint must be added; one degree for each year of life up to a maximum of 30 degrees. The younger spine is more mobile and adaptable to compensate for loss of movements at the hip joint.
d. In *healed status of disease,* operations may be indicated in certain patients. Depending on the socio-economic status of the patient and facilities available following alternatives are available: (i) upper femoral corrective osteotomy to correct severe flexion-adduction deformity; (ii) upper femoral displacement-cum-corrective osteotomy in a case of fibrous ankylosis with gross deformity to correct the deformity and hopefully to convert fibrous ankylosis to bony fusion; (iii) conversion of a painful ankylosis to a sound arthrodesis by intra-articular or extra-articular or panarticular arthrodesis of the hip joint; and (iv) conversion of an ankylosed hip to a mobile state by Girdlestone's type excisional arthroplasty **(Fig. 8.28)** or by total joint replacement in selected cases.
e. *Joint replacement, in active disease* is being considered these days (Sidhu et al. 2009, Wang et al. 2010, Neogi et al. 2010, Kim et al. 2013). The author, however, does not feel justified in recommending replacement arthroplasty in the presence of active infection. One may try total joint arthroplasty 2–3 years or more after complete healing of infection (Eskola 1998, Caparros et al. 1999, Saraf et al. 2015). It is mandatory to administer modern antitubercular drugs for 3–5 months after any replacement procedure. Between 2000 to 2013 we had to remove the implants and accept pseudarthrosis like arthroplasty in 4 patients because of persisting active infection and sinuses after joint replacement despite years of postoperative antitubercular drugs.

SURGICAL APPROACHES TO THE HIP JOINT

The Anterior Iliofemoral Approach or Anterolateral Approach (Fig. 8.29)

As described by Smith-Petersen and modified by various workers should be considered almost as a universal surgical approach for any operative procedure for tuberculous disease of the hip joint. This incision can be extended proximally and/or distally depending upon the extent of surgical procedure and the deformities present in the joint.

With the patient supine and toward the edge of the table, give 20 degrees tilt to the opposite side by placing sandbags behind the sacrum. The extremity to be operated is always draped free to permit intra-operative manipulations and rotations. Make the incision along the outer lip

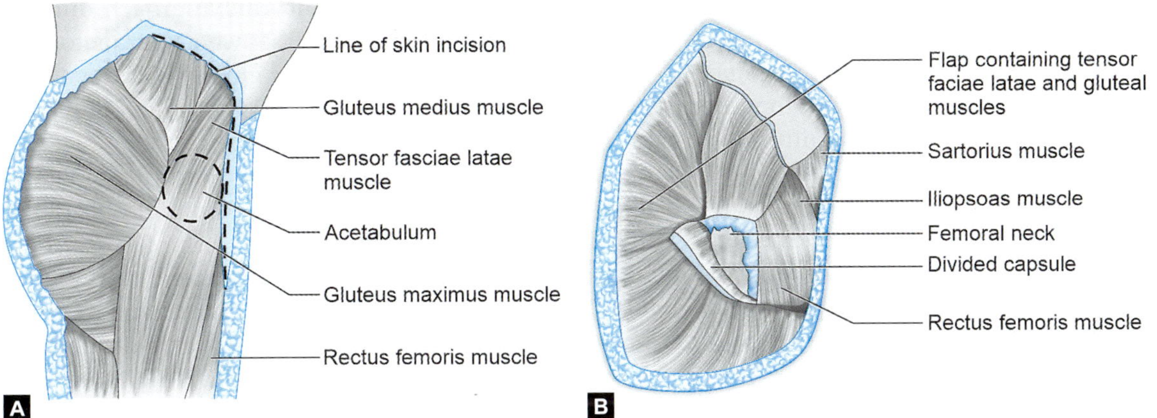

Figs. 8.29A and B: Diagrammatic representation of conventional anterolateral exposure to the right hip joint. This is like a universal approach for any surgical procedure like synovectomy, debridement, relocation of a displaced head, intra-articular arthrodesis of the hip joint, or for excisional arthroplasty.

of the anterior one-third of the iliac crest coming up to the anterosuperior iliac spine, then carry it distally for 8–10 cm in the direction of the lateral border of patella. The vertical limb of the incision is aimed to stay medial to the medial border of the tensor fasciae latae muscle. Now incise cleanly the deep fascia and the muscles (tensor fasciae latae and gluteus medius) along with the periosteum from the outer surface of the iliac bone leaving behind about 1.5–2 cm of muscles attached to the outer lip of the iliac crest. Using a broad chissel and large sponges, reflect these muscles and gluteus minimus as a continuous structure distally and laterally subperiosteally up to the superior, anterior and posterior margins of acetabulum.

Pack tightly the space between the outer surface of the iliac bone and the periosteo-muscular flap. Now carry the fascial incision in the deep fascia distally between the tensor fasciae latae and iliotibial band laterally, and sartorius, rectus femoris and vastus lateralis medially. Develop this plane working disto-proximally as there is more space and areolar tissue in the distal part. In the proximal part of the plane, about 5 cm distal to the hip joint, one may find a leash of blood vessels (from lateral femoral circumflex artery) entering into the medial surface of tensor fasciae latae muscle. These require to be identified, double ligated, cauterized and cut. The lateral femoral cutaneous nerve usually passes over the sartorius muscle and can be saved by retracting the nerve and muscle medially. The packing between the iliac bone and the reflected muscles would have controlled the bleeding by this time. If removal of the packs still shows bleeding it should be controlled by cauterization and ligation. In cases of severe flexion deformity of long-standing, the structures at the anterosuperior iliac spine are markedly contracted, 1–2 cm of the "spine" may be osteotomized free and allowed to retract with its attachments (sartorius, inguinal ligament) distally. Retraction of the lateral periosteo-muscular flap (consisting of tensor fasciae latae, gluteus medius and gluteus minimus) laterally, and sartorius and rectus femoris medially exposes the capsule of the hip joint. For better exposure one can pack and use long bone levers (extracapsularly) along the superior and inferior borders of the femoral neck. Incise the capsule (in an L-shaped manner) starting from the infero-medial aspect of the capsular attachment to the acetabular rim, extend it proximally just lateral and parallel to the acetabular labrum to the superoposterior aspect of the capsule, then curve it laterally parallel to the femoral neck coming up to the greater trochanter. A triangular flap of the capsule can now be lifted with a laterally placed base. This incision of the capsule divides the reflected head of the rectus femoris that blends with the capsule at the superior margin of the capsule. Now reposition the long bone levers intracapsularly. The ligamentum teres may be divided with a knife or with a curved scissors, the cut on the capsule may be extended in all the directions (if necessary) and the femoral head dislocated by external rotation of the femur. It is, however, not necessary to dislocate the femoral head in every case, and this maneuver may even be impossible and dangerous in a case with gross ankylosis of the hip joint which may in addition have osteoporotic bones.

Nearly all surgery of the hip joint for various stages of infection can be carried out through this approach. In the presence of gross deformity of long-standing and scarring of soft tissues, there is obliteration of anatomical planes and the surgeon has to be extra-careful for dissection in the deeper regions. The capsule may also be cut transversely or in a cruciate manner. In any surgical technique whenever preservation of the femoral head and neck is contemplated, one should avoid cutting of the capsule along the base of femoral neck to minimize the risk of loss of blood supply to the femoral head.

Transverse Anterior Approach to the Hip Joint

Luck (1955) described a transverse anterior approach to the hip joint. The tensor fasciae latae is divided transversely in its distal one-third and the cut is extended anteriorly into the fascia lata. Pandey (personal communication) suggested modification of this without cutting transversely the tensor fasciae latae **(Fig. 8.30)**. It preserves the integrity of all the muscles. This approach is not advised for extensive reconstructive procedures nor for restoration of anatomy in gross subluxation or dislocation of the hip joint. We have employed this technique since 1986 for selected cases for performing arthrotomy, synovectomy, joint clearance, and for excisional arthroplasty. We would recommend this approach only for limited procedures in cases where the anatomical position of bones is not grossly disturbed, and the joint does not have severe flexion-adduction deformity.

Begin the skin incision over the femoral head just lateral to the palpable femoral pulsations, carry it laterally, parallel to the flexor crease of the groin, up to a point lateral to the most prominent part of the greater trochanter. Dissect the skin and subcutaneous fatty tissue from the underlying fascia lata for 2–4 cm proximal and distal to the line of skin incision, now split the fascia lata vertically using finger or a blunt dissector. The split in the deep fascia is 8–10 cm long, centering on the hip joint. Retract laterally the lateral lip of fascia lata along with tensor fasciae latae. The medial lip is retracted medially along with the sartorius, the rectus femoris and the iliopsoas. The latter may require to be released from its attachments to the underlying capsule of the hip joint. Use of long bone levers along the upper and lower borders of the femoral neck (still covered with the capsule) to retract the muscles in respective directions, offers an adequate view of the entire anterior surface of the capsule of the hip joint. The capsule is cut in the usual manner, bone levers or skids are then inserted between the femoral neck and the capsule. One can now perform synovectomy, joint debridement or excision arthroplasty.

In case of difficulty of exposure, the lateral end of skin incision may be extended proximally or distally, the tensor fasciae latae and fascia lata cut transversely in the distal third of tensor fasciae latae, and the rectus femoris detached from its origin. However, all this is rarely necessary if we have not selected patients with gross displacements and gross deformities of flexion-adduction and internal rotation for this approach. In a usual case, the wound is closed only by stitching the skin. As no muscles are reflected or cut, postoperative mobilization of the hip joint is remarkably painless and easy.

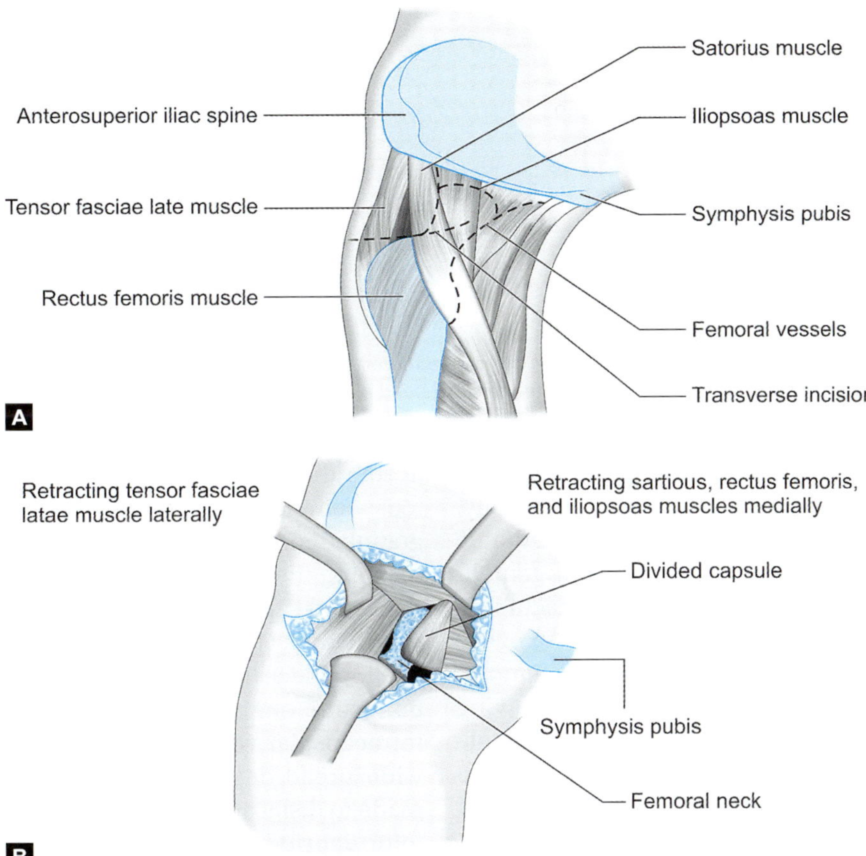

Figs. 8.30A and B: Diagrammatic representation of modified anterior approach to the hip joint. No muscles are cut. The incision in the capsule can be made longitudinally, or in L or T-shaped fashion. The approach is adequate for moderate surgical procedures (arthrotomy, biopsy, synovectomy, debridement, excision arthroplasty) only where the anatomy is not grossly disturbed.

ALTERNATIVE APPROACHES

There are many other approaches to expose the hip joint (Campbell's Operative Orthopedics 1987) which may be rarely necessary in infective lesions. Sometimes, due to infection the femoral head (especially in children) may be sequestrated and lie posterior to the hip joint. Such a sequestrated head can be best removed by making a direct incision centering over the hip joint or over the palpable rounded femoral head. With the patient placed on the sound side with 30–45 degrees flexion of the diseased hip, the skin incision is made in the gluteal region parallel to the direction of fibers of gluteus maximus. Generally, the incision falls on a line from a point 4 cm distal and lateral to the posterosuperior iliac spine to the posterosuperior angle of the greater trochanter. Separate the fibers of gluteus maximus parallel to its own fibers. Relatively little bleeding occurs because the split is through the water-shed of superior gluteal artery (supplying the proximal half of gluteus maximus) and inferior gluteal artery (supplying the distal half). If needed for more extensive procedure, the skin and the insertion of gluteus maximus can be divided further in a longitudinal direction **(Fig. 8.31)** like the vertical limb of the Gibson's or Osborne's

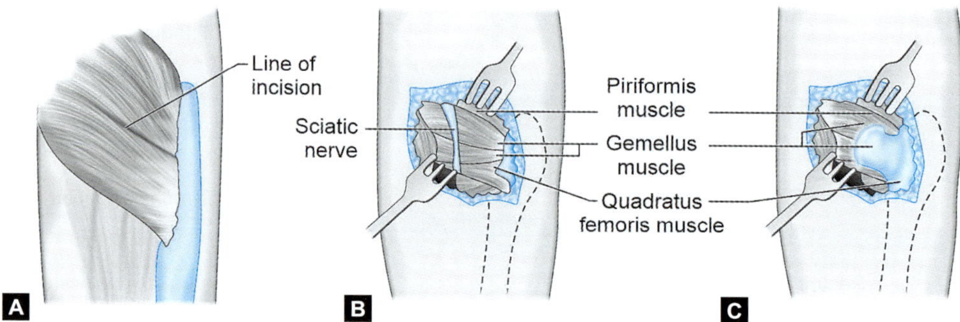

Figs. 8.31A to C: Diagrammatic representation of the conventional posterior approach. It is of special value if there is pathological posterior dislocation or the sequestrated femoral head is lying in the gluteal region.

or Moore's incisions (Campbell's Operative Orthopedics 1987). Rotate the thigh internally, identify and retract the sciatic nerve medially, detach the insertion of piriformis and gemelli muscles from the trochanteric crest, retract them medially and expose the posterior surface of the capsule of hip joint. The sequestrated femoral head generally lies under the muscles having extruded out of the destroyed posterior capsule of the hip joint. If needed, the capsule may be incised to expose the femoral head and neck and to explore the hip joint.

Synovectomy

Having incised the capsule and exposed the hip joint (by any approach) separate the hypertrophied synovium from the inner surface of the capsule and from the synovial reflections near the acetabular rim and on the femoral neck. While working from the inner surface of the capsule, the diseased and thickened capsule may be excised. The diseased synovium from the retinacular reflections on the femoral neck should be gently curetted away. Appropriate rotations of the hip joint permit adequate synovectomy from the deeper parts of the hip joint without deliberately dislocating the hip joint.

Joint Debridement or Joint Clearance

In addition to synovectomy, the destroyed areas in the femoral head and neck and in the acetabulum may require curettage. If there are loosened pieces of articular cartilage, sequestra, granulation tissue and loose bodies/debris within the joint, these should be removed. The diseased thickened capsule may also require to be excised from within. One should refrain from deliberately peeling the articular cartilage off the underlying bone, and one should preserve the retinacular/intracapsular vessels at all cost. Unless there is widespread destruction no attempt should be made to dislocate the hip joint. Synovectomy and joint debridement can be satisfactorily carried out without dislocating the hip joint. Internal and external rotations provide access to the deeper parts of the joint cavity. The synovectomy at best is a subtotal one but nevertheless is adequate.

Possible complications of synovectomy and debridement include avascular necrosis of femoral head, slippage of the proximal femoral epiphysis in children, and fracture of the femoral neck or acetabulum. If curettage of an extra-articular lesion (in the acetabulum, femoral neck, greater trochanter) is required in a patient where the hip joint is not involved, the surgical evacuation should be attempted without arthrotomy.

Arthrodesis

Success of chemotherapy treatment in tuberculous and infectious diseases of the hip joint has almost eliminated the absolute indications for surgical fusion of the hip joint.

Many authors have expressed concern about the effect of arthrodesis of the hip joint on early development of degenerative osteoarthrosis in the lumbosacral spine, ipsilateral knee, and contralateral hip. Compensation **(Figs. 8.3 and 8.4)** for a fused hip involves increased rotation of the pelvis (during sitting and walking), increased flexion of the ipsilateral knee during its stance phase and compensatory ligamentous laxity of the ipsilateral knee (in patients of long-standing).

As far as possible surgical fusion for a hip disease should be offered only for patients whose growth potential of the proximal femur has been completed (>18 years of age). The activities that get maximally limited after fusion of the hip joint are bending, sitting on floor, cross-legged sitting, squatting, kneeling, sports, sexual mechanics (in women), and bicycling. Most of the patients in higher socio-economic strata are able to manage almost normal activities. However, persons from economically weaker strata find it extremely difficult to earn their daily wages, to carry on activities of daily life in their social milieu and to commute by public transport. If a choice was given to the patient between a fused hip and a painless mobile hip, no patient would accept a fused hip. We started offering mobile hip joints to patients suffering from tuberculous arthritis of the hip joint in 1972. Many young adults, especially ladies, who had earlier managed with soundly fused hip joint for 5 to 10 years, reported back to the hospital and asked for a mobile hip joint.

Fusion of the hip joint can be obtained by intra-articular or extra-articular, or by a combined intra-cum extra-articular (pan-articular) arthrodesis. In the presence of adduction deformity ischio-femoral and in the presence of abduction deformity ilio-femoral extra-articular fusions are technically easy to perform **(Figs. 8.32 and 8.33)**. During these procedures, extra-articular upper femoral corrective osteotomy can also be performed to bring the limb into a functional position. In cases where the patient reports with healed disease with a painless fused hip joint in unacceptable deformity, all that is needed to obtain sound fusion is an upper femoral corrective osteotomy. The ideal site for corrective osteotomy is as near the deformed joint as practicable. The best position for fusion of the hip joint is 1–30 degrees of flexion (depending upon age), no abduction or adduction (in adults), and 5–10 degrees of external rotation.

If tuberculous disease in the hip is active, or the joint has a painful fibrous ankylosis, or one requires to obtain the diseased tissue to be sure of the underlying pathology, or whenever in doubt

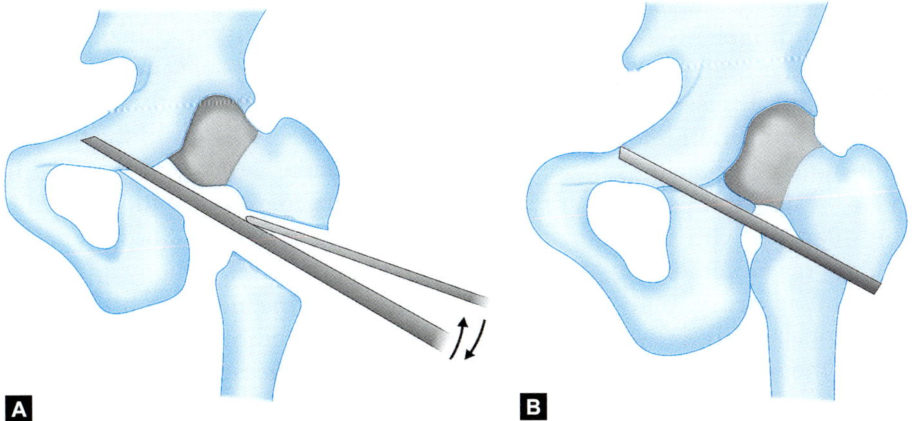

Figs. 8.32A and B: Diagrammatic representation of Brittain's extra-articular operation for tuberculous disease of the hip joint. The upper femoral osteotomy corrected any fixed deformity of the hip joint. The free-bone-graft was fitted between the osteotomy and a slot in the ischium.

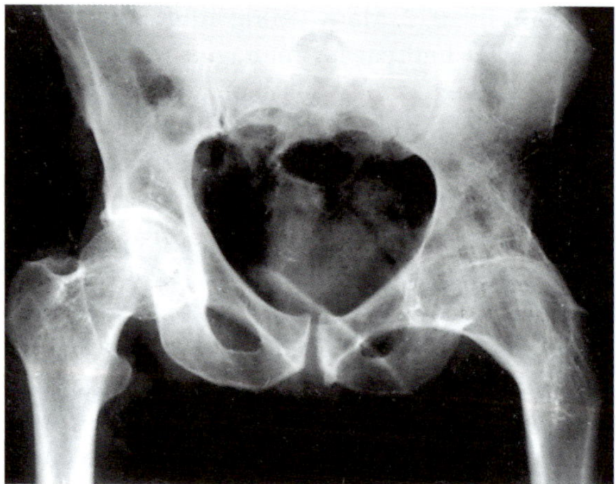

Fig. 8.33: X-ray of surgically performed arthrodesis of left hip joint for tuberculous arthritis at the age of 20 years in 1959. The patient managed normal activities for nearly 40 years. In the year 2000, he presented with moderate pain in the lower back. Sequel of iliofemoral arthrodesis.

about the pathology, it is wise to perform an intra-articular arthrodesis. Intra-articular procedure permits exploration of the joint, excision of the diseased tissues, curettage of the juxta-articular infected cavities, and if needed supplementation with bone grafts to obtain fusion.

Operative Technique of Intra-articular Arthrodesis

For intra-articular arthrodesis approach the hip joint, through the standard antero-lateral incision or any familiar approach. Grossly diseased capsule and synovium are removed. Carefully dislocate the hip joint. Excise the cartilage and subchondral bone from the femoral head and acetabulum down to the cancellous bone. Curet any juxta-articular cavities; the large ones should preferably be filled up with cancellous bone grafts. Repose the rawed femoral head into the freshened acetabular cavity, place cancellous bone grafts (from iliac crest) all around the joint line, approximate the remaining capsule and soft tissues over the site of fusion, hold the hip joint in the best functional position, insert 2 or 3 long Steinmann's pins from the base of the greater trochanter through the femoral neck and head going into the acetabulum. Now close the wound in layers over a suction drain, and apply a single hip spica.

After 6–8 weeks, Steinmann's pins (whose ends may be left out of the skin) and stitches are removed, and a well moulded single hip spica in the desired position is given. Immobilization and weight bearing in the single hip spica is continued for 4–6 months until there is radiological evidence of bone fusion. The hip joint is further protected with crutches for one year, after removal of the plaster.

With availability of options for total hip replacement or excisional arthroplasty, currently arthrodesis is not the preferred option by the patients, this has rendered many complex (Abbot-Lucas 1954) and extra-articular (Brittan 1952) arthrodesis operations **(Fig. 8.32)** for historical education.

Excision Arthroplasty of Hip Joint

Girdlestone (1950) described excision of the femoral head, neck, proximal part of trochanter and the acetabular rim for chronic deep seated infections of hip joint. He advised loose packing of the raw area (left after excision) by petroleum gauze, and emphasized postoperative prevention of proximal displacement of femur by application of plaster cast or by traction.

We expose the hip joint through anterolateral or anterior transverse incision. After liberal incision of the capsule and ligaments, an attempt is made to dislocate the hip joint anteriorly which gives a full view of the diseased area and juxta-articular destroyed areas. It is, however, not mandatory to dislocate the head, this maneuver may be dangerous in fibrous ankylosis of long-standing. In cases of bony ankylosis, and when dislocation was not possible divide the femoral head and acetabular rim obliquely flush with the outer surface of the ileum, divide the femoral neck at its base a little proximal and parallel to the intertrochanteric line. Now remove the femoral head and neck piecemeal, and ensure that an adequate gap (2–4 cm) has been created between the trochanteric line and the pelvis, and no bone is left, especially in the depth. Where anterior dislocation of the hip was possible it allows easy excision of femoral head and neck. The line of bone section was kept parallel to and a little proximal to the intertrochanteric line. One can err to make the bone section a little more horizontal, but it is unwise to err to make it more vertical.

We have been doing this operation since 1972, when due to the efficacy of modern antitubercular drugs we were convinced that the chance of recrudescence of tuberculous infection is no more after excision arthroplasty than in an unsoundly ankylosed hip. On completion of the operation, it was ensured that there was no projecting bone proximally and distally. The raw surfaces of the bones were cauterized. No deliberate attempt was made to interpose soft tissues between the pelvis and the femur. Antibiotics were instilled locally and the wound closed in layers on low suction drainage. Skeletal traction was applied as a rule through the upper part of tibia.

Postoperatively traction in 30–50 degrees of abduction was maintained for 2–3 months. The patient **(Fig. 8.35)** was encouraged to sit soon after the operation, and repetitive active assisted movements of the hip and knee were started during the first week. During the period of traction, active and assisted physiotherapy helped to develop good muscle power, maximal range of hip movements, and encouraged the patients to place the operated limb in the tailor's position and squatting posture. After 3 months of operation, the patients were encouraged to walk using a walker or crutches. The crutches were usually discarded 6–9 months after the operation and the patient was advised to use a walking stick generally in the contralateral hand.

The objective in the use of traction and bracing are basically threefold. If the cut upper end of femur and the outer surface of acetabulum are held apart from one another, an adequate layer of fibrous tissue is more likely to form over both, thereby providing more ideal surfaces for a pseudarthrosis. The shortening can be minimized if the limb is held as far distally as possible during the maturation and contracture of the soft tissues around the operated hip joint. The mean loss of length by this technique is 1.5 cm. For optimum results, regimen of postoperative care is essential **(Figs. 8.35 and 8.36)**.

Some degree of shortening and instability are virtually unavoidable. The pain-free satisfactory movement does not generally deteriorate with passage of time. The walking and standing tolerance vary from patient to patient. Some degree of telescoping of the limb and a tendency toward external rotation are not uncommon. Many a times the degree of function is pleasantly/surprisingly good **(Fig. 8.28)**.

Instability in Excision Arthroplasty: Biological Options

Excision arthroplasty may rarely leave behind a very unstable hip joint. If the assessment, one year after operation, reveals a very unstable hip joint, supplementary operations are suggested, especially for the young patients. Where the disease has healed with minimal fibrosis and scarring of the capsule and soft tissues, the surgeon can anticipate gross instability. In such cases, hip stabilization procedures may be done concurrently or 3–6 months after the excisional operation. After applying skeletal traction for about 3 weeks, a pelvic support osteotomy at the level of ischeal tuberosity (Milch-Bacheolar type) may be done. One may, in addition, provide a shelf at the upper margin of the acetabulum to minimize upward excursion of the femur on weight bearing. One can combine both the procedures in younger patients **(Figs. 8.34 to 8.38)**. As both these procedures are extra-capsular, the movements of the hip are not lost. Pelvic support osteotomy, if done in a growing age, may remodel with decrease of the angle at osteotomy. A well incorporated shelf in fact hypertrophies according to the functional needs of the hip joint. Between 1972 and 1993, we performed pelvic support

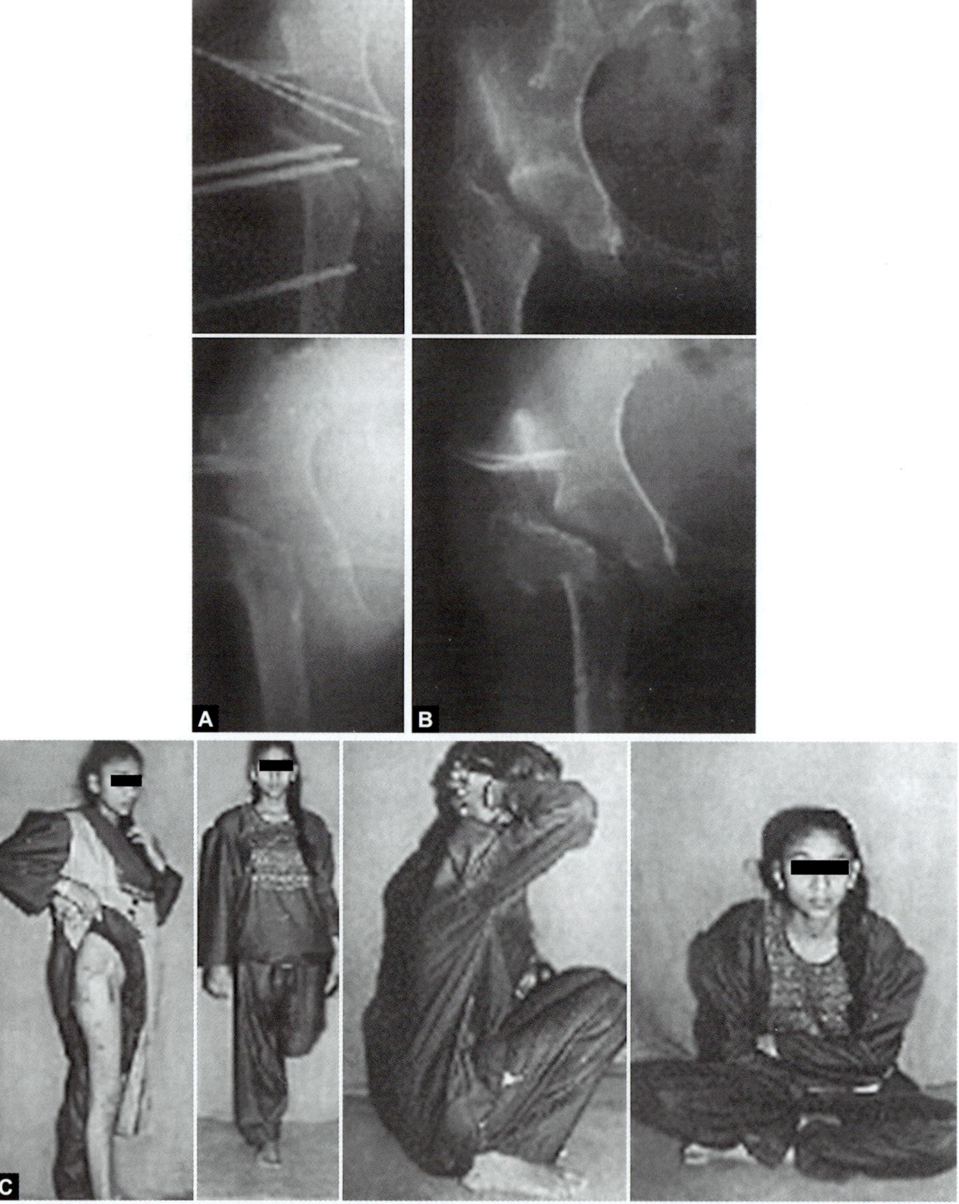

Figs. 8.34A to C: (A) Excisional arthroplasty + pelvis support + shelf operation soon after the procedure, (B) A follow up one year later, (C) Postoperative clinical function the first picture shows multiple scarring around the hip joint. After excisional arthroplasty + shelf operation, note the stability provided along with mobility in a young girl.

osteotomy in 16 patients, supra-acetabular shelf in 7, and the combined procedure in 5 patients for unacceptable instability in young patients who had previous excisional arthroplasty for tuberculous or nontuberculous hip infection. The best results were obtained by the procedure when pelvic support osteotomy was combined with the shelf formation **(Fig. 8.38)**. An interesting technique of interposition arthroplasty employing multilayered amniotic

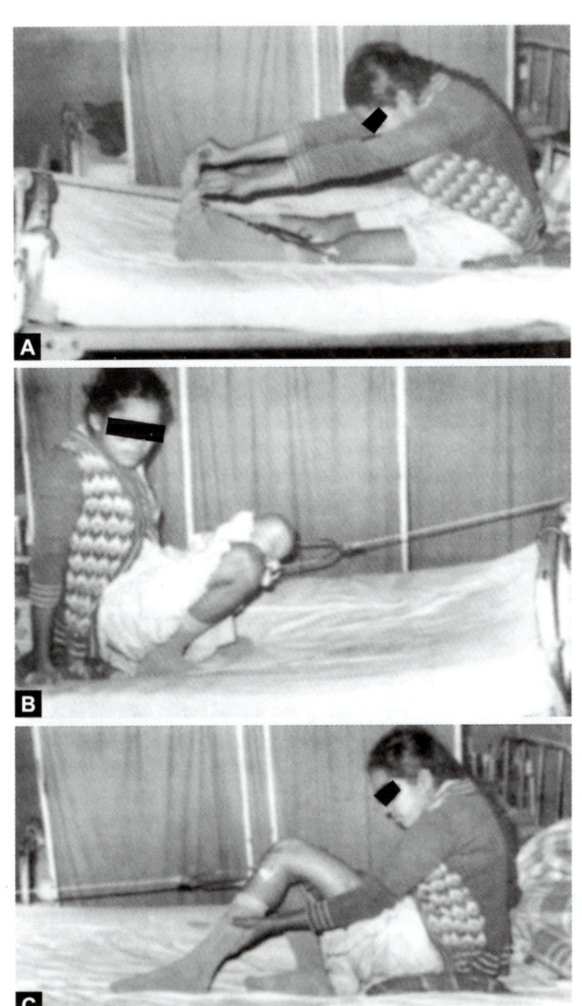

Figs. 8.35A to C: Postoperative traction and exercises done as a routine after excision-arthroplasty of hip joint. Majority of the patients are able to do flexion at hip (A), hip plus knee flexion (B), and external rotation in flexed position (C) without much discomfort by 4th postoperative week.

membrane was reported by Vishwakarma et al. (1986), 25 out of 28 patients were observed by them to have good range of painless movements.

Replacement Arthroplasty

The treatment of tuberculous arthritis of hip joint by replacement arthroplasty is being debated and performed at present in highly selected cases (Kim et al. 1979, 1986, 1987, Harding et al. 1977,

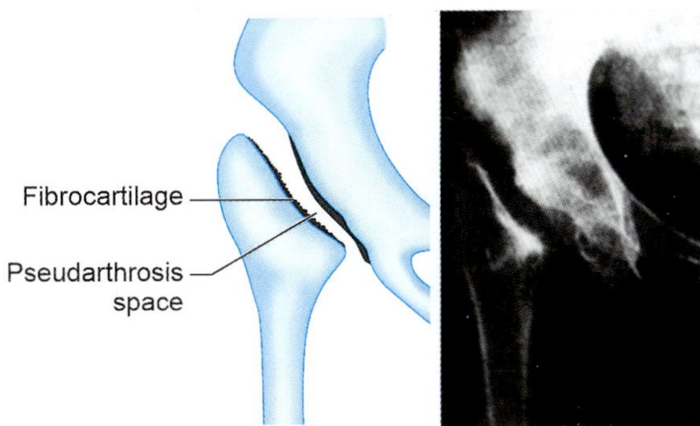

Fig. 8.36: Note the adaptation of the shape of bones at the site of pseudarthrosis. The gap is filled up with newly formed fibrocartilage.

Johnson et al. 1979, Mc Cullough 1977, Hecht et al. 1983, Caparros et al. 1999). Most of the authors suggest this operation at least 3–10 years after the last evidence of active infection or drainage, and majority advise coverage by concomitant antituberculous therapy. However, despite these precautions reactivation of infection after the replacement arthroplasty has been recorded in 10–30% of cases from earlier reports. We feel a minimum of 2–3 years of healed status of infection must be ensured before consideration for joint replacement, and all such procedures must be done under anti-TB drugs umbrella for 3–5 months.

Kim et al. (1988) analyzed the results of 60 patients followed-up for 8–13 years. While operating 8 patients were detected to have active disease in the hip. They stated that the arthroplasty did not result in impressive improvement in hip function but the mobility in general was considerably improved. Santavirta et al. (1988) operated on 14 cases of healed tuberculous arthritis of hip about 43 years after the onset of disease. According to Mayo hip grading at an average follow-up of 8 years, the grading was excellent or good in 8, fair in 3 and poor in 3. None showed reactivation of tuberculosis. Kim et al. (2013) based upon an extensive review suggested use of extensive debridement and postoperative antitubercular medications for 6–15 months. Broad consensus at present is to offer replacement

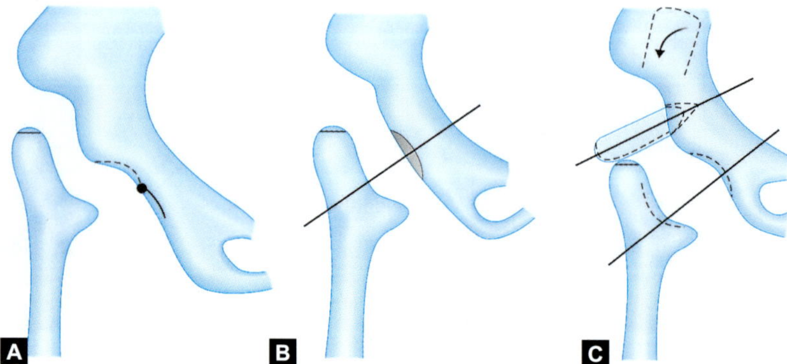

Figs. 8.37A to C: An outline of the pedicled-shelf operation for very unstable hip joint in young patients, (A) Follow-up of excisional arthroplasty, (B) Transfixation of greater trochanter in pulled-down position, (C) Full thickness of iliac bone still covered with gluteus medius muscle has been turned and shifted downwards. The pedicled graft has been fixed in a slot in the supra-acetabular area.

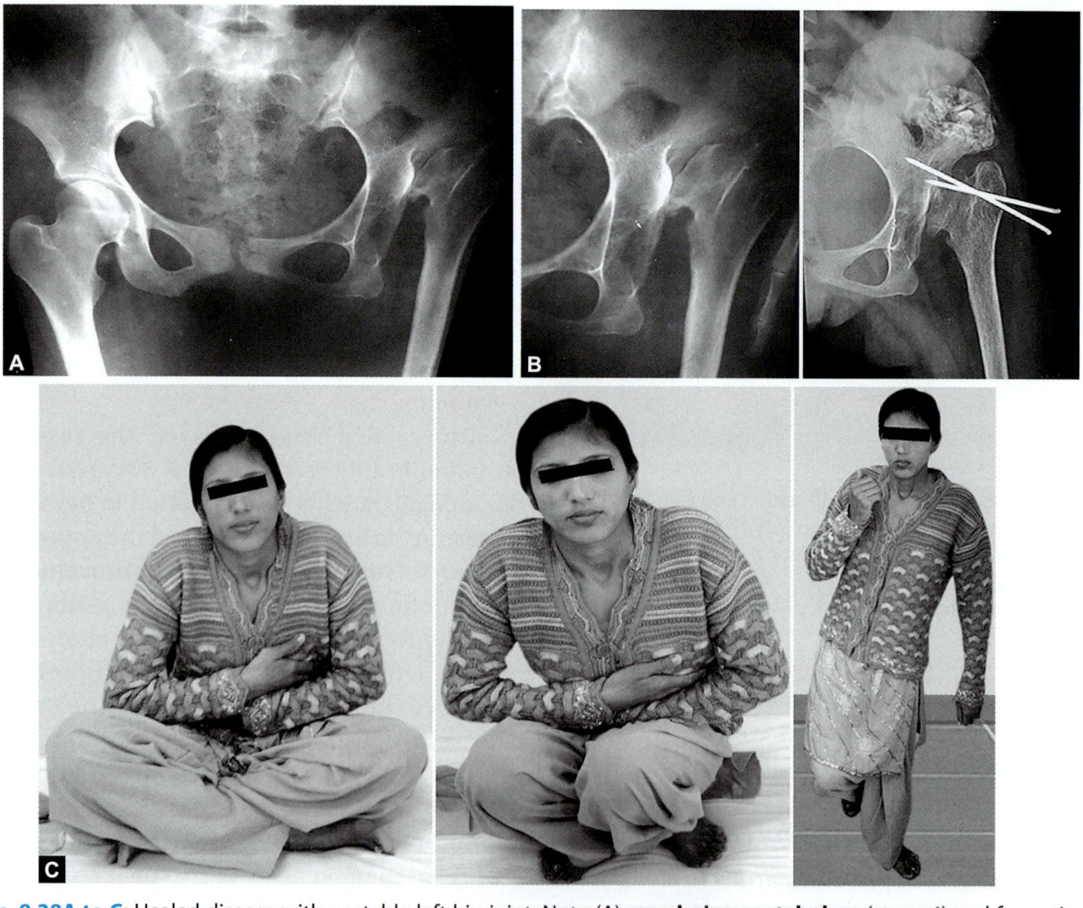

Figs. 8.38A to C: Healed disease with unstable left hip joint. Note (A) **wandering acetabulum** (stage 4) and formation of a **secondary acetabulum** in a young girl of 20 years. (B) Stability of hip was improved by creating a supra-acetabular shelf (tectoplasy). (C) Note the clinical function, she was able to stand on the operated limb with positive Trendelenburg. About 10 years later she reported with active tuberculosis in left wrist.

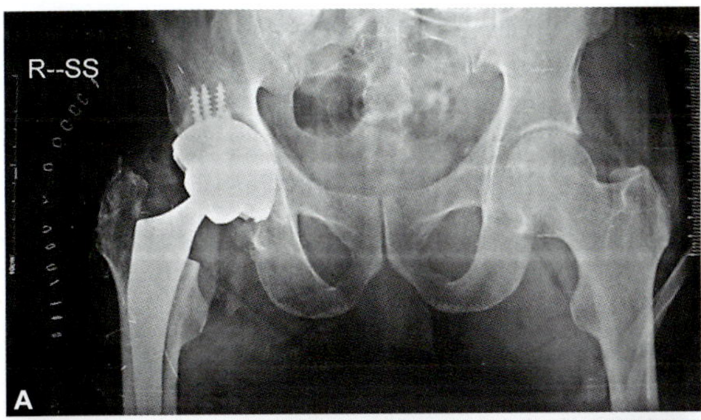

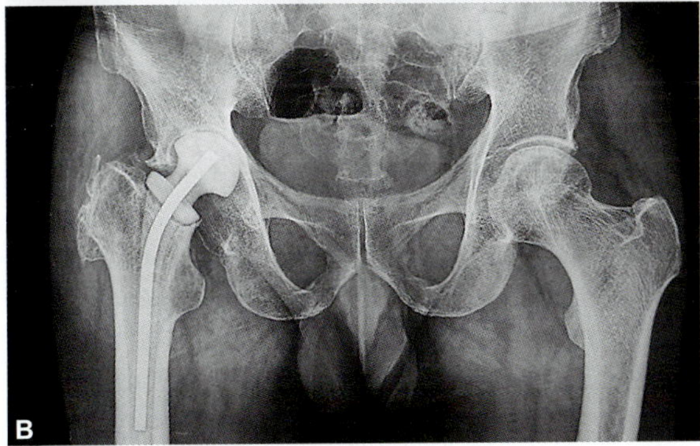

Figs. 8.39A and B: Hip replacement in active tuberculous infection resulted in uncontrolled infection (A). The implant had to be removed, a "spacer" was implanted, anti-TB multidrug therapy was continued for a further period of one year (B) before re-operation.

arthroplasty for patients whose infection in the joint or any other part of body has remained healed for more than 2–3 years after stopping the antituberculous drugs **(Fig. 8.39)**.

RELEVANT SURGICAL ANATOMY OF THE HIP JOINT

The hip joint is a ball and socket type of synovial joint. Fibrocartilaginous labrum attached to the acetabulum makes the socket deeper, however, considerable part of the articular surface of the spherical femoral head remains uncovered. The opening of the acetabulum faces laterally, downwards (about 30 degrees), and forwards (about 30 degrees). Consequently, the femoral neck points medially, upwards and anteriorly. The forward inclination or the angle of anteversion in an adult is 10–30 degrees. The neck-shaft angle is 125 degrees. A neck-shaft angle of <125 degrees is referred to as coxa vara and the angle >125 degrees (i.e., more vertical neck) is called coxa valga. Coxa vara causes limitation of abduction and internal rotation due to mechanical reasons, and due to the reduction of the leverage of abductor muscles (predominantly gluteus medius), the Trendelenburg lurch and sign is present.

During standing and walking, the femoral neck acts as a cantilever. The line of body weight passes medial to the hip joint and is balanced laterally by the lateral pelvifemoral abductor muscles (especially the gluteus medius). The combination of body weight, leverage effect and muscle action makes a great deal of resultant forces transmitted through the hip joint. It is about five times the body weight when walking slowly and much more when running or jumping. While standing on one lower limb, its abductor muscles contract causing the pelvis to tilt downwards on the weight bearing side, and thus balancing the body. Pain at the site of fulcrum (femoral head-acetabulum interface) due to active disease, inflammation or degenerative osteoarthrosis, or change in its location due to wandering acetabulum or dislocation, break or deformation of the lever (the femoral neck and head), weakness of abductor muscles or approximation of the distance between its origin and insertion would result in the failure of this "abductor mechanism" and present as a positive Trendelenburg lurch or sign. This sign, however, becomes unreliable and undemonstrable in the absence of free abduction and adduction movements at the hip joint.

The Femoral Head Receives its Arterial Blood Supply from Three Sources

1. **Intraosseous vessels** running up the neck, which may be damaged by disruption of femoral neck or by a destructive lesion located therein.
2. **Vessels in the retinacula** reflected from the joint capsule onto the neck. These vessels are the upward continuation of the vascular anastomosis that develops around

the trochanteric region. These are broadly arranged as "lateral epiphyseal", "superior metaphyseal" and "inferior metaphyseal". Majority of the retinacular vessels are arranged along the posterior surface of the femoral neck; it may, therefore, be wise to cut through the anterior retinaculum (along the long axis of femoral neck) when the surgeon is impelled to expose the neck of femur. These vessels may be damaged by dislocation of joint, disruption of femoral neck or by pressure of a tense intracapsular effusion.

3. **Vessels in the ligamentum teres**, which are underdeveloped in the early years of life, and even later convey only a meager blood supply. At all ages avascular necrosis is a potential hazard. The femoral head and neck are richly supplied by the venous sinusoids. A rise in intraosseous pressure causes pain because sinusoids are richly supplied by sensory fibers.

The capsule of the hip joint is attached circumferentially around the labrum acetabulare and transverse ligament, whence it passes laterally to be attached to the neck of femur. In front, it is attached to the intertrochanteric line, but posteriorly the attachment is about one cm proximal to the trochanteric crest. Thus, the whole of the anterior half of the femoral neck and the proximal part of its posterior half is intracapsular. From the distal attachment of the capsule the fibers are reflected back (as the retinacular fibers) along the femoral neck, intimately blended with the periosteum, up to the articular margin of the femoral head. The retinacular fibers hold down the nutrient arteries that pass upwards, chiefly from the trochanteric anastomosis, along the neck of the femur to supply the major part of femoral head.

The fibrous capsule is strengthened by three ligaments which spiral around the long axis of femoral neck. According to the point of origin, the ligaments are named as:

1. Iliofemoral ligament (Y-shaped ligament of Bigelow) arising as the stem of the "Y" from the anterior inferior iliac spine and the adjacent superior rim of acetabulum.
2. Pubofemoral ligament arising from iliopubic eminence.
3. Ischiofemoral ligament the weakest of the three ligaments arising from the postero-inferior margin of the acetabulum.

If the hip is flexed and rotated externally so as to attain the fetal position, the fibers of these ligaments are "unwound" and relaxed and parallel to the femoral neck. The opposite movement of extension and internal rotation increases the twist of the ligamentous fibers. A perforation occasionally exists in the anterior capsule between the iliofemoral and pubofemoral ligaments. The perforation permits communication (for cold abscess) between the synovial cavity and the iliac bursa **(Fig 8.40)**. The weakest (thinnest) part of the hip joint capsule is situated posteriorly, and the femoral head is most vulnerable to posterior dislocation in flexion-adduction position of the hip joint.

The synovial membrane like all synovial joints, lines the inner surface of whole of the capsule, and is reflected proximally along the reflection of the capsule investing the retinacular fibers up to the articular margin of the femoral head. The Haversion fat pad (filling the

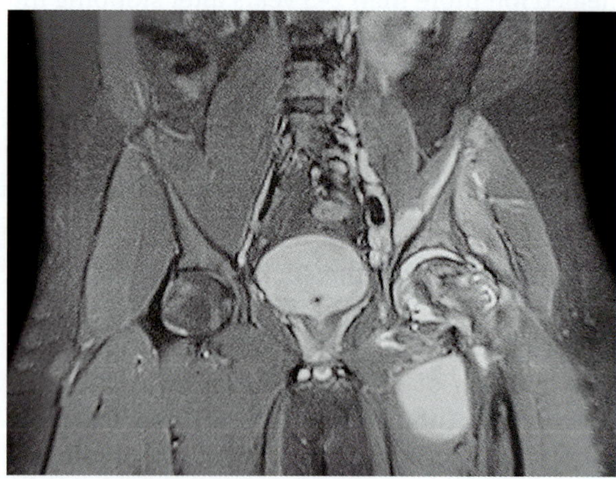

Fig. 8.40: MRI-T2: TB-Left Hip-Transcapsular downwords migration of cold abscess.

nonarticular depression of the acetabulum) and the ligamentum teres are likewise invested in a sleeve of synovial membrane that is attached to the articular margins of the acetabular fossa and of the fovea on the femoral head.

Immediate Relations of the Hip Joint

Anteriorly, the iliac bursa lies over the capsule and extends upwards into the iliac fossa beneath the iliacus muscle. The psoas major tendon and iliacus muscle separate the capsule from the femoral vessels and femoral nerve. Superiorly, there is a cellular space between the capsule and the overhanging gluteus minimus and piriformis muscles. Inferiorly, the obturator externus muscle spirals back around the femoral neck. Posteriorly, the obturator internus and gemelli separate the sciatic nerve from the capsule. Medially, the thin acetabular fossa forms part of the lateral wall of the pelvis.

Tuberculosis of the Knee Joint

The knee joint is the largest joint in the body having the largest intra-articular space. It is the third common site for osteoarticular tuberculosis and accounts for nearly 10% of all skeletal tuberculous lesions.

PATHOLOGY

The initial focus occurring by hematogenous dissemination may start in the synovium, or in the subchondral bone (of distal femur, proximal tibia or patella), or as a juxta-articular osseous focus. The synovial lesion may for many months remain purely as tubercular synovitis. The synovial membrane gets congested, edematous and studded with tubercles. The naked eye examination reveals a pinkish-blue or pinkish-gray appearance. The synovial lining which is normally a single cell layer in thickness becomes hypertrophied and thickened with granulation tissue. The joint fluid in the initial stages is increased, serous, opalescent, turbid, yellowish and may contain fibrinous flakes. **In advanced stage** of the disease, tuberculous process becomes osteoarticular. The tuberculous granulation tissue like the pannus erodes the articular margins, destroys the bones, and involves the cruciate ligaments, periarticular tissues, capsule and ligaments. As a rule, osseous erosion by the pannus starts at the site of synovial reflections, i.e., at the margins of the articular cartilage, and the capsular attachments. The pannus may erode the margins of the articular cartilage, grow between the articular cartilage and the subchondral bone, thus detaching the cartilage from the bone, and may grow over the articular cartilage as a sheet of granulation tissue **(Figs. 9.14 and 9.15)**. Flakes of articular cartilage may sequestrate and lie free in the joint cavities. Nutrition of the articular cartilage is thus interfered. It loses its smooth glistening appearance, there may be fibrillation of its surface, it becomes roughened, pitted and softened, or erosion of the cartilage exposes the subchondral bone like pock-marks.

In cases which start as osseous lesions there may be tuberculous abscess in the subchondral bone, epiphyseal bone, or in the metaphyseal region usually in children **(Fig. 9.1)** leading to various degree of destruction of bone. Abscesses in the epiphyses and metaphyses may sometimes be seen traversing the epiphyseal cartilage plate giving an appearance of a lesion sitting astride the physis **(Fig. 9.1)** The initial tubercular focus may start in the metaphysis in children or the juxta-articular bone in adults.

As the disease advances, large areas at pressure points show osseous destruction, and the whole joint is filled/obliterated with granulation/fibrous tissue, capsular apparatus and ligaments are disrupted and the joint gets a **triple dislocation (triple deformity)**, i.e., flexion of joint, posterior subluxation, lateral subluxation and lateral rotation, and abduction of **upper end of tibia (Figs. 9.2 to 9.4)**.

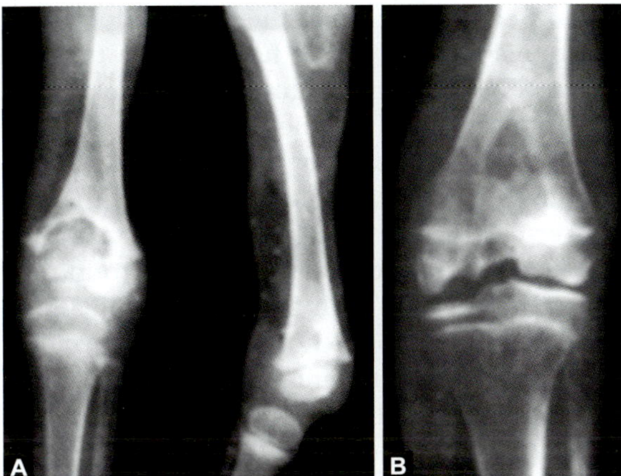

Figs. 9.1A and B: Tuberculosis of the distal end of femur, (A) which has spread to the knee joint. There is a classical tuberculous cavity sitting astride the epiphyseal cartilage plate of femur, the cavity contains a few feathery sequestra. X-ray (B) of the same patient 11 years after treatment by drugs, traction and repetitive knee exercises. The patient retained the healed status of the disease and full range of painless mobility with excellent stability till his last follow-up.

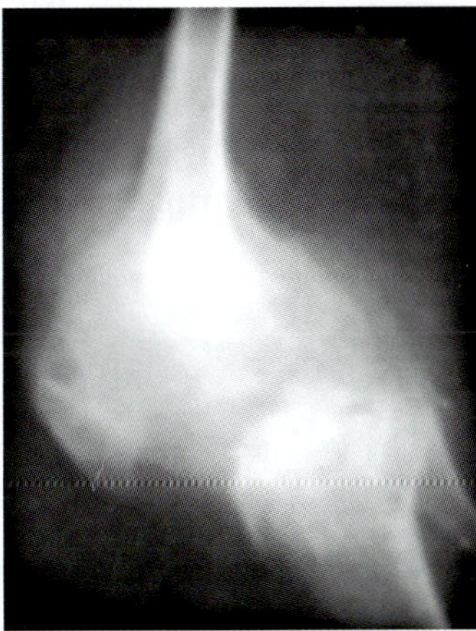

Fig. 9.2: Advanced (Stage IV) active tubercular arthritis of knee with triple deformity. Note soft tissue swelling, flexion deformity and posterior subluxation (of tibia), diminished joint space, fuzzy joint margins, cloudy appearance of bones, and lytic areas in patella.

CLINICAL FEATURES

The onset and course is insidious with usual systemic and local features of tuberculous disease. The knee shows swelling, filling up all

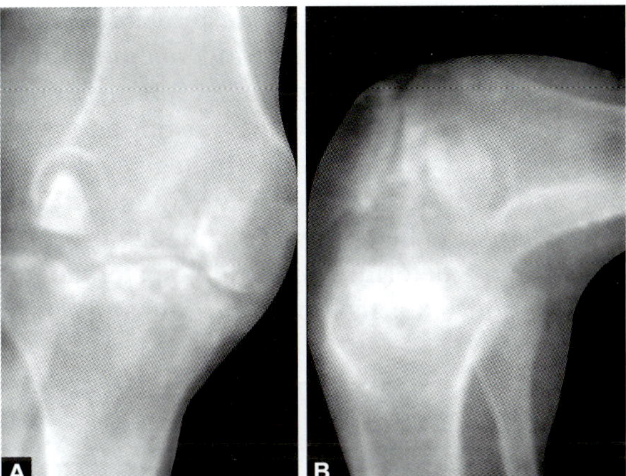

Figs. 9.3A and B: Advanced tubercular arthritis (Stage IV) of the knee joint with triple displacement (i.e., lateral and posterior subluxation and lateral rotation of tibia). Note gross diminution of the joint space, irregularity of articular margins and a coke-like sequestrum contained in a cavity in the lateral femoral condyle. There are destructive kissing lesions in the lateral and medial compartments of the joint. These are the X-rays done one year after the treatment, therefore, the joint margins are quite sharp. The joint aspirate had grown mycobacteria. The patient was a physician, he refused to get an arthrodesis, however, by antitubercular drugs and functional treatment he obtained a healed status with painless range of movements from 10 to 90 degrees. With an above the knee orthosis he continued his normal activities for 15 years when he died of unrelated causes.

parapatellar fossae appreciated earliest in medial parapatellar fossa, suprapatellar pouch, and even popliteal fossa **(Figs. 7.2 and 7.3)**. The swelling is warm, patellar tap is present if the swelling is predominantly due to the synovial effusion, the thickened synovium gives a boggy (doughy or semielastic) feel and can be rolled between the fingers and the underlying femur. It is best palpated on the medial side of knee because vastus medialis remains muscular up to its insertion to patella and gets waisted early. Muscles on lateral side are aponeurotic and these are covered by thick iliotibial band. The skin may be stretched and blanched giving the appearance of a white swelling (tumor alba), and may be edematous. Tenderness to pressure is most marked at the synovial reflections and along the joint line. In the synovial disease, for a long time there may be only terminal restriction of movements **(Fig. 7.3)**.

When arthritis has set in, the movements are grossly restricted, painful and accompanied by muscle spasm (particularly of hamstrings). Quadriceps muscles show gross wasting and there is regional lymphadenopathy. In neglected cases due to the spasm and contracture of hamstrings particularly the biceps femoris, the leg (tibia) is pulled into a deformity of flexion, posterolateral subluxation, external rotation and abduction **(Figs. 9.2 to 9.4)**. Once the flexion deformity is established, the tensor fasciae latae through iliotibial band further exantuates the deformity. Posterior capsule of the knee joint gets contracted in cases of long-standing. Complications from prolonged immobilization employing up to groin plaster-cast or hip spica for one year or more, included premature fusion of physes around the knee ("frame knee") on the affected side. Such complications should not occur now because currently articular tuberculosis is best managed by functional treatment. In the growing child, transient limb lengthening due to chronic juxta-physeal hyperemia may be observed in some cases.

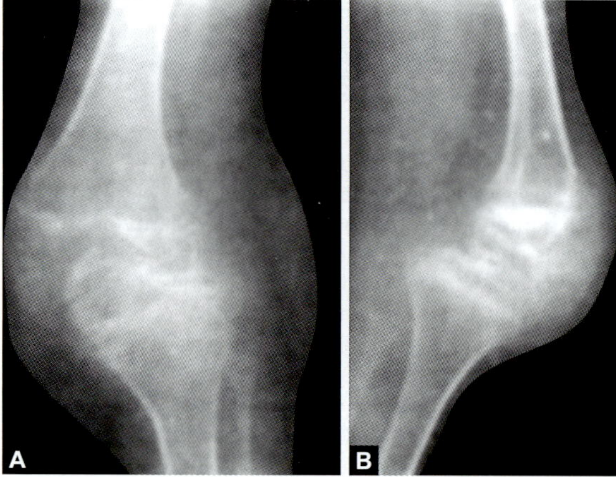

Figs. 9.4A and B: Typical radiological appearance in a child suffering from advanced tuberculous arthritis of the knee joint with "triple deformity". Note flexion of the knee, lateral subluxation and lateral rotation of tibia, and it's posterior subluxation.

Roentgenograms, like other joints, in the **synovial stage** show generalized osteoporosis, and increased soft tissue swelling caused by synovial effusion, thickened synovium and capsule. As **arthritis** sets in the x-rays reveal loss of definition of articular surfaces, marginal erosions, diminution of the joint space and destruction of the bones forming the joint **(Figs. 9.1 to 9.4)**. In **advanced stage** of arthritis, marked diminution of the articular space, gross destruction and deformation of bone ends, osteolytic cavities, tubercular sequestra and triple deformity may be seen **(Figs. 9.2 to 9.6)**.

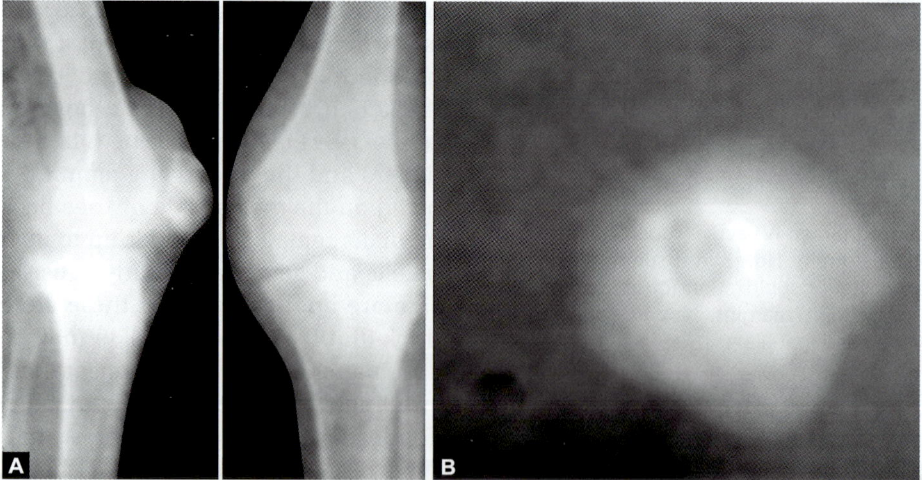

Figs. 9.5A and B: (A) Tubercular arthritis of knee joint. The patella was also involved with multiple cystic (lytic) lesions, (B) X-ray of another case of tuberculosis of patella showing a coke-like sequestrum contained in a cavity.

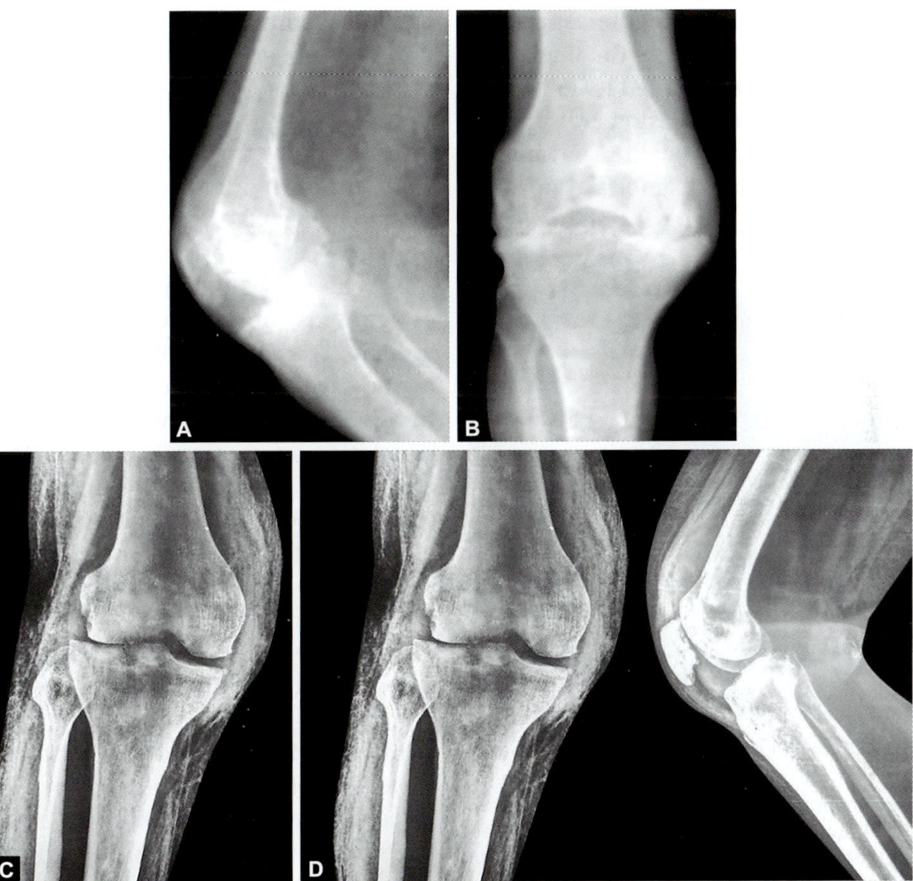

Figs. 9.6A to D: An advanced case of tubercular arthritis of knee joint managed by functional treatment and followed-up for 12 years. Despite irregular joint surfaces the patient maintained a stable, nearly painless and fairly mobile (5–50 degrees) knee joint. The X-rays show a healed status with incongruous congruity and degenerative changes. Stage II—early arthritis of knee showing diminished joint space especially in the lateral compartment and fuzzy joint margins. After 6 months of the "functional treatment", one can appreciate the remineralization of articular margins, she could regain a useful range of motion from full extension to 70 degrees of flexion.

DIFFERENTIAL DIAGNOSIS

Tuberculosis of the knee requires differentiation from other monoarticular affections, such as rheumatic arthritis (in children), chronic traumatic synovitis due to chronic internal derangement of knee (e.g., meniscal tears, loose bodies, osteochondritis dissecans, chondromalacia patellae, discoid semilunar cartilage, etc.), rheumatoid arthritis (in adults), subacute pyogenic arthritis/synovitis, hemarthrosis, dysenteric arthritis, villonodular synovitis, synovial chondromatosis, synovioma, hamartoma/lipoma arborisence, juxta-articular **(Fig. 9.7)** osseous lesion (leading to irritable joint), foreign-body granuloma, etc. Careful history, examination and investigations help arrive at correct diagnosis in majority. In doubtful cases, biopsy for histological, microbiological and PCR investigations is mandatory. In any persistent swelling of the knee of insidious origin, possibility of tuberculous pathology must be entertained, otherwise they would be treated as rheumatoid disease (Su 1985). Inadvertently given intra-articular steroids may flare up the inflammatory signs in a case of tuberculous joint. PCR for mycobacterial infection, fine-needle aspiration cytology and/or a needle biopsy of the thickened synovium **(Fig. 9.10)** or an enlarged lymph node, or a core biopsy of an osseous lesion are some of the semi-invasive outdoor procedures available these days to reach the final diagnosis. A positive PCR may be of immense value (in the presence of clinically inflamed knee), however, a negative PCR does not exclude tuberculous infection.

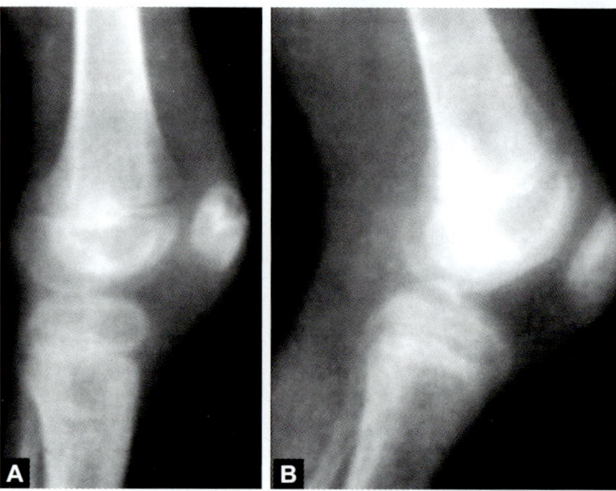

Figs. 9.7A and B: Tuberculosis of proximal pole of patella without involvement of the knee joint. By anti-tubercular drugs and the functional treatment, the destroyed area in the patella got reconstituted within one year, the knee joint did not get affected and the patient made a complete radiological and functional recovery.

PROGNOSIS

With modern methods of management the functional results are directly related to the extent of disease at the onset of antitubercular drugs (Lee et al. 1995, Hoffman et al. 2002). In the stage of synovitis, nonoperative (or operative when indicated) treatment often results in complete healing with an excellent range of movements. In advanced arthritis with subluxation, severe restriction of motion is inevitable, therefore, arthrodesis (in adults) in functioning position (5–10 degree of flexion) was one of the options of treatment (prior to 1987). In early or advanced arthritis (when a patient has been managed by functional treatment), a reasonable range of movements in the functional arc may be the outcome in many cases. The patient may continue to have a painless and a fairly mobile joint **(Figs. 9.1, 9.3 and 9.6)** for many years (5-12 years). Joint replacement in such cases should be deferred to when the joint becomes painful and starts losing movements due to early degenerative arthrosis **(Fig. 9.8)**.

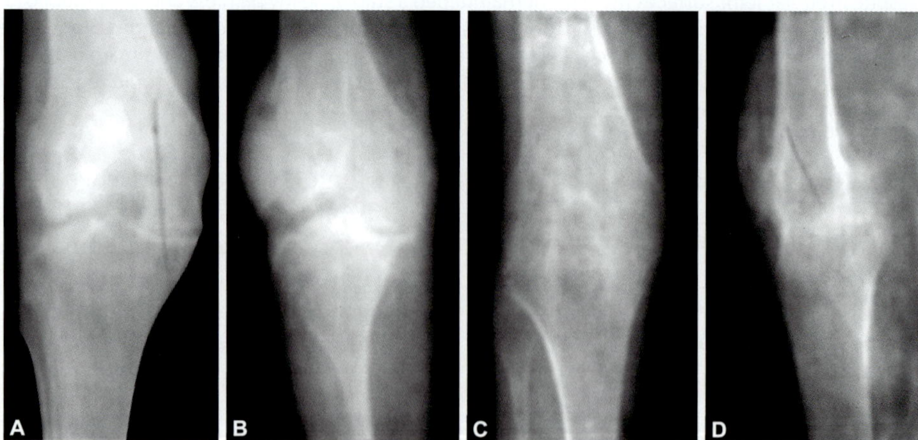

Figs. 9.8A to D: A Sarvodaya social worker presented with advanced tubercular arthritis of right knee. The disease healed (A and B) under the influence of antitubercular chemotherapy with a mobile joint (5–90 degrees). The pain on prolonged walking, however, interfered with his profession. After 2 years of waiting and trial he accepted Charnley's compression arthrodesis (C and D). He was treated 12 years ago for tuberculous infection of fifth toe, thereafter he remained free from any clinical disease. The fresh disease in the knee was probably precipitated because the patient now developed diabetes.

TREATMENT

Nonoperative treatment with antitubercular drugs is employed in tubercular synovitis and in children. Traction is applied to prevent (or correct) flexion and subluxation deformity, and to keep the joint surfaces distracted. In addition to the systemic drugs, the joint may be aspirated (when accompanied by excessive effusion), and streptomycin and isoniazid in solution may be instilled intra-articularly once weekly. With the quiescence of acute local signs, gentle active and assisted knee bending exercises should be carried out intermittently, for 5–10 minutes each half to one hourly. Usually, after 12 weeks of treatment the patient may be permitted ambulation with suitable orthosis and crutches. After 6–12 months of treatment, in cases with favorable response, the crutches or orthosis (caliper) may be discarded. Unprotected weight bearing is usually permitted 9–12 months after the start of treatment. Excellent results are obtained in majority of cases of synovial disease and early arthritis.

In children with arthritis, the deformity and subluxation is corrected/minimized by employing double traction **(Fig. 9.9)** or rarely by corrective plasters. Once the deformity is maximally corrected, the child can be mobilized wearing orthosis. Joint replacement (or arthrodesis) of the grossly destroyed knee in children should be deferred till the completion of growth potential of the distal femur and proximal tibia.

Operative Treatment

In synovial stage, if the disease is not responding favorably or the diagnosis is uncertain even after semi-invasive procedures **(Fig. 9.10)**, arthrotomy and synovectomy should be carried out. In early arthritis, in addition to synovectomy, removal of loose/rice bodies, debris, pannus, loose articular cartilage, and careful curettage of osseous juxta-articular foci should be carried out. Postoperatively, triple drug therapy, traction, intermittent active and assisted exercises, suitable brace ambulation should be continued.

In adults with advanced arthritis or in cases which resulted in painful fibrous ankylosis during the process of healing **(Fig. 9.8)**, the knee joint may be treated by arthrodesis. This operation provides a painless stable knee, prevents recrudescence, corrects deformity, and the patients can do long hours of standing and walking. Healing of the operative incision after synovectomy is seldom a problem. However, operations in cases of advanced arthritis often show wound dehiscence and sinus formation. This is because in advanced disease overlying capsule, subcutaneous tissue and skin may be

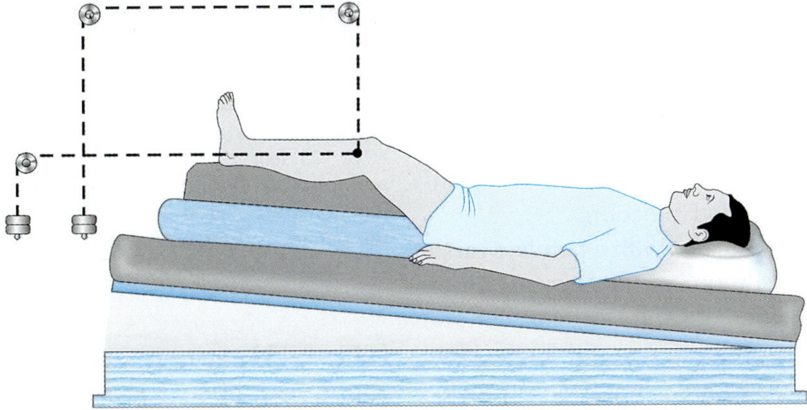

Fig. 9.9: Diagrammatic representation showing the application of "double traction" in cases of triple deformity of knee joint. Correction of such deformities **(Figs. 9.2 and 9.4)** by wedging plasters would increase the posterior displacement further.

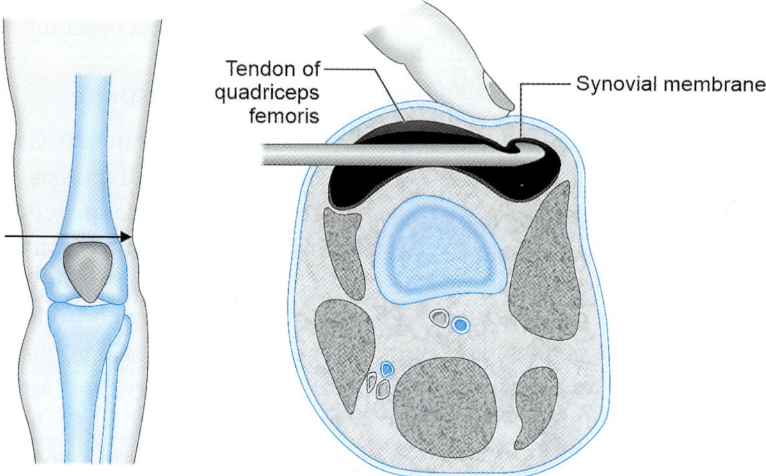

Fig. 9.10: A diagrammatic representation showing the technique of obtaining a piece of inflamed/thickened synovial membrane using a trocar with a catch at its terminal part or by a biopsy punch. The tissue is best obtained from the suprapatellar pouch.

scarred, and may also be affected by the disease process.

Charnley (1953) reluctantly recommended compression arthrodesis in tuberculous disease of the knee joint in children. He advised great caution in clearance of all destroyed areas and caseous debris, and during denuding of the articular cartilage for adequate exposure of the subchondral bone. Arthrodesis of knee joint, however, leads to significant disturbance of kinematics of locomotion over the years. Socially, it entails gross limitations of traveling by public transport and participation in many social functions. Arthroplasty operations are now considered more rational for healed status of advanced disease in adults. Arthrodesis may be considered as a rare indication for post-arthroplasty uncontrolled infection.

If the disease has healed with a painless range of movement (minimum of 20 degrees) in an unacceptable position, a supracondylar femoral osteotomy may be performed to put the residual range of motion of the knee in a position that is functional to the patient. It frequently results in a mobile joint that is useful for another 10–15 years **(Fig. 9.11)**. Osteotomy is also occasionally appropriate where a varus or valgus deformity is associated with relative sparing of one side of the joint and a useful range of movement.

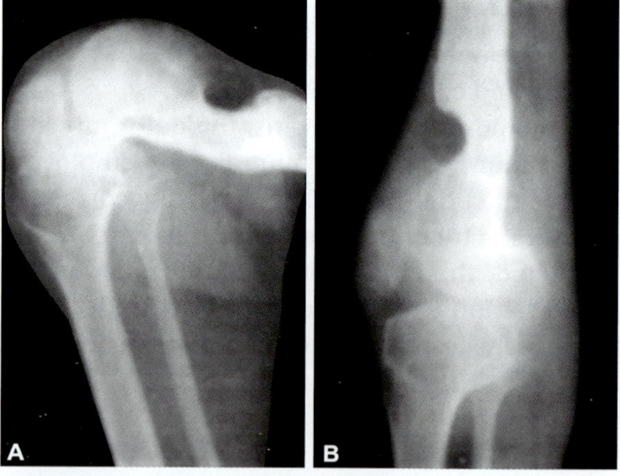

Figs. 9.11A and B: Tuberculosis of left knee joint in this young patient healed with gross limitations of movements. At the age of 15 years, the range of knee motions was from 40 to 105 degrees. A supracondylar femoral osteotomy was performed to bring/transfer the joint movements in the functional arc. Seventeen years after, at 32 years of age, the patient had a painless range of movements from 0 to 100 degrees. Note the adaptive changes in the knee. (A) in maximum flexion and (B) in maximum extension.

SURGICAL TECHNIQUES

Synovectomy of Knee Joint

The operating surgeon is free to modify the approach according to the extent of pathology and local needs. Though "total synovectomy" is desirable but for all practical purposes most of the synovectomies are subtotal. A 15–20 cm curvilinear parapatellar incision **(Fig. 9.12)** may be made along the lateral or medial border of patella. After cutting skin, superficial fascia, deep fascia, one would cut through the quadriceps expansion about 0.5–1 cm away from the patella. The exposure extends proximally to the suprapatellar pouch and distally to the insertion of ligamentum patellae. By sharp dissection a plane of cleavage is developed between the quadriceps expansion and suprapatellar synovial pouch. Starting from its proximal borders the suprapatellar pouch and the thickened synovial membrane surrounding the articular margins of femoral and tibial condyles are excised. The knee joint is now flexed **(Fig. 9.13)** to 90 degrees and inspected from front, and any loose bodies are

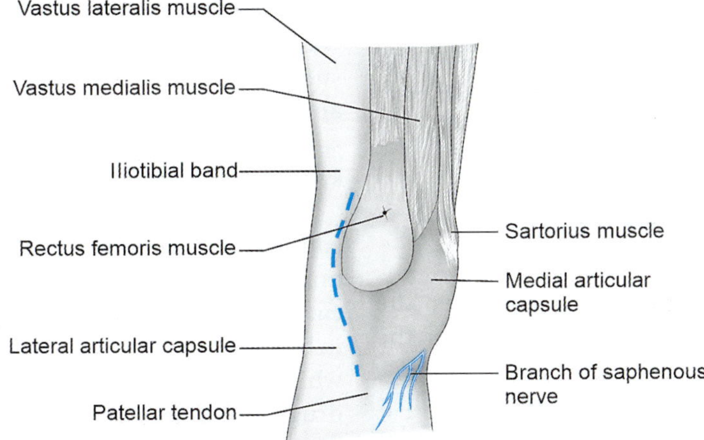

Fig. 9.12: The diagram shows the superficial anatomical landmarks for major operations (synovectomy, debridement, arthrodesis, etc.) on the knee joint. The exposure may be made employing medial or lateral parapatellar incision. Flexion of the knee to 90 degrees permits inspection of intracapsular structures **(Fig. 9.13)**.

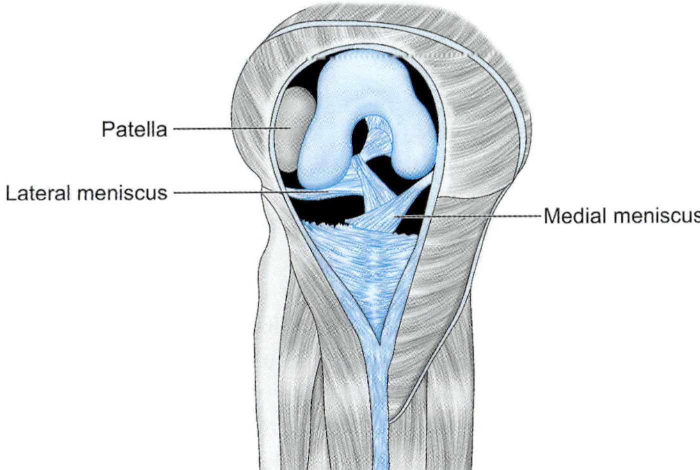

Fig. 9.13: Intracapsular structures visible on flexion of the knee joint which was exposed through the medial parapatellar incision.

removed. The unhealthy synovial membrane is removed as far as possible from the cruciate ligaments and intercondylar fossa. Rotational movements of the tibia with knee in flexion would help access for excision of considerable part of synovial membrane of the posterior compartment. This maneuver also helps inspection of menisci. The surgeon before closure should test if one can achieve at least 90 degrees of flexion of the knee joint easily. Any obstructing intra-articular lesion or extra-articular adhesions should be cut carefully, capsulectomy or capsulotomy performed, to obtain the desired flexion on the operation table. This completes the synovectomy. Antibiotics are instilled locally, suction drainage is introduced and located in the suprapatellar region. The capsule and the quadriceps are then closed with interrupted sutures.

Synovectomy with Debridement (Joint Clearance)

In cases of early tubercular arthritis when the disease has spread beyond the extent of the synovial membrane, in addition to synovectomy, joint clearance is advised. The pannus when present is stripped off the underlying articular surfaces. Smaller areas of destruction are curetted. Larger areas of destruction on articular surfaces and margins are curetted and filled up with cancellous bone grafts obtained from nearby healthy bone, irregular surface and margins are smoothened, destroyed and degenerated menisci, absolutely loose and destroyed articular cartilage, destroyed capsule and ligaments may be carefully removed. If >50% of articular cartilage is destroyed the outcome is likely to be less than half of the normal range of joint motion. The patients must be forewarned about such a prognosis. Before closure, raw areas of bone and areas of prospective bleeding are cauterized. The wound is closed over a suction drainage and postoperative management is similar to that of synovectomy. Where facilities are available, synovectomy and joint debridement can also be done by arthroscopic procedure.

Postoperative Regimen for Synovectomy with or without Debridement

After the closure a well-padded compression bandage is applied and the tourniquet (if used) is released. Postoperatively, the limb is nursed on pillows, below the knee skin traction or tibial pin traction is applied, the limb is elevated and the knee joint kept in about 5–10 degrees of flexion with the help of a rolled towel or a small pillow behind the knee. Exercises at ankle and static quadriceps exercises are started the same evening. Within a day or two of the operation, knee bending exercises are done at hourly basis within the range of the compression bandage. The suction drainage is removed after 48–72 hours and more knee bending is encouraged. The suction drainage system virtually eliminates post-synovectomy hemarthrosis.

Ambulation with the help of weight relieving caliper (orthosis) and crutches is started about one month after the operation when the patient can perform knee flexion to 90 degrees and is able to lift the limb with extended knee against gravity, which-so-ever is later. Appropriate antitubercular drugs and supportive therapy is continued for 12–18 months. Crutches are gradually discarded between 3 and 6 months, and orthosis is gradually discarded between 18 and 24 months depending upon the local progress and healing of the infective process.

Arthrodesis of the Knee Joint

This operation may be indicated in advanced **(Figs. 9.14 and 9.15)** tubercular arthritis (gross limitation of movements, marked diminution of the joint space, destruction of the opposing joint surfaces), tubercular arthritis with triple deformity, cases with gross instability (Friedman and Kapur 1970, Martini 1988) and cases of painful ankylosis after earlier operations like synovectomy and debridement, or in a pationet who failed to heal by drug therapy **(Figs. 9.8, 9.14 and 9.15)** or for patients with failure of prior joint replacement.

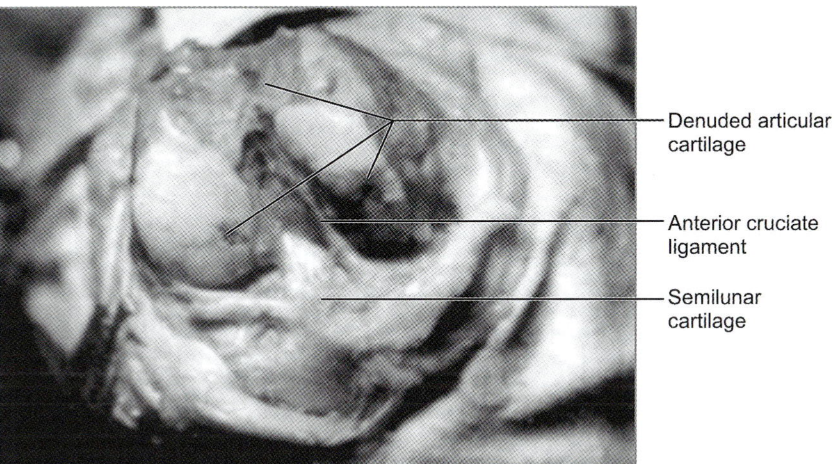

Fig. 9.14: Intraoperative photograph of the right knee joint with advanced tuberculous arthritis and active disease. Note gross destruction of articular cartilage, erosion of subchondral bone, attenuation of anterior cruciate ligament and medial semilunar cartilage, and nodular appearance of the thickened synovium on the medial side.

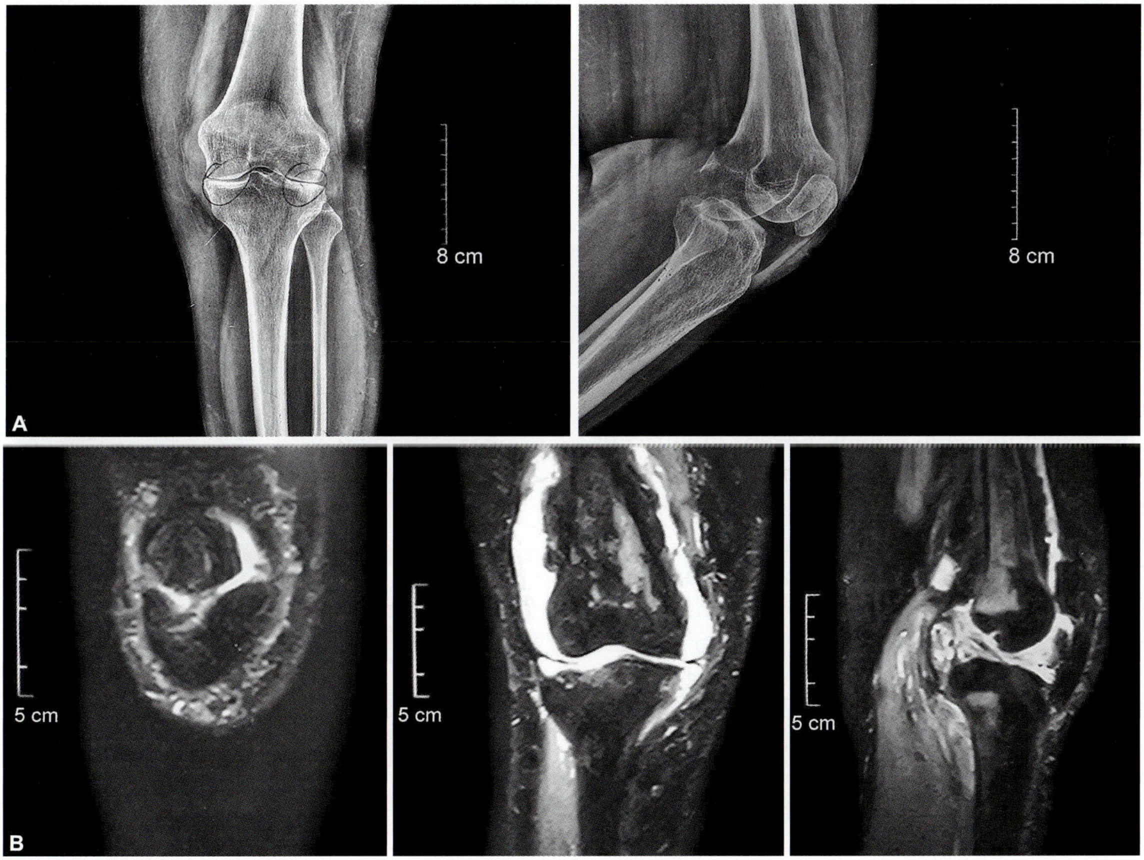

Fig. 9.15: A young male patient presented with painful swelling of left knee. X-ray (A) revealed diminished joint space; aspirated material revealed mycobacteria. At presentation MRIs at presentation (B) showing increased synovial fluid in the joint space, bone edema in distal femur and infected lymph nodes (LN) behind the knee joint.

Acceptability Test for Arthrodesis

Because there is a finality about the loss of movements and restrictions imposed by arthrodesis of the knee joint it is mandatory to explain to the patient and his/her attendants about the resultant domestic, marital, professional, and social limitations. A patient with gross ankylosis (with or without deformity) and pain has nothing to lose except "pain". Whenever in doubt, the "acceptability test" of this operation is advisable by simulating the functional restrictions imposed by arthrodesis of the knee joint. A light above the knee plaster cast is applied to the limb leaving the ankle and foot free for walking. The patient is sent back to his/her social, domestic and professional environments. The patient and his family are advised to report back in the hospital after 3–6 weeks, with their mind made up regarding the acceptability of operation.

The operation is performed under tourniquet, with patient supine, toward the edge of the operating table. An anterior curvilinear parapatellar incision is made starting from the suprapatellar pouch extending up to the tibial tubercle. The quadriceps expansion is cut in the same line leaving 0.5–1 cm of muscle attached to the patellar border. The capsule is erased subperiosteally with the help of a sharp chisel and hammer from the medial and lateral tibial and femoral condyles near the articular margins. The knee joint is gradually flexed, quadriceps expansion and patella are reflected to the medial side in case of lateral parapatellar incision (or lateral side in case of medial parapatellar incision). Grossly diseased synovial membrane and bone are excised preserving the healthy bone and its continuity with quadriceps and patellar tendon. With the knee joint in varying degrees of flexion, the articular cartilage and subchondral bone is removed from the upper end of tibia and distal end of femur up to the cancellous bone. The apposing surfaces of tibia and femur are shaped and brought into contact to obtain maximal contact without rotation, gross displacement and angulation. The articular surface of patella is rawed and is apposed at the site of arthrodesis while closing. Grossly diseased bone, sequestera, tuberculous cavities, caseous tissue and granulation tissue are gouged/curetted out from the end of the bones. The resultant cavities are filled up with cancellous bone chips obtained from nearby healthy bone. Toward the end of bone resection one must ensure good apposition of the largest possible areas of bone. No more than a few degrees (5–15 degrees) of flexed position of arthrodesis is desirable. There should be no lateral angulation at the level of knee. The neutral position in the long axis of leg is achieved by the screw-home movement of the tibia, placing the tibial tubercle a little lateral to the midline of thigh (giving 5–7 degrees of external rotation). The stability at the site of arthrodesis is obtained generally by employing Charnley's compression clamps. We have as a rule employed Charnley's compression apparatus for >30 years **(Fig. 9.16)** with universal success. In cases with long-standing disease and severe osteoporosis, it is advisable to insert Steinmann pins well away from the line of arthrodesis through the area of lesser osteoporosis.

Antibiotics are instilled locally, suction drainage is introduced and the wound closed in

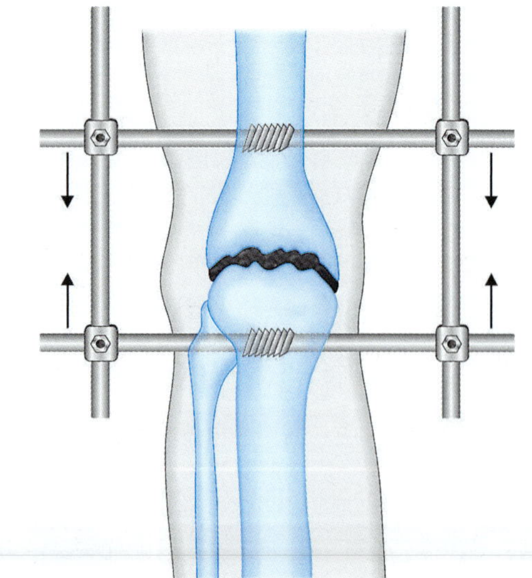

Fig. 9.16: Diagrammatic representation of Charnley's compression arthrodesis of knee.

layers. Over a thick layer of cotton, compression bandage is applied on the operated area, the tourniquet is released and the limb is supported with mild flexion at the knee level on a strong posterior plaster shell. Axial rotation of the leg is prevented by incorporating a derotation bar in the plaster.

Postoperatively, the limb is kept elevated on pillows. Considerable postoperative blood loss is expected from the raw cancellous bone ends, and it is mandatory to replace one unit of blood (500 mL) soon after the surgery. Appropriate antibiotic and chemotherapy is continued for 12–18 months.

About 72 hours after the operation, the suction-drain is removed, the bandage covering the compression clamps is cut longitudinally and the compression nuts are exposed. The desired degree of compression is maintained by frequent tightening of the screws, initially by one round and later by 1/2 to 1/3 of the round every 24 hourly for about 4–6 weeks, when the compression apparatus and the pins are removed and an up to groin well-fitting plaster cast is applied on stockinet excluding the ankle and foot. Weight bearing in the plaster cast is commenced 5–6 weeks after the operation, and the walking plaster is retained for 3–6 months. Sound fusion, as confirmed by the X-rays **(Fig. 9.8)**, is generally obtained by this time to permit unprotected weight bearing.

In patients with severe flexion deformity (>90 degrees), care must be taken to prevent damage to the neurovascular bundles by sudden correction of deformity. Preoperative skeletal traction in cases of fibrous ankylosis would minimize this risk by reducing the degree of deformity. While operating in the presence of a severe fixed flexion deformity, the soft tissues behind the upper end of tibia should be carefully erased subperiosteally before correcting the deformity. Lateral popliteal nerve should be exposed and released from its surroundings around the neck of fibula and along the medial border of the tendon of biceps femoris. About 8 cm of upper end of fibula may be excised to relieve any tension on the lateral popliteal nerve on straightening the knee. The excised fibula may be used as a bone graft for fillings around the site of arthrodesis.

Arthroplasty for Tuberculous Arthritis

Besser (1980), Wray and Roy (1987) performed arthroplasty inadvertently in the preoperatively unsuspected cases of tuberculosis of the knee. Reactivation of infection after the operation was controlled by modern antituberculous drugs. The range of motion obtained in the knee joint is, however, not clearly mentioned by the authors. Eskola et al. (1988) reported the results of replacement arthroplasty in 6 patients who had the primary disease about 35 years ago. Marked improvement in the function of the knee joint was observed during a follow-up of nearly 6 years. Kim (1988) reported good results after total knee arthroplasty in selected cases of old healed tuberculosis of knee. Gale and Harding (1991) reported a short term result of total knee arthroplasty in the presence of active disease. Koga et al. (1988) reported an interesting series of resection and interposition arthroplasty in 25 patients who had infection of long-standing (tuberculosis in 8 cases). The interposition material was a preremoved and chromatized autogenous graft of fascia lata. During a mean follow-up of 22 years, none had severe pain, 13 had >60 degrees of movements, 12 had a range of 45 degrees or less, and radiographs showed adaptive remodeling of bone ends. This methodology may offer another solution with the adoption of continuous passive, assisted and active motion during the postoperative period.

In a grossly destroyed painful knee joint, with or without deformity, the traditional treatment has been arthodesis in the best functional position. Arthrodesis of knee, however, imposes lot of restrictions in sitting, using public transport, and many other social activities. Indications for arthoplasty for a healed disease may be more justified for the knee than for any other joint. While resecting the bone one must ensure preservation of medial and lateral ligaments of knee, correction of deformity, and placement of inplants in a way to achieve about 5–7 degrees of valgus. Once the knee arthroplasty is infected no satisfactory outcome is achieved by resection arthroplasty, arthrodesis, or revision arthroplasty (Thornhill et al. 1982). Arthrodesis or interval revision arthroplasty in such cases may be the only practical option.

At present, replacement arthroplasty of knee is being offered to selected patients. Most of the authors suggest this operation at least 3–5 years after the last evidence of activity of infection (Eskola et al. 1988, Kim 1988, Gale and Harding 1991). The minimum disease free period prior to arthroplasty procedures must be 2–3 years. It implies to infection in any part or system of body. Prior hip or knee prosthetic joint infection in another joint increases the risk three-fold of prosthetic joint infection after primary total knee arthroplasty (Chalmers 2019). Mandatory coverage by modern antitubercular drugs for about 5 months after replacement surgery is advised.

We should also be aware of development of tuberculous arthritis in patients after replacement knee arthroplasty performed for non-infective pathology. In the last 12 years (1996–2008), the author has observed 10 such patients from well-equipped institutions. The diagnosis of tuberculous pathology was confirmed by histology, microbiology and by PCR **(Fig. 9.17)**.

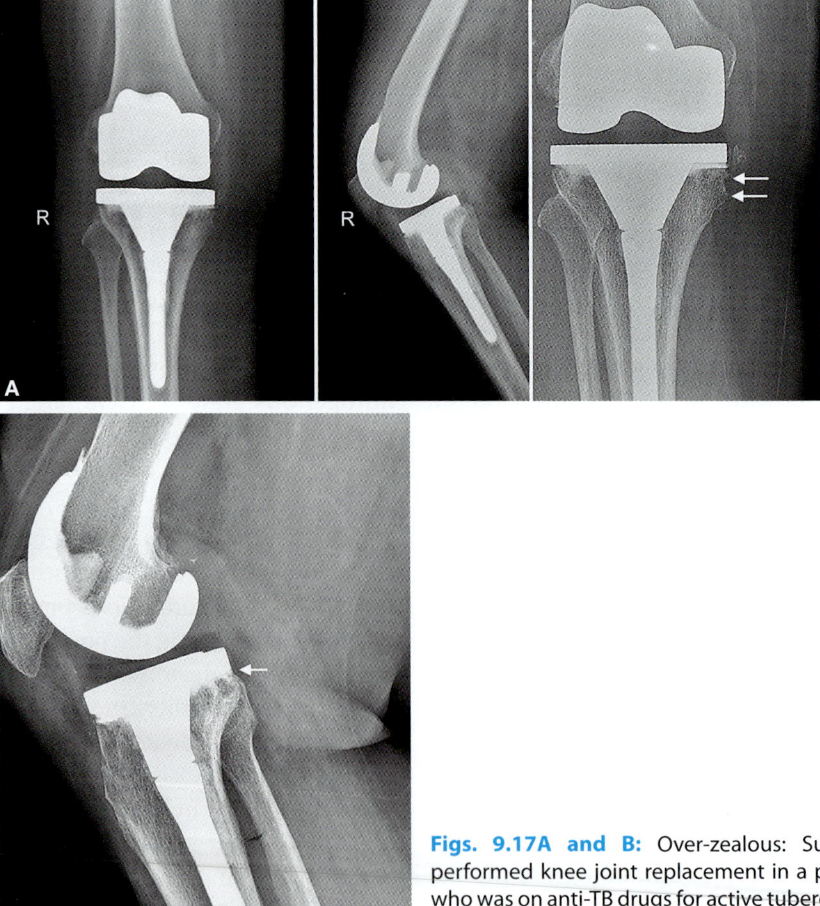

Figs. 9.17A and B: Over-zealous: Surgeon performed knee joint replacement in a patient who was on anti-TB drugs for active tuberculosis of spine. The operated knee is showing erosions on the proximal tibia (arrows).

RELEVANT SURGICAL ANATOMY OF THE KNEE JOINT

The knee joint is the largest articulation in the body. For stability, it depends upon the strength of the capsule, the collateral and cruciate ligaments and the surrounding muscles. The fibrous capsule completely invests the joint particularly on its posterior aspect which is strengthened by the oblique popliteal ligament. Medially and laterally, it is reinforced by collateral ligaments. Forward and backward stability of the tibia on the femur in flexed position is predominantly provided by the anterior and posterior cruciate ligaments, respectively. Gross destruction of the posterior cruciate ligament would result in posterior subluxation of the knee joint. The anterior capsule is replaced by/composed of the quadriceps expansion inserting into the patella, the ligamentum patellae (infrapatellar tendon), and the blending of fibrous aponeuroses from the vasti medialis and lateralis. The "capsule" is thinnest between the ligamentum patellae and the collateral ligaments, up to its attachment to the anterior margin of the tibial plateau.

The synovial membrane lines the inner aspect of the capsule. It extends upwards as the suprapatellar pouch on the anterior aspect of femur under cover of the quadriceps expansion up to the extent of a hands breadth. A diverticulum of synovium is prolonged (or herniated) posteriorly and distally between the proximal part of popliteus and the underlying femur and tibia. Another synovial pouch extends/herniates posteriorly to communicate with a bursa lying between the semimembranosus and the medial head of gastrocnemius. Generally, a bursa beneath the lateral head of gastrocnemius also communicates with the joint **(Fig. 9.18)**. Any disease involving the synovium would easily extend to the communicating synovial prolongations and present as popliteal cysts/swellings. These ramifications also preclude complete surgical excision in an operation

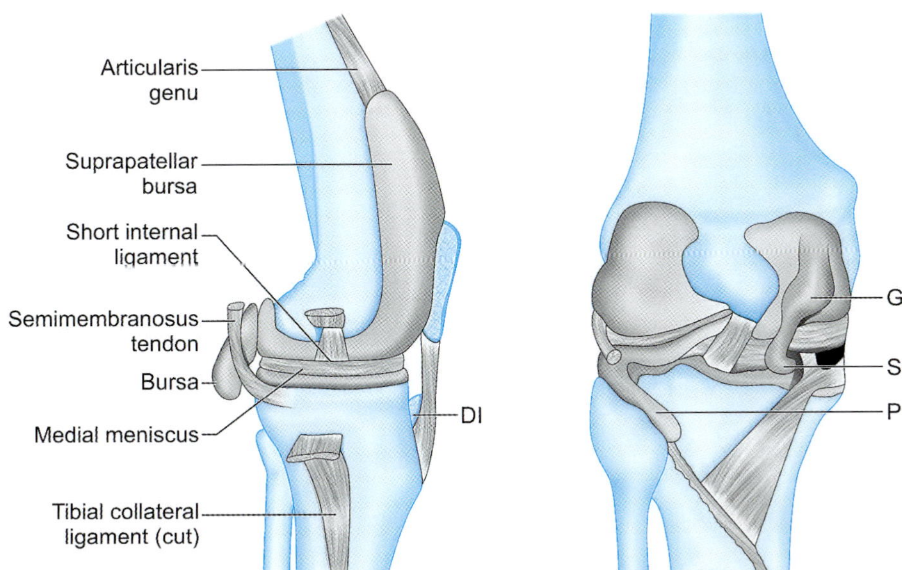

Fig. 9.18: Diagram showing the bursal sheaths and bursal herniations around the knee joint. Any one or many of these may be involved by tuberculous pathology.

(DI: deep infrapatellar, G: bursa related to the medial head of gastrocnemius, P: bursa along the origin of popliteus, S: bursa related to the semimembranosus insertion)

attempted to be a total synovectomy **(Fig. 9.18)**. There are many more unnamed synovial pouches and bursae around the knee joint.

The cruciate ligaments are intracapsular but are not intrasynovial. It is as though they had been herniated into the synovial membrane from behind, carrying forward over their surfaces the synovial fold which invests their anterior, lateral and medial surfaces but leaves their posterior surfaces uncovered. The synovium from the lateral and medial sides of the cruciate ligaments becomes continuous with the synovial lining of the intercondylar notch of the femur. Anteriorly, the synovium is invaginated by the infrapatellar pad of fat which lies extrasynovially distal to the patella up to the anterior margins of medial and lateral tibial condyles.

On the lateral aspect of knee joint, the head of fibula has attachment of fibular collateral ligaments extending from the fibular head to the lateral epicondyle and condyle of femur. The tendon of biceps femoris is inserted into the head of fibula, splitting into two parts to enclose the fibular collateral ligament. The common peroneal (lateral popliteal) nerve lies just behind the biceps tendon insertion and passes distally to wind around the neck of fibula under the peroneus longus muscle, clinically the nerve is palpable medial to the tendon of biceps and on the neck of fibula. This nerve is likely to be damaged by stretching or rough handling while correcting a severe flexion deformity (90 degrees or more) of long-standing. A bursa exists in between and around the conjoint insertion of sartorius, gracilis, and semitendinosus (pes anserinus) on the proximal medial aspect of tibia medial to the tibial tubercle. Bursa pes anserinus may rarely get involved by tuberculosis.

CHAPTER 10

Tuberculosis of the Ankle and Foot

TUBERCULOSIS OF ANKLE

Tuberculous disease of the ankle is relatively uncommon. The initial focus may start in the synovium, especially in children, or as an erosion in the distal end of tibia **(Fig. 10.1)**, malleoli **(Figs. 10.2 and 10.3)** or talus. Rarely, tuberculosis of calcaneum may reach the ankle joint after involvement of subtaloid joint and the talus. The incidence of ankle tuberculosis is <5% of all osteoarticular tuberculosis (Silva 1980, Martini 1988, Dhillon et al. 2012).

Clinical Features

Pain, limp and swelling are the earliest features. The swelling is evident in front of the joint and there is fullness around the malleoli and tendo-Achilles insertion. The ankle joint is usually held in plantar flexion. In cases of long-standing with gross destruction of bones and ligaments, the ankle joint may show pathological anterior subluxation/dislocation. Radiologically, during active stage, marked osteoporosis **(Fig. 10.3)** is seen with or without areas of osseous erosions

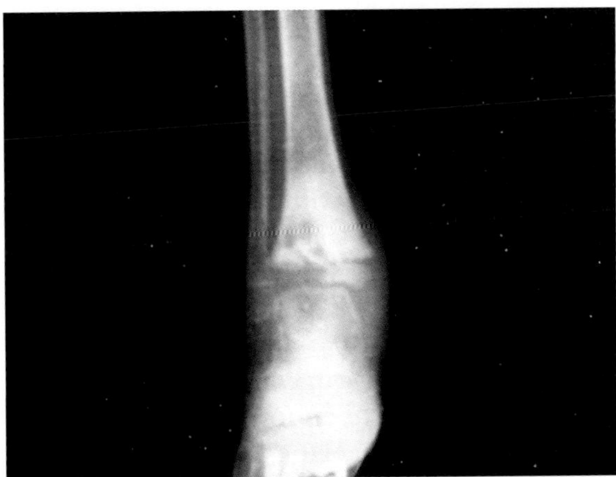

Fig. 10.1: X-ray of an active tuberculous arthritis of ankle joint in a child. The disease probably started in the tibial metaphyseal region, penetrated the physis, epiphysis and entered the joint cavity. Note a lytic cavity sitting astride the physis, opening into the joint, the cavity contains a soft sequestrum. The ankle joint space is diminished and there is circumferential soft tissue swelling.

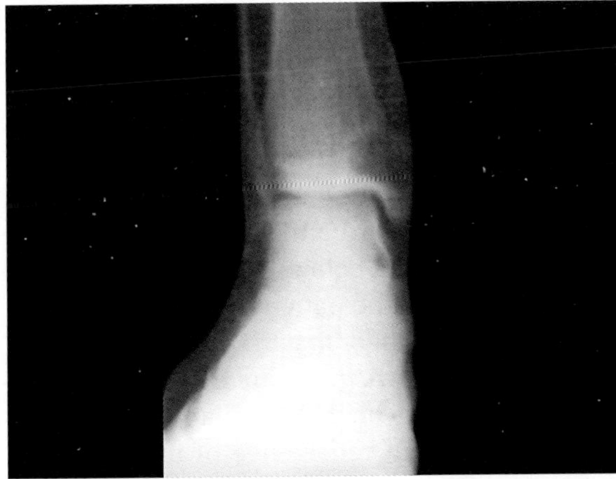

Fig. 10.2: A juxta-articular lytic lesion at the base of medial malleolus. Histology proved it to be tuberculous in nature. The disease healed with complete restoration of osseous architecture and retention of ankle movements.

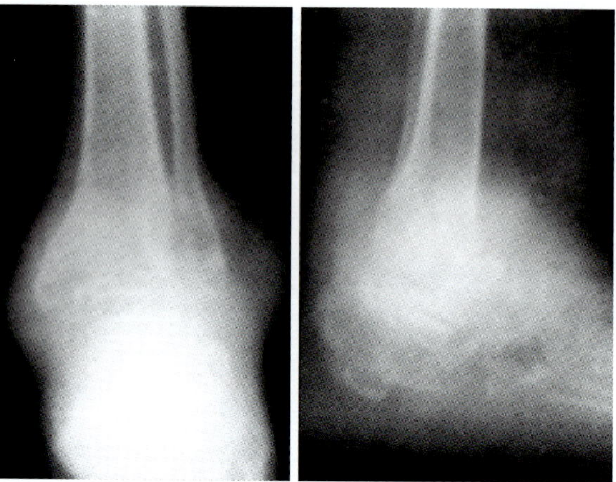

Fig. 10.3: Advanced tubercular arthritis of ankle joint. The disease probably started in the body of talus, however, at present there is destruction and involvement of ankle joint, subtaloid joint, lower ends of tibia and fibula, calcaneum and tarsal bones. Note marked soft tissue swelling. The expected result on healing would be sound ankylosis in functioning position.

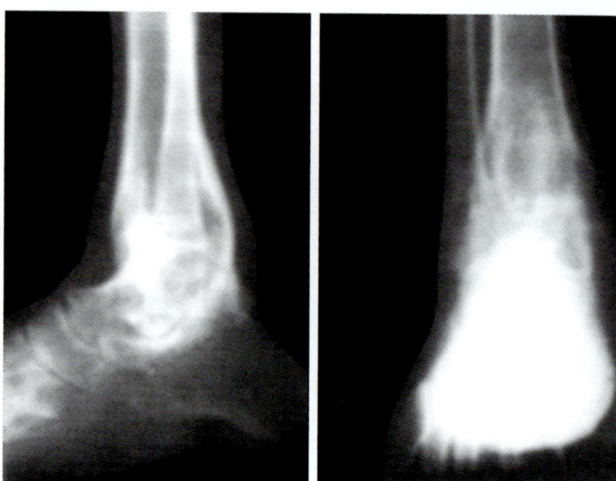

Fig. 10.4: Spontaneous bony fusion of tuberculosis of the ankle joint in a case who had discharging sinuses at presentation. The patient was treated by plaster immobilization and drugs.

or destruction in the bones. Sinus formation with concomitant secondary infection is not an unusual feature (Dhillon 2001).

Management

The ankle is a complex joint with high degree of weight bearing and locomotion. Fortunately, isolated ankylosis of ankle joint causes little or no disability in normal activities. A painless ankylosis of the joint in neutral position (i.e., plantigrade position) is the aim of treatment (in advanced arthritis), which can be achieved in majority of the cases by standard antitubercular drugs and immobilization in a below-knee plaster cast or a suitable orthosis. The patient is ambulatory with the help of crutches for first 8–12 weeks, thereafter guarded weight bearing is encouraged with the plaster or orthosis on. The appliance is worn for 2 years to prevent recurrence of infection and deformity. On completion of treatment, out of an unselected group nearly 50% would heal with almost full range of movements, 30% with useful range of pain-free motion, and 20% with painless gross ankylosis. Patients who had secondary infection with gross destruction of joint ended up with gross ankylosis or spontaneous osseous fusion **(Fig. 10.4)**. Generally patients are satisfied with a painless ankle in neutral position even if there is gross stiffness. Early disease of ankle and foot (stage of synovitis or early arthritis) is best treated by "functional treatment" and multidrug therapy. Most of these patients would heal with retention of a useful range of motion.

Operative Treatment

Surgery is indicated for cases that are not responding to antitubercular drugs and rest to the part, or when the diagnosis is in doubt. Synovectomy with or without joint debridement is performed for the stage of synovitis and early arthritis. When surgery is indicated for advanced disease **(Fig. 10.3)** or for painful ankylosis or in the presence of pathological subluxation/dislocation, or in case of concomitant secondary infection it is wise to perform arthrodesis (with prior explicit consent of the patient) following the joint clearance. Arthrodesis should be restricted to cases with persistent clinical disability and never solely for the radiological evidence of joint damage (Martini 1988). Rarely, a patient may present with ankylosis in an awkward position, arthrodesis in neutral (plantigrade) position should be performed with suitable wedge resection of bones. Though the position of choice for fusion is 90 degrees (plantigrade), some women habituated to wear high heels would prefer fusion with 5 degrees of plantar flexion.

Surgical Technique

Exposure of Ankle Joint

Anterolateral approach is simple and can be extended distally to expose tarsal joints if necessary. Make 8–10 cm long incision lateral to the tendon of extensor digitorum centering in front of the ankle joint. Cut subcutaneous tissues, extensor retinaculum and expose the capsule of the ankle by retracting medially the tendons in front of the joint. Avoid cutting the anterior tibial artery and nerve situated between the tendons of extensor digitorum laterally and tibialis anterior medially. Cut the capsule transversely and expose the articular surfaces of the joint. Remove the diseased synovium and loose articular cartilage and any debris within the joint cavity. Attempted plantar flexion, and inversion/eversion helps to reach the deeper areas of the joint to achieve subtotal synovectomy with or without joint debridement. If the disease is at a stage of advanced arthritis and patients functional demands are heavy, one should proceed ahead with arthrodesis in adults.

For *arthrodesis* remove any visible articular cartilage till bleeding raw surfaces of lower end of tibia, articular surfaces of medial and lateral malleoli, medial, lateral and upper surfaces of the body of talus are clearly exposed. Removal of bone should be minimum to preserve as much bone stock as is possible. Hold the foot in the desired plantigrade position, fill up any gaps around the site of fusion by bone grafts, and insert Steinmann's pins transversely one each through the distal part of tibia and through the body of talus **(Fig. 10.5)**. Close the wound over suction drainage and apply compression device on the pins. Support the position of the limb by a strong posterior plaster cast. Maintain the compression (as for knee arthrodesis Chapter 9) for 4–6 weeks, when the compression device is removed and a well fitting below the knee full plaster cast is applied. Now encourage the patient to walk with full weight bearing with the plaster on. The plaster protection is necessary for 3–5 months, till solid osseous fusion is evident on X-rays.

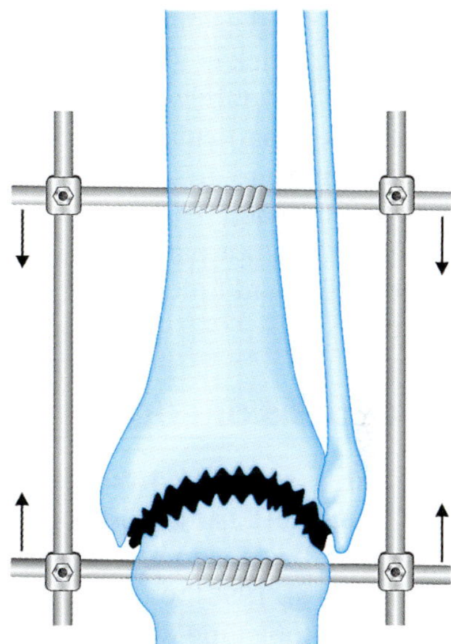

Fig. 10.5: Diagrammatic representation of Charnley's type compression arthrodesis of ankle joint.

Pantalar Fusion

If there is concomitant involvement of subtaloid joint **(Fig. 10.3)**, its fusion, in addition to the ankle is indicated in the same sitting. Extend the incision distally as required, invert the foot to open the subtaloid joint (from the lateral side) and clear away all the diseased and destroyed tissues. Remove the articular cartilage and freshen the opposing surfaces of talus and calcaneum, pack any gaps with bone grafts, and insert the distal compression pin through the calcaneum (instead of the body of talus). Now apply the compression clamps to exert compression forces at the ankle as well as the talocalcaneal joint. The remaining postoperative management is the same as for ankle arthrodesis. The ideal position of fusion of ankle is recommended as neutral flexion, slight (1–5 degrees) valgus angulation of the hind part of foot, and 5–10 degrees of external rotation at the level of ankle (Buck et al., 1987). Below the knee amputation may rarely be indicated where destruction is severe, particularly in older patients, or if the tarsal joints are grossly deformed (Silva 1980, Newton et al. 1986). We, however, never had such an indication in our patients, every sensate foot can heel with good function, amputation is seldom needed.

TUBERCULOSIS OF FOOT

The commoner sites of involvement are calcaneum, subtaloid, and mid-tarsal joints. Sometimes the disease may remain limited (Garela-Perrua et al. 1998) to the central part of a tarsal bone for a long time without extension to the neighboring joints. The order in decreasing frequency of such lesions is calcaneum, talus **(Figs. 10.6, 10.8 and 10.9)**, first metatarsal, navicular, first and second cuneiforms, cuboid and other bones (Mittal 1999, Gupta et al. 2000, Dhillon 2002). Endarteritis of the nutrient artery in such lesions is common and many would show a cavity with or without a typical coke-like sequestrum on the X-rays **(Fig. 10.7)**. Once the intertarsal joint is involved from the synovium, or from the superficial lesions of tarsals or penetration from the deeper lesions, the tuberculous process spreads rapidly to many parts because of intercommunicating synovial channels or cavities of these joints. Isolated lesions of one joint or one tarsal or metatarsal bone are exceptions. In general, the symptoms are less pronounced, therefore, it is seldom that a patient at an early stage of disease reports to the hospital. Diagnosis is easily made by the presence of pain, swelling, tenderness and cold abscess/sinuses. X-rays reveal osteoporosis, areas of bone destruction and cavitation. In the initial active disease, it may be difficult to localize the lesion because of extensive and intense osteoporosis. Comparative X-rays of both feet are of great help. Low grade pyogenic infection and rare

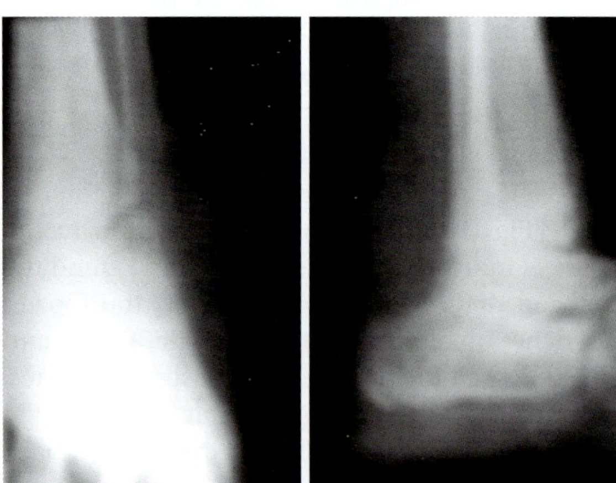

Fig. 10.6: This child was treated 4 years ago by antitubercular drugs, splintage in plantigrade position, and repetitive active and assisted exercises of the ankle. Clinically, at present, the patient has a healed status and is fully active. The present X-rays show a flattened dome of the body of talus, and ill-formed talar head and its trabeculae. The ankle and subtaloid joints show reduced cartilage space. Lateral part of the lower end of tibia shows a clean defect. It is expected that this young patient will continue to have a painless mobile ankle and foot for many years.

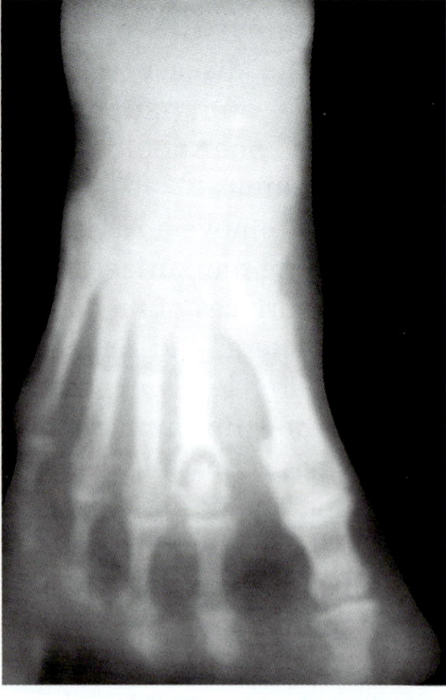

Fig. 10.7: Tuberculosis of second metatarsal showing a coke-like sequestrum in a cavity in the second metatarsal head.

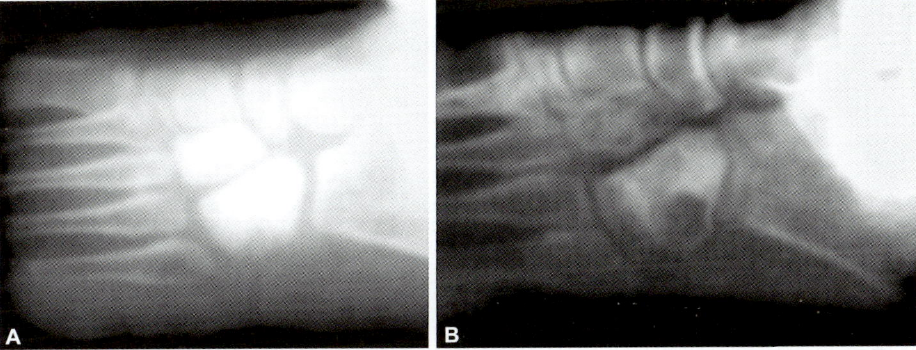

Figs. 10.8A and B: Histologically proved tuberculosis of tarsal bones (A) in a young girl of 6 years. The disease healed under the influence of antitubercular chemotherapy. However, at 12 years of age she reported again with recrudescence of disease. Note deformed lateral cuneiform bone and cavitations in the cuboid (B).

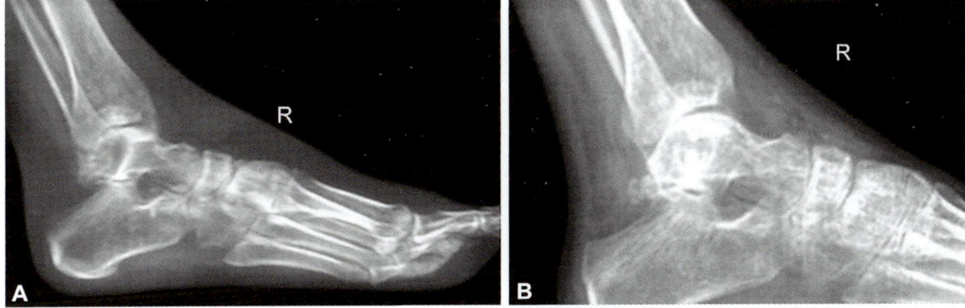

Figs. 10.9A and B: A cystic lesion in the body of talus on histological examination turned out to be tuberculosis (A). As tuberculosis can mimic any pathology, therefore it is mandatory to obtain tissue for diagnosis whenever in doubt. The follow up X-ray (B) shows healed lesion.

granulomatous conditions (mycosis, brucellosis, sarcoidosis, etc.) have to be considered in differential diagnosis.

Conservative treatment with below knee plaster cast or a below knee orthosis with a fixed ankle combined with antitubercular drugs is as a rule effective in majority. As the healing progresses, spontaneous bony fusion may occur in the involved joints, especially in cases with superadded infection **(Fig. 10.4)**. Surgical excision of a large isolated osseous lesion (e.g., in calcaneum) to prevent involvement of adjacent joints, or debridement and curettage may be indicated in nonhealing lesions. Resection of a destroyed or sequestrated phalanx or metatarsal may be required only in rare cases (Martini 1988). If surgical treatment is indicated in a joint involvement the operation should be combined with deliberate arthrodesis. If talocalcaneonavicular joints are involved, a standard triple arthrodesis is necessary. If involvement is of ankle, subtaloid and midtarsal joints concomitantly, pantalar arthrodesis is justified. Whenever the diagnosis is in doubt the diseased tissue should be obtained for microbiological, serological and histological studies by core biopsy or by open biopsy **(Figs. 10.8 and 10.10)**. Like osteoarticular tuberculosis in general isolation of acid fast bacilli is uncommon. Dhillon and Nagi (2002) reported 2 positive cultures out of the 17 cases tested. Once the disease is healed, the gait and function for normal activities are not restricted.

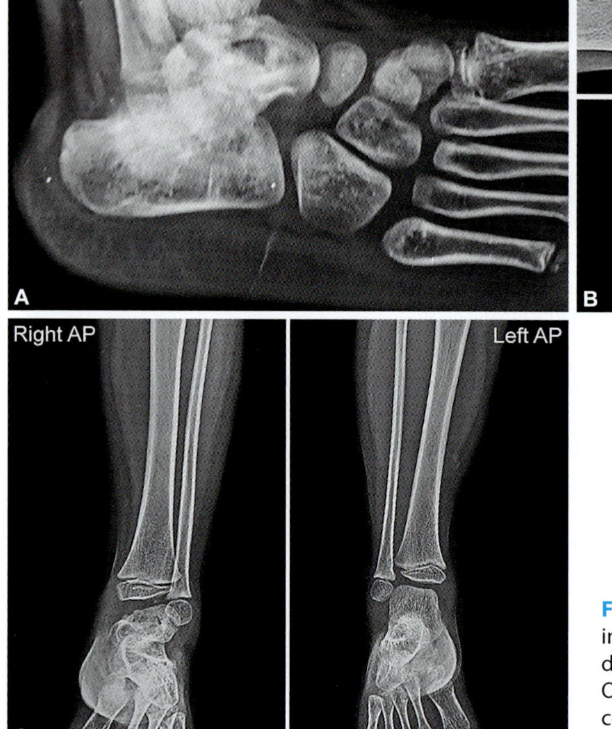

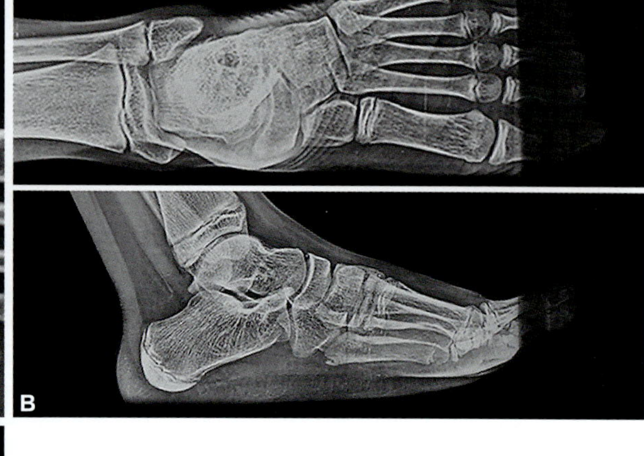

Fig. 10.10: X-rays reveal gross destruction of right-talus in a child aged 3 years (A). Patient was treated by anti-TB drugs, rest to the ankle and standard functional treatment. Observe the healing potential in growing years (B). X-ray (C) compares the healed (right) ankle and the normal ankle at age 14 years.

RELEVANT SURGICAL ANATOMY OF THE ANKLE AND FOOT

The ankle and foot generally function as an integrated unit and together provide a stable support, proprioception, mobility and balance. The ankle is a hinge joint in which the body of the talus fits into a mortise or socket formed by the distal ends of tibia and fibula. The mortise is deepened posteriorly by the transverse tibiofibular ligament. The lower ends of tibia and fibula are held together by the interosseous ligament, and the anteroinferior and posteroinferior tibiofibular ligaments.

The capsule of the ankle joint is composed of various ligaments joined together. The anterior ligament is wide, membranous, extending from the distal anterior part of tibia to the neck of talus. The posterior ligament is short and thin extending from the distal posterior surface of tibia to the posterior surface of talus. Medially deltoid ligament is attached above to the medial malleolus and distally radiates anteriorly to the tuberosity of navicular, the spring ligament and the neck of talus; directly below to the sustentaculum tali, and posteriorly to the body of talus. The lateral ligament has 3 thickened bands: the anterior and the posterior talofibular ligaments getting attached to the respective parts of talus, and between them the calcaneofibular ligament extending from the tip of the lateral malleolus to the lateral surface of calcaneum. The ankle allows movements in the sagittal plane only, i.e., plantar flexion and dorsiflexion. Synovial membrane lines the inner surface of the capsule and as usual is attached to the articular margins. Intracapsular part of neck of talus is clothed with the synovium. Occasionally, the synovial cavity may extend a little upward into the inferior tibiofibular articulation.

The talus forms a gliding synovial joint with the calcaneum, a strong interosseous ligament holds the two bones firmly together. The distal end of talus articulates in a socket in the navicular. The calcaneocuboid joint lies lateral to but in the same transverse plane as the talonavicular joint; together these are described as "transverse tarsal or midtarsal joint". Medial to the cuboid and distal to the navicular are situated the cuneiform bones and their articulations. At all the intertarsal joints the principle movement is gliding to provide plantar flexion and dorsiflexion of the distal part of foot. Inversion and eversion movements occur mostly at talocalcaneal, talonavicular, and calcaneocuboid joints. Fusion of these 3 joints "triple arthrodesis", is considered necessary by majority to obtain a stable hind-foot.

A synovial-lined cavity exists between each pair of tarsal bones, and these joints frequently communicate with one another. This explains the ease with which an infective lesion spreads to many tarsal joints.

Tuberculosis of the Shoulder

Tuberculous disease of the shoulder is rare constituting nearly 1–2% of skeletal tuberculosis. It is more frequent in adults and the incidence of concomitant pulmonary tuberculosis is high. The disease originates in the head of the humerus, glenoid of the scapula, or rarely from the synovium. It is extremely uncommon for the disease to present at the stage of synovitis. Painful limitations of abduction and external rotation occur early and there is marked wasting of the deltoid, supraspinatus and other muscles. As the disease progresses, there is marked destruction and atrophy of upper end of the humerus and glenoid **(Figs. 11.1 and 11.4)** and the shoulder undergoes fibrous ankylosis. The common variety is a dry atrophic form (caries sicca), very rarely there may be swelling and cold abscess (caries exudata) or sinus formation presenting in the deltoid region, along the biceps tendon, in the axilla or in the supraspinous fossa. In unattended cases, the scapulohumeral muscles contract, pull the humeral head against the glenoid and fix the shoulder in adduction **(Figs 11.2 and 11.4)**.

While making observations (during 1977–1988) on osteoarticular tuberculosis in children, Srivastava and Singh (1987) found only one case of tuberculosis of shoulder (aged 16 years) amongst 104 patients below the age of 18 years. During the last four decades since 1960, tuberculosis of the shoulder has been rarely reported (Tang et al. 1983, Martini 1988, Antti-Poika 1991, Patel et al. 2003). At the present time, tuberculosis occurs almost exclusively in adults. All the patients reported by Martini were >20 years, and half of his patients were older than 60 years. Though dry type of lesion is the common variety, in our institution one-third of the patients were observed to have abscess formation with or without sinuses **(Fig. 5.9)**.

A case of adhesive capsulitis (frozen shoulder or periarthritis) with a coexisting pulmonary

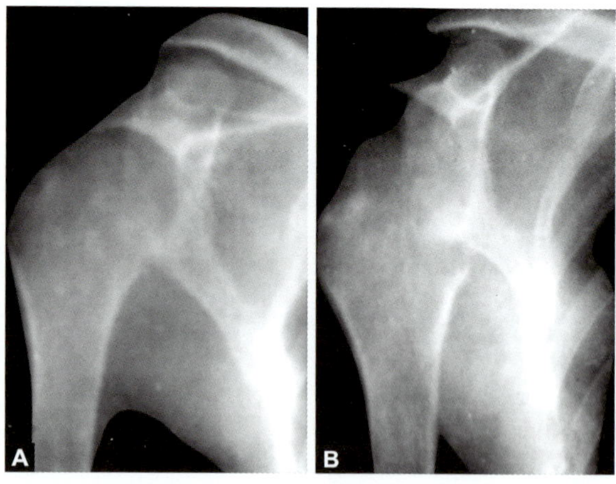

Figs. 11.1A and B: X-rays of a patient with active tuberculous disease of right shoulder, (A) was the appearance in June 1988 and (B) in February 1989. Localized osteoporosis, cloudy appearance of the glenoid and humeral head, fuzzy articular margins, destruction of the humeral head, and pathological subluxation of the joint (B) are obvious. The patient had discharging sinuses along the anterior border of deltoid muscle in the course of biceps tendon. He was not on treatment, note the deterioration in 7 months from (A) to (B).

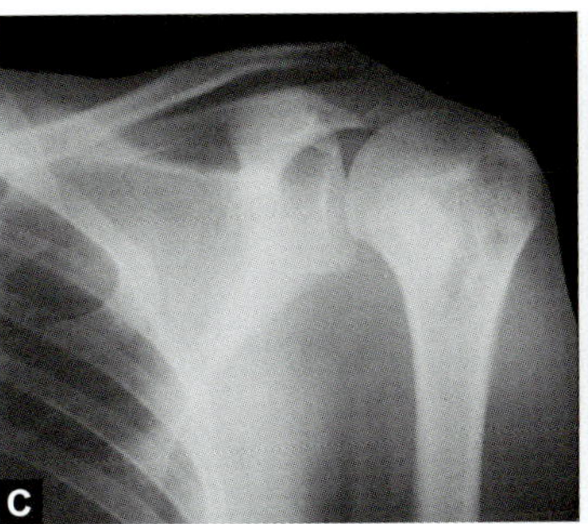

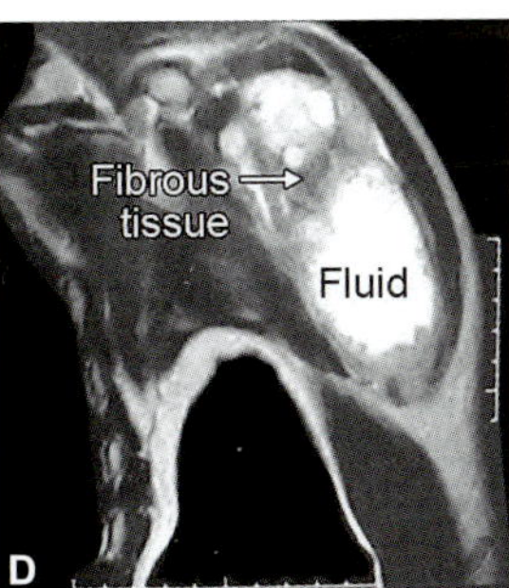

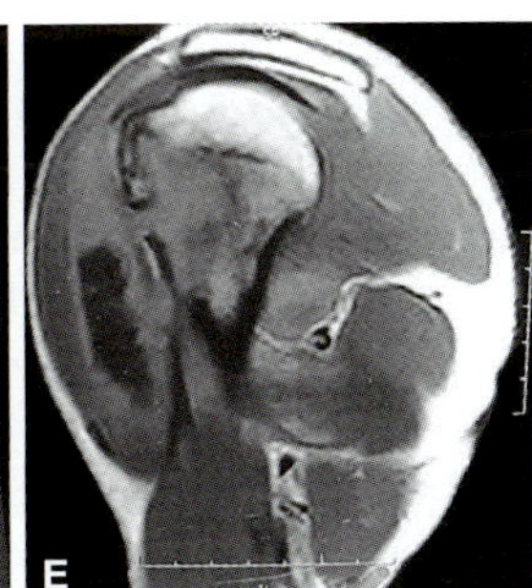

Figs. 11.1C to E: Another patient showing multiple lytic lesions in the upper end of humerus as seen in the X-ray (C), one can also appreciate the soft tissue collection (cold abscess). The MRIs (D and E) show the changing signal in T1 and T2 sequences according to the contents of the cold abscess.

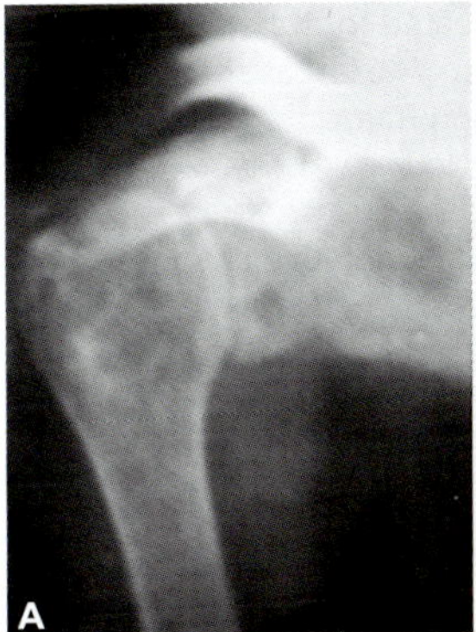

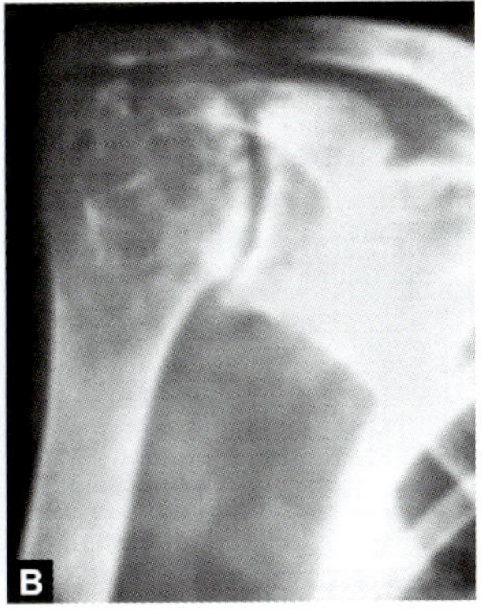

Figs. 11.2A and B: Advanced tubercular arthritis of right shoulder showing gross diminution of the joint space, irregular destruction of the joint margins and tuberculous cavities in the proximal humerus and scapular neck (A). The disease in (B) is in the process of healing as suggested by the lack of osteoporosis. The glenohumeral articulation is, however, developing ankylosis in a position of adduction; the long axis of humerus and the lateral border of scapula are forming an angle of 60 degrees despite attempted abduction while taking the X-ray

tuberculosis may be misdiagnosed as "caries sicca". Rheumatoid arthritis of the shoulder joint usually presents with marked soft tissue swelling and synovial effusion. Whenever there is doubt about the diagnosis the proof should be obtained by subjecting the biopsy of the diseased tissue, to bacteriological, histological and serological examination.

Radiologically, generalized rarefaction of bones is present with varying degree of erosion of articular margins or actual destruction of upper end of humerus or the glenoid. In a disease of long-standing one may observe concomitant destructive lesion is coracoid process and acromio-clavicular articulation **(Fig. 6)**. In the absence of sinus formation, little periosteal reaction is seen. In advanced cases, inferior subluxation of the humeral head may occur **(Fig. 11.1)**.

MANAGEMENT

In addition to the general treatment for skeletal tuberculosis, in adults with advanced disease the shoulder is immobilized by an abduction frame (orthosis) in 70–90 degrees of abduction, 30 degrees forward flexion and about 30 degrees of internal rotation (saluting position). Gross ankylosis of shoulder is expected on healing in patients with advanced disease. After about 3 months the abduction frame may be replaced by an arm-pouch sling and repetitive active/assisted movements of shoulder are encouraged. In an advanced disease when ankylosis is expected, the abduction orthrosis would achieve the angle between the lateral border of scapula and the long axis of humerus nearly 90–110 degrees in the X-rays taken in attempted abductions. After healed status most of such patients can manage all activities of daily living. If diagnosed at an early stage, one may obviate the use of abduction frame, arm-pouch sling provides relief of pain and permits functional range of exercises.

As a rule sufficient compensatory movements develop at the scapulothoracic articulation to permit all routine activities **(Figs. 11.3 and 11.4)**. Some patients with active lifestyle may develop symptomatic secondary osteoarthrosis during their middle-age **(Fig. 11.3)**. Generally, a sound fibrous ankylosis of the shoulder is obtained with a fair range of painless motion retained. Being a nonweight bearing joint a sound fibrous ankylosis is acceptable. If the ankylosis is painful or the disease is uncontrolled or in case of recurrence, excision-arthroplasty may be considered under exceptional circumstances.

Response to chemotherapy and splintage is as a rule favorable. Of the 12 shoulders treated by Martini et al. (1986), abduction obtained was <60 degrees in 3 cases, and 60 degrees or more in the remainder. One patient treated by excision did not gain more movement than others who were

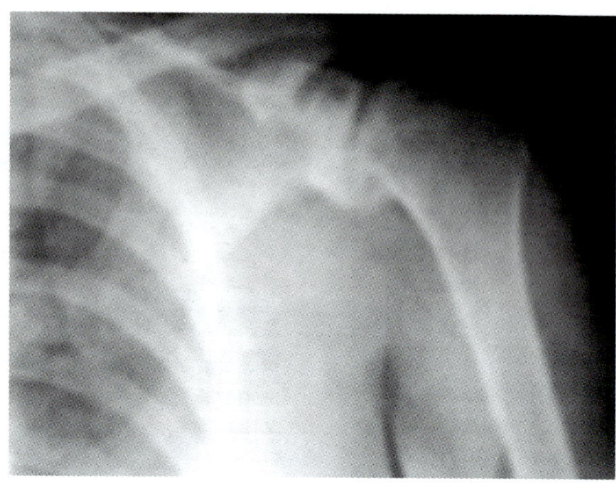

Fig. 11.3: A young man was treated for tuberculosis of left shoulder joint about 25 years ago. The disease had healed by drugs and splintage in abduction frame. He leads an active life as a travelling sales man. Now at 41 years he started having dull pain in the shoulder and the X-ray showed a healed status with secondary degenerative changes in the joint.

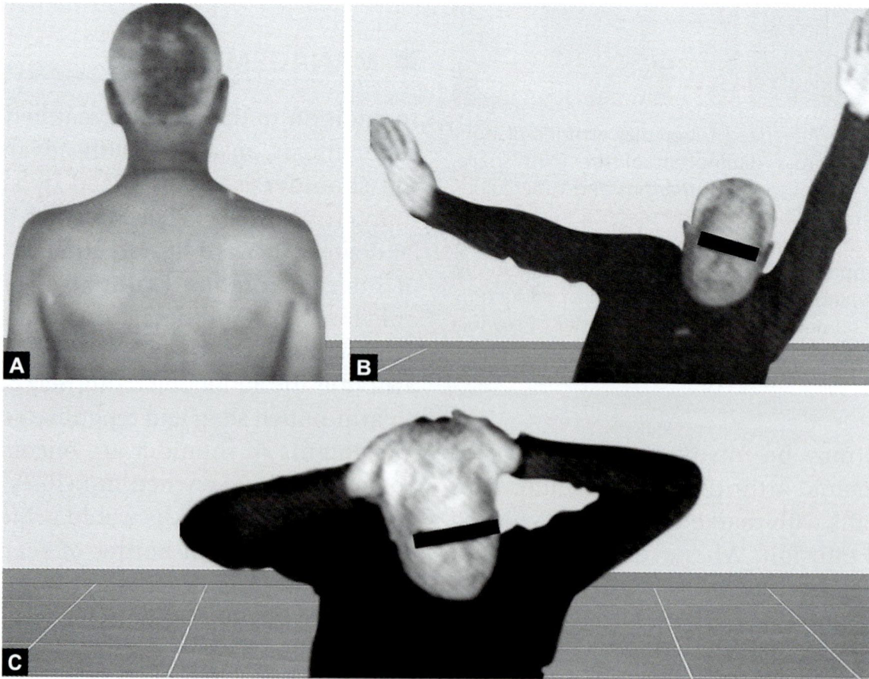

Figs. 11.4A to E: *Continued*

Continued

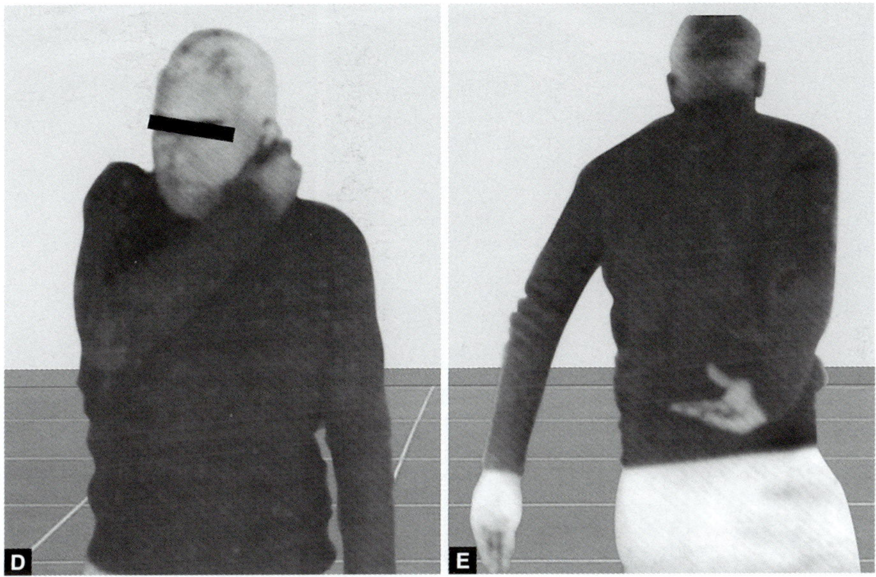

Figs. 11.4A to E: Clinical picture of tubercular arthritis of right shoulder treated by antitubercular drugs and abduction frame. Note (A) marked wasting of deltoid, supraspinatus and infraspinatus muscles, (B and C) Nearly 80 degrees of functional abduction, and very useful external rotation, (D) Internal rotation and adduction to reach face and opposite shoulder and (E) Partial capability of reaching the back of the trunk.

treated conservatively. Tang and Chow (1983) described 5 patients treated by chemotherapy alone. All achieved a healed status with satisfactory mobility of shoulder. Return of movements in the elderly is less **(Fig. 11.4)** as compared to younger patients, and in general external rotation remains limited beyond 20 degrees. During a period of 25 years (1965–1990), in 3 patients we had to revise the clinico-radiological diagnosis of tuberculosis of shoulder to neuropathic joint, villonodular synovitis and rheumatoid disease in one case each. Arthrodesis of shoulder is now indicated extremely rarely. Any palpable cold abscess may be aspirated with instillation of local streptomycin **(Figs. 11.5 and 11.6)**.

ARTHRODESIS OF SHOULDER

Extra-articular Arthrodesis

Before the availability of effective antitubercular drugs, bony fusion of the joint was obtained by an extra-articular operation carried out by inserting an autologous tibial strut graft (12–15 cm) between the scapula and humerus through a posterior approach. The angle formed by the axillary border of scapula and the humerus should be about 90–110 degrees. After the snug fit of the graft is assured, the limb is held in the desired position with the help of shoulder spica for 3–4 months.

Intra-articular Arthrodesis

With the availability of facilities for early diagnosis and effective drugs, indications for arthrodesis for tuberculosis of shoulder is currently seldom required. A brief description of the approach (Charnley and Houston 1964) is described here for the sake of completion. Position the patient in semi-reclining and semi-lateral position on the edge of the table. The incision is shaped like an inverted U, beginning anteriorly 4 cm inferior to the acromioclavicular joint. The incision passes upward along the anterior fibers of the deltoid muscle over the acromioclavicular joint and then posteriorly downward over the posterior

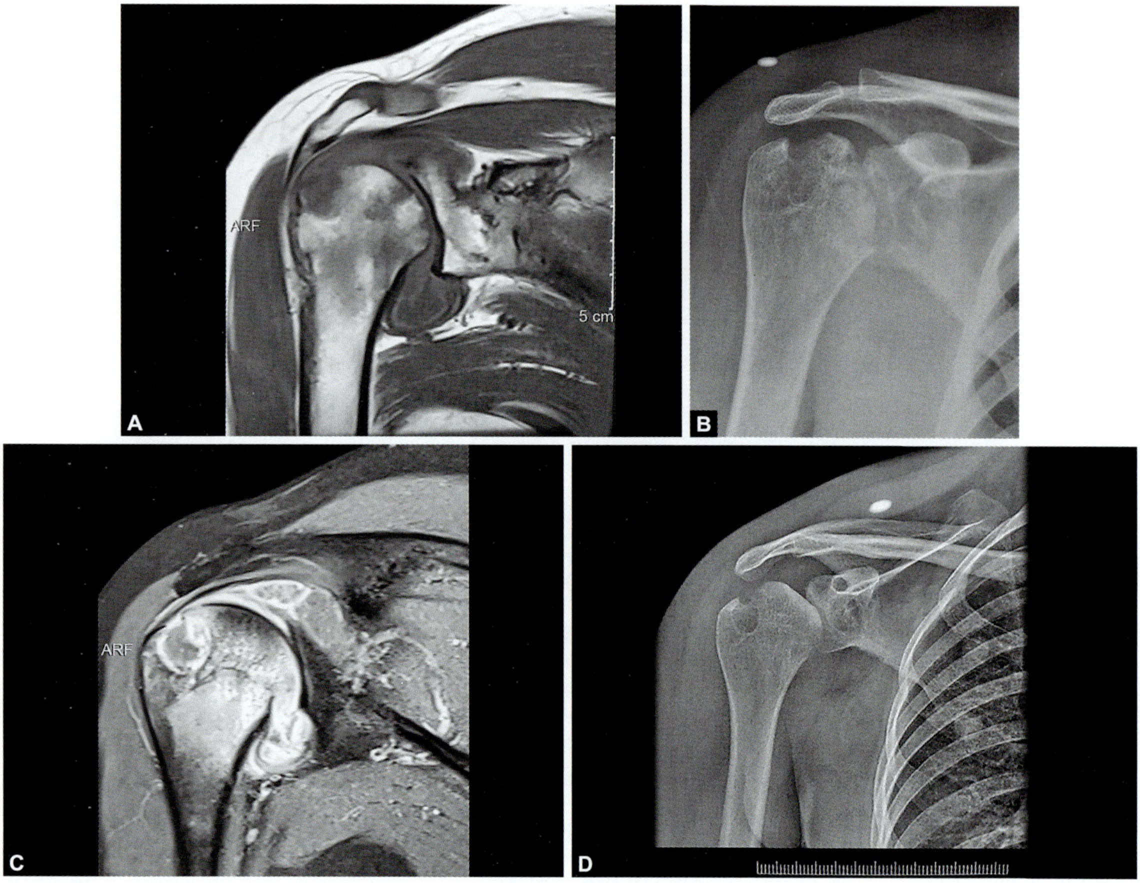

Fig. 11.5: (A) Tuberculosis of the right shoulder at presentation: Observe periarticular osteoporosis, eroded articular margins, destructive lesions in upper end of humerus and scapular neck area. MRIs (B and C) show destructive areas in upper end of humerus, scapular neck, and glenoid margins. Inflamed synovial membrane and fluid collection can be appreciated maximum in the inferior joint space. (D) One can appreciate the progressive healing when comparing with X-ray (A) at presentation. Clinical function on healing of infection **(Fig. 11.6)**.

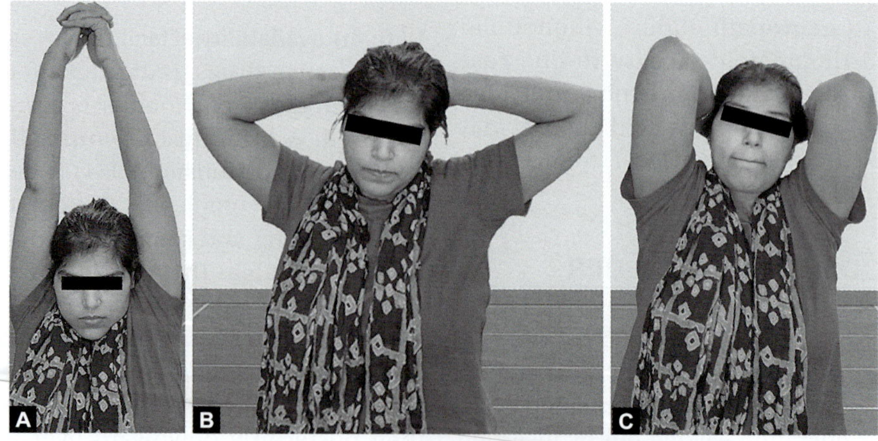

Fig. 11.6: Functional outcome of the patient with tuberculosis of her right shoulder. (A) Over-head flexion; (B) Abduction and external rotation; and (C) Adduction.

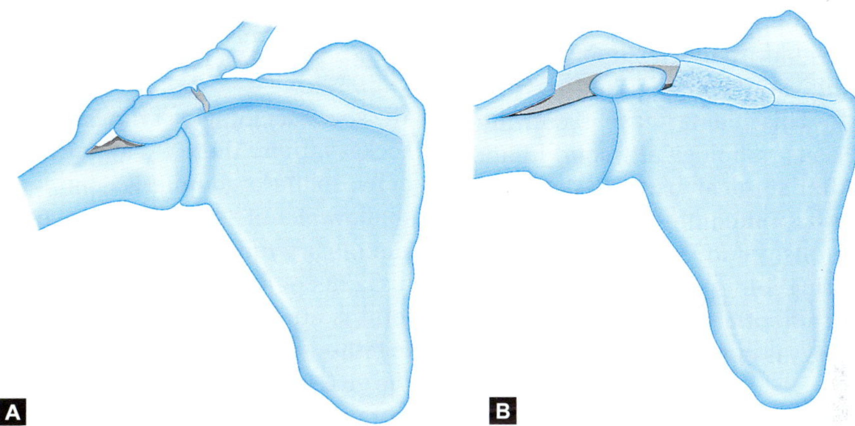

Figs. 11.7A and B: Diagrammatic representation of arthrodesis of shoulder as seen from the back. Note intra-articular arthrodesis supplemented by the osteotomized lateral ends of clavicle and acromion shoved into the slot made in the proximal humerus (A). The shoulder should be held in abduction with the long axis of the scapular spine and the long axis of humeral shaft almost parallel to each other (B).

fibers of the deltoid. A large flap of skin along with subcutaneous tissues is reflected laterally and backward to expose the deltoid muscle. The deltoid is cut near its origin and reflected distally. Osteotomize through the acromioclavicular articulation and freshen both the surfaces of the acromion up to its attachment to the scapular spine. Cut the capsule of shoulder joint transversely. Extend the incision on the capsule anteriorly and posteriorly while doing lateral and medial rotations of the humerus. To expose the humeral head, and the glenoid cavity, one may have to cut the insertions of supraspinatus, infraspinatus and subscapularis tendons. Denude the articular cartilage from the humeral head and the glenoid fossa and position the bones into the desired position for fusion **(Fig. 11.7)**.

Curet away any infective cavities in the exposed bones. With an osteotome split the upper end of humerus medial to the greater tuberosity to receive the acromion at a later stage. Now cut the acromion from the scapular spine without detaching the muscles and periosteum. Bring the humeral head into the desired position in the glenoid fossa, shove the acromion process into the slot made in the humeral head. Similarly, lateral third of the clavicle may also be freshened, osteotomized and shoved into the humeral head **(Fig. 11.5)**. While holding the shoulder in the desired position, insert two 4 mm Steinmann's pins, antero-posteriorly one through the neck of scapula and the other through the surgical neck of humerus, respectively. Connect the pins to the compression device for arthrodesis. If desired, additional bone grafts may be placed at the site of fusion. The wound is closed in layers over the suction tubes and the previously made shoulder spica cast is applied. Compression device is tightened daily for 3–4 weeks. At 4–5 weeks the pins, fixator, and stitches are removed and a new well-moulded shoulder spica in the optimum position is applied in standing posture of the patient.

The position of the shoulder for arthrodesis should be such as to allow the hand to reach the midline of the body in front and behind, to reach the face and ipsilateral trouser pocket (with the elbow flexed). Because of difficulty in measuring the exact position of scapula in relation to humerus at the time of surgery, a wide range of abduction (50–90°), forward flexion (20–90°) and rotations (internal rotation 25–90° by Wild et al. 1987, and external rotation 30–60° by Charnley 1953) have been advised **(Table 11.1)**. Holding the hand in saluting position, with the elbow in front of the trunk, and the long axis of arm almost in line or parallel with the long axis of the scapular spine offers a practical guide to the position of shoulder while operating, and while giving definitive shoulder spica. This plaster cast is continued until arthrodesis is radiologically solid in about 4–6 months. After surgical arthrodesis, osseous fusion is the usual outcome, however, in cases of failures a fibrous union is acceptable, being a nonweight bearing joint patients can do almost all work. Replacement arthroplasty for infective shoulder pathology is not advisable **(Fig. 11.8)**.

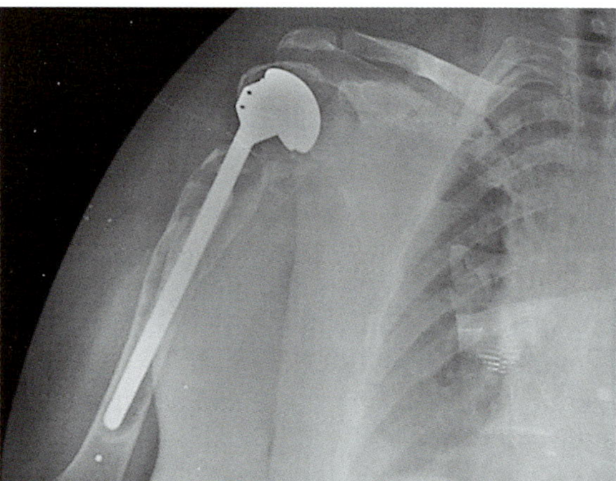

Fig. 11.8: Replacement arthroplasty performed in active disease resulted in perpetuation of infection. The infection spread to the whole of humerus. It is rational not to consider joint replacement earlier than 1–3 years of healed status of infection.

RELEVANT SURGICAL ANATOMY OF THE SHOULDER JOINT

The shoulder joint is a synovial joint of the ball and socket variety. There is a four to one disproportion between the large spherical humeral head and the shallow glenoid fossa. A ring of fibrocartilage, the glenoid labrum, attached to the margin of glenoid fossa deepens its depression. The capsule of the joint is attached to the scapula beyond (medial to) the supraglenoid tubercle (thus making the origin of the long head of biceps brachii intracapsular) and the margins of the labrum. On the proximal end of humerus, the capsule is attached around the articular margins of the head except inferomedially where its attachment is to the neck of the humerus 1 cm below the articular margin, thus making a part of the proximal humeral metaphysial region intracapsular. The capsule is thick and strong but very lax to permit freedom of movements. Near the humeral attachments, the capsule is greatly thickened by fusion of the tendons of subscapularis anteriorly, supraspinatus superiorly, infraspinatus and teres minor posteriorly (jointly forming rotator cuff). A gap in the anterior part of the capsule allows communication between the synovial membrane and the subscapularis bursa. A similar gap often present posteriorly permits communication with the infraspinatus bursa. The synovial membrane

Table 11.1: Recommended positions of shoulder arthrodesis.

Authors	*Abduction degrees*	*Flexion degrees*	*Rotation degrees*
Charnley (1953)	45	45	45 (ER)
Charnley and Houston (1964)	45	45	45 (IR)
May (1962)	65	60	40 (ER)
Raunio (1985)	30	30	30 (IR)
Rowe (1983, 1998)	20	30	40–50 (IR)
Johnson (1989)	20–30	20–30	20–30 (IR)

In clinical practice, holding the limb in saluting position provides a satisfactory guide to the "functional position" of the shoulder.
(ER: external rotation; IR: internal rotation)

lining the inner surface of the capsule, is attached around the glenoid labrum and to the articular margin of the humeral head, covers the bare area of the humeral shaft that lies within the capsule, and extends (up to the bicipital groove) as a sleeve along the long head of biceps tendon. A large subacromial (or subdeltoid) bursa lies under the coracoacromial ligament, it extends beyond the lateral border of acromion to lie under the deltoid with the arm at the side (or when the bursa is distended due to large effusion), but is withdrawn under the acromion when the arm is abducted. Any disease involving the synovium would easily extend to the communicating synovial prolongations and bursae.

The functional movements of the shoulder are the outcome of synchronous movements occurring at the glenohumeral and scapulothoracic articulations along with the consequential gliding movements of the clavicle. The "rotator cuff", long head of biceps and long head of triceps add stability to the joint, especially during movements. It is wise to appreciate that the medial epicondyle of humerus faces in the same direction (and a little backward) as the articular surface of the humeral head. Contrary to the femoral head the humeral head is retroverted by 30 degrees. The major movements that occur at the shoulder are flexion-extension, abduction adduction, rotations, and circumduction (the combination of all the above movements). Very broadly speaking, during the first 90 degrees of abduction-adduction and flexion-extension for every 3 degrees of movement at glenohumeral articulation one degree of movement is occurring at scapulothoracic articulation. The ratio is almost reversed for the movements beyond 90 degrees. With the glenohumeral articulation fused in the ideal position nearly 40% of the functional movements in all the directions can be carried out, at the scapulothoracic articulation, by the motor power of scapulothoracic muscles predominantly trapezius, serratus anterior and rhomboideus.

CHAPTER

12 Tuberculosis of the Elbow Joint

Tuberculous disease of the elbow constitutes nearly 2–5% of all cases of skeletal tuberculosis (Dhillon et al. 2012). The disease commonly starts from the olecranon or the lower end of humerus, sometimes the onset is synovial or from the upper end of radius. In developing countries, the diagnosis can be readily made on clinicoradiological bases. When in doubt the diagnosis requires to be confirmed by examination of the diseased tissue (Parkinson 1990).

The onset is generally insidious accompanied by pain, swelling and limitation of movements of the joint. In active stage, the joint is held in flexion, looks swollen **(Fig. 17.8D)**, is warm and tender. Swelling is maximally appreciated at the back of the elbow on both sides of olecranon and the triceps insertion. Movements are accompanied by pain and muscle spasm. Marked wasting of arm and forearm muscles is obvious. In our institution one of the consecutive 44 patients of tuberculous infection of elbow had bilateral involvement (Srivastava 1983). Supratrochlear and/or axillary lymph nodes are enlarged in nearly one-third of the patients. Sinuses or ulcers connected with the joint may form rarely. Nearly 5% of cases may present at a stage when the disease is synovial. Because of gravity the involved elbow joint may sometimes be held in extension.

Radiologically, areas of destruction can be seen commonly in the olecranon and/or lower end of humerus **(Figs. 12.1 and 12.2)**. During active stage, bones of the joint show generalized demineralization and fuzziness of joint margins. The changes in the X-rays may not be consistent with the degree of loss of movements **(Figs. 12.1 and 12.3)**. Some patients with or without sinuses may show subperiosteal new bone formation **(Figs. 12.1 and 14.1)** on the upper part of ulna (resembling spina ventosa), lower humerus or upper radius. Rarely due to marked destruction of ligaments and bone the elbow may develop a pathological posterior subluxation. In early stage of disease, the clinicoradiological features

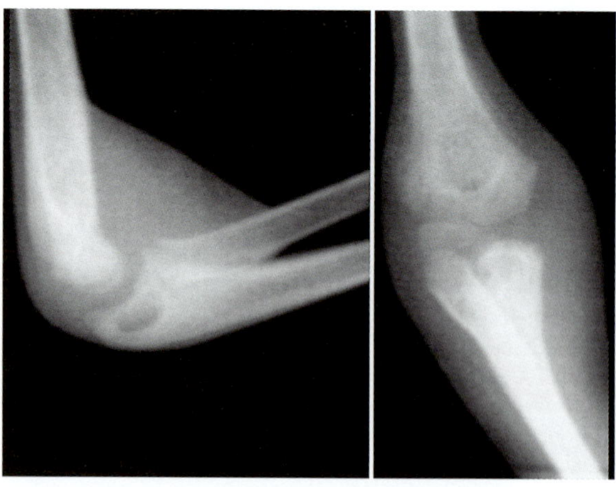

Fig. 12.1: Tuberculosis of the elbow showing slight irregularity of the articular margins, soft tissue swelling around the elbow, a lytic lesion in the olecranon, eroded radial head and mild subperiosteal bone formation on the distal humerus. The disease probably originated from the olecranon. The range of motion at presentation was 10 to 90 degrees of flexion.

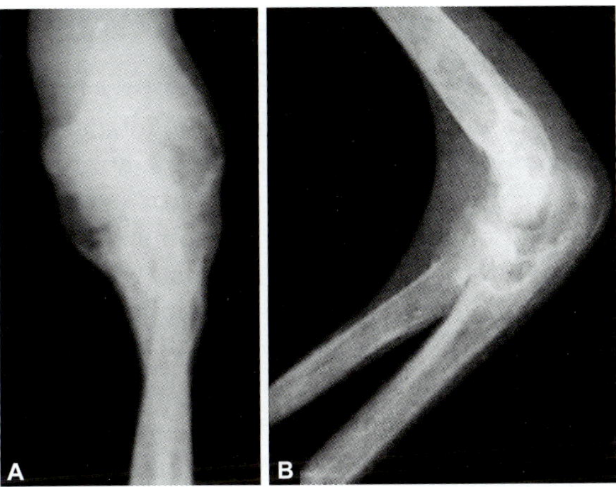

Figs. 12.2A and B: Tuberculosis of the elbow showing lytic lesions in the lateral condyle of humerus (A), Upper part of ulna and radius (B), Joint space is markedly reduced and there is some new bone formation on the medial side of ulna probably a result of superimposed pyogenic infection.

resemble any inflammatory condition. Whenever there is doubt in diagnosis examination of the diseased tissue is imperative.

MANAGEMENT

In addition to general treatment and systemic antitubercular drugs, the elbow is given rest in the best functional position. In a unilateral case, 90 degrees of flexion and midprone position of the forearm is advisable. If a patient with active disease presents with the elbow in extended or any awkward position, the joint should be gradually brought to neutral position by change of plaster at weekly intervals or by change of position under light anesthesia. In the initial stages one may use a strong removable plaster gutter which may be later replaced by removable polythene or metallic splint. As soon as the pain in elbow permits, active, assisted, repetitive flexion-extension and pronation-supination exercises are started. The splint (with the elbow held in 90 degrees and forearm in midprone position) is worn for 6–9 months in between the exercises and at bed time. After the removal of splint, one should avoid overuse of the joint for another 6–9 months.

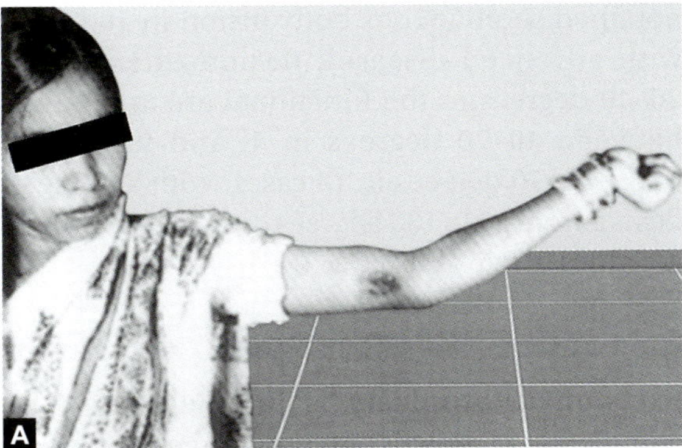

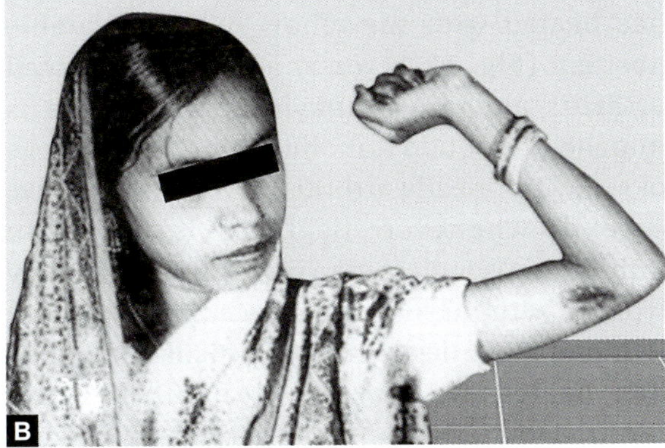

Figs. 12.3A and B: Clinical photographs of the same patient as in **Figure 12.2**. The patient was treated by removable posterior splint, repetitive active and assisted exercises in conjunction with antituberculous chemotherapy. The ulcer (abscess drained outside) and disease healed by 12 months with the range of movements from 30 to 120 degrees.

Functionally satisfactory results **(Fig. 12.3)** are obtained in a large majority with retention of good range of movements in the functional arc of the elbow (Martini et al. 1980, 1986, Srivastava 1983, Vohra 1995). Results are much better in cases of synovial disease, unicompartmental disease, or those of early arthritis. In advanced arthritis with involvement of all compartments of elbow, the end result is usually a gross fibrous ankylosis. In an unselected series, nearly 10% of cases would end up in a healed state with a range of movements that is <20 degrees. Of the 30 patients treated by a regimen of splintage, modern antitubercular drugs, and active repetitive exercises, Martini and Gottesman (1980) obtained spontaneous bony fusion in 10 (cases with advanced disease), flexion-extension of 20–40 degrees in the functional arc in 4, range between 40–70 degrees in 4, and functional range of >70 degrees in 18 cases. With a range of flexion from 30 to 130 degrees one can perform all activities of daily life.

Role of Operative Treatment

Excision arthroplasty is justified after the completion of growth potential when the disease has healed with the elbow in unacceptable position **(Fig. 12.4)**, or in a case of advanced arthritis and gross ankylosis where one is impelled to obtain a mobile joint. At the stage of synovitis or early arthritis, in a nonresponsive case or whenever diagnosis is uncertain arthrotomy is indicated to perform synovectomy with or without joint clearance. If the disease (without gross destruction of articular margins) has healed with gross fibrous ankylosis, "arthrolysis" (excision of contracted capsule and fibrous adhesions) may restore a useful arc of motion. Very rarely arthrodesis of the elbow is justified for heavy manual work.

OPERATIVE TECHNIQUES FOR TUBERCULOUS ELBOW

Elbow can be approached from the medial side, lateral side or through a posterior approach. In a badly ankylosed elbow with extensive destruction or disturbed anatomy, one can use simultaneously 2 incisions placed laterally and medially. It is wise to remember that the flexion crease of the elbow is 2–3 cm proximal to the actual level of elbow joint. The lateral and medial incisions are made in the line of the respective supracondylar ridges. Barring limited arthrotomy, synovectomy or operation essentially for a disease localized in the lateral compartment, a medial incision is preferred. The ulnar nerve should always be identified, exposed and retracted for protection during surgery, and anteriorly transplanted before closure.

Place the patient supine with the affected limb prepped and draped free. After exsanguination, tourniquet may be applied and a posteromedial longitudinal incision is made from about 4–5 cm proximal to and 5–6 cm distal to the tip of olecranon. The skin incision is curvilinear in the middle of the back of arm, on the medial border of

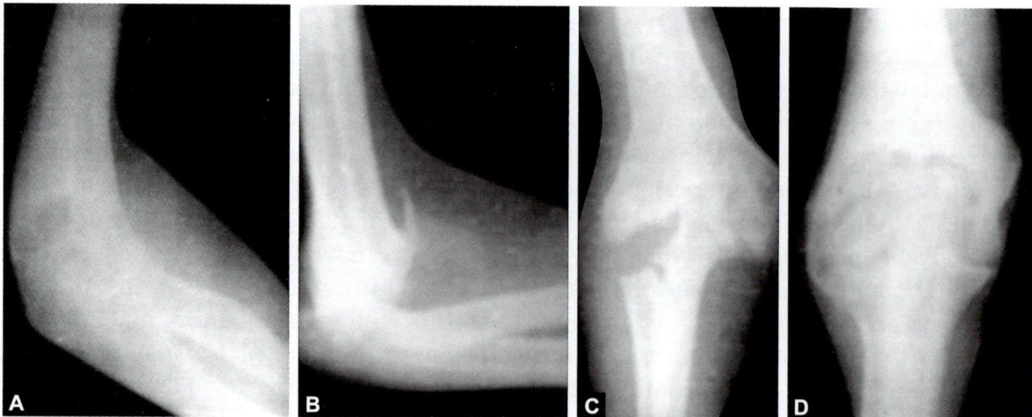

Figs. 12.4A to D: X-rays of an adult suffering from tuberculosis of right elbow. (A) At the time of presentation. (B) One year after antitubercular drugs, note radiological healing of the infection. The elbow, however, achieved fibrous ankylosis with a 10 degrees range from 80 to 90 degrees. Patient was keen to get a mobile elbow, an inverted-V excision arthroplasty was performed under antitubercular drugs umbrella. One year after the operation the patient obtained a range from 10 to 90 degrees (C and D).

the olecranon and along the dorsal border of the ulna. Skin flaps are retracted and the ulnar nerve exposed and protected on the medial side. Cut the triceps longitudinally in the middle up to the bone. Distally, reflect the triceps from its insertion on the ulna maintaining its continuity with the periosteum as a sheath. Reflect the triceps muscle medially and laterally subperiosteally exposing the lower end of humerus and upper ends of ulna and radius. Protect the anterior structures in the cubital fossa by inserting bone levers and/or large packs subperiosteally. Preserve medial and lateral collateral ligaments and the attached muscles as far as possible. Rotational movements of the forearm in various degrees of flexion of elbow would help access to considerable part of the joint. Remove diseased synovium, debris and sequestra, and curet the destroyed areas. This completes the operation of synovectomy with or without debridement. If it is an advanced disease with unacceptable ankylosis one should proceed with excisional arthroplasty.

Excisional Arthroplasty

Remove an inverted V-shaped segment of the lower end of humerus with apex of V reaching the olecranon fossa on the humerus, and preserving the supracondylar ridges, epicondyles, and collateral ligaments on medial and lateral sides **(Fig. 12.5)**. Upper end of ulna (rarely upper end of radius) should be sparingly trimmed of the diseased areas. Permit the proximal ends of radius and ulna to slide in the "inverted V of humerus". Close the wound under suction drainage and hold the joint in 90 degrees flexion and midprone position of forearm. We should

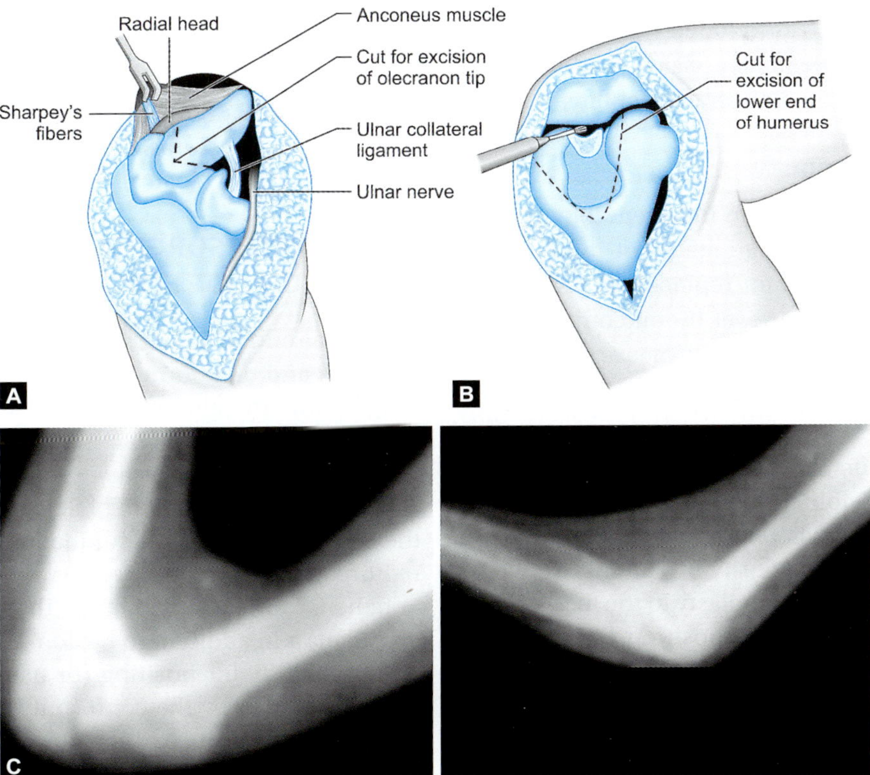

Figs. 12.5A to C: Inverted V-shaped excision-arthroplasty of the elbow. Note the anteriorly transposed ulnar nerve, the spared medial and lateral pillars (epicondyles, condyles, and supracondylar ridges) of lower humerus and limited resection of the upper end of ulna (A, and B). The operation is performed through the posterior approach with the elbow held across the chest. Two years after excisional arthroplasty the range of movements of the elbow joint was maintained from 45 to 130 degrees (C).

hold the ulna in some degree of distraction using a stout Kirschner wire inserted from the medial epicondyle through the upper part of ulna into the lateral supracondylar ridge. Kirschner wire and stitches are removed after 3–4 weeks. After 7–10 days of the removal, start intermittent repetitive active assisted flexion-extension and pronation-supination exercises. The use of splint for night wear must continue for 3–4 months. Permit light work with free elbow 2–3 months after surgery.

During 1965–1998, we performed the above described "inverted-V excision arthroplasty" in 10 adults (6 males and 4 females). The patients were followed up for 2–6 years, most of them maintained the healed status of disease and obtained a range of painless motion in the functional arc. Five had an average range of motion of 65 degrees, and 4 had the average range of 80 degrees. One developed reankylosis of the joint (due to inadequate excision) and none had flail joint due to mediolateral instability.

Elbow Arthroplasty

For gross ankylosis in an unacceptable position in an adult with healed status of infection for >1–3 years, elbow joint replacement is another option. In general, however, the outcome is not like the success stories of hip and knee arthroplasty.

Arthrodesis

Operative fusion of the elbow (essentially ulnohumeral joint) in tuberculous arthritis is rarely indicated where heavy manual strength is the primary aim, majority of patients, however, prefer a resection arthroplasty to the fused elbow. For unilateral disease a position of 90 degrees flexion is desirable. For a rare bilateral case, one elbow should be placed at 110 degrees flexion to reach the mouth and face and the other at 65 degrees to attend to personal body hygiene. The optimum position according to the occupation of the patient is best decided by the patient, by a "trial immobilization" of his elbow (for a few weeks) in the desired position with the help of a plaster cast before surgery.

Expose the elbow through a posterior incision as for excision arthroplasty and protect the ulnar nerve with tapes. Excise diseased and destroyed synovium, capsule and bone. Remove only the minimal amount of bone to retain adequate bone stock. Dislocate the ulnohumeral articulation and decorticate 4–6 mm of distal end of humerus. Excise the radial head proximal to the biceps tuberosity (to permit postoperative pronation-supination). Do appropriate trimming of the lower end of humerus and upper end of ulna to provide maximum contact of the rawed surfaces. Hold the elbow in the desired position and pack bone grafts in gaps around the site of fusion, one may insert two Kirschner wires (through humerus and ulna) for additional support. Transpose the ulnar nerve anteriorly, close the wound in layers over suction drainage.

Postoperatively, the limb is held in a strong posterior plaster slab for 3–4 weeks, sutures are then removed and a fresh elbow plaster cast in the best functional position is continued till the fusion is solid radiologically in 4–6 months.

RELEVANT SURGICAL ANATOMY OF ELBOW JOINT

The distal end of humerus and the upper ends of radius and ulna form the articulation that is a hinge joint. The elbow joint needs to provide a facility for the hand to reach upwards on the face and head, and downwards to the perineum and feet. A varied combination of flexion-extension of the elbow and pronation-supination of forearm is required to carry out a variety of working positions at bench, wall, table and farm. The humeroulnar articulation in addition to flexion-extension, also needs stability for pushing (or using crutches). This is provided by the conformity of the pulley-shaped trochlea which articulates with the moon-shaped concavoconvex deep trochlear notch of the upper end of ulna. The capitulum shaped like a portion of a sphere is situated on the lateral part of the distal end of humerus. It articulates with the proximal surface of the radial head during flexion-extension. The radial head is disc-shaped, covered with articular cartilage, concave on the upper surface, and lies completely within the synovial cavity. The periphery of the radial head articulates with the lateral surface of ulna at the radial notch during pronation and supination.

The capsule is attached to the distal humerus at the margins of the articular surfaces of capitulum and trochlea, but in front and behind it is carried upwards over the bone above the coronoid and olecranon fossae. Distally, it is attached to the margins of the articular cartilage of the trochlear notch of ulna, and to the annular ligament of the superior radioulnar joint.

The capsule and annular ligament are lined with synovial membrane, which is attached to the articular margins of all the 3 bones. The synovium thus floors in the coronoid and olecranon fossae on the distal end of humerus, bridges the gap between the radial notch of ulna and the neck of radius, thus establishing the communication between the elbow and superior radioulnar joints.

Immediately above the condyles on the medial and lateral aspects of the humerus are the epicondyles. The flexor-pronator muscle group originates from the medial epicondyle and medial supracondylar ridge. The extensor supinator group arises from the lateral epicondyle and lateral supracondylar ridge. Both the epicondyles are outside the synovial cavity and give attachment to respective collateral ligaments which provide stability by preventing mediolateral movements at the elbow joint.

The ulnar nerve runs posteriorly in a shallow groove behind the medial epicondyle of humerus, closely applied to the elbow capsule. Distally, it enters the forearm between the humeral and ulnar heads of the flexor carpi ulnaris, and proximally it runs upwards and enters the front of the arm through the medial intermuscular septum at the lower third of the arm. Ulnar nerve requires to be dissected and protected on a tape during any extensive surgical procedure on the elbow. During anterior transposition of the ulnar nerve, it is important to divide the lower end of the medial intermuscular septum, in the arm, otherwise the nerve may get kinked.

On the lateral side of the elbow, the radial nerve crosses the lateral supracondylar ridge about 8 cm proximal to the lateral epicondyle, then it runs distally in the interval between the brachioradialis (laterally) and the brachialis (medially). About 3–4 cm above the elbow joint, the radial nerve divides into two parts. Before dividing, the nerve supplies branches to the brachioradialis and the extensor carpi radialis longus. One division courses distally as the sensory nerve (radial nerve) and the other one named as posterior interosseous nerve passes distally between the superficial and deep bellies of the supinator muscle (about 1 cm distal to the radial head) to reach the dorsal aspect of the forearm. The radial nerve and particularly its posterior interosseous branch is vulnerable to ill-advised surgical exposures around the radial head and neck, resulting in paralysis of the long extensors of the fingers and thumb, and the extensors of wrist. Radial nerve must be dissected and protected on a tape during any extensive surgery on the lateral side of elbow. In front of the elbow, lies the brachialis muscle. Anterior to the brachialis muscle one can see and palpate biceps tendon proceeding distally to its insertion on the radial tuberosity. Medial to the biceps tendon is the neurovascular bundle consisting of the brachial artery and veins and more medially the median nerve. Relationships of these important structures must be borne in mind during any extensive surgical procedure on the elbow. Some degree of distortion of normal anatomy should be anticipated in cases with gross scarring and pathological dislocation or prior operations of the joint.

Two bursae lie in relation to the triceps insertion, one lies anterior to the triceps insertion between it and the upper surface of olecranon. The other lies superficially between the skin and the posterior surface of upper part of ulna. Other bursae have been described around the lateral collateral ligament. All or any of these bursae can get swollen and involved by infection, inflammatory or traumatic conditions.

CHAPTER 13

Tuberculosis of the Wrist

Tuberculosis of the wrist is a rare localization, it is more frequent in adults. The disease may start in the synovium but very soon gets disseminated in the whole carpus. A patient would rarely present before the disease has progressed to arthritis. Common sites for the primary osseous focus are the os capitatum or the distal end of radius **(Figs. 13.1 to 13.3)**. In addition to generalized carpal dissemination, the disease may spread to the neighboring flexor tendon sheaths or in extensor tendon sheaths. Most of the workers feel that the concomitant involvement of the flexor or extensor tendon sheaths is secondary to the tuberculous disease of the wrist. However, tuberculosis of the wrist joint secondary to the spread from tuberculous tenosynovitis also has been suggested by Martini (1988) and Leung (1978). Abscess and sinus formation, and regional lymph node enlargement are common.

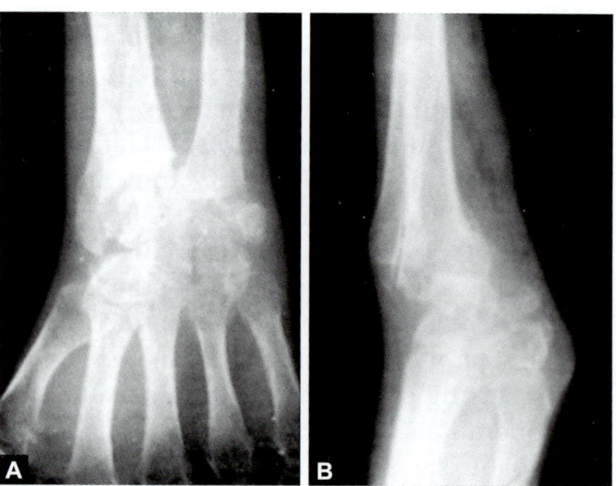

Figs. 13.1A and B: Tuberculosis of the wrist joint (Stage IV). Note gross destruction of all carpal bones, lower end of radius and inferior radioulnar joint. There is marked diminution of the radiocarpal and intercarpal joints, fuzziness of the joint margins and anterior subluxation of the wrist.

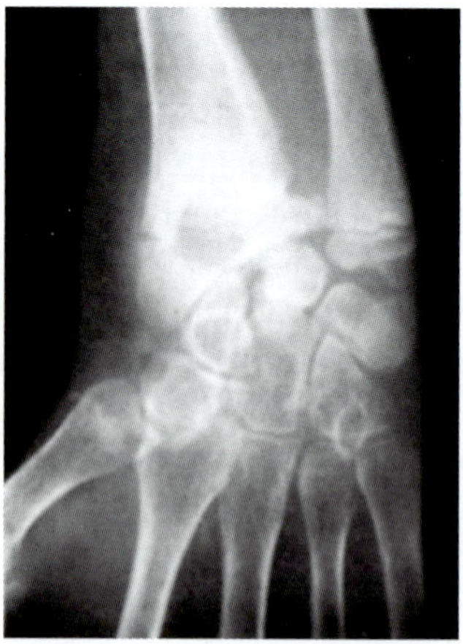

Fig. 13.2: A young lady presented with swelling around the wrist and this X-ray. On suspecting it to be a neoplastic lesion, biopsy was done in another institution which on histology proved to be tuberculous in nature. Note a classical lytic lesion sitting astride the epiphyseal cartilage plate, erosion on the ulnar border of radius and involvement of radiocarpal articulation. The patient achieved a healed status by drugs and splintage.

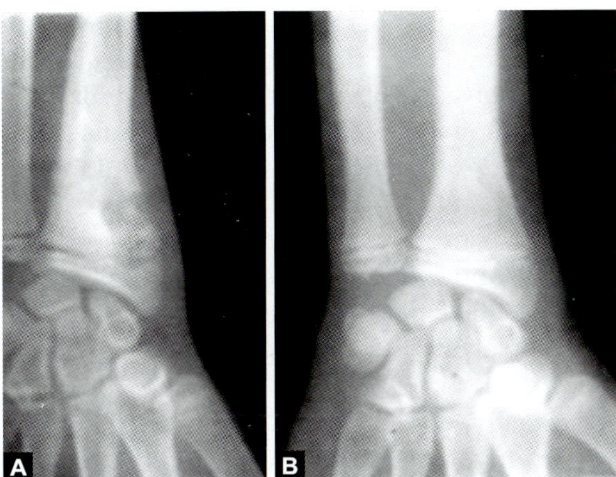

Figs. 13.3A and B: Juxta-articular tuberculous lesion in the distal radius. The lytic lesion is sitting astride the physis (A). There was complete resolution (B) of the lesion within 12 months by the use of antitubercular drugs.

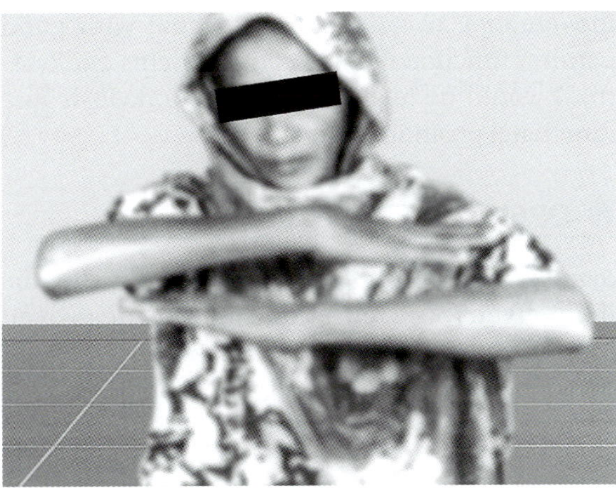

Fig. 13.4: Clinical photograph of the patient of tubercular arthritis of right wrist with anterior subluxation of the wrist joint (patient **Fig. 13.1**).

CLINICAL FEATURES

Clinical features as usual are pain, limitation of movements, swelling, tenderness, and usually a palmar flexion deformity. With the extension of disease into the distal radioulnar joint, pronation and supination is also limited. Further destruction of bones and ligaments leads to an anterior subluxation/dislocation at the radiocarpal articulation **(Figs. 13.1 and 13.4)**. Enlargement of supratrochlear and/or axillary lymph nodes is highly suggestive of an infective pathology. A case of monoarticular rheumatoid arthritis may strongly resemble tuberculosis. Rheumatoid disease may sometimes have regional reactive lymphadenopathy. Extremely rarely a patient may present at a very early stage when the X-rays may reveal (on comparison with the normal wrist) demineralization, marginal erosions and slight diminution of the joint space. Postero-anterior (PA view) X-rays of both wrists with ulnar deviation provide us maximum information especially in early stages of any disease/disorder. Confirmation of the diagnosis from the diseased tissue is mandatory whenever there is doubt about the nature of pathology.

MANAGEMENT

The treatment is essentially chemotherapy, correction of deformity and splintage of the wrist in 10–15 degrees of dorsiflexion and forearm in midprone position. Immobilization in the initial active stages of disease may be by a plaster of Paris cast which may be replaced by a leather/plastic/metallic corset. In the tuberculous disease without subluxation/dislocation, intermittent active exercises for the wrist, hand, and forearm should be encouraged out of the splint as soon as the pain permits. The splintage is continued in between the exercises and at bed time for about 12 months to minimize collapse of bones and to avoid deformity. Heavy physical work like hammering, weight-lifting, kneading should be avoided for about 2 years. In patients with subluxation/dislocation, the anticipated result is a healed status with gross ankylosis. In such patients, a well-fitting splintage ensuring 10–15 degrees of dorsiflexion and midprone position of forearm should be continued for 12–18 months or till the development of ankylosis, whichsoever is earlier. In unselected patients treated by modern anti-tuberculous drugs and functional movements, two-thirds would heal with good painless functional range of movements and one-third would be healed with gross ankylosis in a functional position.

OPERATIVE TREATMENT

Synovectomy of the joint (and tendon sheaths if involved) and curettage of the destroyed areas may be indicated in nonresponsive cases or whenever there is doubt in diagnosis. In a case of advanced disease having ankylosis in an awkward position, or when the ankylosis is painful, or if there is a history of recrudescence of infection, arthrodesis of the wrist in the optimum functioning position (10–15 degrees of dorsiflexion, 5 degrees of radial deviation and midprone position of forearm) is the treatment of choice. With the availability of effective antitubercular drugs and application of sound orthopedic splintage, surgical intervention is rarely indicated (Hodgson 1972, Leung 1978).

WRIST ARTHRODESIS

With the upper limb resting on an arm-board, 6–8 cm long incision is made on the dorsum of the wrist centering over the lower end of radius, carpus and the third metacarpal. Subcutaneous tissue and extensor tendons are retracted, periosteum and capsule cut to expose the underlying bones. The diseased tissue, synovium, and articular cartilage are removed as far as possible and a gutter/trough is made on the dorsal surface of radius, lunate, capitate, and proximal part of the third metacarpal. It is wise to excise 1.5–2 cm of distal shaft of ulna, proximal to the inferior radioulnar joint to create a gap pseudarthrosis in distal fourth of ulna by performing Darrach's like procedure; this helps maintain a useful painless range of pronation-supination even after the fusion of wrist joint. Distal articular end (1–2 cm) of ulna is left in situ to retain the shape of wrist joint. About 5 cm long cortico-cancellous bone graft removed from the iliac crest is snuggly fitted into the gutter. The convex edge of the graft is slotted into the prepared bed to fix the wrist in 10–15 degrees of dorsiflexion and 5 degrees of radial deviation. This may be supplemented by additional grafts (from ulna) and fixation devices if needed. The wound is sutured and the wrist is plastered in functional position in an above the elbow plaster for nearly 2 months. Above elbow plaster is then replaced by a below elbow plaster cast or polythene/metallic wrist corset till clear radiological evidence of bony ankylosis.

RELEVANT SURGICAL ANATOMY OF THE WRIST

The wrist joint is formed by the proximal row of carpal bones scaphoid, lunate, triquetral (from lateral to medial) and the distal surface of radius. The fibrocartilage between the radius and ulna is within the joint. The synovial space between the radiocarpal, intercarpal and carpometacarpal articulations should be considered as continuous freely intercommunicating channels. The anatomical snuff box is formed by abductor pollicis longus and extensor pollicis brevis anterolaterally, and extensor pollicis longus posteromedially. Tenderness in the distal part of snuff box incriminates the first carpometacarpal joint and the trapezium, the tenderness in the proximal part, especially with the wrist in ulnar deviation incriminates scaphoid. The oblique course of extensor pollicis longus around the radial tubercle makes it vulnerable to a careless operative incision on the dorsum of wrist. In flexion-extension movements, the functional movements of the hand are dorsiflexion about 45 degrees and palmar flexion about 90 degrees, approximately first two-thirds occur at radiocarpal joint and the final one-third occur at midcarpal joint. Os capitatum situated in the distal row of carpus is the largest carpal bone which may explain its most frequent involvement by the tuberculous infection. Stability of the wrist depends not only upon the conformity of bones but also upon the capsule and ligaments. The volar radiocarpal ligaments are the most important, and if destroyed by the infective process anterior subluxation/dislocation of the wrist occurs **(Figs. 13.1 and 13.4)**.

It is worth recalling that the most useful movement of the wrist is one of dorsiflexion combined with radial deviation, and of palmar flexion combined with ulnar deviation. Everyday activities like hammering, eating, washing, writing, etc., illustrate these facts. The strongest grip is made with 10–15 degrees of dorsiflexion combined with 5–10 degrees of radial deviation.

On their anterior aspect, the carpal bones form a concavity roofed over by the carpal ligament/flexor retinaculum. The carpal tunnel, thus formed, permits passage to the tendons of flexor digitorum superficialis and profundus, and tendons of flexor carpi radialis and flexor pollicis longus. The median nerve passes between flexor digitorum superficialis (medially) and flexor carpi radialis (laterally). The palmar branch of the median nerve (to the thenar muscles) is in danger if during section of the flexor retinaculum the incision is taken too far radial-wards. Marked inflammatory edema in front of the wrist, tense swelling of flexor tendon sheaths and pathological subluxation/dislocation of the wrist joint may cause symptoms of median nerve irritation. The position of ulnar nerve on the radial side of pisiform bone must be borne in mind while operating in that region.

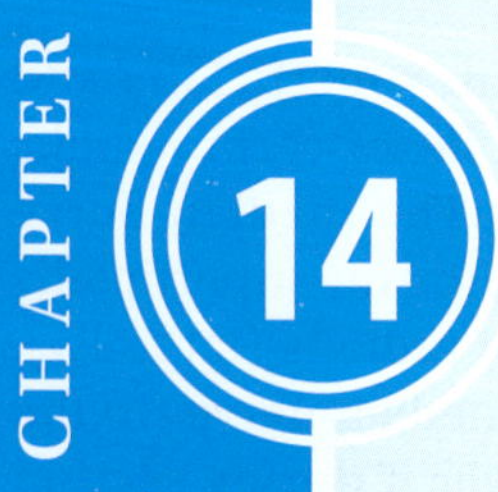

Tuberculosis of Short Tubular Bones

Tuberculosis of the metacarpals, metatarsals, and phalanges is uncommon after the age of 5 years. In children, the disease may occur in more than one short tubular bone at a time. Tuberculous infection of metacarpals, metatarsals, and phalanges of hands and feet is also known as tuberculous dactylitis. The description here is applicable to all cases of tuberculous dactylitis. The hand is more frequently involved than the foot. There are not many reports devoted to tuberculous dactylitis (Benkeddache and Gottesman 1982, Leung 1978, Martini 1988, Bavadekar 1982).

During childhood, these short tubular bones have a lavish blood supply through a large nutrient artery entering almost in the middle of the bone. The first inoculum of the infection is lodged in the center of the marrow cavity and the interior of the short tubular bone is converted virtually into a tuberculous granuloma. This leads to a spindle-shaped expansion **(Fig. 14.1)** of the bone (*spina ventosa). With occlusion of the nutrient artery of the involved bone and the destruction of internal lamellae (or formation of sequestra), there is endosteal destruction and concomitant subperiosteal new bone formation; successive layers of subperiosteal new bone formation are deposited over the involved bone. Abscess and sinus formation is quite common leading to secondary infection and further thickening of bone **(Fig. 14.2)**. In the natural course, the disease heals with shortening of the involved bone (when the physis is damaged) and deformity of the neighboring joint. Radiologically, the affected bone appears expanded with a lytic lesion in the middle and subperiosteal new bone deposited along the involved bone. The cavity may contain soft coke-like sequestra. Radiologically, in spina ventosa the bone may take the shape of honey combing, diffuse uniform infiltration, or of a cystic lesion, or rarely the involved bone may show atrophy.

DIFFERENTIAL DIAGNOSIS

Tuberculous dactylitis requires to be differentiated on one hand from chronic pyogenic osteomyelitis and syphilitic dactylitis, and on the other hand from neoplastic conditions with lytic lesions (e.g., enchondromata or fibrous defects). Other rare granulomatous conditions which may mimic tuberculous infection are mycotic infections, sarcoidosis, and brucellosis. Whenever in doubt serological, histological, and bacteriological investigations are mandatory to confirm the pathology.

*Spina ventosa is a Latin expression; spina = short bone, ventosa = inflated with air.

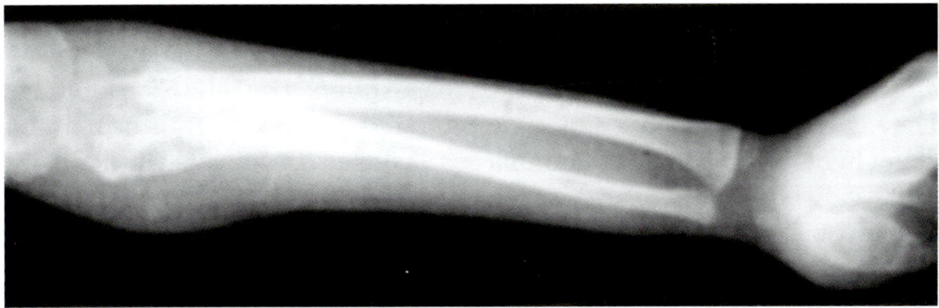

Fig. 14.1: Tuberculosis of fifth metacarpal in a child. There is also involvement of proximal ulna. Note the cystic lesions, central lucency, expansion of bone and soft tissue swellings. Multiple cystic type of tuberculosis was described by Jungling as "osteitis tuberculosa multiplex cystoides".

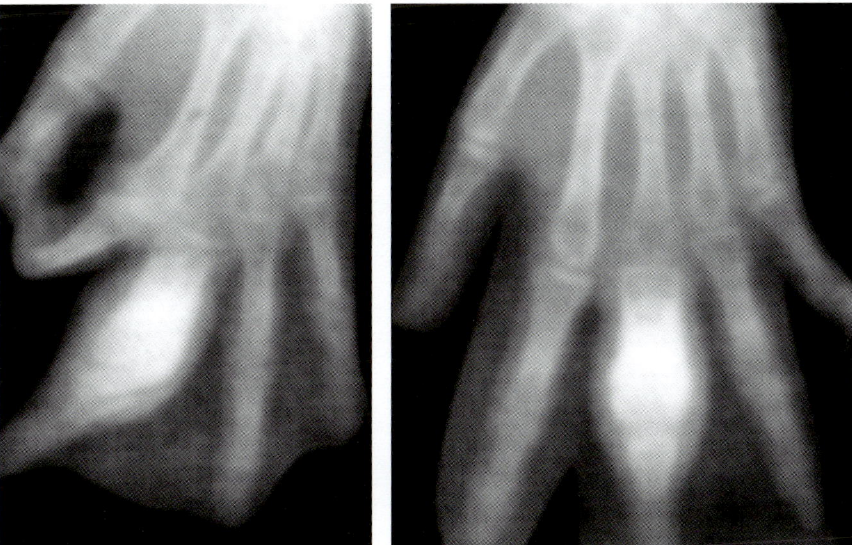

Fig. 14.2: Tuberculous dactylitis of middle finger involving its proximal and middle phalanges, showing cystic cavity (wind-blown widening) and involvement of intervening joint. Thickening and sclerosis of bone was accentuated due to sinus formation and secondary infection.

TUBERCULOSIS OF THE JOINTS OF FINGERS AND TOES

The lesion may develop either in the juxta-articular bone or in the synovium. Primary lesion in the bone seems more frequent. Involvement of the finger joints is more common than those of toe joints, and in general metacarpophalangeal/ metatarsophalangeal joints are involved more frequently than the distal joints.

Like tubercular arthritis in general the clinical development of the disease is slow and insidious. The patient presents with a spindle-shaped swelling of the joint and flexion deformity; the swelling is boggy, warm and tender, movements of the joint are restricted. Enlarged regional lymph nodes, cold abscess and sinuses (usually on dorsal aspect) may be present. Radiologically, in addition to the changes in the bones, the articular ends may show osteoporosis, erosion of joint margins, destruction of bones and subluxation. Destruction of physis and pathological fracture are not unusual.

Subacute pyogenic arthritis or rheumatoid arthritis have to be considered in differential diagnosis. In countries where typical mycobacterial disease is disappearing, atypical (non-typical) mycobacterial infections due to *Mycobacterium kansasii* or *marinum* have been reported (Chow et al. 1987, Lacy et al. 1989). Such lesions are relatively frequent in hand, and history of trauma from marine life can be obtained on leading questions in majority of such patients.

Management is essentially by antitubercular drugs, rest to the part in functioning position and early active exercises of the involved parts or joints. In patients with unfavorable response or with recurrence of infection, surgical debridement is justified. If a metacarpophalangeal, metatarsophalangeal or interphalangeal joint is ankylosed in an awkward position, excision arthroplasty or corrective osteotomy is indicated. Rarely if a finger has ankylosis of more than one joint, is grossly deformed, scarred and interfering with the normal functioning of the adjacent rays, it may be wise to amputate the finger.

Tuberculosis of the Sacroiliac Joints and Sacrum

Sacroiliac joint is a true synovial joint, and therefore subject to tuberculous infection like any other joint. The disease may originate in the lateral masses of sacrum, from the ilium or from the synovial membrane. Rarely the disease may spread from or coexist with tuberculosis of lower lumbar vertebrae or ipsilateral hip disease. Children are seldom affected; however, the disease is relatively more common in women of child-bearing age. In patients with poor nutritional status, the disease may be not infrequently bilateral. The overall frequency varies between 1–5% (Silva 1980, Shanmugasundaram 1983, Martini 1988, Ramlakan and Govender 2007). In an analysis of 69 cases of tuberculosis of sacroiliac joints (Tuli and Sinha 1969), the female to male ratio was 5:2, and associated tuberculous foci (as observed by conventional X-rays) were present in 50% of patients. The mortality rate was 33% before the availability of antituberculous drugs.

CLINICAL FEATURES

The disease takes an insidious course and the patient has persistent pain localized to the diseased area. Rarely the pain may present with a sciatic radiation. The pain is more on prolonged walking and sitting, and worse while sleeping supine or turning in bed. The pain on sitting and standing gets relieved on shifting the weight (leaning away) to the contralateral normal buttock or normal leg, respectively. **Goldthwait's sign** is positive, i.e., in recumbent position, distraction of both sacroiliac joints by simultaneous pressure exerted on both anterosuperior iliac spines causes pain, in majority of the cases with active disease. Stressing the sacroiliac joint with forced flexion, abduction and external rotation of the ipsilateral hip joint **(Faber test)** is another method to elicit sacroiliac pain.

Local examination reveals moderately increased temperature, tenderness to local pressure or percussion, and there may be an abscess or a sinus present. Rarely the abscess or sinus may present in the gluteal region, iliac fossa, groin or track down in front of the sacrum to present in the perineal region, or the abscess may spread through the greater sciatic notch following the course of sciatic nerve. Before the availability of modern imaging modalities the diagnosis was often delayed and tuberculosis of sacroiliac joint was considered a serious disease with a high mortality, and such patients looked ill.

Radiographs are not helpful in early stages, but in due course would show fuzziness and erosions of the joint margins, osseous destruction and thickening in the adjacent sacrum and/or iliac bones and widening of joint space. Tomography or modern imaging techniques are particularly of value in detecting early joint erosions and cavitations in the region of sacroiliac joints **(Figs. 15.1 to 15.5)**. Comparative X-rays, tomograms or MRIs of both the sides are imperative in the initial stages. Ankylosing

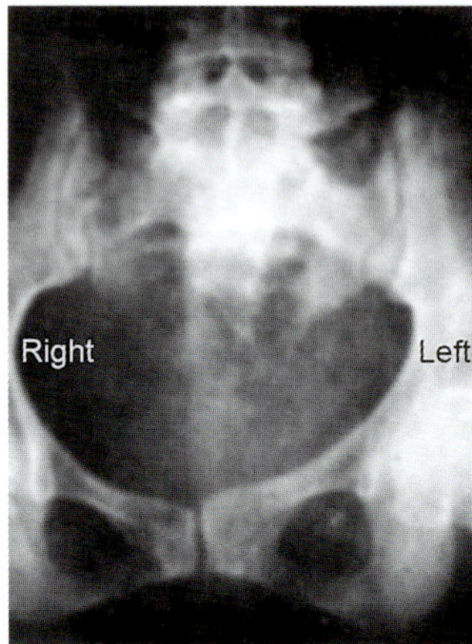

Fig. 15.1: A large destructive lesion due to tuberculosis in the left half of sacrum. The patient had cold abscess at the back of sacrum. Small lesions are best diagnosed by CT scan and MRI.

spondylitis in early stages, rheumatoid disease, pyogenic infection, and juxta-articular neoplastic lesions should be considered in differential diagnosis. In patients with concomitant involvement of symphysis pubis, the pelvic bone may show upward subluxation. Pouchot et al. (1988) emphasized that high suspicion index must be maintained to diagnose this supposedly uncommon disease in the affluent society. While analyzing 11 consecutive patients the disease was confirmed by closed needle biopsy in 9 cases, by histology and/or microbiology.

MANAGEMENT

Conservative treatment as for lower lumbar disease gives satisfactory outcome. In early stages

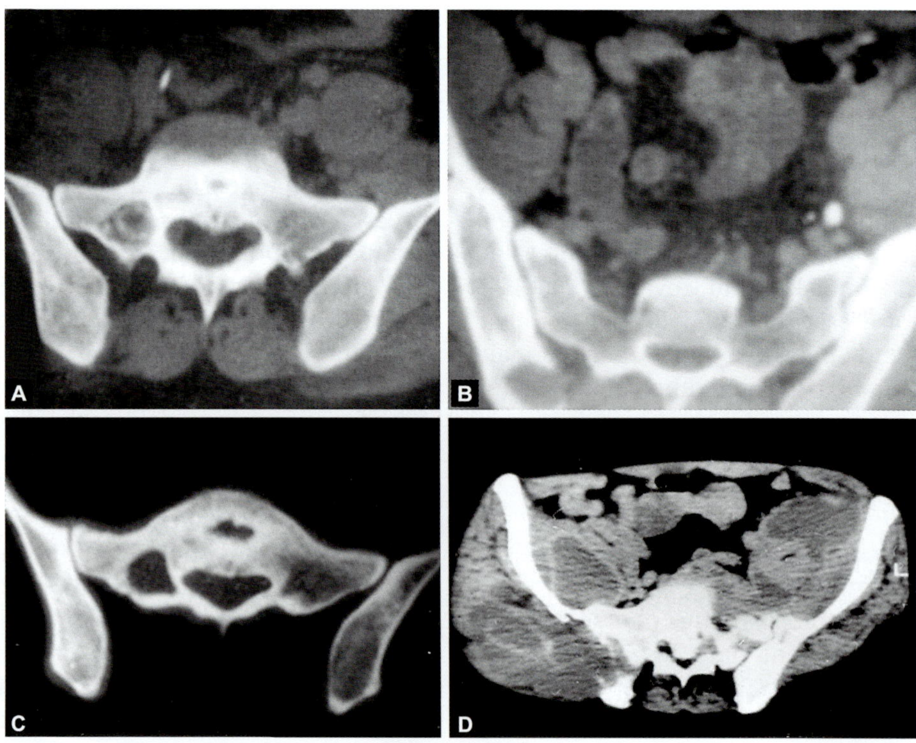

Figs. 15.2A to D: The CT-scan appearance of tuberculosis of sacroiliac region. Note the destructive cavities in the right ala of sacrum (A), posterior end of right iliac bone (B), and the body and right part of sacrum (C). Destruction of left half of sacrum with cold abscesses on the anterior aspect; and destruction of posterior part of right iliac bone with cold abscesses in front and back (D).

when the disease is active and painful, antitubercular drugs and recumbency is indicated. With relief of pain the patient is permitted ambulation wearing a low lumbosacral brace or a corset. The brace and antitubercular drugs are continued for 18–24 months. Most cases heal within this period by spontaneous bony fusion or a sound fibrous healing. With clinical awareness and availability of modern imaging modalities extensive surgery is seldom indicated. Operative treatment has been suggested by Tian et al. 2022.

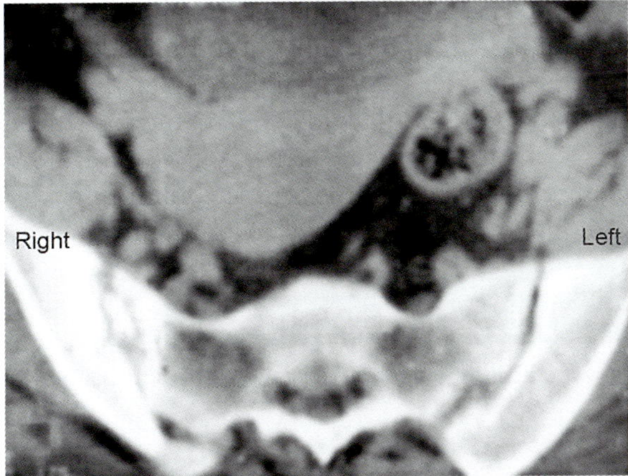

Fig. 15.3: Clinically and radiologically suspected case of tuberculosis of right sacroiliac joint. The CT scan confirms the diagnosis of tuberculous process, note the destruction of sacral and iliac joint surfaces on the right side, irregularity and sclerosis of the joint margins and a soft sequestrum contained within the destroyed area.

Operative Debridement and Arthrodesis of Sacroiliac Joint

Operative treatment is only indicated in refractory cases, in cases of recrudescence, or whenever the diagnosis is in doubt. With the patient in prone, or lateral position with the diseased side upward, make a semilunar incision along the posterior one-third of the iliac crest. Cut skin and subcutaneous tissues and expose about 8 cm of posterior part of the iliac bone by reflecting the fibers of gluteus maximus. After retraction of the skin margins, incise up to the bone the origin of gluteus maximus muscle from the iliac crest, the aponeurosis of the sacrospinalis from the sacrum, and reflect it (gluteus maximus) laterally and distally to expose the posterior aspect of the ilium. With an osteotome or an oscillating saw cut 1–2 cm wide full thickness quadrangular segment of the ilium, beginning at its posterior border between the posterosuperior and posteroinferior iliac spines. The length of the segment is 3–5 cm laterally and slightly cephalad. The inferior border of this section is almost parallel to the superior border of the sciatic notch. Avoid entering the sciatic notch. Reflect the bone block laterally, if

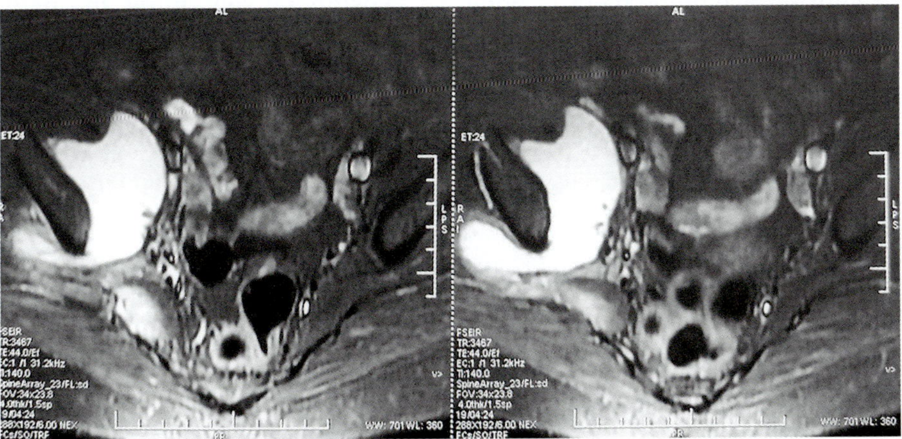

Fig. 15.4: Typical MRI images of a patient having tuberculosis of right sacroiliac joint, cold abscess can be seen on both surfaces of iliac bone.

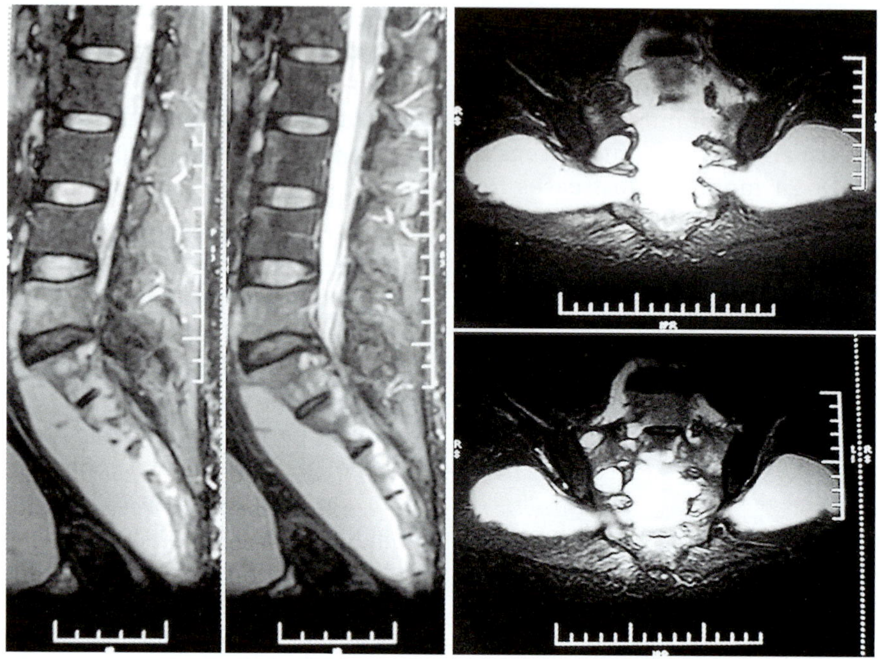

Fig. 15.5: Cold abscess from tuberculous infection of sacrum showing its location in presacral area and it's tracking both sides through the greater sciatic foramina.

possible on a muscular pedicle. All tuberculous material from the sacroiliac joint now exposed is removed with the help of sharp curette, gouges and nibblers. Any remaining articular cartilage, synovium, ligaments from the joint surfaces are removed from the sacral surface of the joint and also from the joint surface of the block of bone reflected laterally. Freshen the surfaces on the sacrum, counter-sink the iliac block of bone into the prepared bed on the sacrum. Osteotomize the edges of the window and turn the fragments inward as rose-petals to cover the margins of the reposed iliac block of bone. If there are gaps between the iliac block of bone and its bed in the sacrum, pack the gaps with cancellous bone grafts obtained from the neighboring iliac crest. Stitch the soft tissues in layers.

Postoperatively, nurse the patient on firm bed for 6–8 weeks. The patient may be permitted limited ambulation wearing a moulded brace as the pain subsides. The brace is worn till clear osseous fusion of the joint is seen radiologically.

Tuberculosis of Rare Sites, Girdle and Flat Bones

Infection of sacroiliac, hip and shoulder joints are described in appropriate sections. However, other bones and joints of the girdle regions also get involved by tuberculosis rarely (Manjul 2000, Babhulkar 2002). At early stage of infection, prior to the formation of a cold abscess or sinuses, the disease can be suspected only by MRI or CT scan.

STERNOCLAVICULAR JOINT

It is an extremely rare location. The condition usually starts from the medial end of clavicle. The patient presents with a painful swelling of insidious onset in the sternoclavicular joint. The swelling is warm, tender and boggy. There may be a cold abscess or sinus formation. Radiologic signs are not easy to discern. Tomograms or MRI of the diseased and normal side for comparison may be able to show osseous destruction of clavicle, and sternum, and soft tissue collection. Whenever in doubt, examination of the aspirate or surgically excised diseased tissue is of great help. Common conditions in differential diagnosis are low grade pyogenic infection, rheumatoid disease, myeloma, or secondary deposits. Treatment is essentially by antituberculous chemotherapy.

ACROMIOCLAVICULAR JOINT

This location is extremely uncommon. The disease may start from the lateral extremity of the clavicle or from the tip of the acromion. The signs, symptoms, differential diagnosis and treatment is like that of sternoclavicular joint **(Fig. 16.1)**.

TUBERCULOSIS OF CLAVICLE

Tuberculosis of the clavicle without involvement of the neighboring joints can be seen rarely. Most of the patients are children presenting with painful swelling of the clavicle associated with formation of cold abscess or sinuses. X-rays may show diffuse thickening and honeycombing, or multiple cystic cavities, or sequestration not unlike pyogenic infections **(Figs. 16.1 and 16.2)**. Treatment is essentially antitubercular drugs. Surgical excision may be rarely justified when diagnosis is uncertain, or disease is unresponsive or for removal of a large sequestrum. Large parts of clavicle can be excised without loss of function (Srivastava et al. 1974).

We had an opportunity to observe 7 patients of tuberculosis of clavicle with or without the involvement of the neighboring joint (Tuli and Sinha 1969). The incidence of involvement worked out to be <1% of all skeletal tuberculosis. The location was sternal end in 4, diaphyseal segment in 2, and acromial end in one case.

TUBERCULOSIS OF SCAPULA

Isolated involvement of scapula without involvement of shoulder joint can be rarely

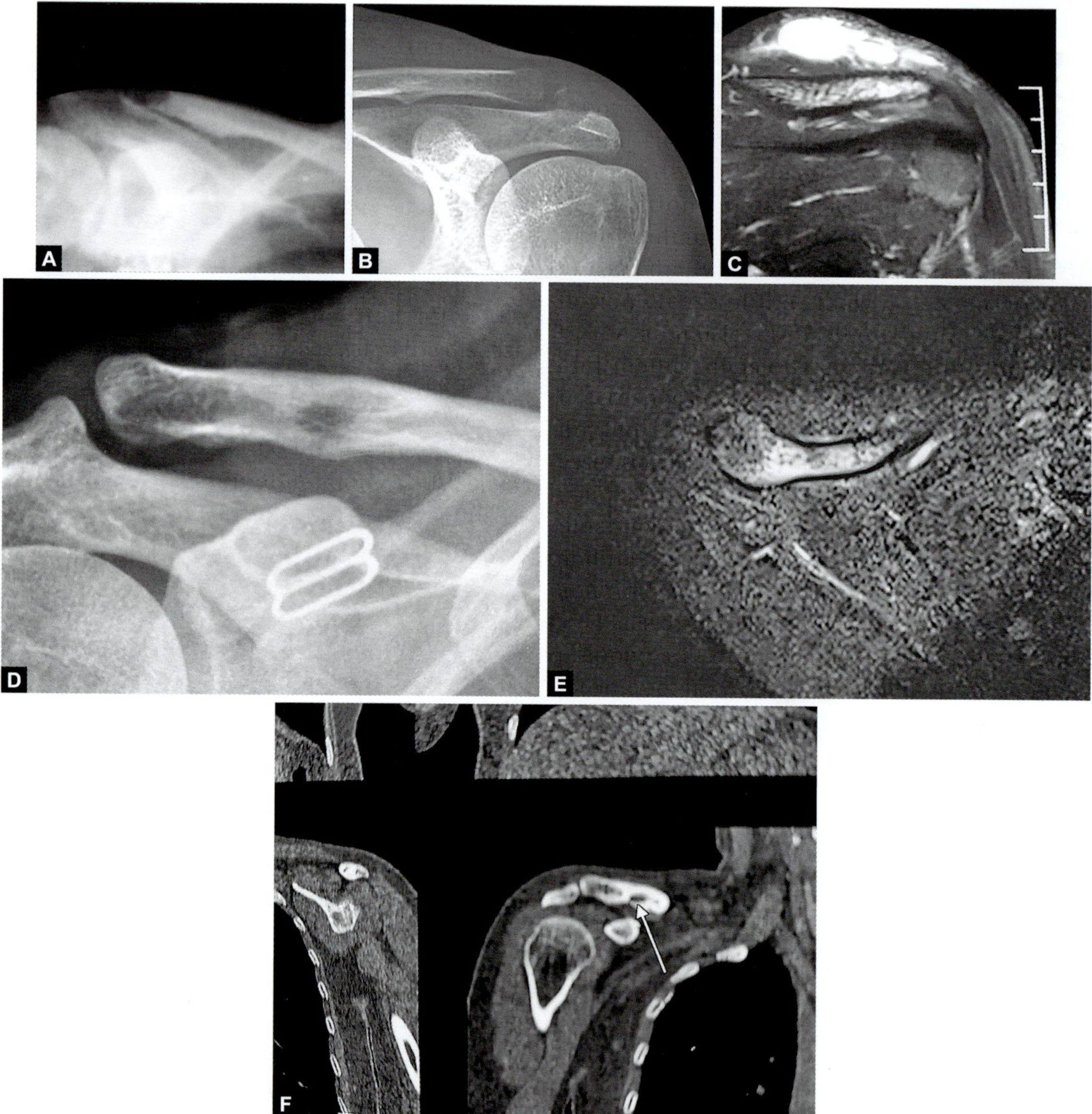

Figs. 16.1A to C: (A) Tuberculosis of the lateral end of right clavicle involving the acromioclavicular joint. Note a lytic lesion without any new bone formation. (B and C) Another patient showing tuberculosis of the lateral end of left clavicle. The cold abscess can be appreciated as soft tissue collection in (B) the X-ray, as well as (C) MRI. Tuberculosis of lateral part of clavicle: Observe the cavity in X-ray (D), MRI (E), and CT scan (F).

encountered (Mohan et al. 1991, **Fig. 16.3**). The patient would present with mild pain and swelling and/or sinuses in supraspinous fossa, infraspinous fossa, along the scapular spine, on the inferior angle or the vertebral border. We had an opportunity to observe seven cases of tuberculosis of scapula (Tuli and Sinha 1969) giving an incidence of <1%. The osseous lesion was detected in the angle of acromian, scapular spine, inferior or superior angle of scapula, or in the neck of scapula. Lasting healed status of the disease is achieved essentially by drugs.

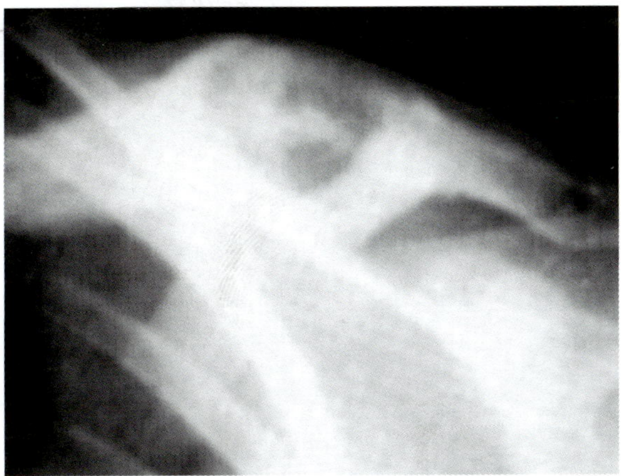

Fig. 16.2: Tuberculosis of clavicle with expansion of bone, and a cavity containing a feathery sequestrum.

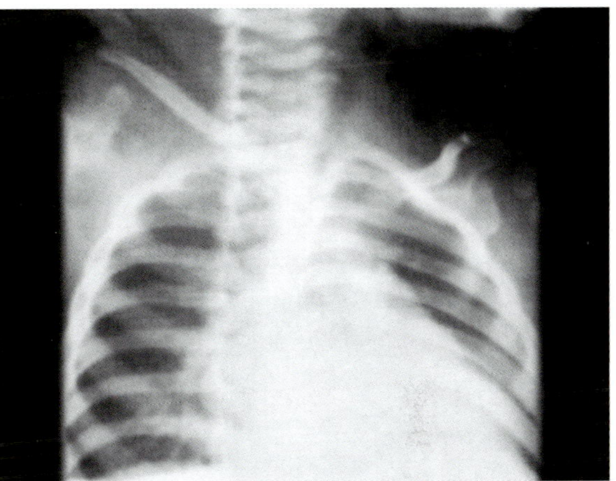

Fig. 16.3: Tuberculosis of the right scapula. Practically, the whole of scapula is involved, however, the shoulder joint was spared.

TUBERCULOSIS OF SYMPHYSIS PUBIS

It is a rare location (<1%) for the disease. We analyzed 6 patients (Tuli and Sinha 1969); all at the time of presentation had abscess formation and discharging sinuses in the upper part of thigh and perineum, 5 were females of the reproductive age. The disease probably starts in the pubic bone and then spreads to the symphysis. Radiologically, one may find destruction of symphysis and pubic bones **(Figs. 16.4 and 16.5)**. If one is aware of the condition, diagnosis is not difficult (Bayrakci et al. 2006, Lal et al. 2013). Chemotherapy heals the lesions. Cold abscesses may require aspiration. Associated lesions in the sacroiliac joints are not uncommon, and some of these cases may exhibit displacement at the symphysis.

Isolated tuberculous lesions may rarely occur in the iliac bone, ischial tuberosity **(Figs. 16.4 to 16.8)**, and ischiopubic ramus. Clinically, these patients present with swelling, pain, tenderness, local abscess and discharging sinuses. Radiologically, the lesion may show varying number of lytic cavities, some cavities may contain feathery sequestra. Depending upon the superimposed pyogenic infection, there may be sclerosis and new bone formation surrounding the lytic areas. Awareness of the disease helps detect cases on presentation. Treatment is by antitubercular drugs (Bayrakci et al. 2006, Lal et al. 2013). Surgery is indicated in doubtful diagnosis, refractory cases or those who have recurred despite adequate drug therapy.

TUBERCULOSIS OF SKULL AND FASCIAL BONES

Amongst 940 patients we came across 3 cases of tuberculosis of skull **(Fig. 16.8)** and 2 of facial bones (Tuli and Sinha 1969). During 1964–1988 we had diagnosed and treated tuberculous lesions of frontal, occipital, parietal, zygomatic and other fascial bones. Majority of these patients have concomitant tubercular foci in other parts of skeleton or other regions of body. In the initial stages we always proved the diagnosis by histological examination of the diseased tissue. However, with familiarity clinico-radiological diagnosis is reliable. These patients present as multiple discharging sinuses and puckered adherent scars. Radiologically, irregular punched out lytic areas are seen in the involved bone. All patients recover quickly with antitubercular drugs. There are a few case reports of mandibular involvement (Sepheriadou-Mavropoulou 1986). Their reported case was from Athens, the patient had a chronic swelling with fluctuations and

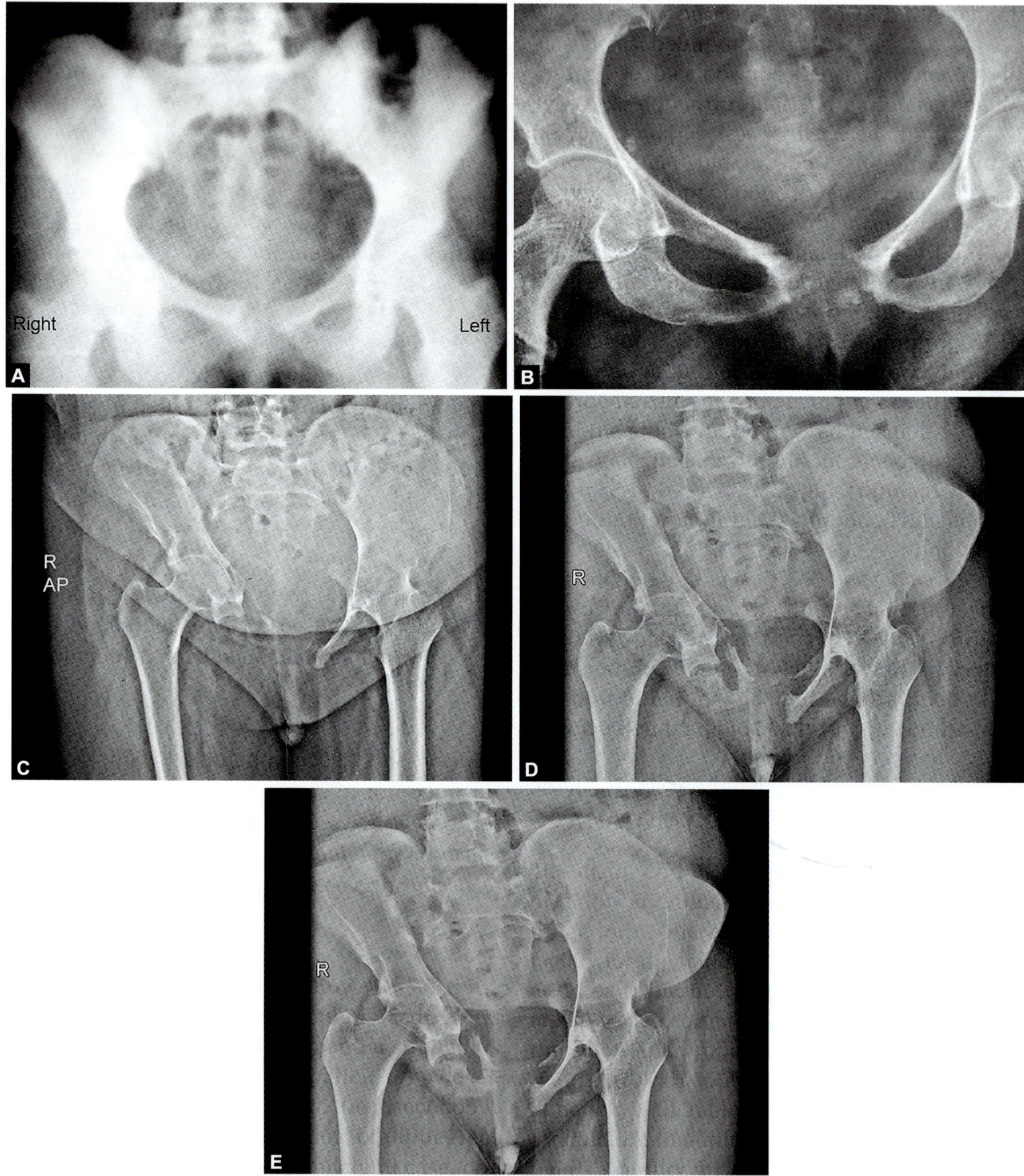

Figs. 16.4A and B: (A) A young lady presented with multiple discharging sinuses in the region of symphysis pubis and along the left vulva. X-ray showed destructive change in the symphysis pubis and left inferior pubic ramus. Note faintly visible dystrophic calcification in the soft tissues on the left side. Complete healing of sinuses took place by antitubercular drugs. (B) Another patient showing the changes in symphysis pubis. Disseminated tuberculosis of pelvis in a female patient presenting with perineal descharging sinuses (C) at presentation. (D) Observe the involvement of right sacroiliac joint distraction of bones around symphysis pubis, old healed tuberculous left hip joint. (E) Under the influence of anti-TB drugs many bones not visible at presentation are now visible in a process of healing.

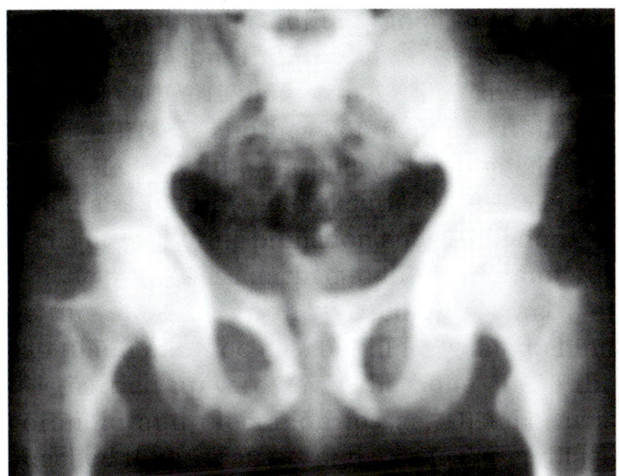

Fig. 16.5: X-ray showing irregular destruction of the bones constituting symphysis pubis. The patient had multiple discharging sinuses on each side of the scrotum. Tuberculous pathology was confirmed by tissue histology. There was excellent healing of disease on multidrug therapy.

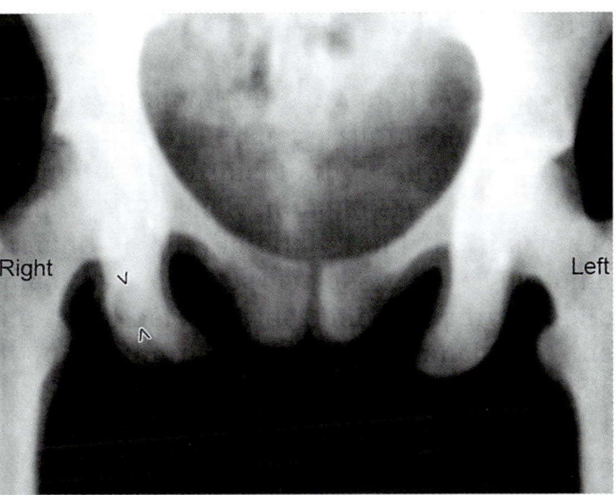

Fig. 16.6: X-ray of another young lady who presented with pain, swelling and a discharging sinus in right buttock. Note a classical tuberculous lesion showing a soft coke like sequestrum contained in a cavity in the right ischial tuberosity.

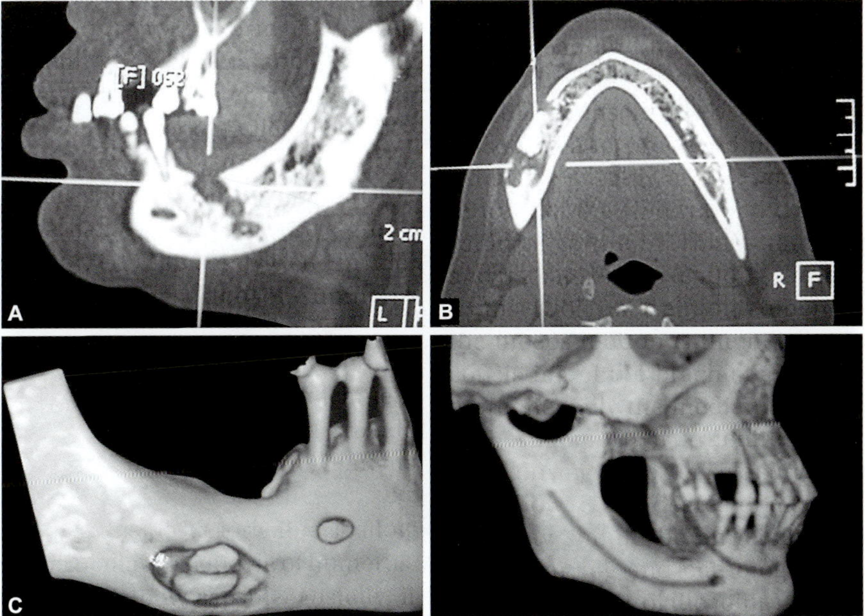

Figs. 16.7A to C: Tuberculosis of the mandible is very rare localization. This patient developed a non-healing ulcer on the lateral surface of right mandible after a dental procedure. Histology from the margin of the ulcer proved the diagnosis of tuberculous pathology. The ulcer and the destructive lesion healed under the influence of antitubercular drugs. (A) The destructive lesion in CT scans, (B) the cavity in the X-rays, (C) the resolving destructive lesion after antitubercular therapy.

trismus. Radiologically, a rarefied area with ill-defined borders was found at the mandibular angle. We encountered in 2010, a 40-year-old lady presenting with an ulcer on the mandible preceded by a history of tooth ache **(Fig. 16.7)**. Clinical examination revealed an ulcer with undermined edges and an irregular visible bone. Histological diagnosis of the tissue from

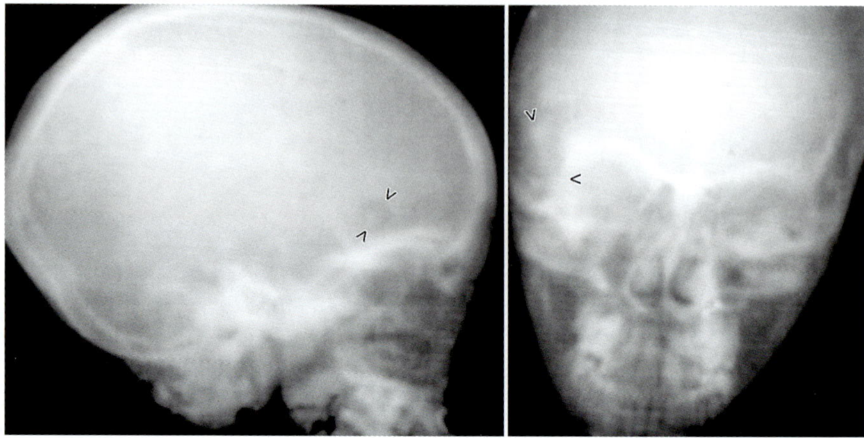

Fig. 16.8: Tuberculosis of right temporal bone in a young boy. Note the area of destruction behind and above the right orbit and a soft sequestrum contained in a cavity.

the ulcer proved the tuberculous pathology. Under the influence of antitubercular drugs, the ulcer healed with restitution of the bone texture. This patient was on a long course of steroids (2007–2009) for suspected sarcoidosis of lungs. Steroids induced lowered cell mediated immunity probably predisposed this patient to tuberculous osteomyelitis.

TUBERCULOSIS OF STERNUM AND RIBS

Tuberculous localization in the thoracic cage is rare (Khan et al. 2007). Amongst the 980 patients suffering from osteoarticular tuberculosis, 19 (2%) had lesions in the ribs and 14 (1.5%) in the sternum. Sternal tuberculosis has been observed in a few patients after cardiopulmonary operations. Nearly one-third of these patients had detectable tuberculous lesion in other parts of the skeleton or in the lungs (Tuli and Sinha 1969). Positive X-ray signs occur much later than the presenting clinical features. Abscess or sinuses are present before the focus can be detected radiologically **(Figs. 16.9 to 16.11)**. Sternal disease is seen as irregular destructive areas or cavities. The diseased rib may show thickening or expansion with punched out erosions; rarely there may be sequestrum formation of a segment of rib. All such cases would heal under the influence of antitubercular drugs. Surgical treatment may be rarely justified for a doubtful diagnosis, a nonresponsive case or for removal of a large sequestrum. The most common cause of chronic osteomyelitis of a rib in TB endemic areas is tuberculosis.

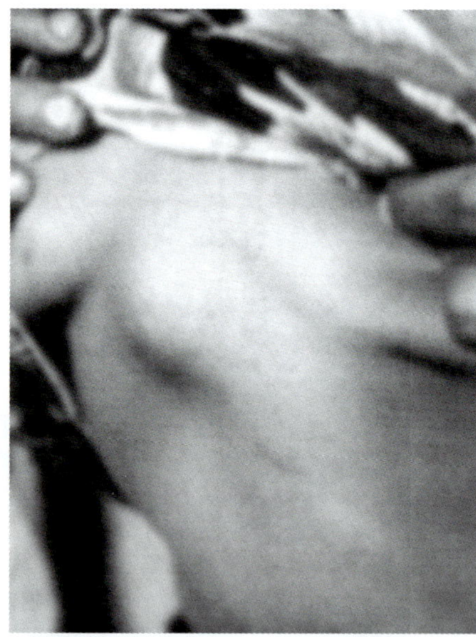

Fig. 16.9: A case of tuberculosis of the body of sternum. Note a cold abscess in front of lower sternum between the breasts.

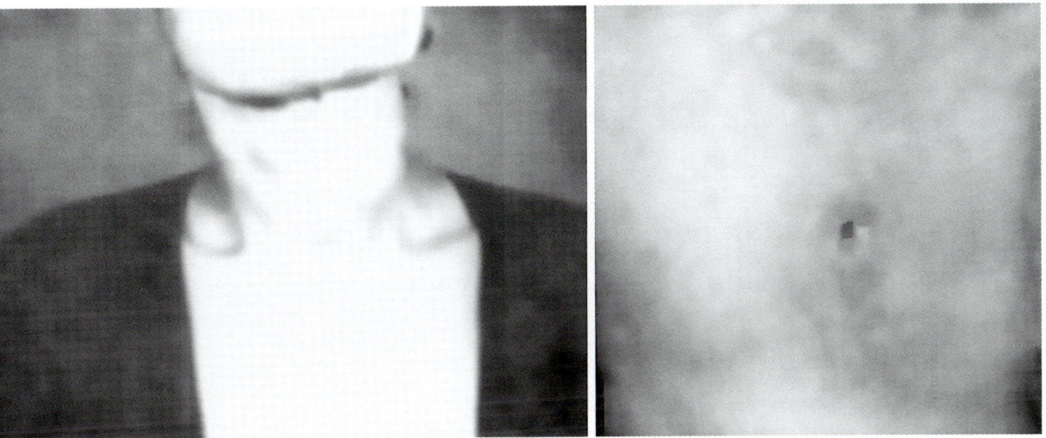

Fig. 16.10: Clinical features of a healed case of tuberculosis of the sternum. Note healed ulcers (puckered scar) on the manubrium stemi and the body of sternum.

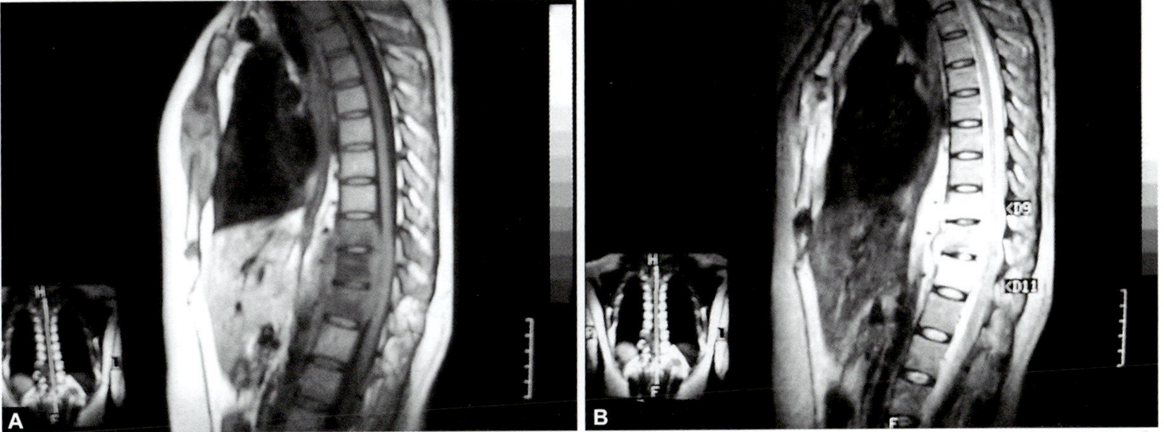

Figs. 16.11A and B: MRI showing tuberculosis of sternum along with tuberculosis of D9 to D11 vertebrae, (A) T1 shadow, (B) T2 shadow. Observe cold abscess around anterior and posterior aspects of the sternum and vertebral bodies.

Tuberculous Osteomyelitis

Pathologically, the onset of tuberculous focus is always located within the bone. In children, the disease develops differently, especially in short tubular bones. Because of the deficient anastomoses of the osseous arteries in childhood, thrombosis caused by the tuberculous pathology may lead to sequestration of a major part of the diaphysis. The infected and necrosed diaphysis becomes surrounded by newly formed subperiosteal bone not unlike pyogenic chronic hematogenous osteomyelitis. If rigorous histological and microbiological tests were performed in all atypical cases of hematogenous osteomyelitis **(Fig. 5.3)**, a large number of them may turn out to be tuberculous in pathology (Tuli 1969, Martini 1988).

TUBERCULOUS OSTEOMYELITIS WITHOUT JOINT INVOLVEMENT

Isolated bone involvement without spreading to the joint occurs commonly in ribs, metacarpals, metatarsals, calcaneum, femur, tibia, fibula, radius, humerus, sternum, fascial bones, pelvis and skull. In a long series, any type of bone can be seen to be involved. However, tuberculous osteomyelitis (without involvement of joints), especially of long tubular bones, is so infrequent that it often fails to attract the attention of the clinician. The incidence reported is 2–3% of all cases of osteoarticular tuberculosis (Tuli and Sinha 1969, Silva 1980, Halsey et al. 1982, Martini et al. 1986). Nearly 7% of these cases may have involvement of more than one site **(Figs. 14.1, 17.1 to 17.4, 17.7 to 17.9)**. Because of low suspicion index and mild local symptoms, there is always delay in the diagnosis. The common presenting features are pain, swelling of bone with warmth and tenderness, overlying boggy swelling of soft tissues, abscess or sinus formation, and enlargement of regional lymph nodes. High suspicion index and detection of typical (undermined edges) tubercular sinuses, ulcers or cold abscesses are of great clinical significance.

X-rays may reveal irregular cavities and areas of destruction in the bone with little surrounding sclerosis (honeycomb appearance), and there may be soft tissue swelling. The cavities may contain soft feathery sequestra, and the bone may show subperiosteal new bone formation (spina ventosa type). If complicated by sinus formation or secondary infection, there may be intense reactive sclerosis and occasionally sequestration of the cortical bone resembling hematogenous osteomyelitis, and rarely there may be a pathological fracture (Tuli and Sinha 1969, Martini et al. 1986). In growing age, the lesion may be typically sitting astride the epiphyseal cartilage plate **(Figs. 10.1, 13.2 and 13.4)** (Ohtera et al. 2007). Such lesions should be treated by multidrug therapy and suitable protective orthosis. Limited operative debridement may be justified to obtain tissue for diagnosis in case of uncertainty. Many of such lesions have a remarkable potential for repair and growth to near normal bone.

The clinicoradiological picture requires to be differentiated from chronic pyogenic osteomyelitis, Brodies abscess, tumorous conditions **(Fig. 17.10)**, or rare granulomatous conditions. "BCG osteomyelitis" of long bones may resemble the clinical features of tuberculous osteomyelitis (Shanmugasundaram 1983, Fellander 1963). Histological, bacteriological and serological investigations help to reach the final diagnosis. Presumptive diagnosis may be confirmed by a favorable response to modern antitubercular drugs.

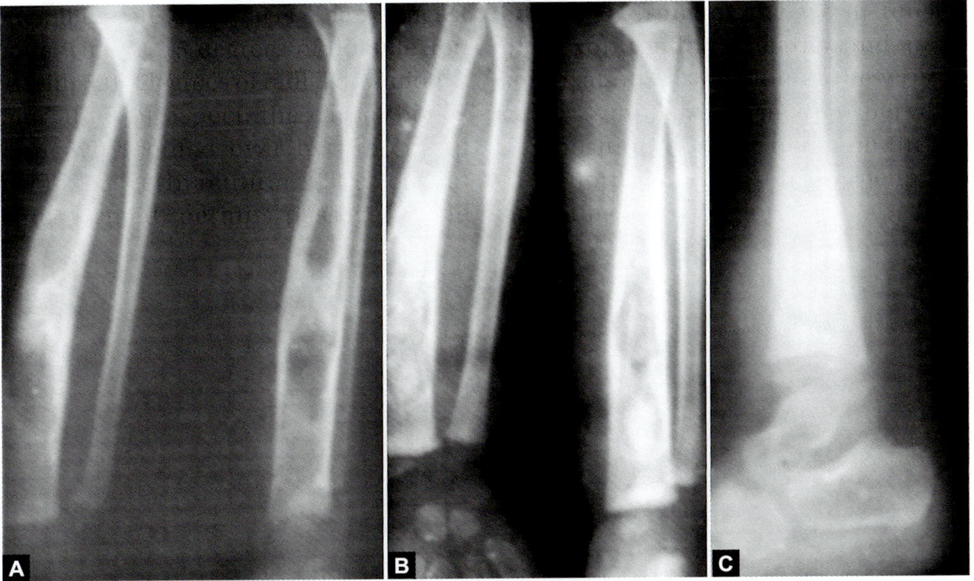

Figs. 17.1A to C: Multiple cystic tuberculosis of the radial diaphysis (A), (B), and distal tibia (C). The diagnosis was confirmed by examination of the tissue. Under the influence of antitubercular drugs the cavities underwent resolution and there was remineralization (B).

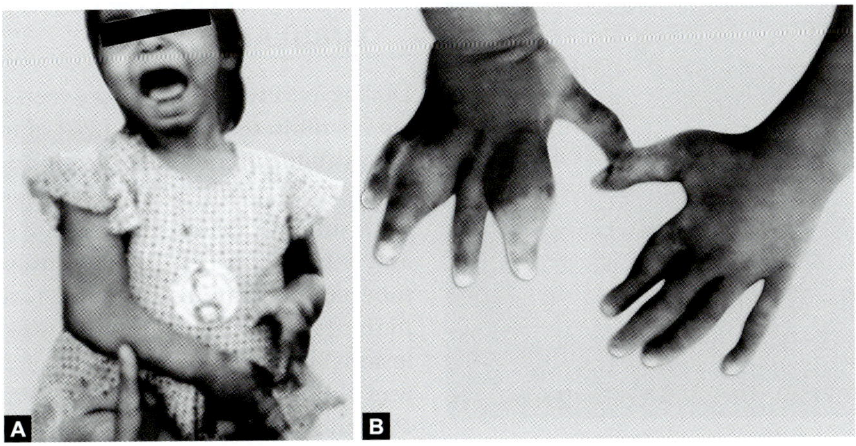

Figs. 17.2A to H: *Continued*

Continued

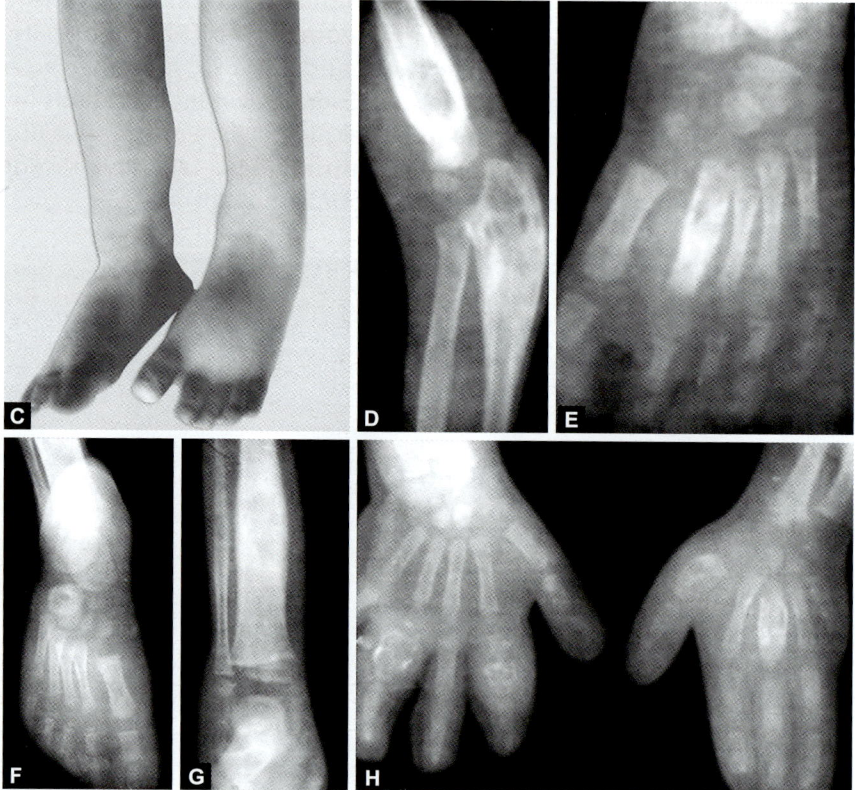

Figs. 17.2A to H: Clinical picture and X-rays of a child suffering from disseminated multiple cystic tuberculosis. Note the typical spindle-shaped swellings of the involved areas—right upper limb: Distal humerus, proximal ulna, second and third fingers; left hand: First and third metacarpals; left lower limb: Tibia and second metatarsal; right foot cuboid.
Courtesy: Professor Jawaharlal Nehru Medical College, Ajmer.

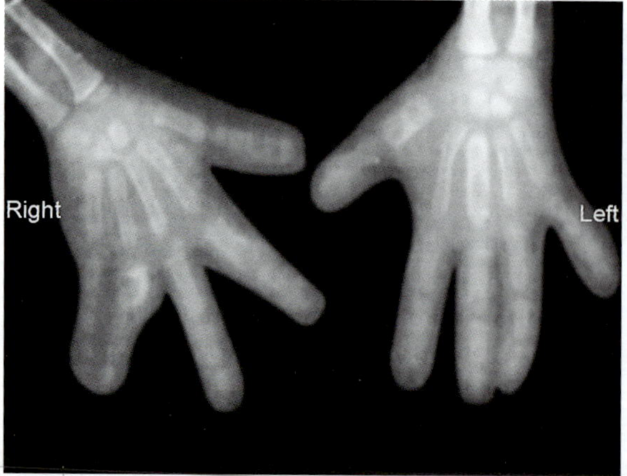

Fig. 17.3: Tuberculosis of small bones of hand: right second and fourth fingers: left first and third metacarpals. This is post-treatment picture of **Figure 17.2H**.

TUBERCULOSIS OF LONG TUBULAR BONES

During a study conducted between 1965 and 1967, we encountered 33 cases (3%) of tuberculosis of long tubular bones. The location in descending order of frequency in this material was tibia (11), ulna (8), radius (6), femur (5), fibula (2), and humerus (one). This was the only obvious tuberculous manifestation in 23 cases, in 10 the patients had other concomitant tuberculous lesions in the body. The radiological appearance was typical spina ventosa in 7 **(Figs. 14.1, 17.1, 17.5 and 17.6)**, resembled Brodie's type of abscess in 12, appeared like low grade hematogenous pyogenic osteomyelitis in 12, and one case of

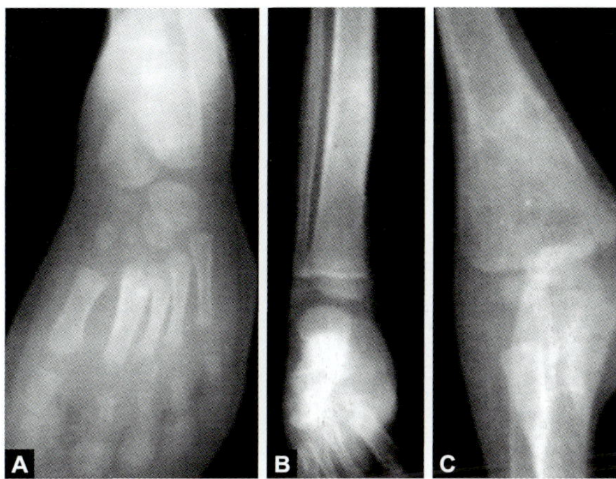

Figs. 17.4A to C: Patient **(Fig. 17.2)** was treated by antitubercular drugs. Note remarkable resolution of the osseous lesions and reconstitution of the diseased bones; (A) Post-treatment of **Figure 17.2F**, (B) Post-treatment of **Figure 17.2G**, (C) Post-treatment of **Figure 17.2D**.

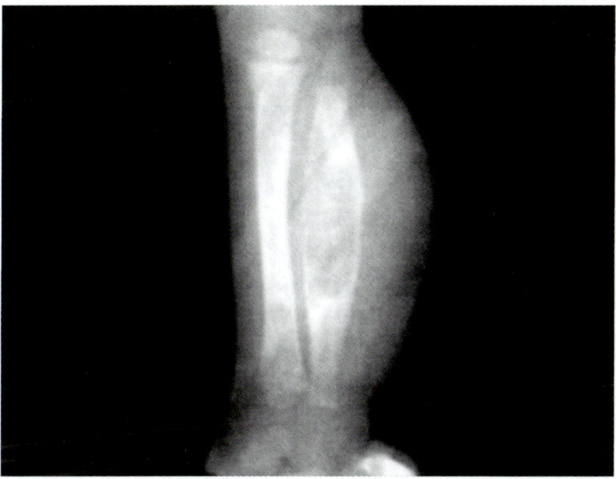

Fig. 17.5: Cystic type of tuberculosis of fibula. Note subperiosteal new bone formation and the soft tissue shadow caused by the cold abscess.

radius resembled a neoplasm **(Fig. 17.10)**. Of all these patients, 16 had the lesion located at metaphysiodiaphyseal junction and 17 were located in the diaphyseal region **(Figs. 17.7 and 17.10)**. The cases analyzed were proved by histopathology.

Disseminated skeletal tuberculosis is considered to be very rare **(Figs. 17.2 and 17.4)**. In our studies (prior to general availability of modern imaging modalities), nearly 7% of cases showed tuberculous lesion in more than one skeletal site **(Figs. 14.1, 17.1, 17.2, 17.6 and 17.8)**. The incidence reported by other workers ranges between 5–10% (Sanchis-Olmos 1948, Kumar and Saxena 1988, Ormerod et al. 1989). Most of these patients are ill-looking and poorly nourished. The pathogenic mechanism is considered two-fold, the hematogenous dissemination that creates one lesion may also create others, whereas in others different lesions may correspond to repeat impregnations at different occasions (Tuli and Sinha 1969). Rarely disseminated lesions during childhood may present as multiple cystic lesions (Sharma 1978, Edeiken et al. 1963) called by Jungling (1936) as "osteitis tuberculosa

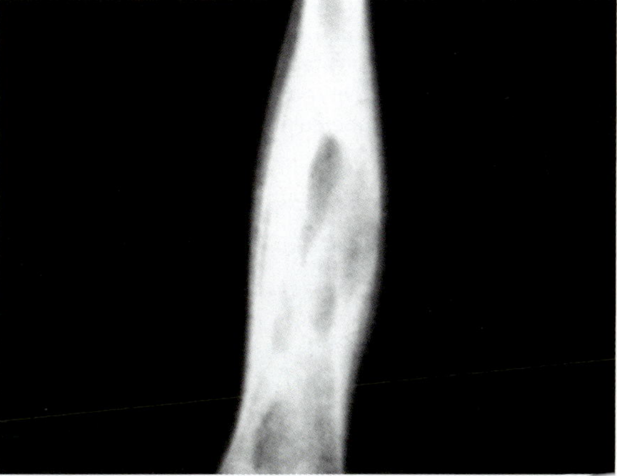

Fig. 17.6: X-ray of femur in a child concomitantly suffering from tuberculosis of spine. The femur shows multiple lytic lesions, expansion, and subperiosteal new bone formation. In regions where tuberculosis is endemic, this is a typical picture of tuberculous involvement of long tubular bones.

multiplex cystoides" **(Figs. 14.2 and 17.2)**. The lesions generally occur in children and appear as rounded or oval radiolucent areas. Rarely they require to be differentiated from pyogenic infection, aneurysmal bone cyst, unicameral bone cyst or cartilaginous tumor (Shannon et al. 1990, Rasool et al. 1994). When imaging modalities (MRIs or isotope bone scans) are employed to

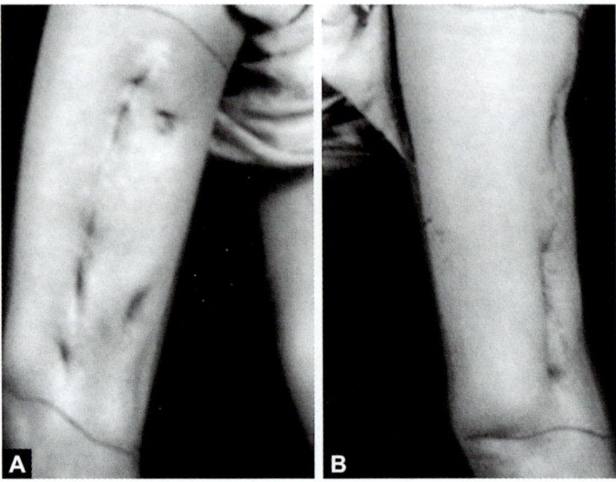

Figs. 17.7A and B: Clinical photograph of a young lady who at the age of 21 years was diagnosed clinico-radiologically and by histology to be a case of extensive tuberculosis of right femur. No formal operation was performed. The sinuses and ulcers healed spontaneously under the influence of antitubercular drugs, and she remained symptom free. At the age of 39, she again reported with local signs of activity of disease. Histology reported chronic inflammatory response. Signs of activity again subsided under the influence of newer antitubercular drugs.

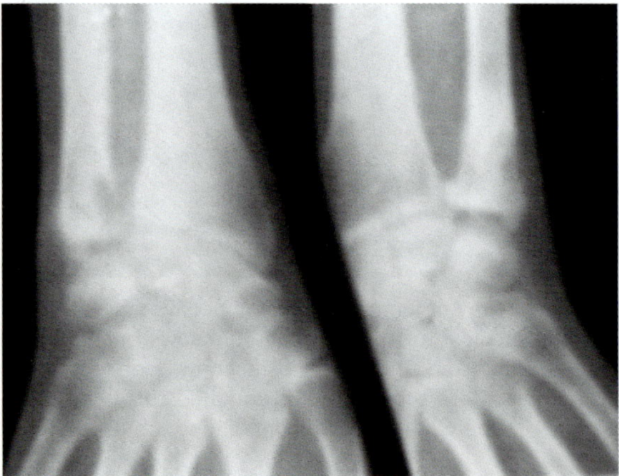

Fig. 17.8: Cystic type of tuberculosis in both ulnae in an adult female.

scan the body, additional (subclinical) active tuberculous foci can be detected in about 40% of patients. Multidrug therapy is successful in most of the cases, rarely a lesion may need curettage for diagnosis and treatment.

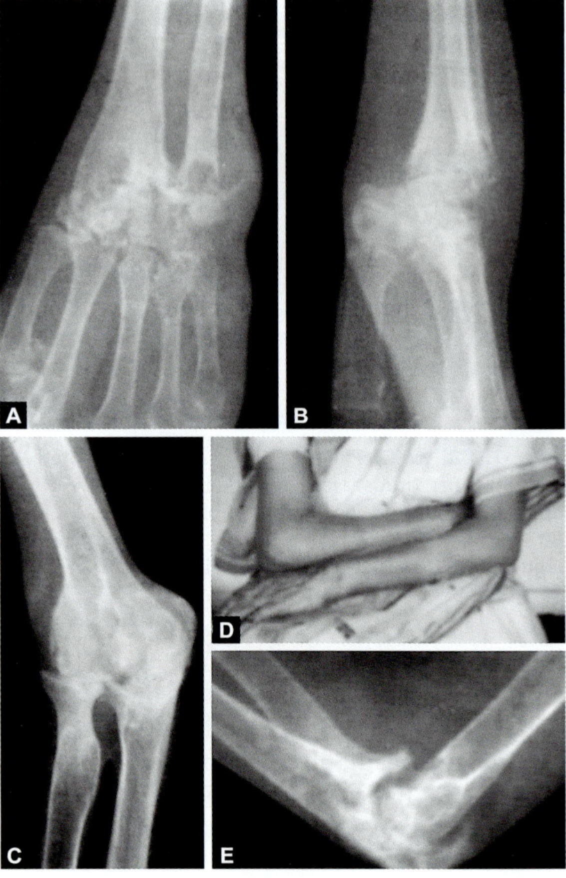

Figs. 17.9A to E: SB 50-year-old lady had involvement of left wrist joint (A and B), right elbow (C to E). Apparently the disease looked like rheumatoid arthritis or multifocal tuberculous arthritis (C). There was gross involvement of elbow joint. The involved left wrist shows anterior subluxation.

TREATMENT

The response to antitubercular drugs is as a rule favorable. The lesions can be observed to undergo healing and resolution by 6 monthly X-rays **(Figs. 17.1 and 17.10)**. Depending upon the stage at which the drugs were started there may be revascularization of sequestra, reincorporation like a graft and near complete restitution of the osseous texture. In refractory cases, or whenever there is doubt in diagnosis, or in the presence of a large abscess in the soft tissues around

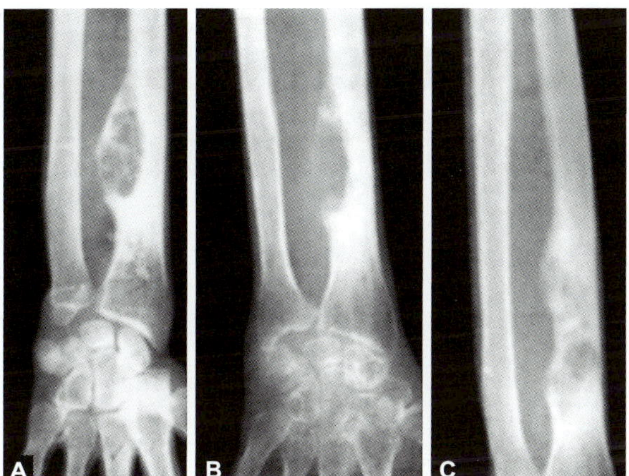

Figs. 17.10A to C: The patient presented as a tumorous condition of the left radius (A). Open biopsy, microscopically and histologically, proved it to be a tuberculous lesion (B). The lesion resolved under antitubercular therapy, (C) One year after the drug therapy.

the involved bone surgical excision is justified. Results of conservative treatment by drugs alone are favorably compared with those obtained by concomitant surgical curettage of the lesions (Lynder 1982, Martini et al. 1981). Coexistence of tuberculous infection and pyogenic infection in the same osseous lesion may cause delay in healing of sinuses and inflammation. Combined newer antimicrobial therapy with or without surgical excision helps heal such lesions on long-term bases.

Tuberculosis of Tendon Sheaths and Bursae

Isolated tuberculous disease of the synovial sheaths or bursae occurs rarely, however, any synovial sheath or bursa can be involved. The disease is thought to reach the synovial/bursal sheaths by direct hematogenous spread, or from the underlying bone/joint disease, or by a gravitational spread from a neighboring diseased area. The infected synovium gets edematous and filled with granulations, becomes hyperplastic, thickened and villous. Excessive synovial fluid may be produced (serous exudate) giving an almost painless swelling. With movements and friction, the broken villi and fibrinous exudate get moulded to resemble rice bodies/melon seeds which may be found in the tendon sheaths as well as in the bursae, closely resembling the rice bodies/melon seeds of rheumatoid disease. Rice bodies or melon seeds are infected villous bodies, their histologic and microbiologic tests would reveal tuberculous pathology. Rarely, necrosis of the underlying tendons may occur. Griffith et al. (2002) suggested ultrasonography as an ideal first-line investigation for tenosynovitis to reveal the degree and extent of involvement of the tendon and its sheath. MRI may reveal juxtaosseous inflammatory collection or abscess formation with concomitant intense edema of the neighboring muscles in cases of bursal tuberculosis.

Tuberculous tenosynovitis is rare and develops insidiously. There is progressive swelling and inflammation of the tendon sheath with limitation of excursion of the involved tendons. The commonest site of involvement is the flexor tendons of the hand (compound palmar ganglion), but other tendon sheaths of fingers and ankle region, radial and ulnar bursae, and extensor tendon sheaths **(Fig. 18.1)** are sometimes affected (Franceschi et al. 2007). Pathologically, both the parietal and visceral tenosynovium is replaced by tuberculous granulations. As the infection progresses, the disease spreads along the sheath to the tendon and its insertion. There is weakness and muscle wasting, rarely a tendon may fray and rupture spontaneously. Clinically, the swelling is doughy with semifluctuations, creaking or crepitations are palpable on movements/fluctuation **(Table 18.1)**.

Treatment is by rest in functioning position, intermittent exercises, and antitubercular drugs. In advanced cases or those not responding favorably, surgical resection of the diseased tissue may be necessary. In the presence of large fluid, aspiration and instillation of streptomycin combined with isoniazid is useful.

Tuberculous tenosynovitis of the common sheath of the forearm flexor tendons distends the sheath proximal and distal to the flexor retinaculum and is classically called "compound palmar ganglion". In addition to the clinical features described above, cross fluctuation is

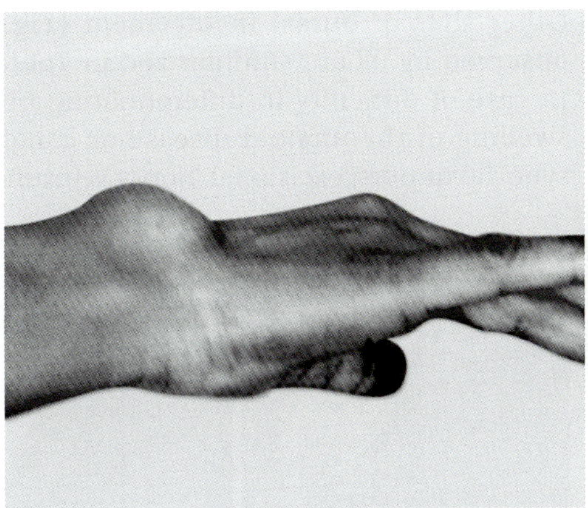
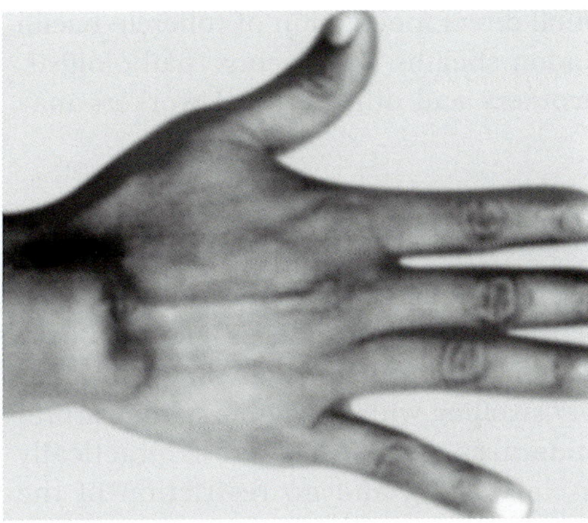

Fig. 18.1: Clinical photograph of tubercular synovitis of the extensor tendon sheaths of wrist. Note distension of the sheath both proximal and distal to the extensor retinaculum (compound extensor ganglion/dumb-bell tenosynovitis). Mycobacteria were isolated in the aspirate of the swelling and from the enlarged lymph nodes in front of elbow.

Table 18.1: Prominent clinical features in tuberculous tenosynovitis observed during 1965–1994 expressed as percentage.

Insidious swelling	100
Mild pain	63
Stiffness	28
"Weakness" of function	32
Local warmth	45
Mild tenderness	27
Boggy on palpation	81
Pseudofluctuation	82
Crepitations/creaking on movements ± fluctuation	63
Local sinus	12
Regional lymphadenitis	74

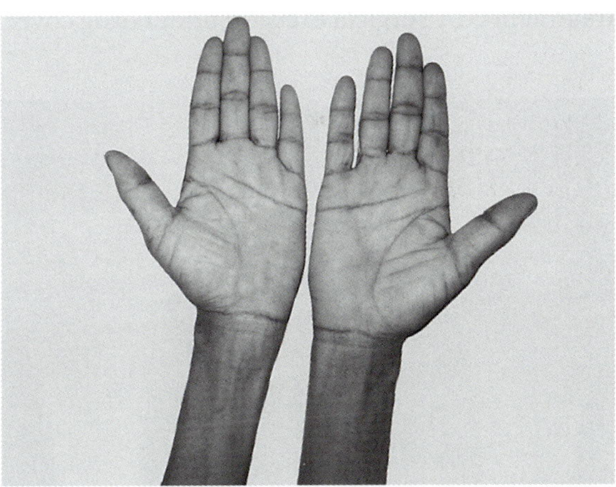

Fig. 18.2: Clinical picture of a compound palmar ganglion caused by tuberculosis of tendon sheaths of flexors of fingers. Note swelling proximal and distal to the flexor retinaculum in the left forearm and wrist. Patient underwent subtotal synovectomy and carpal tunnel release for median nerve symptoms. Histology proved the diagnosis of tuberculosis.

demonstrable between the bulging above and below the flexor retinaculum **(Fig.18.2)**. Pain is not significant but paresthesia due to median nerve compression may be present (Bickel et al. 1953, Arora 1994, Sherwani 2000).

In affluent countries, *Mycobacterium marinum* may cause tenosynovitis of the flexor tendons of hand. The nature of the *Mycobacterium* can be ascertained only from the culture of a suspected material. Fortunately, such cases respond to the newer antitubercular drugs like isoniazid, rifampicin and pyrazinamide which may be combined with surgical excision. Exposure to aquatic environment and trauma by marine life can be obtained on leading questions (Chow et al. 1987, Lacy et al. 1989, Patel 1997). Generally, flexor tendons are involved, however, a third of Chow's (1987) cases had extensor tendon involvement.

Accidental direct inoculation of tubercle bacilli into tendon-sheaths in surgeons, pathologists, dairy workers and other critical workers may occur.

TUBERCULOUS BURSITIS

The least rare (1–2% of all skeletal tuberculosis) site for tuberculous bursitis is gluteal bursa (greater trochanter bursa) **(Fig. 18.3)**. An inflammatory swelling with negligible pain, warmth and tenderness develops. There is practically no muscle wasting and no restriction of the hip joint movements. Almost all cases respond favorably to systemic antitubercular drugs. Large swellings are worth aspirating with instillation of local antitubercular drugs. In refractory cases, treatment is by surgical excision under drug cover.

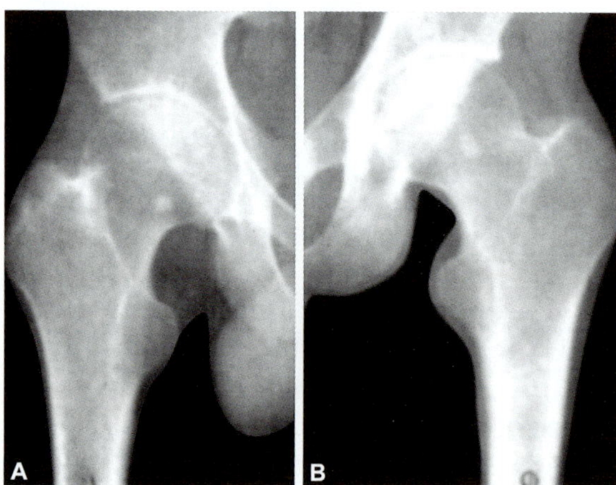

Figs. 18.3A and B: This patient presented with a chronic discharging sinus on the lateral aspect of right thigh (A). Movements of hip joint were normal. The X-ray reveals irregularity of the greater trochanter, erosive lesions and soft tissue swelling behind the hip joint. This is the typical clinico-radiological picture of tuberculosis of the greater trochanter bursa of long-standing; (B) Normal left trochanter for comparison.

Other sites of bursal involvement **(Fig. 18.4)** observed by us are summarized in **Table 18.2**. In case of difficulty in differentiating from the swelling of rheumatoid disease or ganglion or synovial tumors, excisional biopsy is justified.

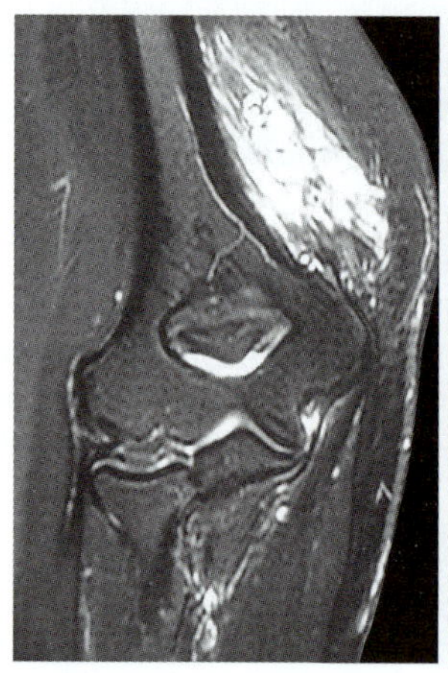

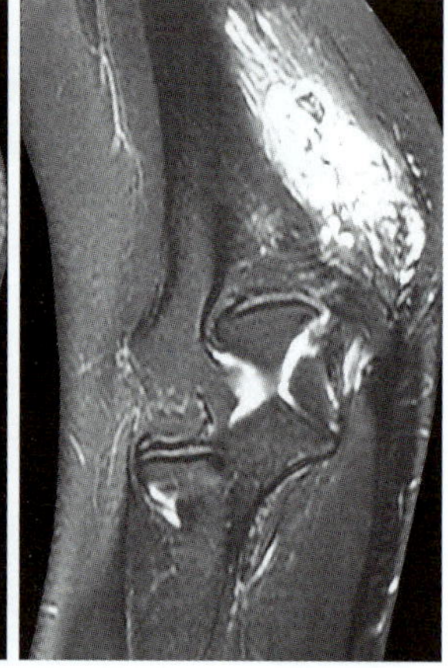

Fig. 18.4: Any bursal sheath can get involved by tuberculous infection. This MRI shows a tuberculous abscess in the intermuscular bursal sheaths on the medical side of arm.

Table 18.2: Location of tuberculosis of bursal sheaths during 1965–1994.

Location	Number
Trochanteric bursa	29
Bursa anserinus	21
Compound palmar bursa	18
Radial long flexor sheath	14
Ulnar long flexor sheath	10
Deltoid bursa	14
Wrist extensor tendons	1
Ankle flexor tendons	8
Peroneal tendons	4
Ankle extensor tendons	2
Miscellaneous intermuscular bursae	26

SECTION 3

Tuberculosis of the Spine

Clinical Features

Vertebral tuberculosis is the commonest form of skeletal tuberculosis and it constitutes about 50% of all cases of tuberculosis of bones and joints. The vertebrae have a rich blood supply and large growth plates, the infection spreads from lungs (or other organs and lymph nodes) along arteries, Batson's paravertebral venous plexus or through lymphatic drainage through para-aortic lymph nodes.

AGE AND SEX

What is true of osteoarticular tuberculosis in general is also true of spinal tuberculosis. It is most common during first three decades, clinically the patients have reported to us with the disease starting at any age between 1 to 80 years. The disease is equally distributed among both sexes. **Table 19.1** shows the age distribution of the patients observed by us. Of the total patients, 52% were males and 48% were females. The figures of other workers regarding age and sex distribution are almost similar (Konstam 1962, Sevastikoglou 1953, Shaw 1963, Wilkinson 1949, Paus 1964, Friedman 1966, Hahn 1977, Martin 1970, Bavadekar 1982, Lifeso 1985, Jain et al. 2014). Schmorl and Junghanns (1959) stated that it occurred in first decade of life in 50% of all cases and in only 25% did it appear after the age of 20. More recent Western figures indicate that at present spinal tuberculosis in the affluent countries is a disease of adults rather than of children (Hayes et al. 1996). During the last two decades, we have been observing another peak of such cases above the age of 60 years probably because of increase in the population of senior citizens and those with compromised immune status and concomitant comorbidities (Jain 2024).

SYMPTOMS AND SIGNS

Active Stage

Symptoms of tuberculosis of the spine are commonly insidious, but sometimes these may be acute. The usual clinical symptoms in active

Table 19.1: Age distribution at the time of presentation of vertebral tuberculosis (1965–1974: at BHU).

	Percentage of patients		
Age in years	*Male*	*Female*	*Total*
1–10	20	9	29
11–20	11	12	23
21–30	7	14	21
31–40	4	6	10
41–50	3	5	8
51–60	4	1	5
61–70	3	–	3
71–80	–	1	1
	52%	48%	

stage of the disease are malaise, loss of weight, loss of appetite, night sweats and evening rise of temperature. The spine is stiff and painful on movements with localized kyphotic deformity which would be tender on percussion. Spasm of the vertebral muscles is present. During sleep, the muscle spasm relaxes permitting movement between the inflamed surfaces resulting in the typical night cries. A cold abscess may be present palpable clinically. However, several of these symptoms and signs may be absent in early stage even in cases of active vertebral disease. A history of tuberculosis in the patient or his family should raise suspicion of tubercular nature of the spinal disease. If the clinician makes it a routine to palpate the spinous processes by sliding his fingertips from the cervical spine to the sacrum, he would be able to detect even a small knuckle kyphosis by palpation of a step or a prominence, thus diagnosing a case before gross destruction has taken place.

Healed Stage

When the disease has healed, the patient neither looks ill nor feels ill, he regains his normal appetite and lost weight, there is no evening rise of temperature or night sweating. There is no pain or tenderness in the spine and the spasm of the vertebral muscles is absent. The deformity that occurred during active stage, however, persists. Erythrocyte sedimentation rate falls and there is radiological evidence of bone healing in serial X-rays.

Unusual Clinical Features

Tuberculosis as a cause of persistent backache must be remembered if we aim at diagnosing the condition early. Rarely caries spine may be responsible for pain referred to the trunk resembling fibrofascitis, cervicodorsal spondylosis or disc syndrome. Pain referred to abdomen may need differentiation from appendicitis, cholecystitis, pancreatitis or renal disease. Sometimes a case of vertebral tuberculosis may present as "spinal tumor syndrome" with neural deficit. In economically underdeveloped countries, where tuberculosis is quite common, a case having a pulmonary lesion with pain in the spine may be a case of ankylosing spondylitis and requires to be differentiated from tubercular spondylitis. Ankylosing spondylitis with concomitant pulmonary tuberculosis is not an uncommon association, especially in those countries where tuberculous infection is almost endemic **(Fig. 21.4)**. Rarely, the first presenting symptom may be neurological deficit. On the other hand, with the availability of MRI and CT scans some patients with localized persistent backache may demonstrate the infective vertebral lesions while their conventional X-rays and laboratory findings may be within normal limits.

ABSCESSES AND SINUSES

Abscesses or sinuses from the cervical or dorsal regions can present themselves far away from the vertebral column along the fascial planes or course of neurovascular bundles. Thus, they may present in the paraspinal regions at the back, in the posterior/anterior cervical triangles, along the brachial plexus in the axilla, and/or along the intercostal spaces on the chest wall. Abscesses from the dorsolumbar and lumbar spine follow the well-known pattern of tracking down the psoas sheath. These abscesses may be palpable in the iliac fossa, in the lumbar triangle, in the upper part of the thigh below the inguinal ligament or even track downwards up to the knee. Sometimes a bilateral psoas abscess **(Figs. 20.11 and 20.12)** may be palpable which may rarely exhibit cross fluctuation across the midline. Psoas abscess can lead to pitfalls in diagnosis; it can give rise to "hip flexion deformity" the so-called **"pseudo-hip" flexion deformity**. The flexion deformity of the hip joint due to spasm of iliopsoas muscle does not show any limitation of external and internal rotations of the hip joint when tested in the position of flexion deformity. A patient may present as "lump in the iliac fossa" or as swelling or sinuses in regions far away from the lumbar spine. Psoas abscess is as a rule associated with detectable tuberculous disease of the vertebral column from dorsal 10th vertebra to the sacrum, or disease of sacroiliac joint, pelvic bones and hip joint. The osseous lesion may not be discernable clinico-radiologically in initial stages (Seber et al. 1993). What is generally expressed as clinically palpable "psoas abscess" in reality is an iliac abscess contained in the sheath of ilio-psoas muscle. The abscess that has tracked down in the psoas sheath penetrates through the iliacus muscle sheath and becomes palpable as a mass in the iliac fossa. The abscess that remains confined to psoas sheath may not be palpable clinically. An iliac abscess may be formed by an abscess from innominate bone, sacroiliac joint, sacrum or hip joint and it may not be associated with an abscess in the psoas sheath. However, possibility of suppuration of retroperitoneal lymph nodes producing a clinical psoas abscess (Berges 1981, Perros 1988) must also be kept in mind. Unfamiliarity with the disease may lead to mistaken diagnosis and inappropriate treatment (Humphries et al. 1986).

ANALYSIS OF CLINICAL MATERIAL

Certain clinical features of spinal tuberculosis based upon observations of nearly 600 cases in our series are summarized in **Table 19.2**. In a series of 100 patients (assessed by conventional radiographs), 68 cases had a large abscess shadow, 25 had a small shadow, while nothing definite could be said about abscess shadows in 7 cases.

Majority of the patients in our series reached the hospital late when the disease was fairly advanced. The duration of symptoms of the illness at the time of presentation in the hospital varied from a few months to a few years. Less than 20% of patients attended within first 3 months of the onset of symptoms. The delay may be due to socioeconomic factors and due to ignorance regarding the gravity of their ailments.

Table 19.2: Showing certain clinical features of spinal tuberculosis in our series (1965–1974 pre-MRI era) expressed as percentage: (BHU stydy).

Feature	%
Clinical kyphosis	95
Palpable cold abscesses	20
Radiological perivertebral abscesses	21
Tuberculous sinuses (active/healed)	13
Associated extra-spinal skeletal foci	12
Associated visceral or glandular foci	12
Neurological involvement	20
Lateral shift (radiological)	5
Skipped lesion in the spine	7

A large number of patients seek the advice only when there is severe pain, marked deformity or when the patient has developed neurological complications. 95% of patients reporting in the BHU hospital between 1965 to 1974, had varying degrees of kyphosis **(Fig. 19.1)** at presentation.

REGIONAL DISTRIBUTION OF TUBERCULOUS LESIONS IN THE VERTEBRAL COLUMN (IN THE PRE-MRI ERA—OBSERVED BY CONVENTIONAL X-RAYS)

Any part of the spinal column may be affected but it is most commonly found in the lower thoracic and thoracolumbar region. The order of frequency in Paus' (1964) series of 141 cases has been lumbar (50), dorsal (35), dorsolumbar (25), lumbosacral (22), cervicodorsal (8), sacral (1) and cervical (nil). In Cleveland's (1942) series, the peak incidence was at the 11th thoracic vertebra, the incidence curve falling away more or less smoothly in each direction along the vertebral column. In Hodgson's series (1969), the peak incidence was observed at L1 and the curve had a uniform fall proximal and distal to this level. He suggested that the peak incidence at lumbar one vertebra was possibly due to spread of infection to the spine directly from neighboring infected kidneys.

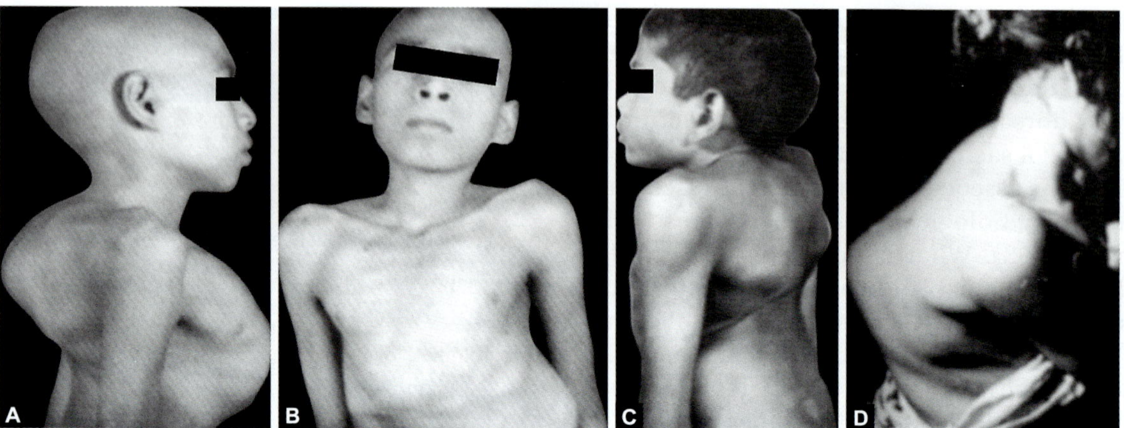

Figs. 19.1A to D: Clinical pictures (A to D) showing severe kyphotic deformity due to involvement of a large number of thoracic vertebrae during the growing age. Note resultant severe deformity of the thoracic cage (A to D)

The incidence of involvement of various regions of spine in our series is shown in **Table 19.3**. The order of frequency has been dorsal, lumbar, cervical and sacral. There were 7% patients who had involvement of more than one region of spine, each region being separated by two or three normal vertebrae **(Fig. 22.9)**. Friedman (1966) described 84 spinal lesions in 64 of his patients of tuberculosis of the spine. The overall higher incidence of cervical spine involvement in our series may be explained on the basis of large number of children suffering from spinal tuberculosis; cervical spine tuberculosis being more common in children. During a period of 25 years, we observed 2 patients having three skipped lesions in their spine. Involvement of the distal part of vertebral column is quite rare (Patel et al. 2000).

Table 19.3: Regional distribution of tuberculous lesions in vertebral column (1965-74) expressed as percentage in pre-MRI era

Cervical (including atlanto-occipital)	12
Cervicodorsal	5
Dorsal	42
Dorsolumbar	12
Lumbar	26
Lumbosacral (including sacrum)	3

VERTEBRAL LESION

By conventional radiology in the majority of patients there are the typical paradiscal lesions **(Fig. 19.2)** characterized by destruction of the adjacent bone end plates of the vertebral bodies and diminution of the intervening disc space **(Fig. 20.1)**. The following uncommon varieties (Rahman 1980) were encountered in the present series which may show (<2% of all spinal lesions) radiologically intact disc spaces. These were the anterior type [involvement of anterior surface of vertebral bodies **(Fig. 8.22)**],

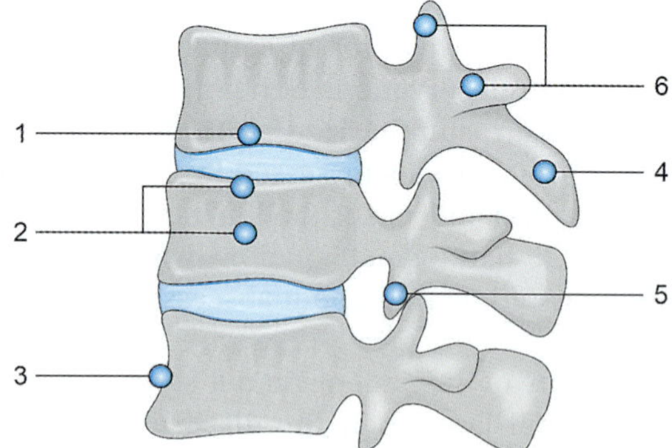

Fig. 19.2: Common sites for initiation of vertebral tuberculosis (1) commonest paradiscal vertebral bodies (6) transverse processes and pedicles: least common.

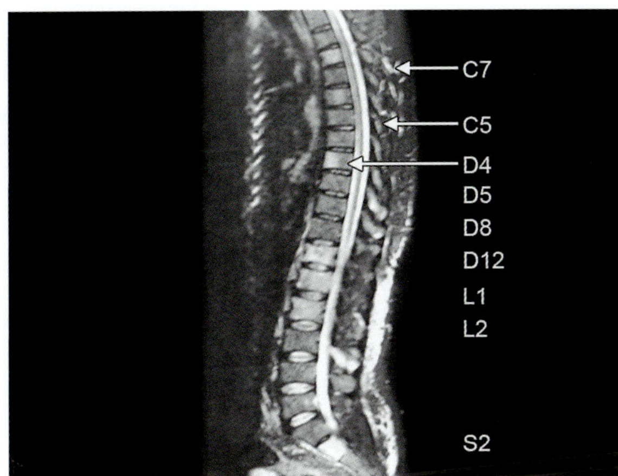

Fig. 19.3: MRI of a patient who presented with dorsolumbar pain. The screening of the whole spine revealed many more subclinical active foci of tuberculosis in the vertebral bodies and the sacrum, seven vertebrae showing involvement.

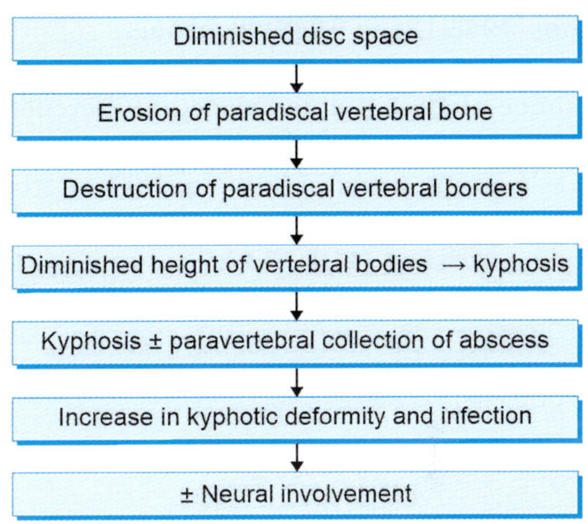

Flowchart 19.1: Usual cascade of tuberculous infection in vertebrae.

posterior spinal disease (involvement of pedicles, transverse processes, laminae or spinous process) **(Fig. 20.18)**, and the central cystic type of tuberculosis of the vertebral body (radiologically a lytic lesion in the centrum or concentric-vertebra plana (collapse) **(Figs. 20.14 to 20.16)**. Tuberculosis of vertebral arches is very rare and Schmorl (1959) quoted the figures of Novak showing such involvement in only 8 of 2,202 cases of vertebral tuberculosis. Isolated involvement of vertebral arches and/or vertebral processes was observed in <2% of our cases of tubercular involvement of the vertebral column. Kumar (1985) suggested that nearly 5% of spinal tuberculosis could be located in the posterior elements, many of them would present with an abscess or a sinus in midline or paramedian region posteriorly. Rarely tuberculous process may be in the form of a tuberculous synovitis of posterior vertebral (apophyseal) articulations, atlanto-occipital or atlantoaxial joints. If every patient diagnosed as spinal tuberculosis by X-rays, were subjected to MRI or CT scan, or isotop bone scan the extent of disease demonstrated would be far greater than suggested radiologically **(Fig. 19.3)**.

Modern imaging modalities may change the figures of site of involvement as mentioned in the pre-MRI era literature. Early tuberculous disease of cranio-vertebral region, cervicodorsal area, sacrum and coccyx may not be discernable in conventional X-rays. The cascade of vertebral involvement is shown in **Flowchart 19.1**.

ASSOCIATED EXTRA-SPINAL TUBERCULAR LESIONS

Spinal tuberculosis is always the result of a hematogenous dissemination from a primary focus; the detection of the primary focus or an associated visceral tubercular lesion, however, depends largely upon the amount of effort put into the investigation. In the present series, a pulmonary and/or visceral and/or glandular tubercular lesions could be detected in 12% of patients. The detection of an apparently small number of associated tuberculous lesions in the viscera in our series is explained because of lack of facilities for mass radiography of different systems for a very large number of patients. 12% of cases of spinal tuberculosis had associated osteoarticular tuberculous lesions in other regions of the skeletal system **(Table 19.2)**. The detection of associated visceral tuberculous lesions (in lungs, urogenital organs and lymph nodes) in the series of other workers (Konstam 1962, Friedman 1966, Wilkinson 1949, Sanchis-

Olmos 1948, Paus 1964) has been reported to be rather high, between 40 and 50%. The presence of disseminated skeletal tuberculosis and association with other visceral tubercular foci is a strong proof of hematogenous spread. Most of such patients are ill-looking and poorly nourished **(Fig. 17.2)**. Presumably, this condition is produced as a result of massive infection in subjects with poor body resistance and nutrition, giving rise to multifocal hematogenous lesions, some more advanced than others. Employing modern imaging techniques would demonstrate an additional sub-clinical skeletal or visceral tuberculous lesion in approximately 40% patients clinically presenting as spinal tuberculosis.

X-ray Appearances and Findings on Modern Imaging

NUMBER OF VERTEBRAE INVOLVED

On an average involvement of 3.4 vertebrae was reported by Hodgson and Stock (1960) in each patient. A figure of 3.8 was given by Mukopadhaya and Mishra (1957). Average number reported in children was 3.4 by Martin (1970). Average number of vertebrae involved in each lesion in our series was 3 for children and 2.5 for adults as judged by X-rays. Spinal tuberculosis is most difficult to recognize radiologically in its early stages. There are mainly 4 sites **(Fig. 20.1)** where tuberculosis occurs in the vertebral column: paradiscal type, central type (central part of the vertebral body), anterior type (involving anterior surface of the vertebral body), and appendiceal type (involving pedicles, laminae, spinous process or transverse processes). 7% of patients may show "skipped lesions" **(Fig. 22.8)**. The largest number of radiologically involved vertebrae observed by us was 10–12 contiguous dorsal vertebrae in 6 patients each, over a period of 35 years of observations. Some of the vertebral bodies were eroded probably by an extensive paravertebral abscess of long-standing. Immunocompromised state, diabetes, and hemoglobinopathies should be suspected in such cases (Pande et al. 1996, 2002).

Paradiscal Type of Lesion

It is **(Figs. 20.2, 20.4, 20.5 and 20.7)** the commonest type of lesion and narrowing of the disc space is often the earliest radiological finding. Any reduction in disc space, if it is associated with a loss of definition of paradiscal margins of the vertebrae, must invite the suspicion of tuberculosis. Radiologically, disc space narrowing is observed before the appearance of osseous destructive changes. Although the small necrotic foci are easily recognized in an anatomic specimen and CT scans, they are

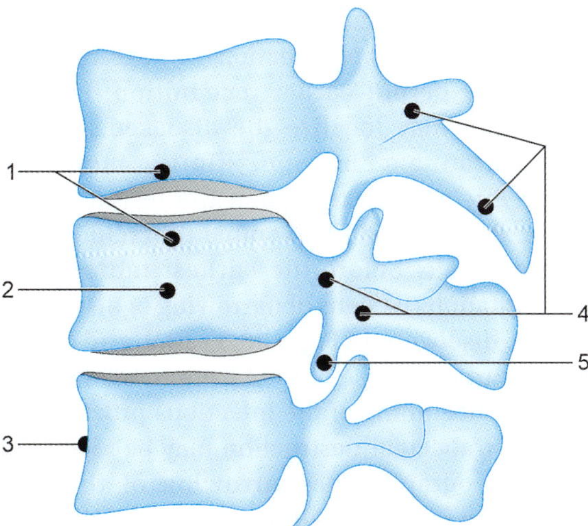

Fig. 20.1: Diagrammatic representation of the frequency of location of tuberculosis of the vertebral column. The most common (1) variety of tubercular spondylitis (spondylodiscitis) occurs in the paradiscal region, and the least common is synovitis in the posterior facet joints (5). (1) = paradiscal, (2) = central, (3) anterior, (4) = appendiceal, (5) = synovial.

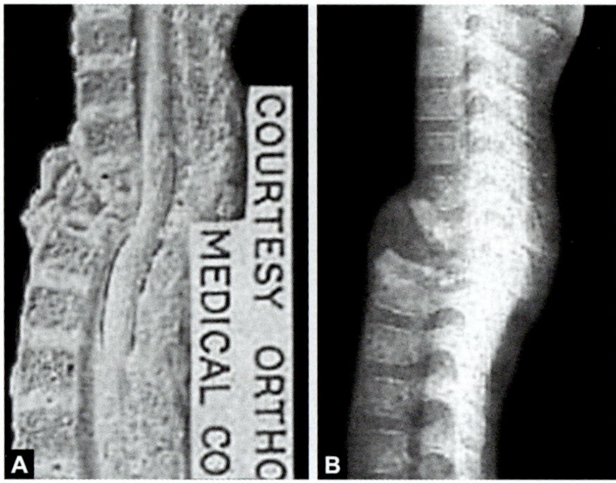

Figs. 20.2A and B: This is a museum specimen of spinal tuberculosis (A) and it's X-ray (B). The destruction is essentially in paradiscal vertebral bodies. Despite gross destruction and deformity the dural tube is intact.

Courtesy: Orthopedic Department Medical College, Patna, Bihar, India.

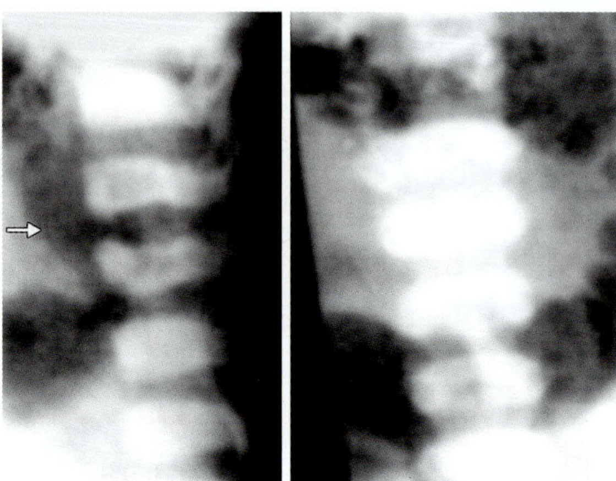

Fig. 20.3: X-rays of a young child showing tuberculosis of lumbar 3 and 4 vertebrae. The apposing metaphyseal regions of these vertebrae due to disease have been softened and the turgid disc has protruded proximally and distally giving it a ballooned out appearance. In due course, the nutrition of the intervertebral disc will be cut off and the space would appear diminished radiologically.

difficult to identify in the radiographs. It has been shown by various workers that foci of <1.5 cm in diameter are not demonstrable in conventional radiographs (Schmorl and Junghanns 1959, Boxer et al. 1992). 30–40% of calcium must be removed from a particular area to show a radiolucent region on X-rays. Planographic section (tomograms/CAT scan) may permit earlier recognition. Isotope bone scan may localize the diseased area by demonstrating a "hot spot" (in the metabolic hyperemic zone) even when the lesion size is 5 mm. Patients have had spinal tuberculosis for several weeks before the earliest radiological manifestations or signs of narrowing of disc space can be discovered **(Figs. 20.3, 20.5 and 20.6)**. It is not until a lapse of time from 3 to 5 months after the beginning of the infectious process that the first trabecular destruction may be identified in a radiograph. The narrowing of the disc space may represent either atrophy of the disc tissue due to lack of nutrition or prolapse of the nucleus pulposus into the soft necrotic vertebral bodies now often observed in MRI studies. In the uncommon varieties of vertebral tuberculosis (central type, anterior type, posterior appendiceal type), the disc space may remain radiologically intact for a long time. MRI findings may help clinch the diagnosis or tissue must be obtained for histological confirmation.

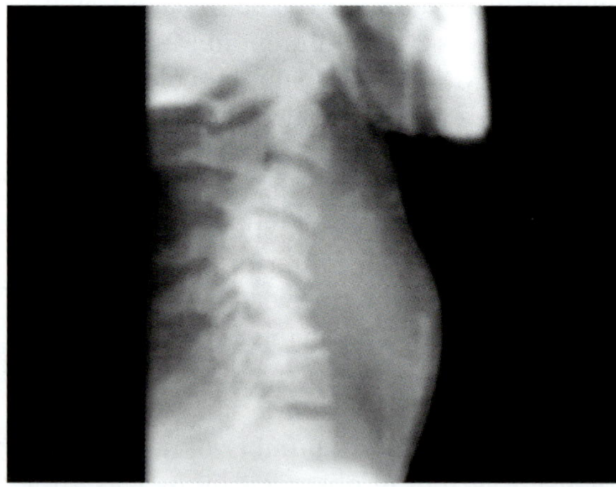

Fig. 20.4: Typical radiological picture of an established case of tuberculosis of cervical spine. Note diminished intervertebral disc spaces between C4 to C7, destruction of paradiscal borders, marked destruction of C5 vertebral body, kyphotic deformity and increased prevertebral soft tissue shadow (tubercular abscess posterior to the trachea).

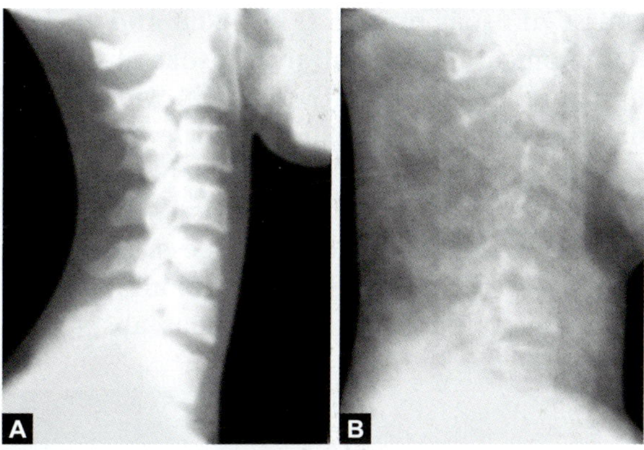

Figs. 20.5A and B: This lateral view (A) of the cervical spine on a casual examination could have passed as "normal". However, a repeat lateral view (B) done after 8 weeks revealed the tuberculous lesion clearly showing diminution of disc spaces (C4–C5 and C5–C6), destructive lesion of cervical fifth vertebral body, and a suspicious increase in the prevertebral shadow.

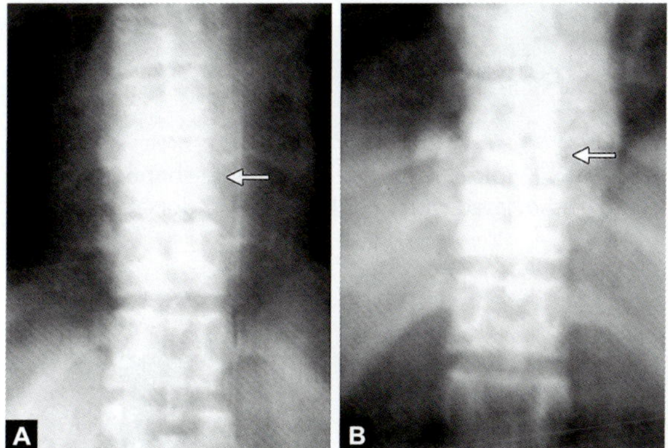

Figs. 20.6A and B: A young lady presented in 1982 with persistent pain in the lower dorsal spine. The routine X-rays (A) were passed as "within-normal-limits". The patient was kept under observation and a repeat X-ray (B) revealed classical tuberculous lesion of dorsal 9–10 vertebrae with a paravertebral shadow. Note diminished disc space (D9–D10) and marked collapse of D10 vertebral body. If more sophisticated investigations are not available one must repeat the X-ray after 2–4 months for comparison with the earlier X-rays.

Paravertebral Shadows

Paravertebral shadow is produced by extension of tuberculous granulation tissue and the collection of an abscess in the paravertebral region. Abscess

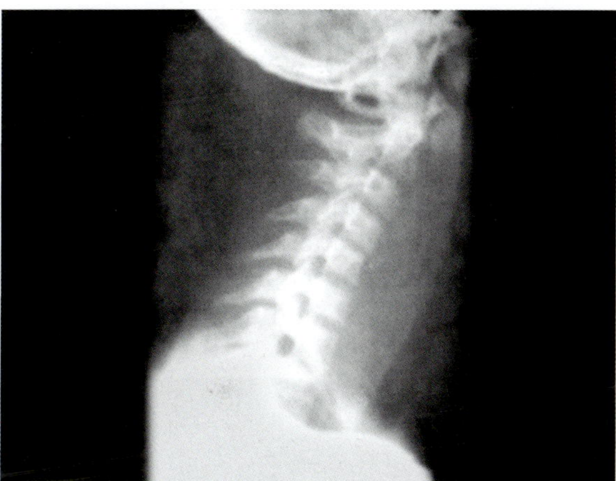

Fig. 20.7: Early tubercular disease between cervical 4th and 5th vertebrae with a huge prevertebral soft tissue shadow. Note diminution of the intervening disc space with erosion and fuzziness of the paradiscal margins. The size of the cold abscess is not necessarily proportionate to the osseous destruction.

in the cervical region usually presents as a soft tissue shadow between the vertebral bodies and pharynx and trachea **(Figs. 20.4, 20.5 and 20.7)**. On an average, the normal space between the pharynx and spine above the level of cricoid cartilage is 0.5 cm and below this level it is 1.5 cm. The upper thoracic abscess in the anteroposterior X-rays cast a V-shaped shadow stripping the lung apices laterally and downward, or when it is small the superior mediastinum shows only squaring of its borders **(Fig. 20.24)**. Abscesses in the region of seventh cervical to fourth dorsal vertebrae require good quality X-rays to be diagnosed at an early stage. Even good quality X-rays may not reveal the destruction of vertebral bodies from cervical seventh to dorsal fourth vertebrae. Careful observation of the tracheal shadow (Jain et al. 1994) can point toward the underlying disease warranting investigations by modern imaging techniques. In the lateral view, normally the tracheal shadow is concave anteriorly (parallel to the upper dorsal vertebrae), if there is a change in the normal contour and/or its distance is >8 mm from the vertebrae it is a strong indicator of the disease from C7 to D4 vertebrae. Abscesses below the level of fourth dorsal vertebrae produce typical fusiform-shape **(Figs. 20.9 and 20.11)** (bird nest appearance), however, when the size of the abscess is too large it may take the shape of a generalized broadening of the mediastinum. An abscess under tension may assume a globular-shape **(Figs. 20.10 and 20.11)**. Abscesses formed above the vertebral attachment of diaphragm tend to remain within the thorax, those arising below the diaphragm tend to extend along the course of psoas muscle **(Figs. 20.8 and 20.12)**. Radiological manifestation of psoas abscess is unilateral or infrequently bilateral widening of the psoas shadow **(Fig. 20.12)**. However, it needs an excellent quality X-rays to detect any bulging of the lateral border of the psoas. MRI and CT scan may demonstrate an abscess contained within the psoas sheath much before it can be clinically palpated as an iliopsoas abscess in

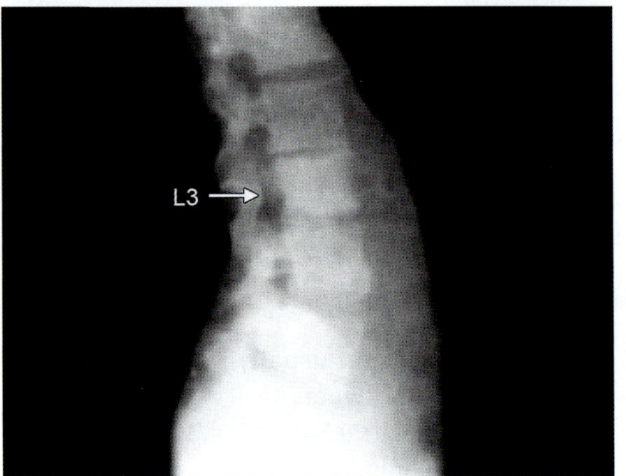

Fig. 20.8: Lateral X-ray of a case of tuberculosis of lumbar 2nd, 3rd and 4th vertebrae. The patient had bilateral cross fluctuant psoas abscesses. The continuity of the abscess across the front of vertebral bodies is shown by a large prevertebral soft tissue shadow.

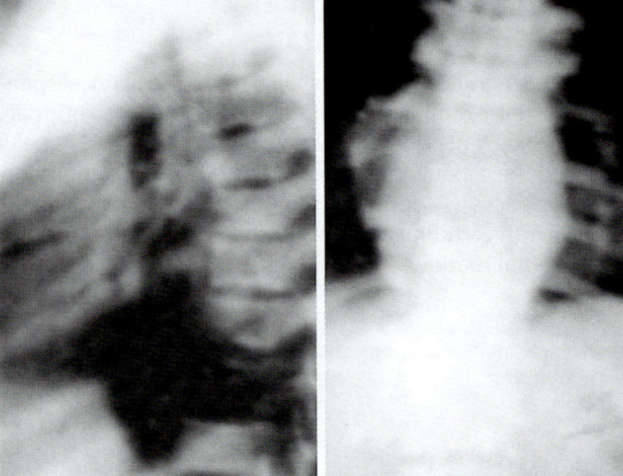

Fig. 20.9: Typical fusiform or spindle-shaped abscess shadow associated with middle and lower dorsal lesions.

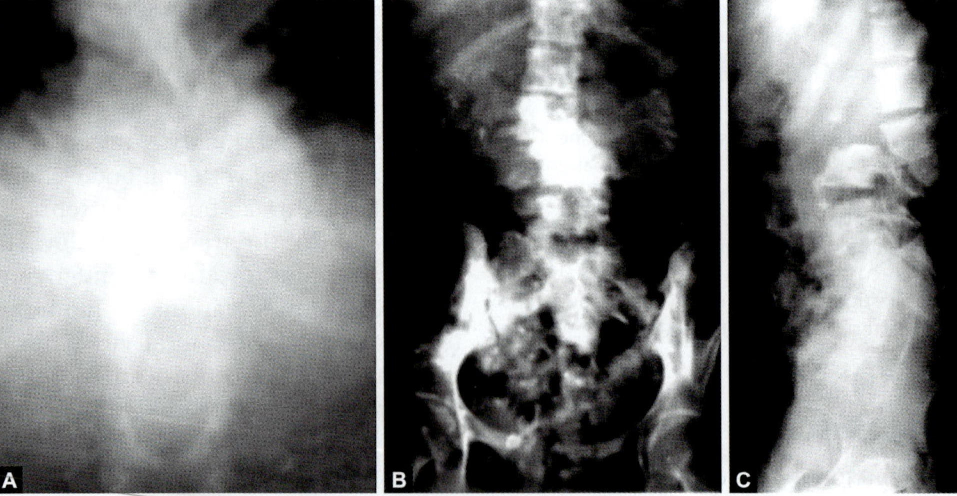

Figs. 20.10A to C: (A) Anteroposterior X-ray of panvertebral tuberculous disease of lower dorsal spine. Note "lateral shift", and a globular paravertebral shadow with calcification in its wall on the left side. (B and C) Show extensive destruction in a case of panvertebral tuberculosis of L2–L4 with gross lateral and anteroposterior dislocation.

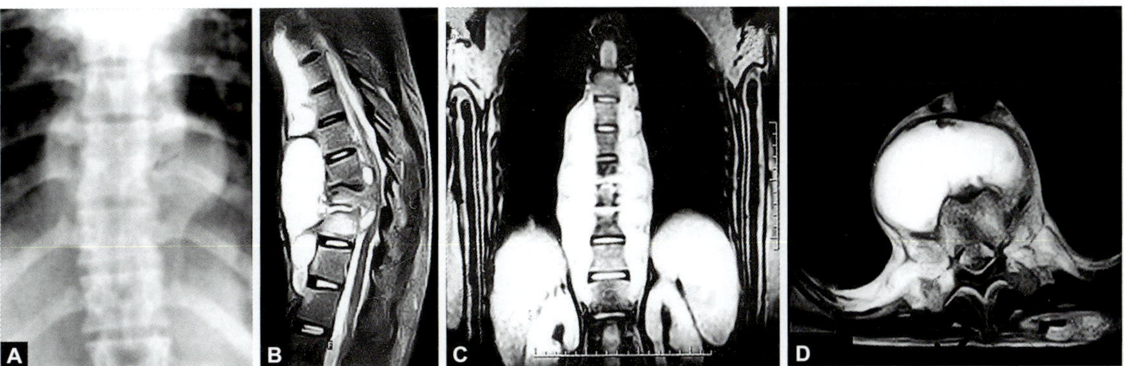

Figs. 20.11A to D: (A) Typical globular, probably tense, paravertebral shadow due to tuberculosis of D9–D10 vertebrae: the patient was operated because she had paraplegia. Nearly 150 mL of liquid pus was drained out. (B to D) show typical MRI appearance of a large paravertebral liquid abscess originating from tuberculous disease of D6–D8. Note the loculated appearance.

the iliac fossa **(Fig. 20.12)**. For the abscess to be clinically palpable in the iliac fossa, the abscess must permeate through the psoas sheath to enter into iliacus sheath **(Fig. 20.28)**, a palpable "psoas" abscess in reality is an "iliopsoas" collection. A "psoas abscess" can be aspirated through the Petit's triangle, whereas the iliopsoas abscess is aspirable through the Petit's triangle as well as through the iliac fossa. Diagnosis of an abscess only on roentgenographic findings is less accurate as many of the densities giving a radiological diagnosis of an abscess may be only absorbed abscesses replaced by fibrous tissue, calcified inspissated **(Fig. 20.10)** matter or granulation tissue. Amongst 100 operated cases reported by Paus (1964) no abscess was found on operation in 5 cases out of 68 with a large paravertebral shadow on the radiographs and in 8 cases out of 25 with a small shadow. In the region of thoracic spine tense paravertebral abscesses of long-standing may show a scalloping effect (aneurysmal phenomenon) as concave erosions along the anterior margins of the vertebral bodies. The healthy discs because of their elasticity in young patients are spared and they stand out to give a "saw tooth" appearance radiologically **(Figs. 20.19 and 20.20)**. Rarely, a small and thin perivertebral abscess may not cast any shadow radiologically.

KYPHOTIC DEFORMITY (ANGULATION OF SPINE WITH CONVEXITY POSTERIORLY)

In a typical tubercular spondylitis of some standing, besides the diminution of disc space, the paradiscal vertebral bodies show areas of destruction and one or more bodies are usually wedged (collapse of bone due to hyperemia, softening or infection) with forward angulation. Involvement of a large number of adjacent vertebrae would produce a severe kyphotic deformity **(Figs. 20.13, 20.14, 20.18 and 20.28)**. Forward wedging of one or 2 vertebral bodies would produce a small kyphos (**knuckle kyphosis**), wedge collapse of 3 or more vertebral bodies would produce an **angular kyphosis**, and moderate wedging of a large number of vertebrae would create a **round kyphosis,** not unlike osteoporotic kyphos. Gibbus deformity and kyphotic deformity are used as interchangeable expressions.

Examining a thoracic spine with Pott's disease which had healed with ankylosis and appreciable kyphosis, there may be considerable increase in the height of the vertebral bodies of the lumbar spine, sometimes amounting to an increase of one-third in vertical height. These "tall vertebrae" can develop only when the

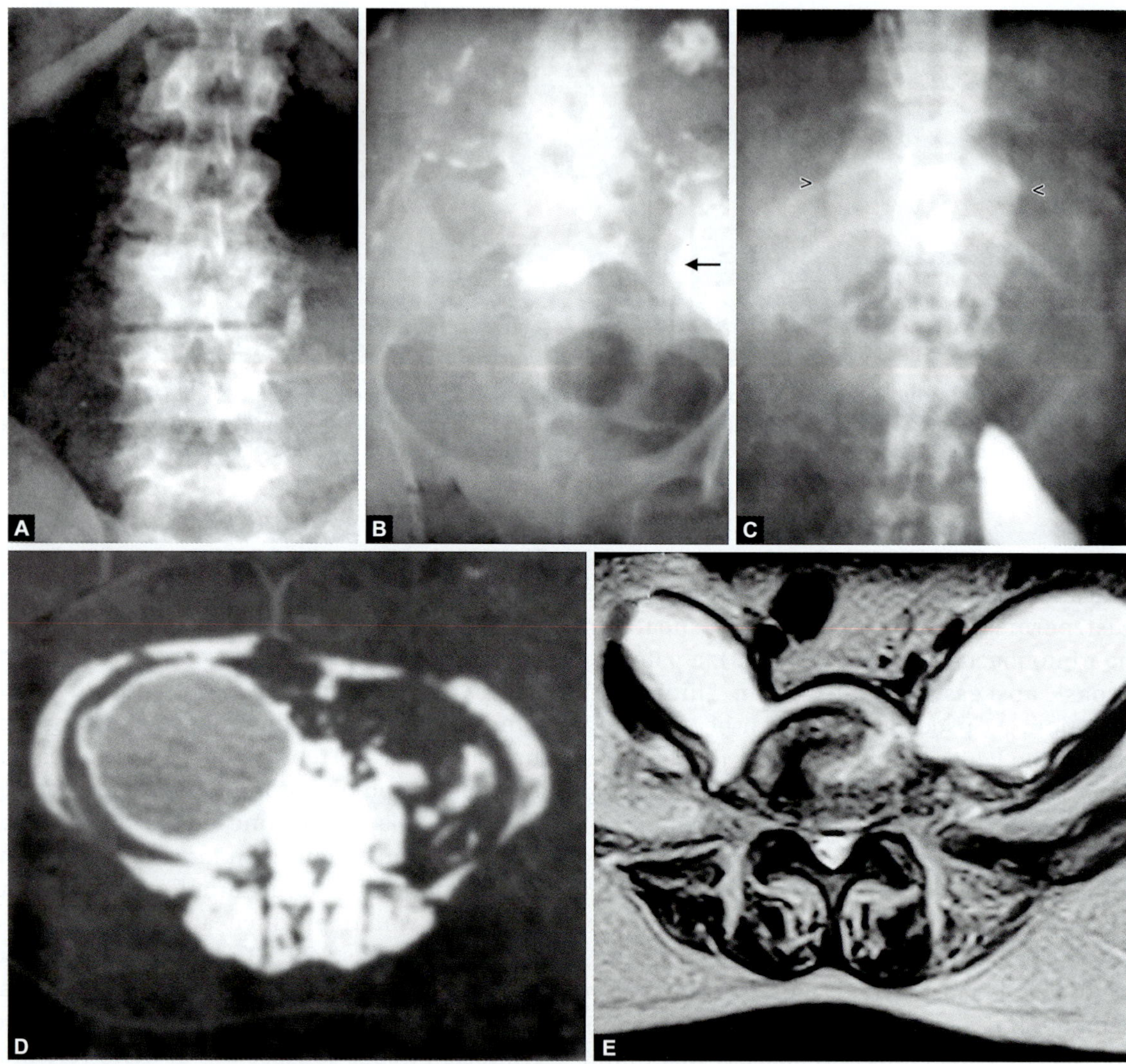

Figs. 20.12A to E: X-rays showing shadows of paravertebral abscesses associated with tuberculosis of dorsolumbar or lumbar regions, (A) Bilateral bulging of the psoas shadows (tuberculosis L2–4), (B and C) Psoas abscesses outlined by an injection of sodium iodide solution [a technique used (1970) prior to availability of CT scans and MRIs]. Note the spread of the dye from the left psoas abscess to the right (B). In (C) note a rounded paravertebral shadow above the region of diaphragm (> <) in addition to a psoas abscess (enhanced by sodium iodide solution) related to tuberculosis of L1–L2. (D) CT scan showing a right psoas abscess from a lumbar lesion. (E) MRI showing the continuity between the left and right psoas abscesses, deep to the anterior longitudinal ligaments. Note the communication of the abscess with the cavity within the vertebral body.

disease occurred during the growth period, i.e., before the disappearance of the growth zones. This phenomenon was first described by Menard, however, later on other workers also reported such observations (Schmorl and Junghanns 1959, Hodgson 1969, Tuli 1970). Because of pre-existing lordosis and large size of vertebral bodies, severe kyphotic deformity in the lumbar spine is rare. However, gross destruction of anterior growth plates of a large number of vertebrae

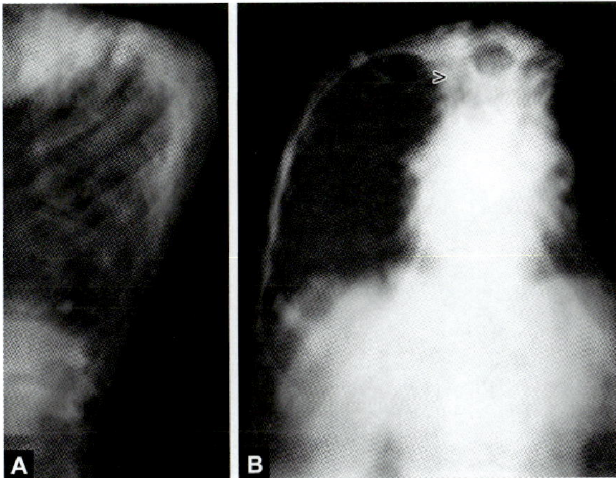

Figs. 20.13A and B: X-rays of a case of severe kyphotic deformity due to tuberculous disease of dorsal 4th to 8th vertebrae. (A) The angle of kyphosis is 110 degrees due to which the "end on view" (B) of the proximal vertebral canal is visible in the anteroposterior view.

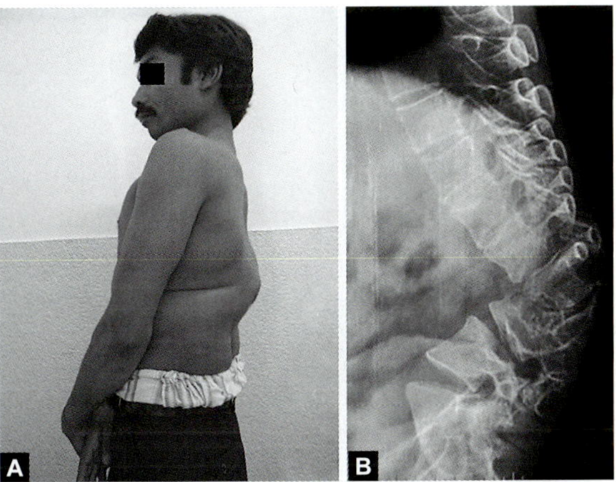

Figs. 20.14A and B: Clinical picture (A) and X-ray (B) of a case of severe kyphotic deformity due to tuberculous disease of 4 lumbar vertebrae. The patient has reached adulthood without neural deficit. Distal to lumbar one vertebra dural tube contents (cauda quina) can tolerate gradually progressive gross deformities retaining neural functions.

with unrestricted growth of posterior elements would result in severe kyphosis. As the deformity develops gradually, the neural elements tolerate the progressive kyphosis for many years. Several patients reach adulthood with intact neural status **(Fig. 20.14)**.

CENTRAL TYPE OF LESION (TUBERCULOSIS OF THE CENTRUM OF VERTEBRAL BODY)

The central disease arises as a result of infection which starts from the center of the vertebral body, the infection probably reaches the center through Batson's venous plexus or through the branches of the posterior vertebral artery. The diseased vertebral body loses the normal bony trabeculae and may show areas of destruction **(Fig. 20.15)**, or the body may be expanded or ballooned out like a tumor. Toward the later stages the diseased vertebral body, however, shows a concentric collapse almost resembling vertebra plana **(Fig. 20.16)**. Diminution of the disc space is minimal and paravertebral shadow is usually not well-marked. In the absence of a paravertebral shadow, this type of lesion is very difficult to differentiate radiologically from vertebral collapse due to Calve's disease or due to a neoplastic condition **(Figs. 20.17 and 20.19)**. Tuberculous nature of the disease is suggested by the presence of local pain, tenderness, spasm, and systemic features when present. Longer follow-up of such patients tends to show diminution of the adjacent disc space in many cases. In TB endemic areas the most common cause of vertebra plana appearance is tuberculous pathology.

Skipped Lesions

Sometimes more than one tuberculous lesion may be present in the vertebral column with one or more of healthy vertebrae in between the two lesions **(Fig. 22.8)**. The average incidence on routine radiology in any large series is 7%. However, if patients were subjected to modern imaging modalities (MRI/CT scan), many more small lesions in the vertebral column have been detected, nearly 40% of patients may show an additional subclinical active or old healed infection.

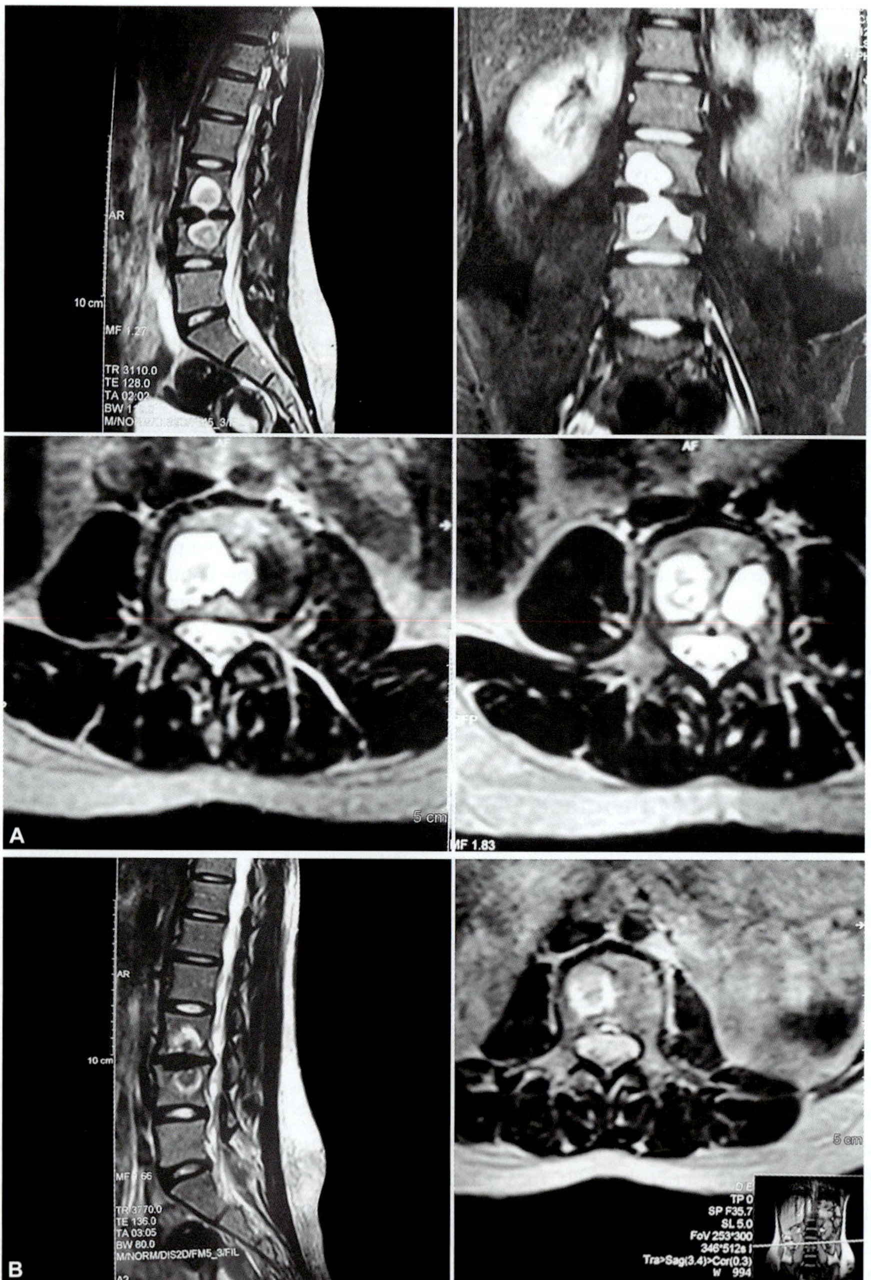

Figs. 20.15A and B: MRIs of a cyst-like tuberculous lesions in 2 adjacent lumbar vertebral bodies (A) is pretreatment. One can observe the reduction in the size of abscess, (B) Post-treatment, under the influence of antitubercular drugs. The lesion in L3 and L4 may be addressed as "kissing lesions".

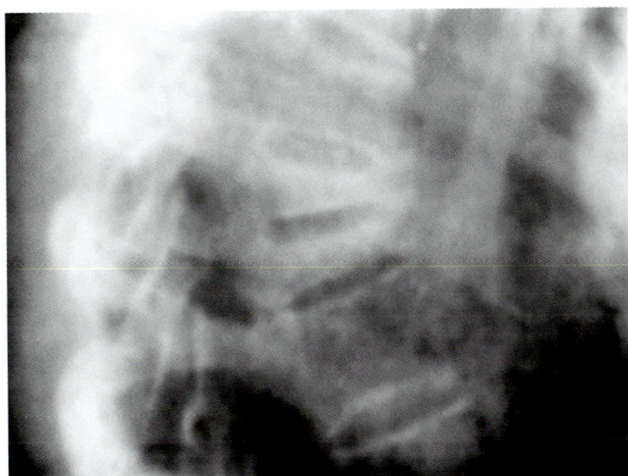

Fig. 20.16: Lateral view of the dorsal spine showing vertebra plana like collapse of two vertebral bodies. Note that intervening disc space is practically unchanged.

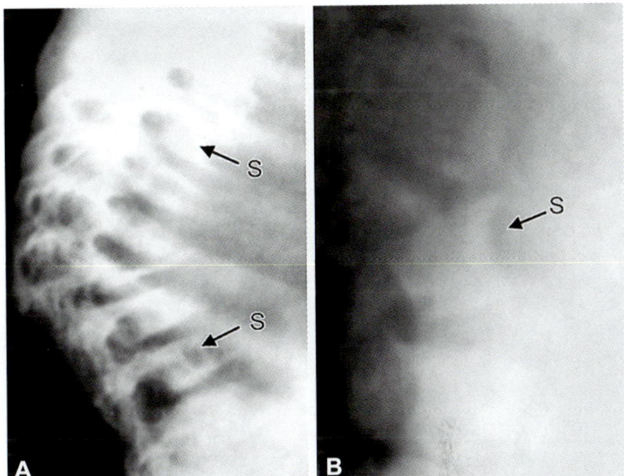

Figs. 20.18A and B: X-rays showing the "scalloping effect" or "aneurysmal phenomenon" or "saw-tooth appearance" in tuberculosis of the spine. The scalloping effect is caused by a large tense abscess of long-standing in the proximity of aorta. Note marked diminution of the intervening disc space at the site of the diseased vertebrae, presence of scalloping effect away from the diseased area, and intact disc spaces in the region showing the scalloping effect where only the anterior surface of the vertebral bodies show destruction, (A) in dorsal and (B) in lumbar spine. Arrows show the scalloping defect.

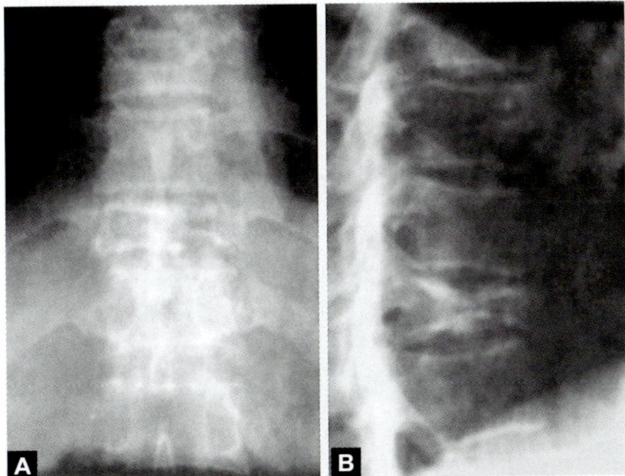

Figs. 20.17A and B: X-rays showing a concentric collapse of dorsal 10 vertebral body with a paravertebral shadow and fairly intact disc spaces. Because of paralysis the lesion was surgically approached and the cord was decompressed through anterolateral extrapleural operation. Examination of the tissues macroscopically as well as by histology proved it to be tuberculosis. The patient made an uneventful recovery.

Anterior Type of Lesion

This lesion occurs when the infection starts beneath the anterior longitudinal ligament and the periosteum. The peripheral portion of the vertebral body (in front and on the sides) shows erosions in lateral view or oblique views as shallow excavations. Collapse of the vertebral body and diminution of the disc space is usually minimal and occurs late. This lesion is relatively more common in thoracic spine in children. These radiologically visible shallow erosions of the anterior surface of the vertebral bodies are to be differentiated, from aneurysmal phenomenon observed in cases of tense paravertebral abscesses of long-standing associated with the usual paradiscal type of tuberculous lesions **(Fig. 20.18)**. Probably the erosion caused in the later is primarily of mechanical nature—a tense paravertebral abscess strips and lifts the anterior longitudinal ligament and the periosteum and thus, causes erosion on the surface of the vertebral bodies. More erosion is caused wherever aorta is in close proximity with the paravertebral abscess (thoracic and thoracolumbar regions) thereby permitting transmission of aortic pulsations to the abscess. Stripping of the periosteum from the underlying bone deprives the bone of its periosteal blood supply which makes the bone more liable to

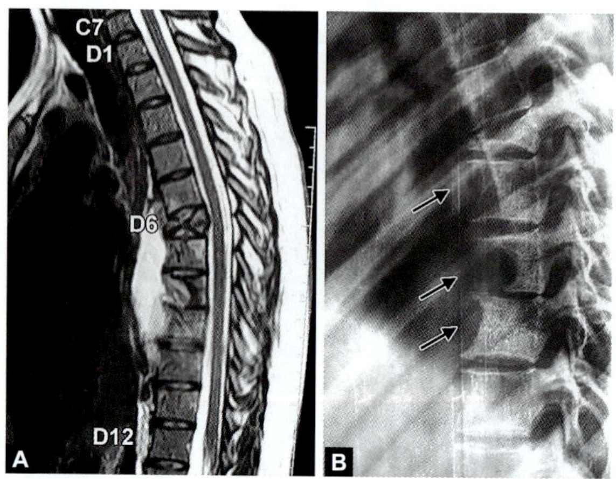

Figs. 20.19A and B: MRI (A) and (B) X-ray of a case of tuberculosis of mid-dorsal spine. Note a paravertebral cold abscess, concentric collapse (vertebrae plana) of D6, and various degree of scalloping effect seen in D7, D8 and D9 vertebral bodies.

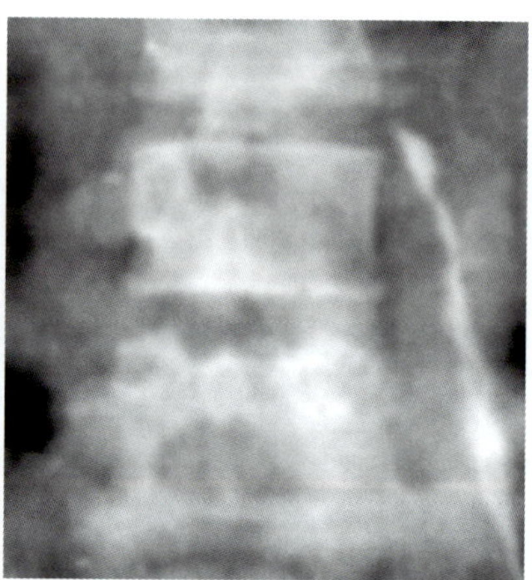

Fig. 20.20: A lady presented with a chronic persistent discharging sinus in the perianal region. The source of the sinus was not detectable clinically. X-rays of the lumbar spine revealed absence of the left pedicle, and destruction of the left transverse process of lumbar 4 vertebra, the sinogram proved the origin to be tuberculosis of the posterior elements.

destructive changes and scalloping effect due to infection and aortic pulsations **(Fig. 20.19)**.

Appendiceal Type of Lesion

Isolated tuberculous infection of the pedicles and laminae (neural arch), transverse processes, and spinous process does occur but uncommonly **(Fig. 20.20)**. Tomographic views are most helpful in detecting these lesions. Radiographically, these lesions may be appreciated by erosive lesions, paravertebral shadows and intact disc space (Rahman 1980). Rarely tuberculous process may be in the form of a tuberculous synovitis of posterior vertebral articulations, atlanto-occipital or atlanto-axial joints. Appendiceal type of tuberculous lesions of the vertebral column occurring in isolation or in conjunction with the typical paradiscal tuberculosis were considered to be very rare (<5 %). However, with the employment of CT scan or MRI nearly 30% of cases of typical paradiscal tubercular spondylitis showed concomitant involvement of posterior elements in our patients (Arora 2012).

At present, CT scan and/or MRI are the best imaging modalities to make diagnosis of isolated appendiceal type of tuberculosis, especially in early stages **(Fig. 20.21)**.

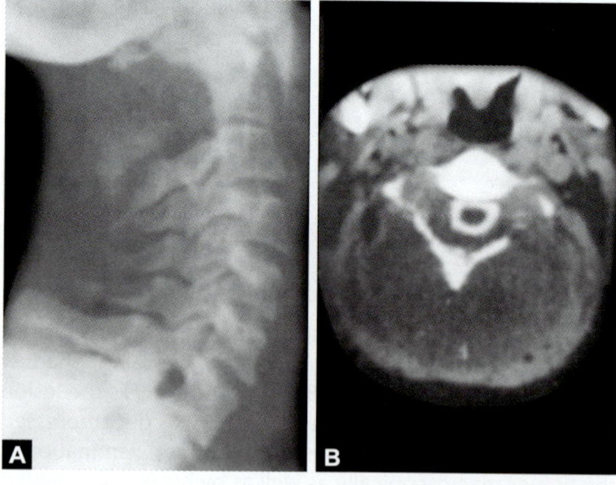

Figs. 20.21A and B: A young lady presented with pain at craniovertebral junction, swelling in the upper part of back of neck and quadriparesis. X-ray (A) revealed destruction of posterior arches of C1 and C2 vertebrae, a soft tissue mass in the back of neck and undisturbed soft tissue shadows anteriorly. The CT scan (B) revealed destruction of the posterior elements as well as the lateral mass of C2, there was a huge soft tissue mass (abscess) in the retrovertebral area and around the dural sheath. The patient made an uneventful neural recovery and healing of disease by drainage of abscess, skull traction, four-post collar and antitubercular drugs.

LATERAL SHIFT AND SCOLIOSIS

A lateral curvature and lateral deviation has been recognized as one of the rare deformities of Pott's disease. It has been explained by various workers to be a combination of lateral deviation as well as rotation (Hodgson 1969). Hodgson explained it on the basis of more destruction of vertebral body on one side, thus resulting in lateral deviation similar to that caused by a hemivertebra. Almost all such cases occurred in the lower dorsal and lumbar spine, and they were associated with marked destruction of vertebral bodies and the intervening disc space.

We had an opportunity to analyze (Gupta et al. 1973) the lateral shift in 15 cases. The site of vertebral involvement was lower dorsal and lumbar spine **(Fig. 20.22)**. The highest level observed in these cases was 10th dorsal. In 10 out of 15 cases, the lateral shift was associated with some degree of rotation. In most of the cases, there was marked reduction of disc space and destruction of bodies of vertebrae **(Fig. 20.22)**. The lateral shift occurs in those cases of tuberculosis of the spine in whom there is involvement of posterior spinal articulations in addition to the usual paradiscal lesions (**panvertebral** or circumferential disease). We had an opportunity to verify this fact at operation on a few cases with lateral shift. The involvement of posterior spinal joints is not easily detected on routine roentgenograms. Majority of the cases observed by us did not have neurological complications.

NATURAL COURSE OF THE DISEASE

Before the availability of modern antitubercular drugs, the mortality rate of the patients, followed-up for a period varying from 1 to 10 years, was about 30% in various series (Harris 1952). A large number of these patients developed severe crippling deformities, cold abscesses, multiple discharging sinuses, spread of tuberculous infection to other parts of the body, paraplegia with all its complications and amyloidosis. Schmorl and Junghanns (1959) quoted Boerema's (1931) statistical studies which demonstrated that 53% of patients with tuberculous spondylitis died within 10 years after the onset of the disease, nearly always from pulmonary tuberculosis. Results of any treatment, operative or orthodox conservative, were on the whole poor before the availability of antitubercular drugs.

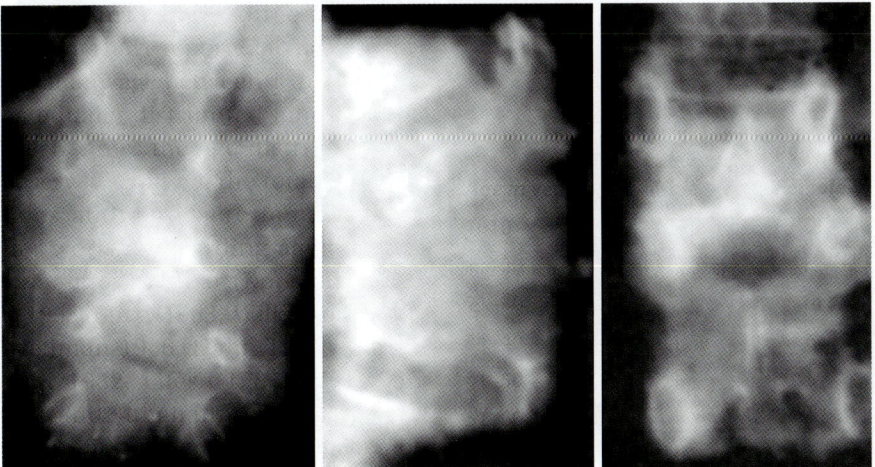

Fig. 20.22: X-rays showing "lateral shift" or lateral translation in tuberculous disease of the spine. Note marked diminution of the disc space, marked destruction of paradiscal vertebral bodies and their posterior elements, and moderate degree of rotational element. Despite gross destruction the disease healed under the influence of antitubercular drugs without surgery with retention of neural functions.

The use of modern antitubercular drugs has, however, changed the outcome of the treatment. When a paradiscal lesion is diagnosed early (predestructive stage) and treated adequately, healing may take place leaving behind no radiological deformity or defect except a moderately diminished disc space **(Fig. 23.6)**. In early stage of healing, the disease focus in some cases may be surrounded by sclerotic bone, giving rise to an "ivory vertebra", and as healing progresses a normal trabecular pattern appears. One of the early radiological signs of healing is sharpening of the fuzzy paradiscal margins, and reappearance and mineralization of trabeculae which had earlier been absorbed. Under the influence of modern antitubercular drugs, remarkable regeneration **(Fig. 20.23)** of the destroyed vertebrae may be observed **(Fig. 23.16)** radiologically. If several vertebral bodies are destroyed and a large gap is produced during the process of healing, the repair takes place by fibrous or fibro-osseous tissues. If the disc space is completely destroyed and the gap is obliterated by the collapse of the vertebrae and by telescopy, healing may take place by bony ankylosis or bone-block formation (intercorporeal bony fusion). Sometimes new bone formation may occur as a result of secondary infection usually associated with sinus formation giving an appearance of "ivory vertebra".

MODERN IMAGING TECHNIQUES

CT scan is a useful tool in assessing the destructive lesions of the vertebral column. It is of special help for posterior spinal disease, tuberculosis of craniovertebral and cervicodorsal region, sacroiliac joints, and of the sacrum where early lesions do not show in routine X-rays **(Figs. 20.24 and 20.26)** (Amouz 1981, Bell et al. 1990, Desai 1994). As the CT scan displays the transectional view **(Fig. 20.25)** of the vertebral column and

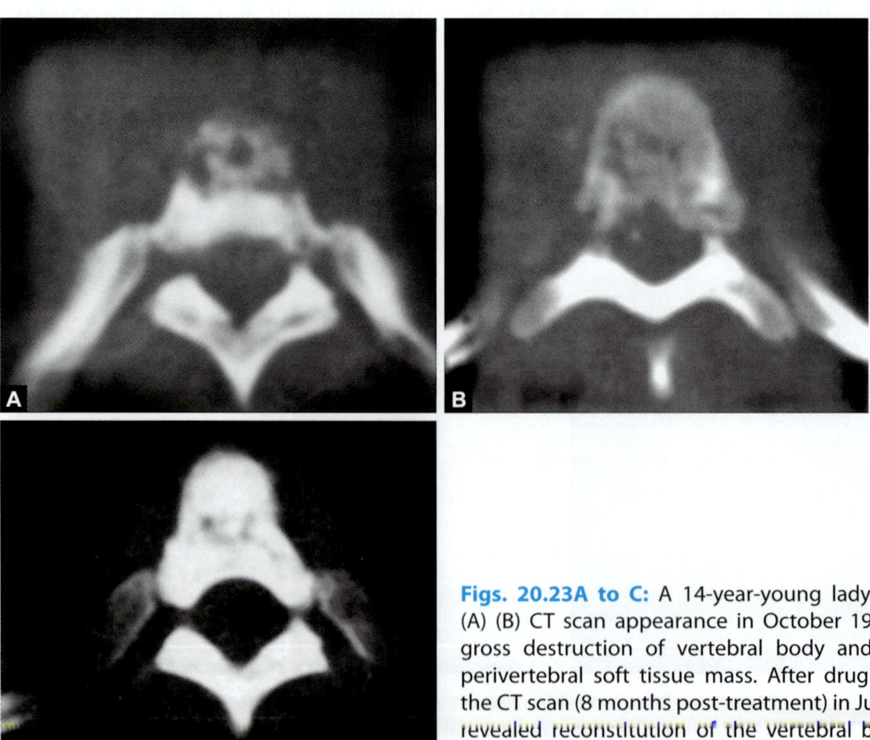

Figs. 20.23A to C: A 14-year-young lady showed (A) (B) CT scan appearance in October 1993. Note gross destruction of vertebral body and a large perivertebral soft tissue mass. After drug therapy, the CT scan (8 months post-treatment) in June 1994, revealed reconstitution of the vertebral body and nearly complete resolution of the perivertebral soft tissue mass (C).

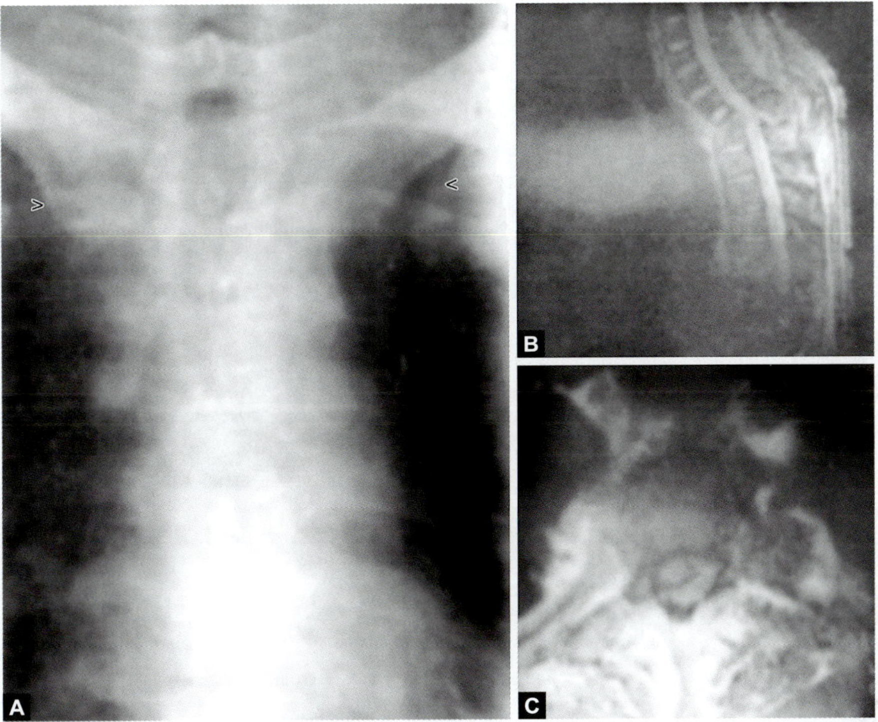

Figs. 20.24A to C: Tuberculous lesions in the region of C7 to D4 vertebrae are very difficult to be visualized in conventional X-rays, suspicion should arise if you observe "widening" of the superior mediastinum (A). CT scan of the suspected area or MRI (B) are of great help in the diagnosis. This MRI shows a destructive lesion of the vertebral bodies of C7, D1, D2. The kyphotic deformity, obliteration of the disc spaces between C7–D1 and D1–D2 and prevertebral soft tissue shadow is clearly visible. The axial section of MRI shows a thick layer of granulation tissue surrounding the cord and shifting it to the right (C).

its neighboring soft tissues, the specialists must localize the suspected area of disease for this investigation **(Fig. 20.25)** to minimize the radiation exposure (Mohanty et al. 2000). Various patterns of destruction of vertebral bodies in tuberculosis are shown in **Figure 20.25**. Delineation of the shape, extent and the route of spread of a cold abscess can also be very well visualized by CT scan **(Fig. 20.27)**.

Magnetic resonance imaging (MRI) has been found to be extremely useful in the diagnosis of tuberculous infection of difficult and rare sites, like craniovertebral region, cervicodorsal region **(Fig. 20.24)**, disease of the posterior elements and vertebral appendages **(Fig. 20.29)**, infections of the sacroiliac region, sacrum and coccyx (de Roos et al. 1989, Smith et al. 1989). Interpretation of common MRI findings particularly in cases of spinal tuberculosis have been outlined in **Table 20.1**. MRI and CT scans should, however, be limited to doubtful cases or the disease in difficult areas **(Figs. 20.21, 20.24, 20.26 and 20.29)**. The role of MRI in the study of cord is described in Chapter 22. MRI is an excellent modality to judge the health of the cord **(Fig. 20.28)** (Jain et al. 2000, Anley et al. 2012, Gupta et al. 2014). If MRI could be done in all radiologically suspected cases of spinal tuberculosis, concomitant or additional involvement of transverse processes, pedicles, spinous processes and adjacent and distant vertebral bodies could be detected in >40% of cases.

Ultrasound echographs have been employed to diagnose the presence of tubercular abscesses in lumbar vertebral disease. We have been able to assess the composition (solid or fluid) of

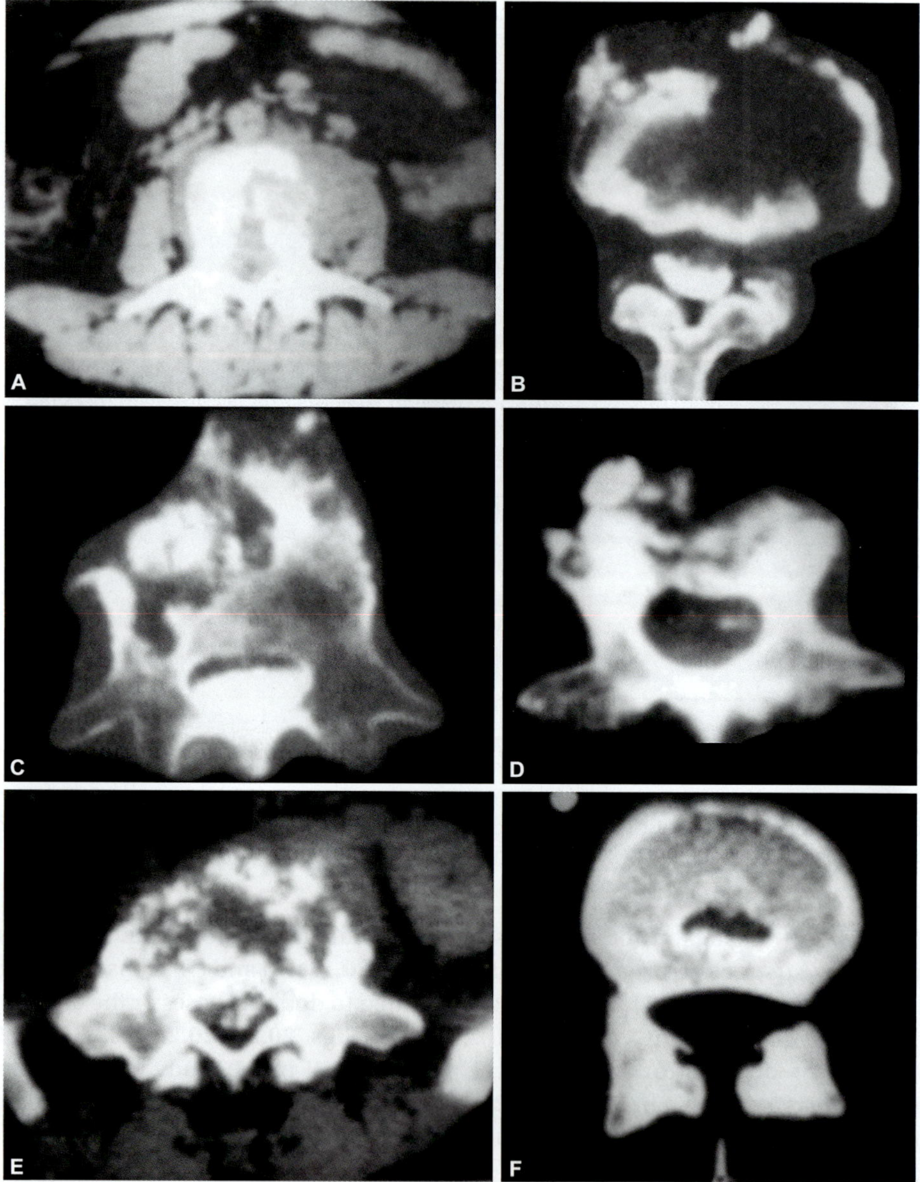

Figs. 20.25A to F: The CT scan essentially gives the information about the geographical configuration of the cavitations and the anatomical extent of the disease process. (A) Shows a large cavity in the left half of vertebral body, the cavity contains soft sequestra and is opening into the vertebral canal as well as into the left psoas sheath. (B) Shows destruction of left half of vertebral body with calcification in the paravertebral soft tissues. (C and D) Show cavitations and destructive changes predominantly in the anterior half of vertebral bodies with extrusion of sequestrae and dystrophic calcification in the paravertebral soft tissues. (E) Shows destruction and fragmentation of the vertebral body. (F) Appearance of a healed cavity in the vertebral body, note sharp and dense margins.

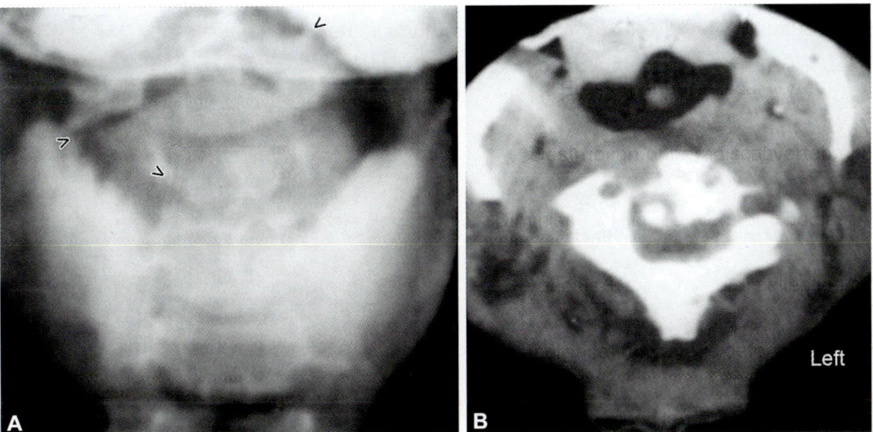

Figs. 20.26A and B: Open mouth view of conventional X-rays showing destruction of left atlantoaxial articulation resulting in right-sided subluxation of atlas over axis. Note the decreased space between the odontoid process and the left lateral mass of atlas, and the step formation (> <) between the right lateral mass of atlas on axis. Changes are best demonstrated in the CT scan which shows gross destruction of anterior arch and left lateral mass of axis. Note increased soft tissue swelling anteriorly on the left side.

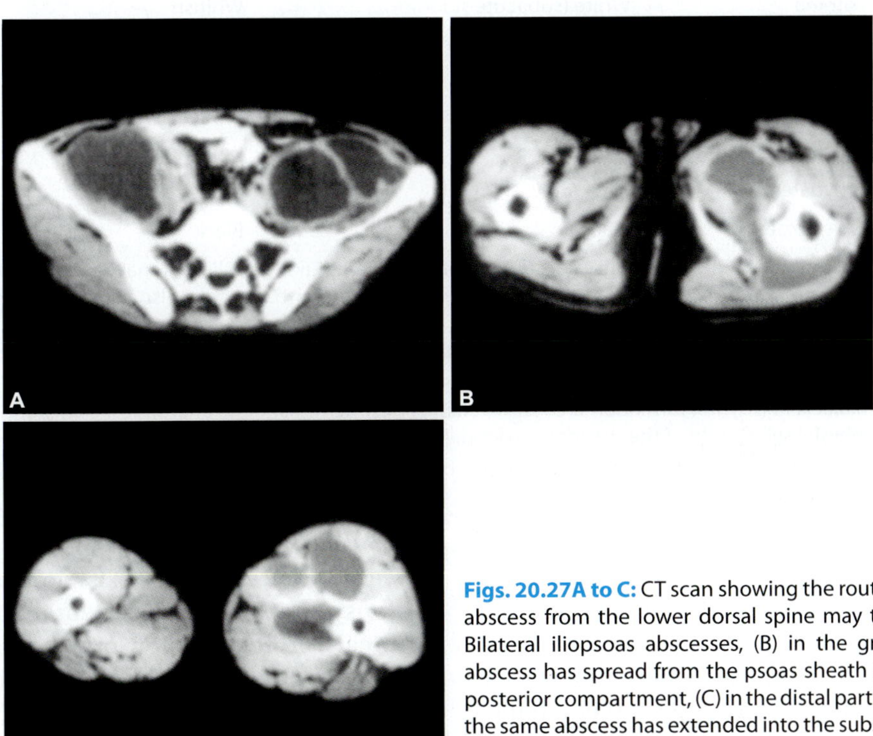

Figs. 20.27A to C: CT scan showing the route a cold abscess from the lower dorsal spine may take: (A) Bilateral iliopsoas abscesses, (B) in the groin the abscess has spread from the psoas sheath into the posterior compartment, (C) in the distal part of thigh the same abscess has extended into the subsartorial canal and in the posterior compartment, probably along the perforating vessels.

Table 20.1: Broad guidelines for interpretation of magnetic resonance images as related to tuberculous infection of the skeletal system.

Tissue/Fluids	*T1 image*	*T2 image*
Fat in marrow or cancellous bone or degenerated areas	White	Grayish-white
Muscles	Gray	Gray
CSF or clear fluid or water in tissues	Black	White
White matter brain/spine	Dark gray	Gray
Gray matter brain/spine	Blackish	Whitish gray
Granulation tissue	Gray	Whitish gray
Air	Black irregular	Black irregular
Bone	Black	Black
Flowing blood	Black	Black
Ligament or capsule (mature fibrous tissue)	Black line/band	Black line/band
Cord contusion or edema (myelitis)	Dark gray	Whitish
Prevertebral hematoma	White (subacute stage)	Whitish
Ischemic/necrosed/sequestrated bone	Gray dead bone surrounded by black zone	Gray dead bone surrounded by white zone
Syrinx	Black cavity in cord	White cavity in cord
Myelomalacia	Dark	White
Nucleus pulposus hydated	Black/gray	White
Nucleus pulposus desiccated	Black	Black

Active inflammation or active infection causes accumulation of edema fluid. Gadolinium may enhance areas of active infection or inflammation to provide better contrast in T2 images. The scar tissue may also show enhancement on T1 images. MRI possibly picks up infective lesions earlier than CT scans. Degenerative changes in the bones may lead to accumulation of fat in bone. MRI shows mineralized bone but not the calcified tissues or the compact borders of bone.

Arachnoiditis is demonstrated as clumping of nerve roots or matted nerve roots. Cord edema (myelitis) is reversible, however, myelomalacia and syrinx formation are not reversible. Despite remarkable anatomical clarity and information about the pathophysiological state of the tissues visualized, MRI is still wisely called an imaging technology.

Imaging specialists expression's "high signal" = white or bright, "low signal" = black or dark, "intermediate (medium) signal" = gray.

iliopsoas mass and the quantity of the liquid material contained therein (Jain et al. 1992) by ultrasonography.

In developing countries where tuberculosis is endemic and resources are scarce, a typical clinical and radiological appearance of tuberculosis may be sufficient reason to begin treatment without biopsy. In case of doubt, however, where facilities exist, for confirmation a biopsy of a small paravertebral abscess or of atypical vertebral lesion may be obtained by core biopsy needle under fluoroscopic control, using the standard techniques (Silverman et al. 1986). Open biopsy with debulking and/ decompression is mandatory if semi-invasive techniques do not prove the pathology.

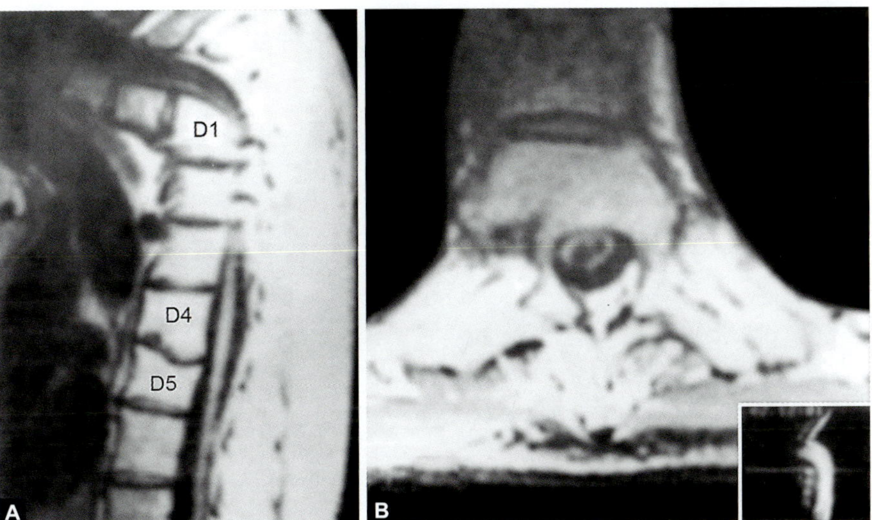

Figs. 20.28A and B: (A and B) MRI of a patient who was treated 26 years ago (aged 12 years) for tuberculosis of dorsal 4th and 5th vertebrae. At the age of 38 years the patient reported with progressively increasing motor weakness. The MRI showed nearly 90 degrees kyphotic deformity at C7–D1 region which was probably missed (without MRI or CT facility at first presentation). The axial T1-weighted image showed syringomyelia in the cord. Presence of syrinx and myelomalacia is an indicator of poor neural recovery even after effective mechanical decompression.

For nearly first 6 months of chemotherapy further bony destruction and collapse can occur as discerned by X-rays and MRI. This may lead to increase in vertebral angulation particularly if significant amount of kyphotic angulation was already present when drugs were started and the spine was not protected by appropriate rest and a suitable brace. Such an appearance should not necessarily cause an alarm because radiological and MRI picture lags behind the biological progress of healing **(Figs. 20.30 and 20.31)**.

CLINICO-RADIOLOGICAL CLASSIFICATION OF TYPICAL TUBERCULAR-SPONDYLITIS

Depending upon the degree of destruction of bone and the angular deformity, Kumar (1988) suggested classification of typical tuberculous spondylitis. Such a classification is important as it permits a more valid comparison of various series. Stage I if diagnosed in time and treated effectively would heal without leaving any defect. Stage II, III, IV and V would also heal but with progressively increasing kyphotic deformity. If neural deficit occurs in Stage V, the chances of complete neural recovery are remote. The outline of the classification is shown in **Table 20.2**.

Biological Healing and Imaging

Radiological and MRI evidence of healing lags behind the biological processes in spinal and skeletal tuberculosis. Despite satisfactory clinical evidence and favorable laboratory findings, X-rays or MRI done up to 5 months after the start of multidrug therapy may show deterioration of the images in most of the patients **(Fig. 20.29)**.

Any repair process involves the penetration of vascular reparative granulations from the perilesional (adjacent tissues) areas. The hypervascular adjacent tissues would show an extended area of "abnormal" signals in **(Figs. 20.30 and 20.32)** the bones as bone-marrow edema and in the adjacent soft tissue

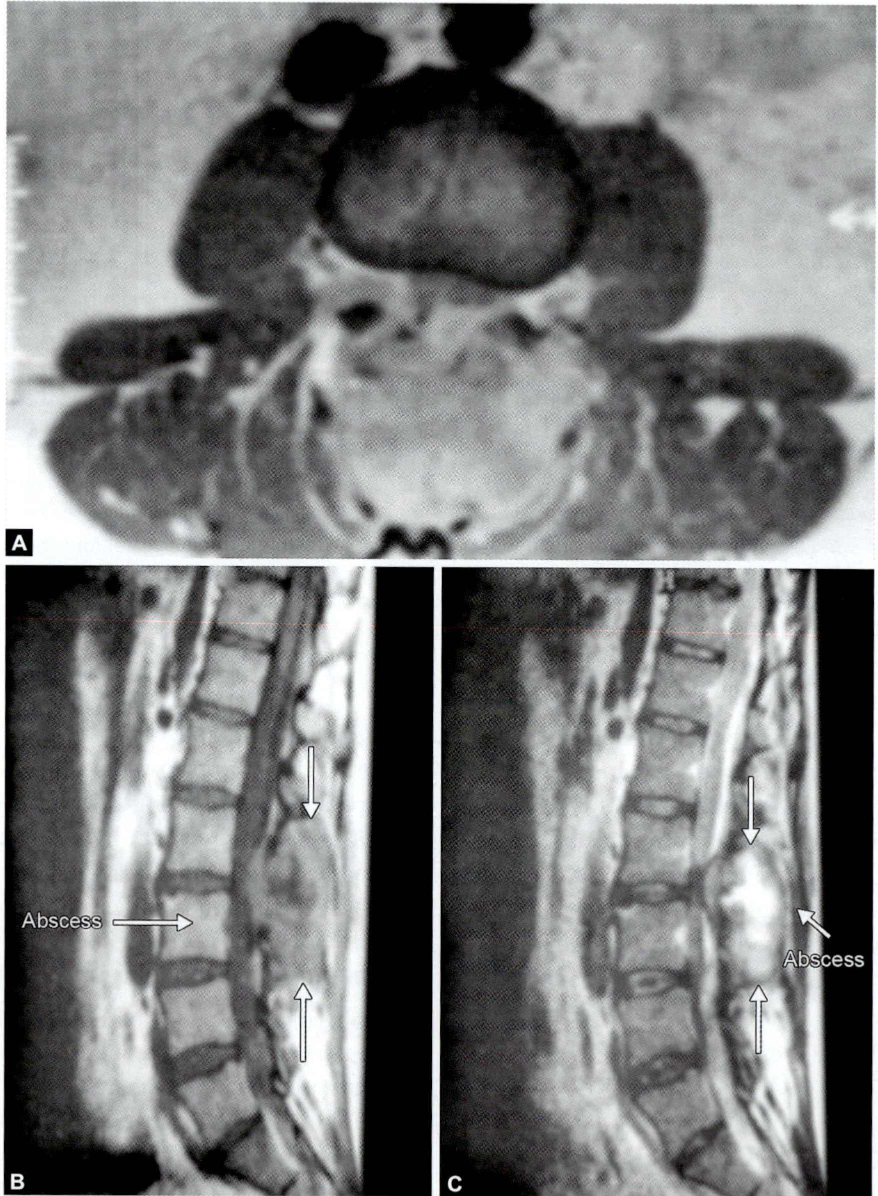

Figs. 20.29A to C: MRI appearance of a case presenting with pain and swelling in the lumbar region. X-ray did not reveal any pathology. The MRI pictures clearly show an abscess in the posterior elements with destruction of bone. The aspirate from the abscess demonstrated acid-fast bacilli on direct smear examination. Note change in the signals in T1 (A), (B) and T2 (C) weighted images.

Table 20.2: Clinico-radiological classification of typical tubercular-spondylitis.

Stage	***Clinico-radiological features***	***Duration of active disease at presentation***
I. Pre-destructive	Straightening of curvatures, spasm of perivertebral muscles, scintiscan would show hyperemia, MRI shows marrow edema	< 3 Months
II. Early-destructive	Diminished disc-space + paradiscal erosion ('Knuckle' <10°) MRI-shows marrow edema and break of osseous margins, CT scan shows marginal erosions or cavitations	2–4 Months
III, IV, V all have vertebral-bodies destruction and collapse + appreciable kyphos:		
III. Mild angular kyphos	2–3 vertebrae involved (K: 10°–30°)	3–9 Months
IV. Moderate angular kyphos	>3 vertebrae involved (K: 30°–60°)	6–24 Months
V. Severe kyphos (Humpback)	>3 vertebrae involved (K: > 60°)	> 2 Years

K is the angle of kyphosis as measured by the technique of Dickson (1967).

Note: In Stage III, IV, V diagnosis is clear on conventional X-rays. CT-scan and MRI would show advanced changes, however, these are unnecessary except for difficult sites (Kumar, 1988).

Nontraumatic symptomatic disc space reduction in young persons needs clinical observations and use of MRIs to exclude tuberculosis infection.

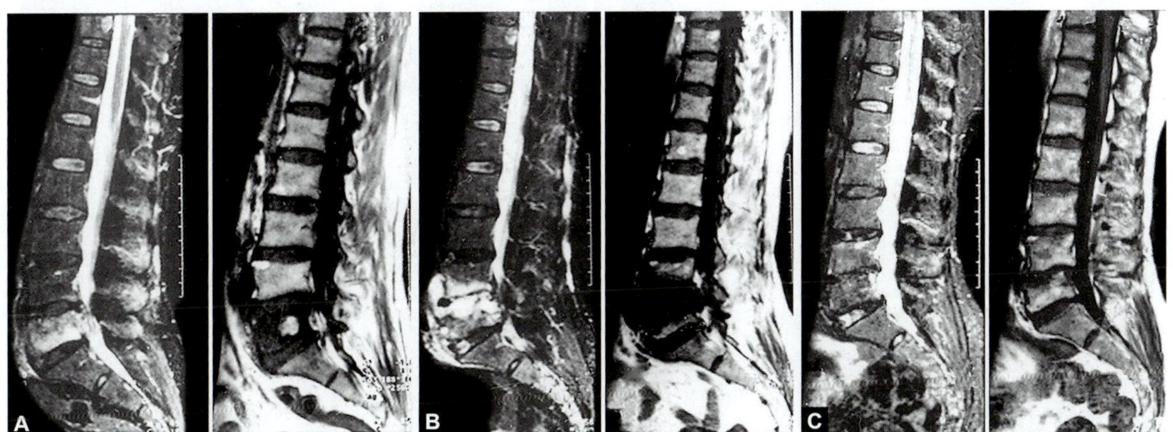

Figs. 20.30A to C: Serial MRI pictures of a lady aged 48 years suffering from tuberculosis of L4-L5 vertebrae. (A) At presentation in May 1999, (B) in November 1999 shows "deterioration" in the appearance despite antitubercular therapy and clinical improvement of her symptoms, (C) in June 2000 there is complete resolution of the diseased area and attempted bone block formation between L4–L5. No operation was done.

as inflammation. This should not create an unnecessary alarm. However, if the images do not show improvement when repeated >6 months after the onset of treatment one should consider the possibility of an alternative pathology or a therapeutically refractory disease. Once the disease has healed, the bony architecture is restored **(Fig. 20.29, 20.32)**. Rarely the healing is accompanied by fat replacement of the healed area **(Fig. 20.31)**.

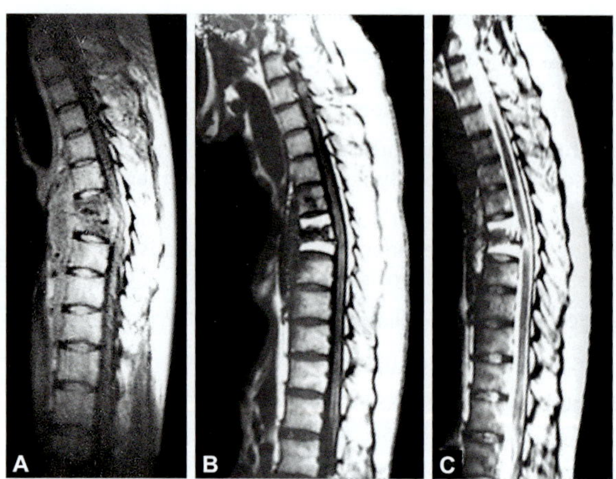

Figs. 20.31A to C: Shows the MRI of a case where the diseased area healed, accompanied by fat replacement, (A) active infection at presentation, (B) T1 image and (C) T2 image at healed status, note the bright signal of fat in both the sequences.

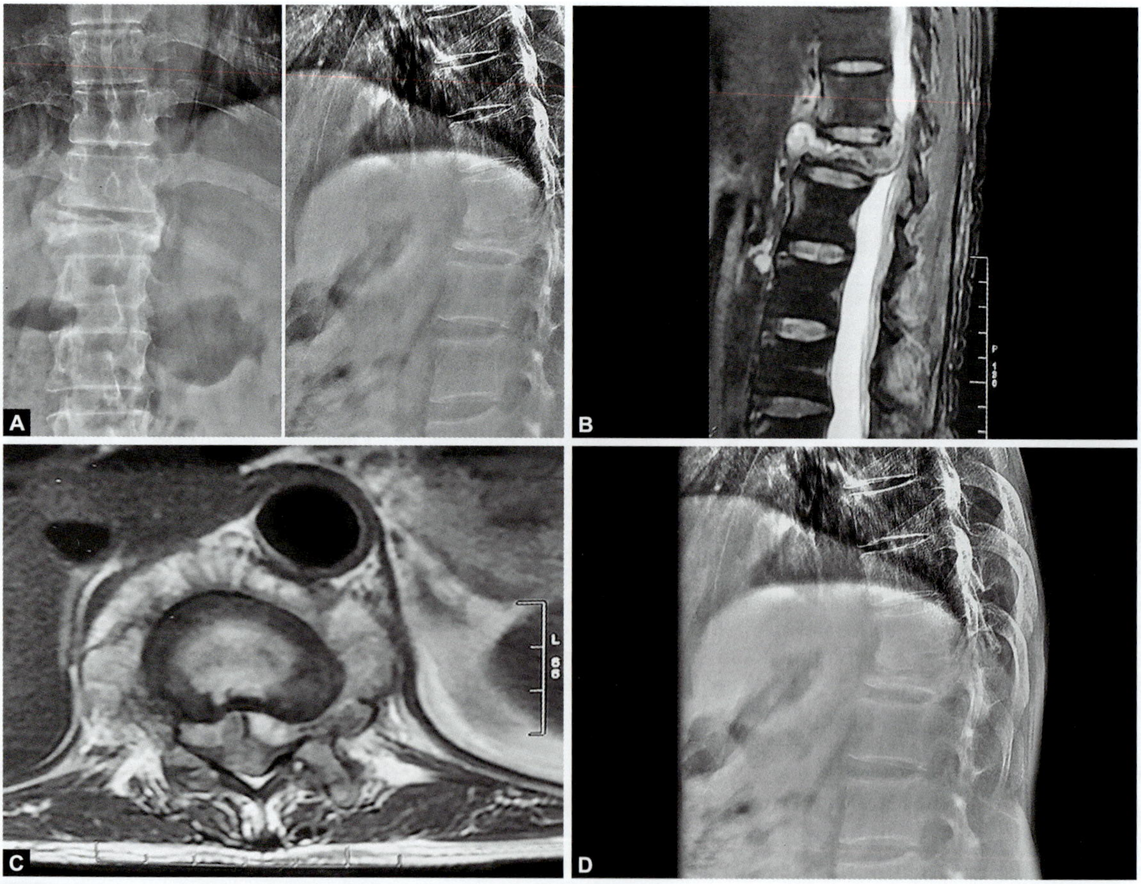

Figs. 20.32A to D: The patient presented with concentric collapse of D12 vertebral body (A) MRIs revealed involvement of D11, D12, and L1 (B). Axial cuts in the MRI (C) reveal a loculated paravertebral collection of pus. (D) The infection has healed with D11-D12 forming a fibro-osseous block.

CHAPTER 21

Differential Diagnosis

The symptoms, signs and radiological findings of tuberculous disease of the vertebral column are often characteristic. In patients with early disease, clinical and radiological re-examinations after 6–12 weeks are of great help in arriving at the final diagnosis. In case of doubt, the exact pathology should be detected by doing a biopsy of the diseased vertebrae and submitting the material for histological, microbiological and serological investigations. In clinical practice, there are some cases whose final diagnosis is revealed only by examination of diseased tissue obtained by operation. There are, however, difficulties in proving the diagnosis in some cases of osseous tuberculosis even from the tissues obtained by biopsy. When biopsy material is submitted for histology and/or culture and/or guinea pig inoculation and/or for PCR, preferably simultaneously, the diagnosis could be proven in 76–91% of the cases (Lakhanpal et al. 1974, Kumar et al. 2014). In an analysis of diseased tissue from tuberculosis of spine during 1989–1997, from Taiwan the authors (Chen et al. 2002) reported that smear was positive for *Mycobacterium* in 15%, histopathology was typical tuberculosis in 60% and compatible with tuberculosis in 36%.

Most of the serology based tests are not highly specific in areas with high incidence of tuberculosis due to common exposure of the populations to asymptomatic latent infection or active disease during growing years and generalized BCG vaccination of children. Serological tests in such people may be falsely positive in tissues or fluids from nontuberculous lesions or healed tuberculous lesions. A positive serology report is of value if the material was obtained from a lesion of clinically active disease/ inflammation. Despite all tests available, in nearly 20% one will have to depend upon the clinical assessment and imaging modalities.

CONSIDERATION OF AGE IN DIAGNOSIS

In young children, congenital defects of the spine and vertebra plana (Calve's disease), and in adolescence Schmorl's disease and Scheuermann's disease may sometimes cause confusion. All these conditions have no constitutional symptoms, have a characteristic radiological appearance and disc space is well maintained. They have negligible or minimal local signs such as pain, spasm and tenderness. In adults and aged people, there may be confusion with primary tumor of the vertebrae or with metastatic carcinomatous deposits. Conditions which may have some resemblance with tuberculous disease of the spine on clinical, radiological and/or MRI examination are as follows.

PYOGENIC INFECTIONS

In acute spinal pyogenic osteomyelitis (spondylitis), the onset is sudden with severe localized pain, spasm and swinging temperature like acute osteomyelitis in any other bone. In early stages, there is bone destruction which is rapidly replaced by bony sclerosis and new bone formation. The sclerosis and new bone formation may be observed radiologically from 8th week onwards. The intervertebral disc space shows varying degree of destruction. Ultimate outcome with healed disease, marked sclerosis of the diseased vertebrae, proliferative bone formation in the vertebrae and ligaments and even bony ankylosis. Low grade pyogenic infection may have an insidious course and onset like tuberculosis (Buchelt 1993).

Pyogenic infection of the spine may follow infection or surgery of urogenital tract, or postabortal or postpartum infections. In such cases, the infection is presumed to spread along the venous plexus to the vertebral column. The causative organism like common pyogenic infection of bone is as a rule *Staphylococcus aureus*, other organisms (aerobic, nonaerobic) may be rarely responsible for spinal osteomyelitis. Antistaphylococcal titer and/or examination of the biopsy material has been suggested to be useful in the final diagnosis. Pyogenic discitis is a rare complication following any operative intervention on the vertebral column. The clinical and radiological behavior is similar to pyogenic infection. MRI demonstrates the inflammatory changes predominantly in the paradiscal parts of bones and the disc space. Persistence of significant pain and elevated ESR beyond 4 weeks after the operative intervention on vertebral column is a strong indicator of pyogenic discitis.

Typhoid Spine

This is a rare complication of enteric fever. Most of the cases present at the time intervals of 4 weeks to a few months after the resolution of clinical features of typhoid fever. Clinically, the condition is manifested by an excruciating pain and muscle spasm. Radiological picture resembles that of tuberculosis and low grade pyogenic spondylitis. Confirmation can be obtained by agglutination tests, therapeutic trial or by biopsy.

Brucella Spondylitis

This can produce changes in the spine which can be very similar to those seen in tuberculosis. History of undulant fever may be suggestive of diagnosis. However, the diagnosis is best established by identification of the causative organisms, agglutination tests or by biopsy (Mousa et al. 1987, Cordero and Sanchez 1991, Benjamin and Khan 1994). *Brucella* infection of spine, skeletal system and synovial sheath is essentially encountered in endemic areas and in communities consuming unboiled/unpasteurized milk. Anti-*Brucella* Coombs test (BS) generally helps in diagnosis.

Mycotic Spondylitis

The most frequent infecting fungi are of the actinomyces group or blastomycosis group. Besides the involvement of the vertebral bodies, involvement of transverse processes and ribs is not infrequent. Radiologically, the changes resemble those seen in tubercular or pyogenic spondylitis (Eismont et al. 1983). In blastomycosis, paravertebral abscess formation is a common feature. In actinomycosis, sclerosis and destruction of bone proceed hand in hand. The anterior and lateral surfaces of several vertebral bodies may be involved and may show an irregular saw-tooth appearance by periosteal new bone formation. Collapse of the vertebrae is rare, sometimes the involved vertebrae may produce an appearance described as "honeycomb" or "lattice-like", and the condition is usually accompanied by multiple sinus formation and involvement of subcutaneous tissues. It is not possible to distinguish one fungus infection from another radiologically.

Confirmation of diagnosis must rely upon demonstration of mycotic organisms from the discharging sinuses, pus or from the diseased bone. During a period of study of 30 years (1965–1995), we came across two histologically proved cases of mycotic spondylitis.

Syphilitic Infection of the Spine

Three main types of syphilitic infection of the spine have been described: (i) Arthralgic type of syphilitic spondylitis, (ii) Gummatous type of syphilitic spondylitis, and (iii) Charcot's disease of the spine. The most common site of involvement is thoracolumbar and lumbar spine. Radiological picture shows a gross disorganization and destruction of the involved vertebrae along with proliferative new bone formation extending into the adjacent paraspinal tissues. When neuroarthropathic changes are present, varying degrees of subluxation of the vertebrae is evident. It is extremely difficult to differentiate this condition on X-rays alone (Hodgson 1969, Johns 1970) from other infectious lesions of the spine. Diagnosis can be confirmed by serological tests, tissue biopsy or by response to antisyphilitic treatment.

Tumorous Conditions

Following primary benign tumorous conditions may clinically and radiologically have some resemblance with spinal tuberculosis:

Hemangioma is one of the most common benign tumors of the vertebral column. Schmorl (1959) found an incidence of 10.7% of angiomas out of 3,829 spinal columns examined, the most common area being from D12 to L4. Most of these cases are asymptomatic and are diagnosed by chance on radiological examination and "pin-head appearance" on axial sections in CT scans and MRIs for other complaints. The involved vertebra shows characteristic coarsening of vertebral trabeculations more prominent in vertical than in horizontal trabeculae (corduroy appearance) or honeycombed appearance.

Giant-cell-tumor and *aneurysmal bone cyst* of the spine produce typical osteolytic expansile and usually eccentric growth on radiological examination. Such an appearance may be confused with an expansile type of central tuberculous lesion in the vertebral body. We have had examples of 5 cases hemangiomas, 4 cases giant-cell tumor, 4 cases aneurysmal bone cyst, and one intraosseous neurilemmoma (lumbar second vertebra) giving rise to typical expansile lesions (between 1965 to 1995). Disc space is not involved in early stages. Repeated X-ray examination at 6–12 weeks intervals, MRI and CT scan of the localized area are of great help in suggesting diagnosis of a tumorous condition. However, final confirmation of the diagnosis can only be made by histology. Response to radiation treatment is observed in hemangiomas and in aneurysmal bone cysts. Intralesional curettage and impaction bone grafting is a rational procedure for giant-cell-tumor and aneurysmal bone cyst.

Primary Malignant Tumors

Primary malignant tumors of the spine are very rare (Weinstein 1987) but Ewing's sarcoma and osteogenic sarcoma occasionally occur. We had an opportunity to observe (1965–1995) 6 cases of Ewing's tumor of vertebrae, 4 cases of Ewing's tumor of the rib with intraspinal extension and paraplegia, and 5 cases of lymphoma, one presenting as a univertebral sclerosis **(Fig. 21.1)**. The vertebral tumors had rapid course of the disease with progressive paraplegia and radiological evidence of destruction of bony trabeculae, soft tissue paravertebral shadow usually on one side and moderate degree of diminution of disc space in late stages. Diagnosis was confirmed only on biopsy from the vertebral bodies. Osteosarcomas, fibrosarcomas and chondrosarcomas are very rarely reported and can be confirmed only on histological examination. Three cases of extensive chondrosarcoma were observed by us, 2 cases in upper dorsal spine and one in the lumbar region. Chordoma is thought

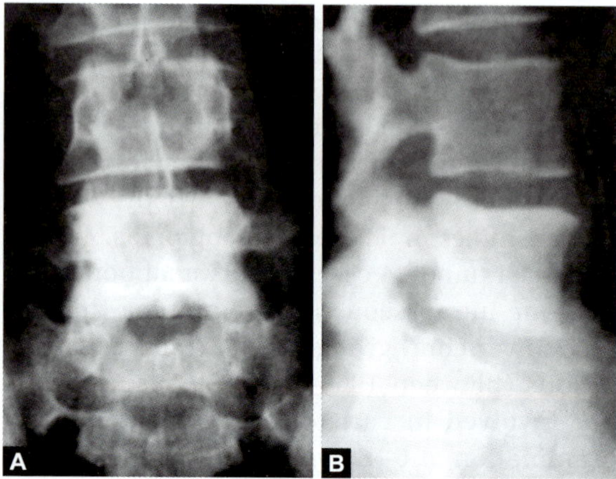

Figs. 21.1A and B: A patient of low backache radiologically revealed a monovertebral sclerosis of the lumbar fifth vertebral body. Noninvasive investigations were none contributory. Biopsy through lumbar transverse vertebrotomy revealed the diagnosis of lymphoma. Two years later the patient showed generalized disease with lymphadenopathy and hepatosplenomegaly.

to arise from the remnants of the notochord. Though it can take place in any part of the spine, most common sites are cephalic and caudal ends of the spinal column. The X-ray appearance is predominantly a lytic and destructive lesion. Two cases of chordoma of sacral region with cauda equina lesion and 3 cases of cervical region with quadriplegia were observed by us between 1965 to 1995 **(Fig. 21.7)**.

Multiple Myeloma (Plasmacytoma)

This is the most common primary malignant tumor of the spine. It may rarely resemble tuberculosis clinically and radiologically, especially if there is involvement of only one or two vertebrae and there is collapse and eccentric destruction. Involvement of multiple bones, high sedimentation rate, anemia, reversal of albumin globulin ratio and myeloma cells detected on bone marrow study are characteristics of this condition. Bence-Jones protein is present in the urine in 60% of such cases. Serum proteins may show typical immunophoretic patterns. One case was clinically diagnosed and treated as tuberculosis of dorsolumbar spine by us because at the time of first presentation there was only a localized lesion. However, later X-rays during follow-up revealed involvement of other vertebrae and other bones. Diagnosis would require confirmation by the presence of myeloma cells in the bone biopsy and presence of M-spike in serum electrophoresis.

Lymphomas

Hodgkin's disease and leukemias may rarely involve the vertebral column **(Fig. 21.1)**. Hodgkin's disease may show deposits in the vertebrae as diffuse sclerosis of bone with disruption of trabecular pattern and paravertebral soft tissue shadows. Leukemias may occasionally present as vague pain in the back associated with collapse of several vertebral bodies and generalized osteoporosis. Enlargement of spleen, liver and lymph nodes with characteristic blood changes help to arrive at the correct diagnosis.

Secondary Neoplastic Deposits

Secondary malignant deposits in the vertebral column constitute the largest number of malignant neoplasms of the spine (Harrington 1986). Symptoms may be similar to those in tuberculous disease but usually the onset is more acute, progress more rapid and local signs more widespread. Radiological and MRI examination usually help to differentiate it from the infective lesions. In infective lesion, if there is collapse of the diseased vertebrae, the intervening disc is generally diminished in size. A secondary deposit nearly always involves a vertebral body which collapses, whereas the discs on either side remain unaffected for a long time. Involvement of other bones and destruction of pedicles suggest a metastatic lesion. Secondary tumors may be osteolytic, osteoblastic or of mixed variety depending upon their density on X-rays. Osteoblastic secondaries are usually from prostate or breast and may resemble the radiological changes of Paget's disease. Secondaries may cause compression paraplegia. In case of doubt, biopsy examination of the diseased bone will reveal the correct diagnosis.

Histiocytosis-X

Lichtenstein (1953) suggested that eosinophilic granuloma (spine-Calvé's disease), Hand-Schüller-Christian disease, and Letterer-Siwe disease should be classified under one heading of histiocytosis-X, as these conditions were considered interrelated. Eosinophilic granuloma may develop in the vertebral body which undergoes an extensive degree of concentric collapse giving rise to the radiological appearance of vertebra plana or Calvé's disease. The discs above and below are unaffected. Rarely other bones in the body may show a similar involvement. Hodgson et al. (1969) mentioned about a case of eosinophilic granuloma of dorsal spine with paravertebral shadow and paraplegia. Usually, the disease occurs between 6 and 12 years of age and the patient complains of local pain without appreciable constitutional symptoms. The disease is self-limiting and during a long follow-up, the vertebral body may return almost to normal size and shape. The most common cause of vertebra plana in developing countries would still be tuberculosis of the centrum of vertebrae.

Local Developmental Abnormalities of the Spine

These may be in the form of hemivertebrae, fusion of two or more vertebral bodies (block vertebra), defects or synostosis of the neural arches and rarely varying degree of narrowing of disc spaces **(Fig. 21.2)**. A careful history, absence of any constitutional reaction or local spasm or tenderness or restriction of mobility, and absence of radiological evidence of paravertebral shadows and disturbance of bone structure usually make the diagnosis clear. The usual deformity in spinal tuberculosis is that of kyphosis whereas kyphoscoliosis is suggestive of congenital hemi-vertebrae. Without a suggestive history it may be difficult to differentiate a healed tuberculous spine with kyphoscoliotic deformity or with formation of block vertebrae from a congenital defect of the spine with similar radiological features. Other differentiating features may be concomitant synostosis of spinous processes and neural arches, irregularities and fusion of adjacent ribs, and other congenital defects associated with

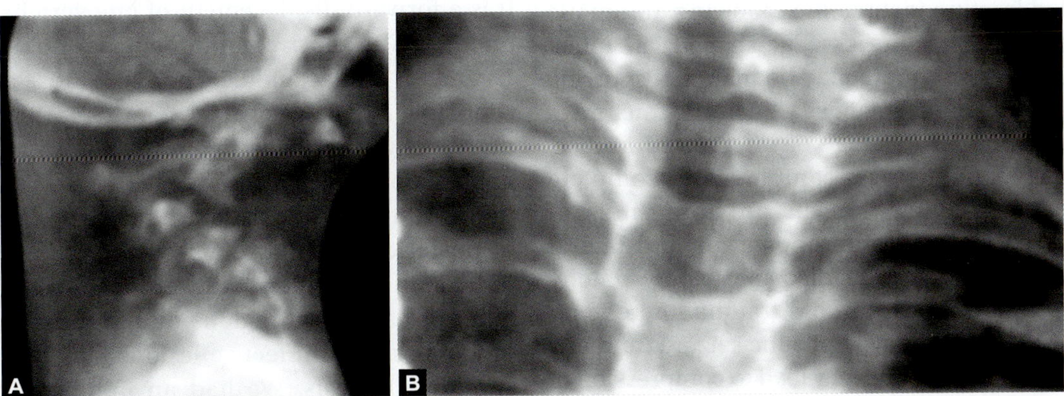

Figs. 21.2A and B: X-rays of a young male child who presented with difficulty in deglutition, tetraparesis, spinal deformity, increased prevertebral soft tissue shadow (A), and shifting of tracheal shadow to right side (B). The picture resembles tuberculosis; careful examination of the patient, however, proved the diagnosis of generalized neurofibromatosis. Abnormal increase of the interpedicular distance in the upper dorsal spine is obvious (B). Increase in the prevertebral retropharyngeal shadows can also be observed in neoplasms of vertebral bodies, recent fractures or fracture-dislocations of cervical spine, soon after anterior operations on the cervical spine, and massive enlargement of thyroid gland.

developmental abnormalities. Congenital fusion of vertebral bodies or acquired fusion in early childhood show a waist formation (constriction) opposite to the fused disc space (fused paradiscal growth plates).

Spinal Osteochondrosis

This is an ischemic lesion of the apophysis of several vertebrae occurring in early adolescence. A rounded kyphosis develops because of fragmentation, and mild wedging of several vertebral bodies. The changes of increased density of epiphyseal plates may be widespread throughout the thoracic region (Scheuermann's disease) or rarely the affection may be of a localized form (usually in lumbar spine). The absence of any constitutional reaction, spasm or any radiological paravertebral shadows and bony destruction, together with minimal local symptoms distinguishes this condition from infective lesions of the spine.

Traumatic Conditions

Careful history, clinical examination and X-rays are almost always able to diagnose a recent case of fracture or fracture dislocation of the spine. The radiological features which favor the diagnosis of healed fracture include the following: traumatic compression fracture is wedge-shaped with intact disc spaces and there may be marginal spurring and spondylolitic changes. When the fracture is associated with damage of intervertebral disc, in long-standing cases complete or incomplete osseous bridging is seen on both sides of the disc space in anteroposterior and lateral roentgenograms. The disc may show patchy calcification. In case of old trauma, there is no paravertebral shadow. Epileptic seizures and any other convulsive state may lead to compression of several vertebral bodies.

Osteoporotic Conditions

Generalized osteoporosis of the vertebral column may be caused by many conditions, a few common are senile osteoporosis, osteogenesis imperfecta, osteomalacia, rickets, Cushing's disease or iatrogenic steroid osteoporosis. Radiological changes of osteoporosis in the spine, of whatever cause are almost alike and are typical. In advanced cases, the trabeculae of the vertebral body are not able to resist the weight of the body. This results in the collapse of the vertebral bodies, upper end-plate is the earliest to yield. In the precollapse stage, the vertical bony trabeculae appear more prominent (because of early resorption of horizontal trabeculae) but there is no evidence of osteolytic destruction. The nucleus pulposus of the intervertebral discs expands because of its elasticity, and the softened vertebral bodies attain a biconcave appearance. The classical radiological picture of biconvex disc and biconcave bodies of the vertebrae may not be present in the aged, as the nucleus pulposus is no more elastic (turgid) because of aging processes and degenerative changes. Osteoporotic conditions can be easily differentiated from tuberculous disease by careful physical examination and radiological changes in other parts of the skeleton.

Spondylolisthesis

It is a forward displacement of one vertebra on another. The most common sites are between L5 and S1, and L4 and L5. The usual cause of the slipping is a deficiency in the pars interarticularis due to congenital defect or due to a stress fracture, or the slipping occurs due to degenerative changes in the posterior articulations. Rarely, destruction of posterior articular elements or destruction of pars interarticularis with or without involvement of paradiscal regions due to tuberculous process or other infective lesions may result in spondylolisthesis. We had an opportunity to observe 6 such cases in the lumbosacral region in the middle-aged patients. The infective pathology was suspected radiologically because of destructive changes in the posterior elements with or without the typical paradiscal lesion.

The tuberculous nature of pathology was proved by surgery and examination of the diseased tissue. Two patients of typical tuberculous spondylodiscitis developed spondylolisthesis (one each at L4/L5 and L5/S1) after ill-advised laminectomy.

Hydatid Disease

Hydatid disease of the spine is a very rare condition. We had an opportunity to observe 4 such cases. First case presented as a multiloculated destructive lesion in the rib with a soft tissue mass in the paraspinal muscles. Exploration revealed the diagnosis of hydatid disease of the rib with extension of the cysts in the muscle mass. Six months after excision of the rib the patient presented again, this time with compression paraplegia due to extension of the hydatid disease within the vertebral canal. Decompression did not recover paraplegia. Another patient (Srivastava and Tuli 1974) presented with a compression paraplegia with a radiological appearance of unilateral paravertebral shadow, moderate degree of diminution of the disc space and moderate collapse of the vertebral body in the region of D7–D8. While doing decompression through anterolateral approach and later through laminectomy, hydatid cysts were removed, however, it did not relieve the patient of paralysis. In retrospective, history of urticaria which was thought to be a drug rash should have guided us to perform a Casoni's test. During follow up, the patient developed hydatidosis of liver and lungs. The third patient had the involvement of lumbar vertebrae **(Figs. 21.3 and 21.8)**. One case of hydatidosis of mid-dorsal spine was diagnosed preoperatively by MRI (Jain et al. 1990).

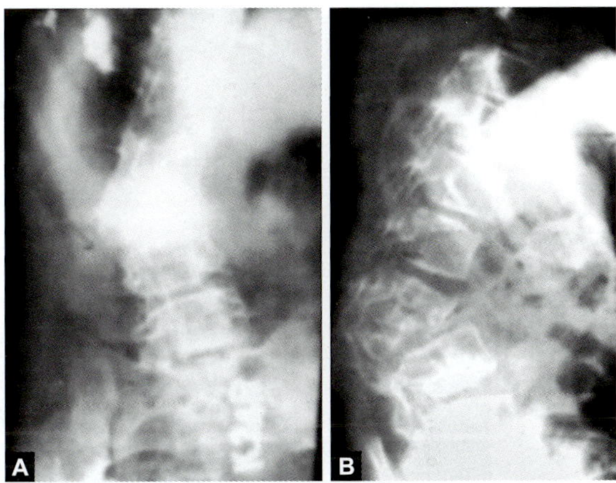

Figs. 21.3A and B: X-rays of a young girl who presented with cauda-equina type of paralysis. Because of gross destruction of lumbar-3 vertebral body and diminution of the disc spaces between L2–L3 and L3–L4, and presence of a soft tissue mass in the left iliac fossa a diagnosis of tuberculosis was made. On operation the condition turned out to be *hydatidoses affecting* the lumbar spine.

Miscellaneous conditions **(Figs. 21.6 and 21.7)** which may rarely resemble tuberculous infection of the spine are spondylolisthesis, ankylosing spondylitis, scoliosis, disc degeneration, osteoarthrosis, aortic aneurysm causing erosion of the vertebral bodies, and Paget's disease of vertebrae. Careful clinical and radiological examination and other relevant investigations help to arrive at a correct diagnosis **(Figs. 21.4 and 21.5)**. CT guided core biopsy or fine-needle aspiration biopsy in expert hands may give a tissue diagnosis in nearly 80% of cases (Mondal 1994). The vertebral bodies that can be approached with minimum risk are lower 4 cervical, lower 4 dorsal and upper 4 lumbar. Ankylosing spondylitis may sometimes be affected by concomitant tuberculous infection. By non-invasive investigation it may be difficult to differentiate between the picture of "pressure osteolysis" (Anderson's lesion) or that of infection. Tissue diagnosis may be required in difficult cases **(Fig. 21.4)**.

An "isolated ivory vertebra" or a monovertebral sclerosis may invite the possibility of a lymphoma, osteoblastic metastasis, Paget's disease, pyogenic osteomyelitis or rarely secondary pyogenic infection in vertebral tuberculous infection. During a span of nearly 40 years, we had three patients of "spinal tuberculosis" operated because of neural deficit in whom the histological observations revealed an **additional pathology**

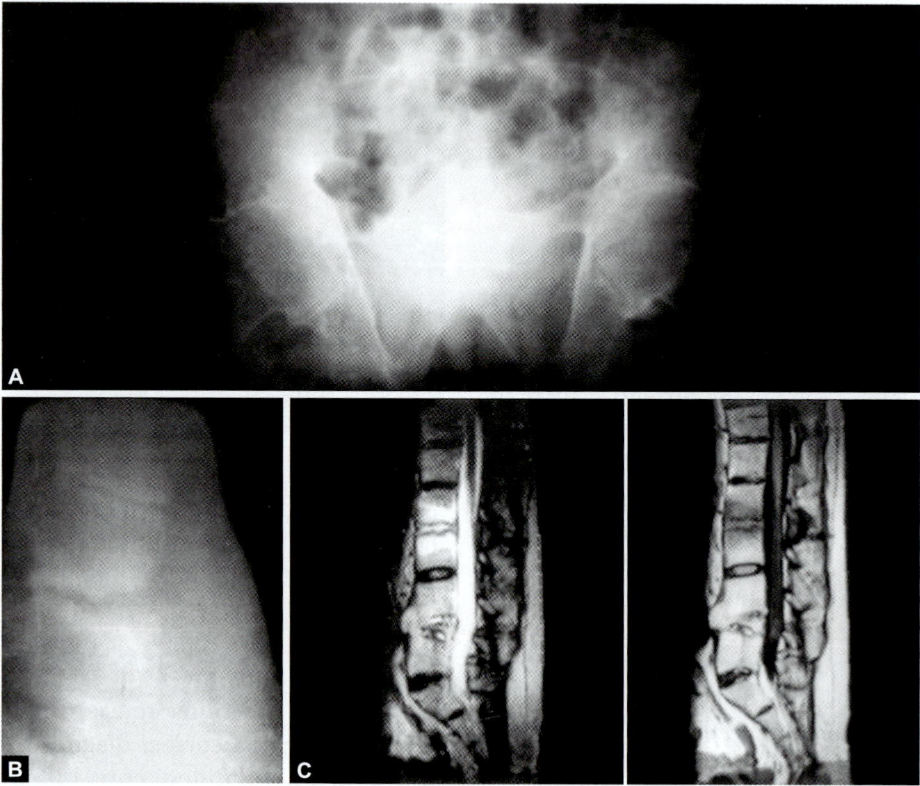

Figs. 21.4A to C: A and B are X-rays of a typical case of ankylosing spondylitis with gross involvement of pelvic joints. The vertebrae at the apex of angulation show irregular destruction of the disc space, sclerosis of the paradiscal margins and fluffy borders of the affected disc. Is it a case of superadded tuberculous infection or a stress resorption/reaction at the apex of angulation? (C) These are the MRI pictures of another classical case of ankylosing spondylitis showing destruction of L4 vertebral body with near complete obliteration of adjacent disc spaces due to old healed tuberculous disease. The reaction between L1 and L2 space may reflect active inflammation due to ankylosing spondylitis or due to infection.

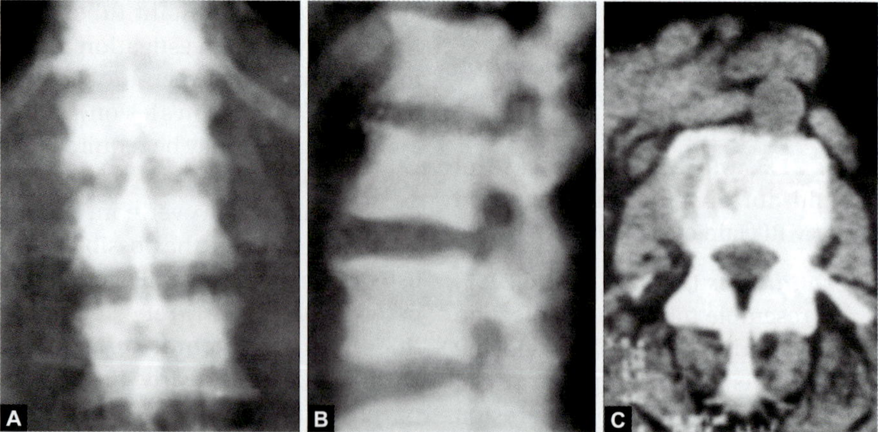

Figs. 21.5A to C: Stiffness of the vertebral column does not necessarily make it immune to the implantation of a tuberculous focus. These X-rays show classical changes of fluorosis of the vertebral column. Note diminution of the disc space between L1–L2, fuzziness and irregularity of the paradiscal margins. The CT scan shows destructive cavities in the vertebral body opening into the right psoas sheath.

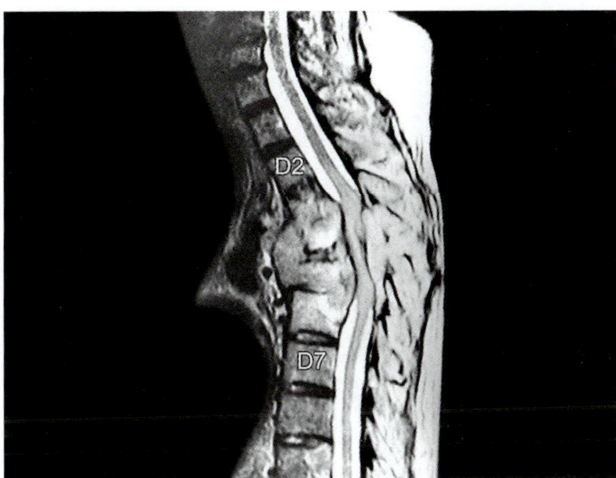

Fig. 21.6: MRI picture does not give tissue diagnosis. This picture shows destructive lesion of D3–D6 vertebrae with perivertebral collection. As the patient did not show a favorable response to antitubercular drugs for 3–4 weeks, an operative decompression and debridement was performed. The tissue diagnosis was *myeloma*.

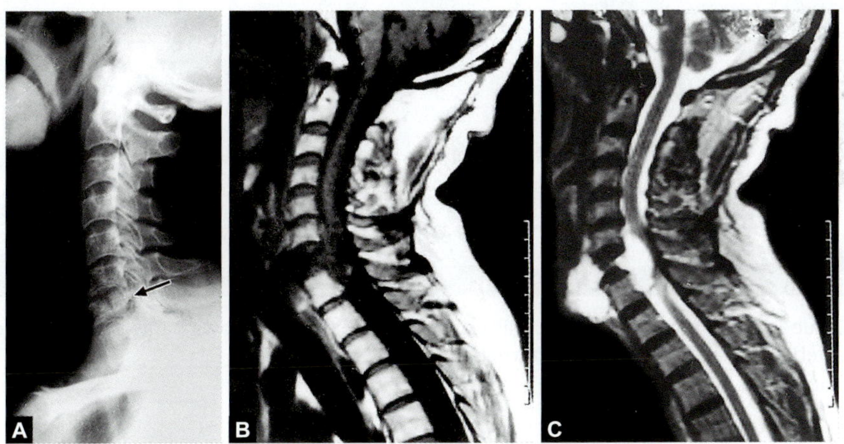

Figs. 21.7A to C: (A) X-ray showed destruction of C7 vertebra with a prevertebral shadow, (B and C) MRI pictures revealed a perivertebral mass in addition to the destruction. Histology of the tissue obtained after debridement, debulking and decompression proved it to be a *chordoma*.

of myeloma (two cases) and metastatic deposit (one case).

In brief the most common tumor of vertebral column is vertebral hemangioma, this also happens to be the most common benign tumor of spine. The most common malignant tumor of the vertebral column is a metastatic deposit and the most common primary malignant tumor is multiple myeloma. Vertebra plana is caused by many pathologies, however in TB endemic populations one of the common cause is tuberculous infection.

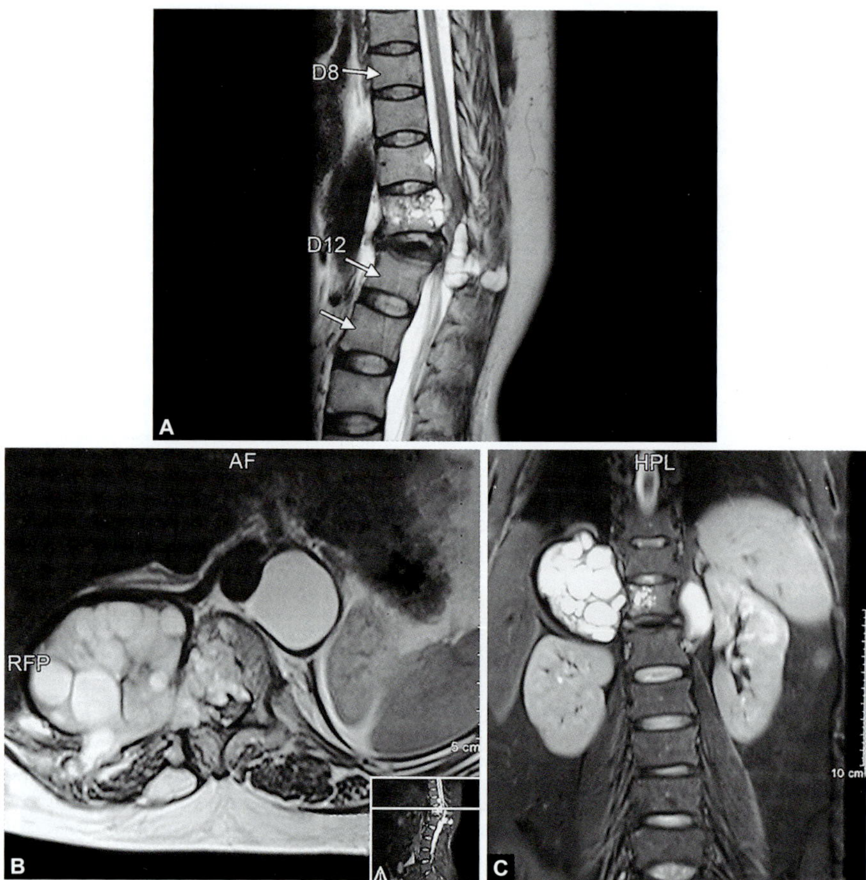

Figs. 21.8A to C: Tuberculosis is a great mimic: MRIs of dorsolumbar spine shows paravertebral collection along with involvement of vertebral bodies. Final pathology turned out as *hydatid disease*.

Courtesy: Dr Dhruv Chatturvedi.

CHAPTER 22

Neurological Complications

INCIDENCE

Neurological complication is the most dreaded and crippling complication of spinal tuberculosis. The overall incidence in various series has been reported to be between 10 and **30%** (Bosworth 1953, Cleveland 1935, Girdlestone 1950, Griffiths 1952, Risko 1963, Ferrand 1967, Lagenskiold 1967, Tuli 1967, 1969, 2007, Jain 2002). Bailay et al. (1972) reported an incidence of 43%. With improvement in medical facilities and awareness about the disease the incidence of neural complications at presentation in the hospital has now reduced to about **10%**. Age incidence of tuberculous paraplegia follows closely the incidence of the tuberculous disease of the vertebral column itself, being more common during first three decades of life. Paraplegia most commonly results from interference with the function of the cord, thus disease below the level of first lumbar vertebra rarely causes paraplegia due to compression of cauda equina. Above the level of first lumbar vertebra the highest incidence of paraplegia is associated with tuberculous disease of the lower thoracic region. **24%** patients of cervical spine tuberculosis showed varying degree of neural deficit (Tuli 1988, Jain 2000).

In affluent countries of the world, it is nowadays extremely rare to see this complication. However, in economically underdeveloped countries, which also happen to be highly populated areas of the world, spinal tuberculosis and its complication, Pott's paraplegia, is still very common. Many patients there reach the hospitals late with advanced neural deficit. During an investigation (1965–1974) of etiology of "compression paraplegia" in Banaras Hindu University (BHU), tuberculous pathology was the etiological factor in nearly **50%** of the cases. Commonest pathology responsible for non-traumatic paraplegia in developing countries still remains tuberculosis. In most of these cases, the vertebral lesions were well-advanced at the time of presentation.

The data on duration of neural involvement, severity of neural involvement and the site of the vertebral lesion observed (in 200 cases) in BHU are summarized in **Tables 22.1 and 22.2**. The youngest patient was a boy, one-year-old, and the oldest was a man, 69-year-old. The data on age and sex in this series are essentially the same as those in other series (Wilkinson 1949, Konstam 1962, Masalawala 1963, Paus 1964, Friedman 1966, Guirguis 1967, Kohli 1967, Martini 1988 and, Jain 2013). Vertebral regions involved in order of frequency in our series were the thoracic, cervical and lumbar. The neurological complication in our cases (1965–1974) was found in 20% of the cases.

CLASSIFICATION OF TUBERCULOUS PARAPLEGIA

Paraplegia due to tuberculosis of the spine had been classified into two main groups (Griffiths, Seddon and Roaf 1956) in preantitubercular era.

Table 22.1: Duration of neural complications at the onset of treatment as related. To the early results (minimum follow-up of 6 months or shorter in cases who died earlier) in 200 cases (1965–1974 = at BHU).

Duration	*Total no.*	*Success*	*Partial success*	*Failure*	*Death*
4 weeks or less	79	64	5	4	6
> 4 weeks to 3 months	67	54	3	3	7
> 3 months to 6 months	32	25	2	2	3
> 6 months	22	14	3	1	4
Total (percent)	200	157 (78)	13 (7)	10 (5)	20 (10)

Table 22.2: Overall results in 200 cases of neural involvement complicating caries of the spine. Results tabulated with a minimum follow-up of 6 months or shorter in cases who died earlier (1965–1974).

Vertebral level	*Severity of neural involvement*	*Mode of treatment*	*Results*	
Cervical = 13	Quadriparesis 10	Conservative 2	S	10
	Quadriplegia 3	Conservative + Traction + Drainage 9	PS	2
		Anterior Decompression 2	F	0
			D	1
Cervicodorsal = 13	Quadriparesis 3	Conservative 2	S	12
	Quadriplegia 10	Conservative + Traction + Drainage 7	PS	1
		Anterior Decompression 4	F	0
			D	0
Dorsal = 139	Paraparesis 29	Conservative 46	S	111
	Paraplegia 110	Decompression 93	PS	5
			F	7
			D	16
Dorsolumbar = 21	Paraparesis 11	Conservative 8	S	18
	Paraplegia 10	Decompression 13	PS	0
			F	2
			D	1
*Lumbar = 10	Paraparesis 7	Conservative 8	S	6
	Paraplegia 3	Decompression 2	PS	2
			F	0
			D	2
*Lumbosacral = 4	Paraparesis 2	Conservative none	S	0
	Paraplegia 2	Decompression 4.	PS	3
			F	1
			D	0

Notes: S–Success, PS–Partial Success, F–Failure, D–Death

* * Cauda equina lesion.
* Paresis = patients had motor weakness but were able to walk without support.
* Plegia = due to advanced motor weakness the patients were unable to walk without support, many had additional paresthesia and/or sphincter disturbances.

Group A "Early-onset Paraplegia"

This occurs during the active phase of the vertebral disease usually within first 2 years of the onset. Underlying pathology in most of such cases is inflammatory edema, tuberculous granulation tissue, tuberculous abscess, tuberculous caseous tissue or rarely ischemic lesion of the cord.

Group B "Late-onset Paraplegia"

This appears many years (>2 years) after the disease has persisted in the vertebral column. Neurological complications may be associated with recrudescence of the disease or due to mechanical pressure on the cord. Underlying pathology in most of these cases is tuberculous caseous tissue, tubercular debris, sequestra from vertebral body and disc, internal gibbus, stenosis of the vertebral canal or severe deformity. The pathology of cord compression resulting from recrudescence of the disease will be similar to those of early onset paraplegia.

A more rational classification is "paraplegia associated with active disease", and "paraplegia associated with healed disease". The purpose of both these classifications is to suggest the basic pathology responsible for compression of the cord. In most of the cases of "early onset paraplegia" and in "paraplegia associated with active disease", the pathological cause of compression is inflammatory edema, granulation tissue, tuberculous pus or caseous tissue. Prognosis regarding recovery of neural deficit is favorable. The basic pathology in most cases of "late onset paraplegia" and in "paraplegia associated with healed disease" is mechanical, like tubercular debris, sequestra from vertebral body/disc, stenosis of the vertebral canal, localized internal gibbus or severe kyphotic deformity. Surgical removal of mechanical causes is mandatory, however, prognosis is less favorable **(Fig. 22.1)**.

The progressive severity of neural deficit due to cord compression is staged by some workers essentially depending upon the degree of motor involvement (Goel 1967, Tuli 1985, Kumar 1988, Jain 2002) **(Table 22.3)**.

Stage I: The patient is able to walk normally and he is not aware of any motor weakness. It is the

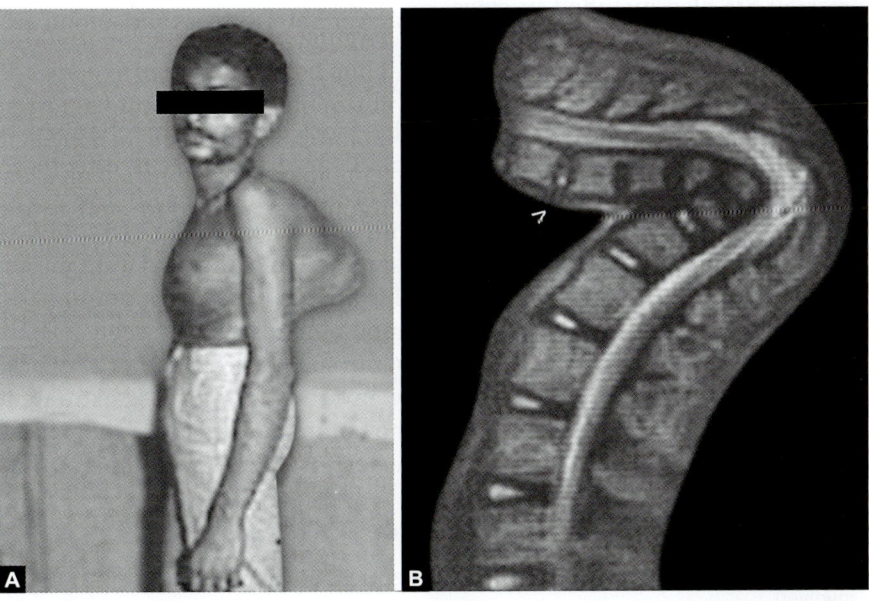

Figs. 22.1A and B: Approximately 3% of patients develop severe kyphotic deformity (internal gibbus), which after 10–20 years may lead to late-onset paraplegia.

attending physician who on clinical examination finds ankle clonus and, extensor plantar response with or without brisk tendon reflexes. Most of these signs may disappear if these patients are re-examined a few hours after rest in recumbent position.

Stage II: The patient presents with the complaints of clumsiness (incoordination) or spasticity or "jumpiness" of the limbs while walking. Though he is aware of the weakness but he is able to manage to walk with or without support. Clinical examination reveals all signs of spastic paresis.

Stage III: The patient is bedridden and cannot walk because of severe weakness. The examination would reveal spastic paraplegia in extension. Sensory deficit, if present, is generally <50%.

Stage IV: The patient has paraplegia with flexor spasms or paraplegia in flexion. A case of paraplegia in extension who develops complications like spontaneous flexor spasms and/>50% of sensory deficit (usually with bed sores) and/or sphincter disturbances also fits into stage IV. Flaccid paralysis due to very severe cord compression (terminal stage of compression), or flaccid paralysis due to sudden compression are also included in stage IV. Disturbances of bladder and bowel sphincters are generally associated with severe compression, however, rarely sphincter dysfunction may occur at an early stage. The higher the stage of paralysis more severe is the compression of cord and poorer the prognosis of recovery of neural deficit. Flaccid paralysis is considered a terminal stage created by progressive compressive myelopathy, many a time associated with concomitant arachnoiditis.

***Table 22.3:** Classification of tuberculous paraplegia/tetraplegia (Predominantly based upon motor weakness).

Stage	Clinical features
I Negligible	Patient unaware of neural deficit, physician detects plantar extensor and/or ankle clonus
II Mild	Patient aware of deficit but manages to walk with support
III Moderate	Nonambulatory because of paralysis (in extension), sensory deficit <50%
IV Severe	III + Flexor spasms/paralysis in flexion/flaccid/sensory deficit >50%/sphincters involved

*Applicable to compression of cord and not cauda equina.

PATHOLOGY OF TUBERCULOUS PARAPLEGIA

The essential pathology of paraplegia associated with tuberculosis of the vertebrae in majority of the cases is pressure on the tissues of the cord, as follows:

Inflammatory Edema

Edema of the spinal cord (in a confined space of vertebral canal) due to vascular stasis and due to toxins from the tuberculous inflammation in the neighboring vertebrae is considered to be a cause of early cases of neurological deficits. This view gets support from the fact that certain cases of paraplegias show quick recovery after a simple procedure like rest in bed or draining a paravertebral abscess and antitubercular drugs.

Extradural Mass

The most common mechanism by which the spinal cord function is affected, is a state of tuberculous osteitis of the vertebral bodies with an abscess in the extradural space causing compression of the cord from the anterior aspect. The abscess may be composed of fluid pus, granulation tissue or caseous material. The effect on the spinal cord is rather similar to that caused by any anteriorly located extramedullary tumor. The nature and extent of the peridural mass can be best visualized by MRI **(Figs. 22.2 and 22.3)**.

Bony Disorders

Sequestra from avascular portions of the diseased vertebral bodies or intervertebral disc may be responsible for narrowing of the spinal canal and

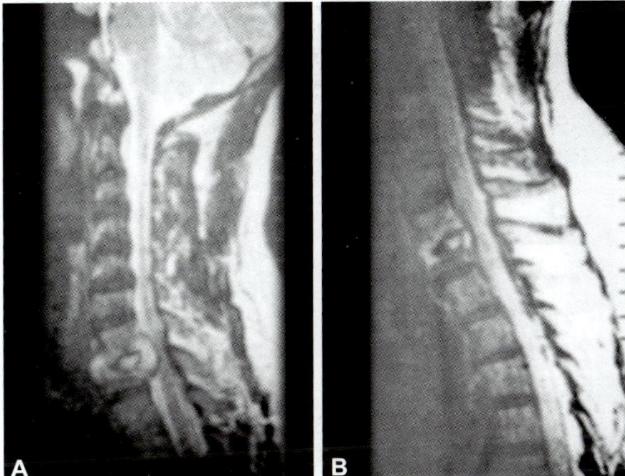

Figs. 22.2A and B: MRI picture of a case of tuberculosis of C7–D1 region showing nearly 60% encroachment of the vertebral canal at presentation (A). The patient had stage I neural signs in lower limbs and slight weakness in the right hand grip. After 6 months of domiciliary treatment with antitubercular drugs and ambulation with braces the patient made near complete neural recovery, resolution of the encroachment (B) and early healing of the vertebral lesion is obvious in the follow-up MRI.

pressure on the cord. Angulation of the diseased spine may lead to the formation of a bony ridge or spur called "internal gibbus" on the anterior wall of the spinal canal. Rarely, a pathological dislocation may damage the neural structures **(Fig. 22.4)**. Jain and associates (1999, 2002) calculated canal encroachment on CT scans from cervical 3 to dorsal 12 vertebral levels and found that up to 70% of vertebral canal encroachment was compatible with intact neural status. However, concomitant mechanical instability can produce neural complications even at lesser encroachment of the canal. Compression causing neurologic complications in tuberculosis is a slowly developing process except in vascular catastrophe or in pathological subluxation or dislocation.

Meningeal Changes

It is a common observation to find a thick layer of tuberculous granulation tissue lying outside the dura. This thickened granulation tissue can be gently pealed-off from the underlying dura which is as a rule not involved and is intact to macroscopic examination. This extradural granulation tissue probably is not an important factor in the causation of the paralysis, however, it may contract and undergo cicatrization in cases of long-standing. This "peridural fibrosis" may be responsible for some cases of recurrence of paraplegia in long-standing disease, which seldom achieve complete neural recovery despite adequate surgical decompression.

Infarction of Spinal Cord

This is an unusual but important cause of paralysis. The infarction is caused by endarteritis, periarteritis or thrombosis of an important tributary to the anterior spinal artery or other spinal arteries, caused by an inflammatory reaction. The paralysis caused by infarction is irreparable. Doing selective spinal angiography, an invasive investigation (Mittal 1990), does not seem to be justified for diagnosing this complication because of its extreme rarity. If one found the obstruction in the spinal arteries it suggests a poorer prognosis for complete neural recovery, however, it does not obviate the necessity of providing decompression at the site of disease with the hope of rare improvement of neural status, like protective sensations. Ischemic necrosis of the cord is seen as an area of high intensity MRI signal in T2 reflecting focal myelopathy (Hoffman et al. 1993). Rarely ischemia of the cord may also result because of surgery or observed postoperatively because of spontaneous thromboembolic phenomenon.

Changes in Spinal Cord

Unrelieved compression of the spinal cord shows loss of neurons and white matter in the damaged segment. The lost cells and fibers are replaced by gliosis and the neural fibers show a gross loss of myelin. Such type of changes may be present in the cord when a chronic grotesque deformity of the spine is complicated by complete paraplegia, or the compression has lasted for many months. In patients who did not recover after adequate surgical decompression, MRI studies have

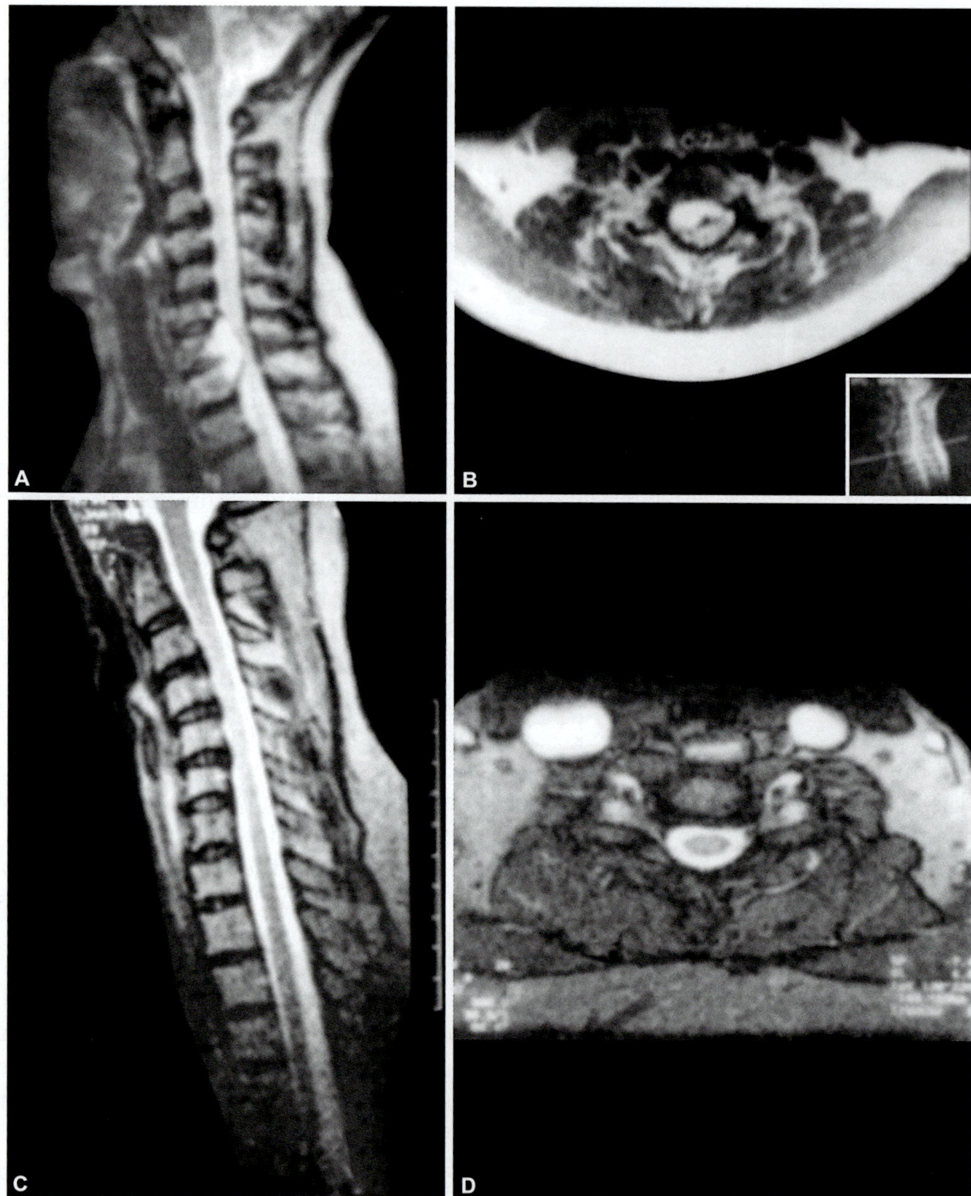

Figs. 22.3A to D: MRI showing encroachment of the vertebral canal in the sagittal (A) as well as in the axial sections (B) due to tuberculosis of C7–T1 region. Patient had stage II paraparesis. She was treated by rest, drugs and bracing at home. She made complete neural recovery and obtained healed status of the vertebral disease. Note spontaneous resolution of the encroachment (C and D) and reconstitution of the diseased vertebrae C7–T1.

revealed myelomalacic and syringomyelic changes (Hughes 1966, Jain et al. 2000) in the cord.

Thinning ("atrophy") of the spinal cord can now be very well visualized by contrast CT or by axial sections of MRI. We have observed that up to 50% reduction in the diameter of the cord substance is often compatible with good cord function. Presumably sufficient number of neurons and the long tracts survive despite thinning of the cord. The surviving undamaged or uninjured neurons and long tracts due to neuronal plasticity ensure adequate neural functions. "Neuronal plasticity" is induced when compression or deformation of the cord takes place slowly over a length of time. A sudden severe compression or gross deformation would almost lead to near transection of the neural elements. Isolated moderate thinning of cord or moderate syringomyelia are not incompatible with intact neural status. However, thinning ("atrophy") of the cord associated with syrinx and/or myelomalacia and/or arachnoiditis has as a rule very poor cord function, and despite mechanical decompression the chances of any worthwhile neural recovery (for ambulation) are remote; protective sensations in the lower limbs may recover to prevent or heal decubitus ulcers.

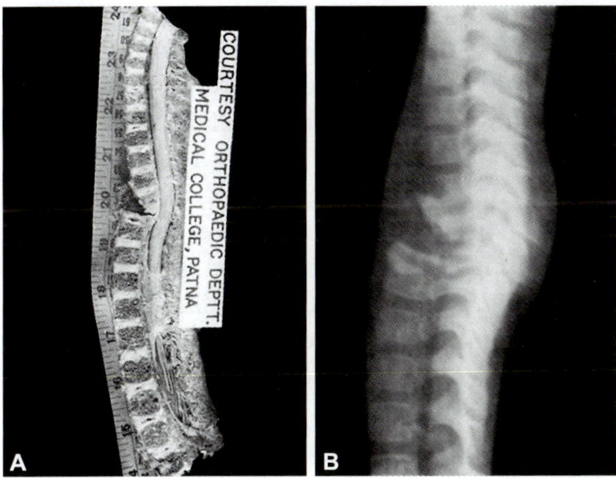

Figs. 22.4A and B: Sagittally sectioned specimen (A) of the vertebral column showing tuberculous disease in the dorsal spine. At the diseased area one can appreciate destruction of 2 vertebral bodies, gross diminution of 2 intervertebral discs, and kyphotic deformity. The cord adjusts itself to the deformed posture without anatomical damage because the deformation occurs slowly. The dura provides a tough barrier to penetration of tuberculous pathology. X-ray (B) of the same specimen is more disturbing because it shows much more destruction, distortion, and pathological dislocation. The gross specimen, however, shows intact spinal cord and dural sheath.

EXTRADURAL GRANULOMA AND TUBERCULOMA

Very rarely a small tuberculoma of the spinal cord **(Figs. 22.5 and 22.6)** or diffuse extradural granuloma **(Fig. 22.7)** of the cord may be responsible for neurological complications without any radiological evidence of tuberculous involvement of the vertebrae. Such cases present as a "spinal tumor syndrome". Sometimes one is able to suspect tuberculous pathology in the presence of previous history of tuberculosis or another evidence of a tuberculous lesion in the patient. We had six cases of extradural granuloma and three of tuberculoma of the cord responsible for paraplegia during a period of 20 years (1965–

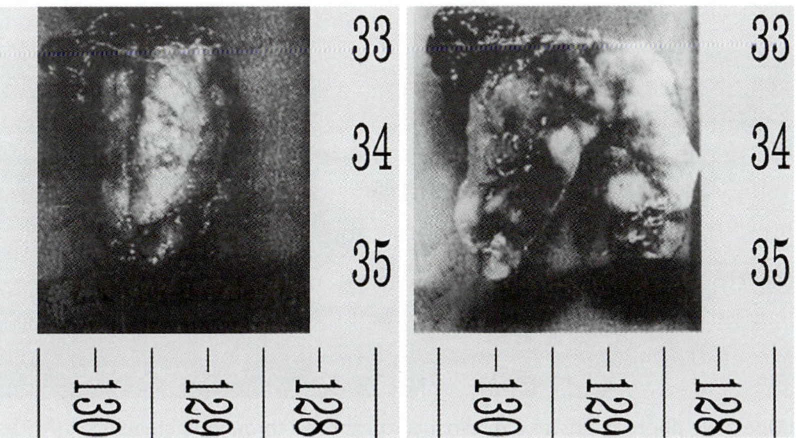

Fig. 22.5: An excised (through durotomy) specimen of an intradural tuberculoma from a female patient who presented with quadriparesis as a case of spinal tumor syndrome. The bisected surface of the specimen shows caseating tubercles, and hemorrhage in the inferior part. Histology confirmed tuberculous nature of pathology.

1985). In developing countries, tuberculoma/granuloma must be kept as one of the possibilities in cases of spinal tumor syndrome (Choksey et al. 1989, Jain et al. 2003, Singh et al. 2005, Kumar et al. 2007). Of all the patients admitted as "spinal tumor syndrome" without an obvious osseous lesion in conventional radiology, in the orthopedic services of teaching hospitals (University Hospitals at Varanasi and Delhi 1965 to 1994), nearly 10% proved to be caused by generalized extradural granuloma or localized intradural tuberculoma.

Figs. 22.6A and B: Sagittal (A) and axial (B) T2-weighted images through the dorsolumbar spine shows expansion of the terminal cord and the conus. There is a well-defined oval intramedullary mass at D11 showing low intense signal with a small central hyperintense signal, the classical MR appearance of tuberculoma. The cord above and below shows edema seen as hyperintense signal.
Courtesy: Dr Praveen Gulati, MR Center, New Delhi.

Tuberculous granuloma and tuberculoma: Extradural granulomas with neural complications have good neural recovery after posterior decompression (not unlike an epidural abscess) and gentle extradural peeling of granulomatous layers. Resolution of intramedullary tuberculoma has been observed with standard antitubercular therapy, however, a deteriorating neurology may warrant a decompression.

For long it has been accepted that dura mater resists **(Fig. 22.4)** tuberculous infiltration, and the spinal meninges and the cord itself are virtually never infected by direct extension. However, autopsy observations by Hodgson (1967) have shown the presence of tubercular myelitis. Biopsy of dura from two patients of tuberculoma in our material showed actual tuberculous infiltration of the dura mater.

Based upon the clinical response of the neurological complications, the radiological findings and the observations at operations in our patients, the usual causes of neurological complications in tuberculosis of the spine, in order of frequency are as shown in **Table 22.4**. The observations in the present series are in general agreement with those reported by others

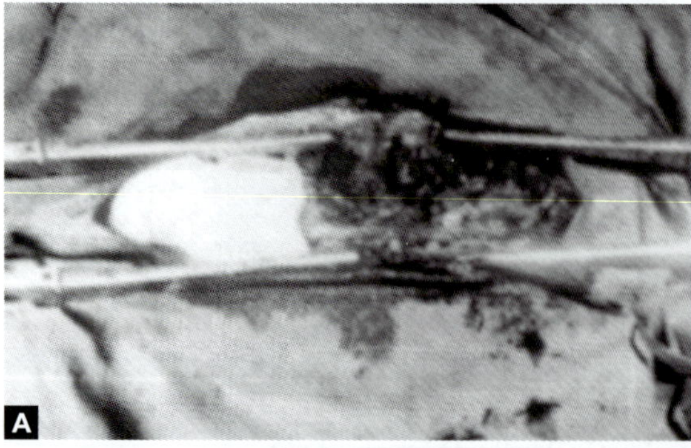
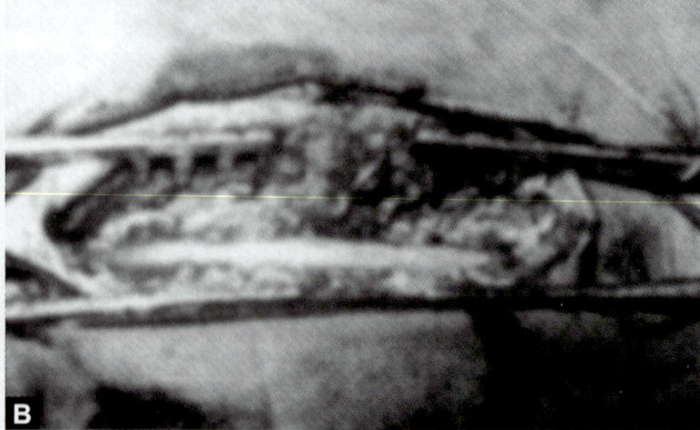

Figs. 22.7A and B: Operative photographs of the spinal cord exposed through laminectomy. (A) The left picture shows the dura (partly cleared) covered by thick granulation tissue. (B) The right picture shows the dura that was cleared off by removing or gently peeling away the granulations. The diagnosis of "spinal tumor syndrome" due to tuberculous granuloma/tuberculoma was suspected preoperatively as there was evidence of old healed tubercular sinuses in the region of neck.

Table 22.4: Usual causes of neurological complications in caries spine.

Inflammatory	
1. Inflammatory cord edema	Recovers by rest and drug therapy
2. Tuberculous granulation tissue	Mostly recovers by rest and drug therapy
3. Tuberculous abscess	Recovers by conservative therapy; rarely requires evacuation and decompression
4. Tuberculous caseous tissue	May subside by conservative therapy; sometimes requires evacuation and decompression
Mechanical	
5. Tubercular debris	Solid debris requires operative removal and decompression
6. Sequestra from vertebral body and disc	Require operative removal and decompression
7. Constriction of cord due to stenosis of vertebral canal	Requires operative decompression (kyphoplasty)
8. Localized pressure due to salient (internal gibbus) along anterior wall of vertebral canal	Requires operative decompression
Intrinsic (cord atrophy)	
9. Prolonged stretching of the cord over a sever deformity	i. Stretched cord may be more vulnerable to other causes, then decompression, release of cord, and anterior transposition may lead to recovery ii. Rarely stretching leads to interstitial gliosis or atrophy of cord (may be visualized by myelo-CT and/or by MRI) which does not recover completely
10. Infective thrombosis/endarteritis of spinal vessels	Difficult to prove/disprove, does not recover appreciably
11. Pathological dislocation of spine	Rare complication, usually results from rough manipulation by masseur or indiscriminate laminectomy for caries spine; irreparable severance of cord
12. Tuberculous meningomyelitis (leptomeningitis)	Difficult to prove/disprove; myelitis does not recover completely
13. Syringomyelic changes	Seen on MRI; poor recovery
Spinal tumor syndrome	
14. Diffuse extradural granuloma or tuberculoma or peridural fibrosis	Present as spinal tumor syndrome, surgical approach is by laminectomy

Notes:

- As a rule more than one cause may be acting in the same case.
- MRI wherever available can demonstrate atrophy of cord, myelomalacia, syringomyelia, tuberculoma and infarction of spinal cord.

(Butler 1935, Garceu 1950, Griffiths et al. 1956, 1986, Seddon 1956, Hodgson et al. 1960, 1964, 1967, Konstam et al. 1962, Paus 1964, Friedman 1966, Tuli 1969, Nand 1972, Bailey 1972, and Jain 2013). It may be pointed out that the deformity of the spine was not a significant cause of paraplegia in our series. There are many patients who have lived with an extreme degree of deformity without any neurological involvement for 10–15 years **(Fig. 21.1)**. As a rule more than one cause may be acting in the same patient. Interstitial gliosis of the cord, infective thrombosis or arteritis of the end arteries of the spinal cord, atrophy of the cord, and meningomyelitis of the cord, are difficult to prove or disprove without CT scan, MRI or autopsy. The patients who did not recover after a satisfactory mechanical decompression may be presumed to have had these factors, or a severance of the cord due to pathological dislocation. In two patients in our series who did not recover, the unfavorable result seemed to be due to pathological dislocation. The exact cause of other failures may only be presumed to be due to infective thrombosis or arteritis of the spinal arteries. Tubercular myelitis, interstitial fibrosis, thinning of the cord or syringomyelic changes are very well seen by MRI studies. Acquired syringomyelia can result from tubercular arachnoiditis many years after its occurrence or it can also result as an effect of severe kyphotic deformity of long-standing.

SIGNS AND SYMPTOMS OF POTT'S PARAPLEGIA ASSOCIATED WITH DISEASE PROXIMAL TO LUMBAR FIRST VERTEBRA

Rarely paraplegia may be the presenting symptom of tuberculosis of the spine. Commonly this is associated with a known lesion of the vertebral column. In a paraplegia of slow onset, the first signs of interference with the conduction of cord may be spontaneous twitching of muscles in the lower limbs and clumsiness while walking, extensor plantar response and exaggerated reflexes. Sustained clonus of ankle and patella may be present. Motor functions are almost always affected before and to a greater extent than the sensory functions because the diseased area in the spine lies anterior to the cord, thus being nearer to the motor tracts. Besides, probably the motor tracts are more sensitive to compression of the cord. The paralysis may pass with varying rapidity through the following stages: Spastic motor paraparesis, spastic paraplegia in extension and later on spastic paraplegia in flexion. As the cord is increasingly compressed, the patient develops uncontrollable flexor spasms which in later stages remain established in flexion, this indicates complete loss of conductivity in the pyramidal and extrapyramidal tracts. In very advanced cases of compression, bladder and anal sphincters may be involved and there may be a varying degree of sensory deficit. Sense of position and vibration are the last to disappear. In extremely severe cases, all spasticity disappears and the paralysis becomes flaccid (areflexic paraplegia) with anesthesia and loss of sphincter control. Exceptionally, the damage to the cord may be so sudden and complete that the patient presents with sudden, complete flaccid paralysis like the clinical picture of "spinal shock", generally associated with traumatic paraplegia. This may later gradually change into spasticity. Sudden complete paralysis may be caused by ischemia of the cord due to thromboembolic phenomenon or transection of the cord due to pathological dislocation or extremely rarely due to rapid accumulation of infected material or iatrogenic damage to cord.

On rare occasions paraplegia of tuberculous etiology may present like a "spinal tumor syndrome" due to a localized tuberculoma or a diffuse granuloma or due to peridural fibrosis. A lumbar puncture myelography (the only investigation available prior to 1987) disclosed evidence of complete or partial block without any gross osseous pathology on conventional X-rays of the spine. Intraspinal tubercular granuloma should be considered in the differential diagnosis when a case of spinal tumor syndrome is encountered in an endemic zone of tuberculosis (Kumar et al. 2007). Currently, MRI is the best available investigation whenever intraspinal tuberculoma or extradural granuloma is suspected. Most of the intramedullary tuberculomas would resolve by antitubercular medicines **(Fig. 22.8)**. Extradural granulomas when associated with significant non-resolving neural signs should be treated by surgical decompression. The thick layer of granulations needs to be peeled off as sheet or in piece meal.

MYELOGRAPHY (NOW REPLACED BY MRIs SINCE 1987 ±)

As a rule there is little difficulty in determining the level of cord compression from clinical, neurological, radiological and MRI examination. In cases of paraplegia without the radiological

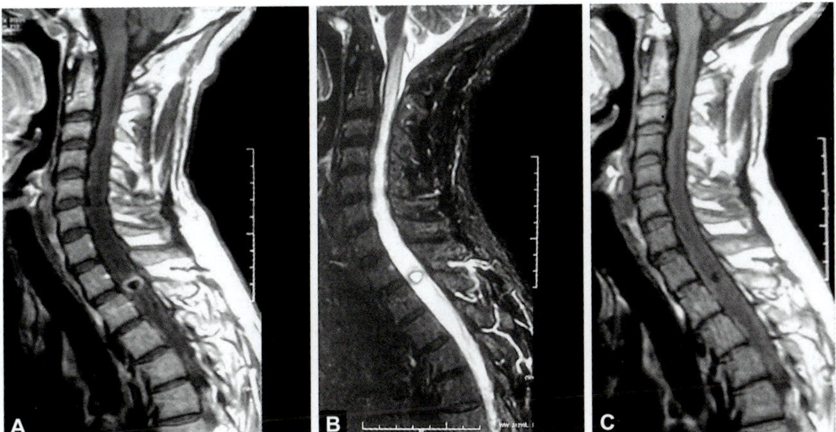

Figs. 22.8A to C: Classical MRI appearance of an intramedullary tuberculoma at the level of D1–D2 vertebral bodies. Note the ring like appearance (A), enhancement of the ring by gadolinium (B), the resolving lesion (C), under the influence of antitubercular drugs. Non-caseating (soft) granuloma (tuberculoma) is hyperintense in T2 (B) and hypointense in T1 (A). Solid caseating granuloma usually is hypointense in both T1 and T2 MRI images.

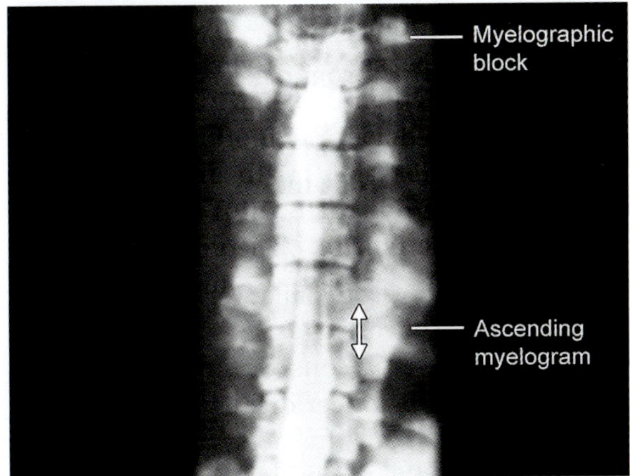

Fig. 22.9: Myelogram performed in a case of tuberculous paraplegia with 2 skipped lesions in the dorsal spine. The die passed upwards clearly opposite the lower dorsal lesion, however, a complete block was observed at the site of the higher lesion. Note broadening of the superior mediastinum at the level of upper lesion.

evidence of disease, as in "spinal tumor syndrome", or in cases with multiple vertebral lesions **(Fig. 22.9)** myelography was helpful in determining the level of obstruction. Another situation when myelography was indicated and useful was when a patient had not recovered after decompression operation. Presence of a myelographic block in such cases indicated inadequate mechanical decompression and warranted a second decompression operation. If a block was not present the cause of failure of recovery was considered an intrinsic damage to the cord such as ischemic infarction, interstitial gliosis, atrophy of the cord, tuberculous myelitis or myelomalacia **(Figs. 22.10, 22.11 and Table 22.5)**.

Hodgson et al. (1969) advocated myelography in all cases of tuberculous paraplegia. We used it only for the indications as mentioned above because in a usual case of tuberculosis of the spine the site of the disease is well demonstrated in plain X-rays. MRI studies in 30 patients with clinico-radiological diagnosis of tuberculous spondylitis did not reveal any observations differentiating the presence or absence of associated neural deficit (Booysen et al. 1989). Conventional myelography has now (since 1990s) been replaced by MRI studies, which give us the level and extent of the vertebral pathology and also delineates the health of the cord parenchyma/substance.

PROGNOSIS FOR RECOVERY OF CORD FUNCTION

The clinical evaluation of prognosis in any particular case depends on many factors

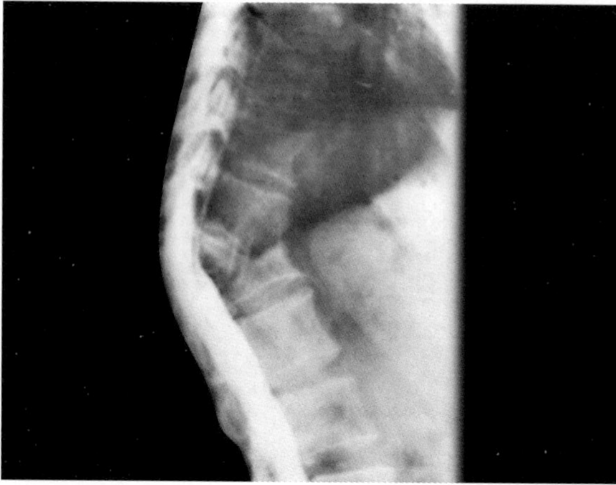

Fig. 22.10: This young engineer was operated 18 years ago (at the age of 22 in 1969) for tuberculous paraplegia. Through anterolateral approach decompression and bone grafting was then performed. The patient made an uneventful postoperative recovery and lead an active life till 1987, when he reported back with gradually progressive spastic paraplegia with no evidence of active disease. Myelogram done in 1987, revealed the die passing freely across the site of healed disease, "intrinsic causes" were presumed to be responsible for the recurred neural complication.

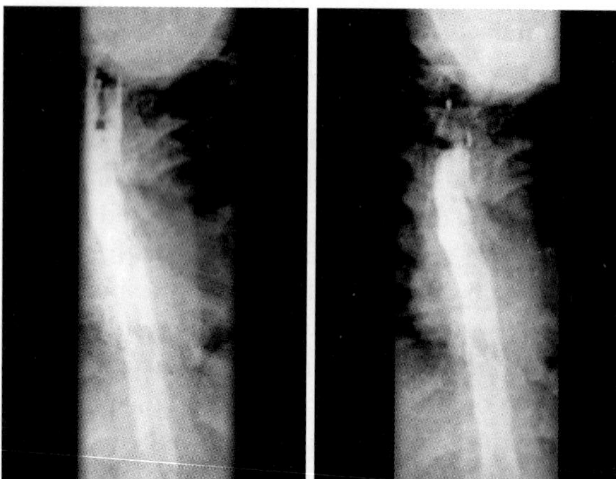

Fig. 22.11: Paraplegia caused by a tuberculous lesion of mid-dorsal spine was treated by anterolateral decompression of D6–D8 region. As the patient did not make appreciable neural recovery, 6 weeks after the decompression a myelogram was done to judge the adequacy of mechanical decompression. The myodil flowed freely past the site of disease and decompression excluding a mechanical pressure. The presumptive pathology in such a case would be intrinsic causes such as ischemia of the cord, tuberculous myelopathy or myelogliosis.

Table 22.5: Clinical factors influencing prognosis in cord involvement.

Cord involvement	*Better prognosis*	*Relatively poor prognosis*
Degree	Partial (stage I, II)	Complete (stage IV)
Duration	Shorter	Longer (> 12 months)
Type	"Early onset"	"Late onset"
Speed of onset	Slow	Rapid
Age	Younger	Older
General condition	Good	Poor
Vertebral disease	Active	Healed
Kyphotic deformity	<60°	>60°
Cord on MRI	Normal	Myelomalacia/ Syrinx
Peroperative	Wet lesion	Dry lesion

(Table 22.5). The prognosis is better if there is only partial cord involvement, the neural complications are of short duration, there is "early onset" cord involvement, the neural complications developed slowly, the patient is young and his general condition is good. Conversely, the prognosis is relatively poor if the cord involvement is complete (severe flexor spasms, flaccid paralysis and gross sensory loss), the neural complication is of longer duration, there is "late onset" involvement, the neural complications developed rapidly, the patient is older, and the general condition of the patient is poor or there are other associated active tuberculous foci or it is a case of multidrug resistance (MDR) or in a patient with HIV infestation. No patient should, however, be considered to have too advanced a disease for treatment. There were many patients with advanced disease in our series who recovered to some extent (providing protective sensation) after a satisfactory mechanical decompression of the cord and antituberculous therapy. The evidence for these statements is summarized in **(Tables 22.1 and 22.2)**. Similar success was also reported by other workers (Donaldson 1965, Goel 1967, Griffiths 1956, Hodgson 1960, Masalawala

1963, Seddon 1935, 1956, Shrivastava 1961, Misra et al. 1996, Moon et al. 1996, Jain et al. 2000, Jain 2002). Irrespective of the mode of treatment, the patients who show neural recovery, various modalities generally recover in the following order: Vibration and joint sensation; temperature, touch, pain; voluntary motor activity, sphincter functions and wasting of muscles.

TREATMENT OF POTT'S PARAPLEGIA

The prevention of paraplegia in tuberculous disease of the spine is of paramount importance, it can be largely achieved by early diagnosis of spinal caries and its prompt and suitable treatment. Every case of neurological complication with tuberculosis of the spine warrants immediate admission and care by a suitable orthopedic center where all facilities for spinal surgery are available. Modern chemotherapy has brought a remarkable revolution in the approach to the treatment of tuberculosis in general. The treatment of tuberculous paraplegia is the treatment of tuberculosis of the spine with the added aim of performing a mechanical decompression of the cord by removing the diseased tissues without compromising stability, in cases who need surgery **(Flowchart 22.1)**. The details of various useful procedures are given in Chapter 24 on Operative Treatment.

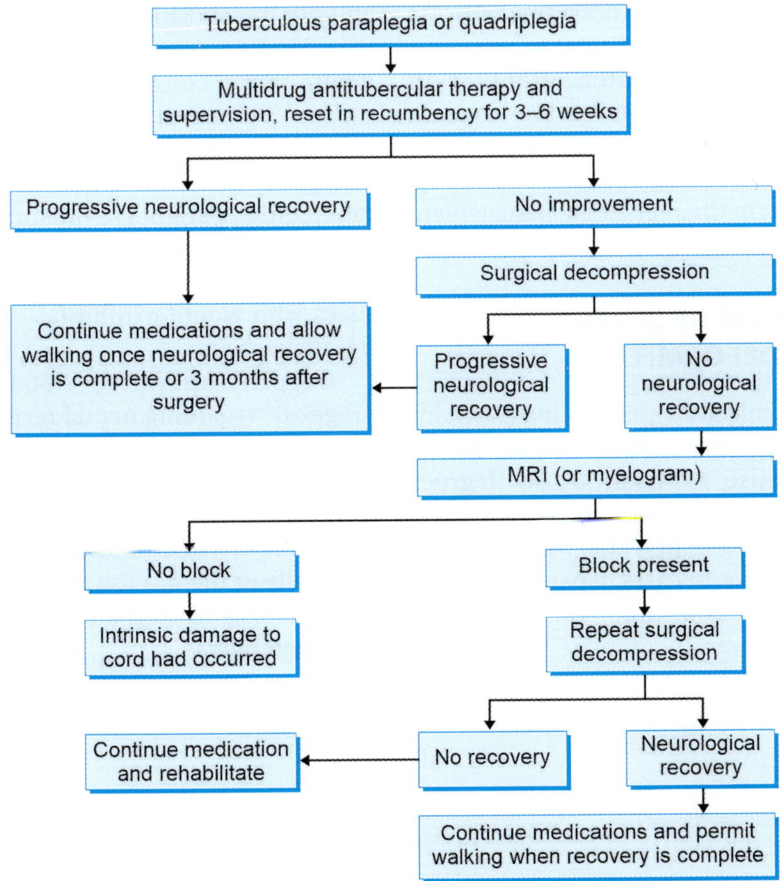

Flowchart 22.1: Suggested algorithm for management of vertebral tuberculosis with neurological complications.

In the usual paradiscal lesion the compression of the cord takes place primarily and maximally anteriorly. Therefore, it is absolutely rational to adequately decompress the cord anteriorly by anterior approach or through an anterolateral approach. Laminectomy for decompression is contraindicated as this procedure is inadequate for decompression of the anterior part of the cord; besides it removes the healthy areas of the vertebrae, thus rendering the vertebral column unstable and liable to pathological dislocation. Deterioration of the neural status and increase in the kyphotic deformity has been recorded after ill-advised laminectomy in patients suffering from paradiscal tubercular spondylitis (Rand and Smith 1989). Role of costotransversectomy is extremely limited; this is good enough to drain fluid abscess but inadequate for removal of solid tuberculous debris, thick caseous matter, granulation tissue, sequestra, bony salient, etc. We have not performed decompression in every case, we have rather advocated a middle path (Tuli 1969, 1970, 1975) as described in Chapter 23 on Management and Results.

DEVELOPMENT OF SEVERE KYPHOTIC DEFORMITY

It should be minimized by performing posterior spinal fusion for extensive spinal disease during childhood, because kyphosis of 60 degrees or more as a rule produces delayed neural complications 10–15 years after the onset of disease and deformity. In cases of paraplegia with kyphosis of 60 degrees or more, removal of the "internal gibbus" (even if comprised by healthy bones) is mandatory permitting the cord complete freedom anteriorly. This may produce some relief in the neural deficit though seldom complete recovery is observed. Prolonged stretching of the cord probably results in atrophy or gliosis of the neural tracts (Griffiths 1956). For patients with neural complications associated with healed disease of long standing, having severe kyphotic deformity (45 degrees or more), over the years we have evolved a philosophy of not to rush in for surgery so long as the patient is able to walk. They are, however, kept under close observation. Deterioration is slow but the moment a patient is unable to walk, anterior decompression and transposition is carried out (Tuli 1995). Anterior decompression, removal of internal kyphos, and anterior transposition of the cord in such patients may lead to transient or permanent neural deterioration converting a "walker" to a "non-walker". Peroperative evoked potential studies have been suggested for objective documentation of sensory and motor deficits in patients with tuberculous paraplegia (Misra 1996, Jain 2002). This may be of some value in very advanced cases of neurological deficit, however there are many cases who would exhibit false positive or false negative results.

Despite operative decompression the prognosis regarding neural recovery in poorer in patients with long duration of neural invovement (6 months or more), with senior age of patients (65 years or more), with concomitant comorbidities (diabetese or immunocompromise), gross deformity at the disease site (kyphosis >60°) and MRI changes of cord atrophy, syringomyelia or leptomeningitis.

CHAPTER 23

Management and Results

EVOLUTION OF TREATMENT

Pre-antitubercular Era: Historical

Like skeletal tuberculosis, in general, the results of orthodox conservative sanatoria treatment **(Table 23.5)** were disappointing. This made it desirable on the part of the attending physicians to evolve surgical approach to the diseased site. Most of the operative procedures were developed either for the treatment or for the prevention of paralysis in tuberculosis of the spine (Tuli 2013).

Artificial Abscess: Pott in 1779 tried the effect on the paralysis, of an artificially produced abscess, somewhere in the region of the deformity for "producing a large discharge of matter and maintaining such a discharge until the patient shall have perfectly recovered the use of his legs".

Laminectomy and Laminotomy: Chipault in 1896 was first to use laminectomy in Pott's paraplegia which was basically an unsound procedure. Fraser later on performed the operation of laminotomy which was mechanically even less adequate than laminectomy and finally in 1937, abandoned the operation altogether as late results were disappointing (quoted by Griffiths et al. 1956).

Costotransversectomy: Menard in 1894 developed costotransversectomy which fell into general disrepute, because of high incidence of sinus formation and of secondary infection and was finally given up even by Menard. Ito et al. in 1934 also reported 10 cases of lesions of the lumbar spine treated by direct surgical curettage with disappointing results.

Posterior Mediastinotomy: Obalinski performed posterior mediastinotomy for the evacuation of tuberculous paravertebral abscesses (quoted by Griffiths et al. 1956).

Calve's Operation: Calve in 1917 devised a method to aspirate the contents of an abscess without sinus formation (quoted by Griffiths et al. 1956).

Lateral Rhachiotomy of Capener: Norman Capener in 1933 devised lateral rhachiotomy, which was a direct attack on the solid compressing agents anterior to theca whereby he excised a part of the lamina and pedicle from one side to enter the spinal canal anteriorly and remove the cause of pressure on the cord. This operation carried a serious risk of lateral subluxation.

Anterolateral Decompression of Dott and Alexander: Ito et al. (1934) devised an approach similar to anterolateral approach for the curettage of the vertebral body for tuberculosis. Dott (1947) along with Alexander evolved the operation of anterolateral decompression, a modification of Capener's operation, the approach being a little more anterior and involving removal of the transverse process, posterior part of rib, a part of pedicle and a part of the body of the vertebra to gain access to the spinal canal, no part of the lamina was removed.

Results of Operations on the Diseased Vertebrae in the Pre-antitubercular Era

Most of the operations on tuberculous lesions resulted in serious sinus formation and death. General outlook regarding surgery, therefore, was aptly summarized by Calot (1930) as, "the surgeon who, so far as tuberculosis is concerned, swears to remove the evil from the very root, will only find one result waiting him—the death of his patient". Identical views were held by Schmieden (1930) and others. Probably because of such a gloomy picture of the results of operation on the diseased parts of the spine, Albee (1911, 1930) and Hibbs (1912, 1918, 1928) introduced the operation of posterior spinal fusion. Such operations were carried out from 1911 onwards and developed by many surgeons (Bosworth 1953, 1956, Campos 1955, Chandler 1940, Cleveland 1958, Girdlestone 1950, Bakalim 1960) to shorten the period of immobilization in bed, and to provide a permanent internal stability to the tuberculous spine to avoid recurrence of the disease and development of paraplegia. Bakalim (1960) found that the interval between the spinal fusion operation and the resumption of work was about one year in most of the operated cases. Kyphosis could develop or increase in spite of fusion operation. Moderate or severe increase of kyphosis was reported by Bierring (1934) in 8 out of 17 children and 10 out of 59 adults after Albee fusion operations. In other series, same degree of increase of kyphosis was observed in about 20% of cases, who had posterior spinal fusion operation for their disease (Alvik 1949, Bakalim 1960, Hallock 1954, Kaplan 1959). Review of the literature showed an appreciable incidence of pseudarthrosis in the spinal fusion operation; 3.3–26.0% was reported by Bakalim (1960). Long follow-up showed that paraplegia could occur in patients who had a posterior spinal fusion done. Hallock and Jones (1954) reported its occurrence in 23 out of 192 cases followed. Spinal fusion operation did not guarantee against recurrence of the vertebral infection. The results of posterior spinal fusion before the use of antitubercular drugs (published between 1917 and 1954) reviewed by Bakalim in 1960 showed that average percentage of patients reported as "healthy and fit" for work were between 40 and 80%, "improved" 60% and "not healed" between 1 and 14% of the survivals. Over the years it became increasingly obvious that posterior fusion did nothing to the diseased area, where pus, debris and necrotic bone remained enmeshed and encysted in dense fibrous tissue, where the organisms remained alive, sometimes mildly active, in other cases dormant, only to flare up at any chance or provocation. The operation had nothing to offer to the paraplegic patient who failed to respond to the standard sanatoria treatment.

The availability of potent antitubercular therapy, however, improved the results of nonoperative conservative treatment, and posterior spinal fusion (Bakalim 1960, Smith 1968, Neville 1971, Jain 2020). At present with effective drugs, practical use of posterior spinal arthrodesis in Pott's disease is considered: (i) to control mechanical instability or pain due to this instability and not due to the grumbling disease (Somerville 1965), (ii) or for arresting the progress of kyphosis during growing age (Tuli 1995), (iii) or during correction of spinal deformity in a panvertebral operation (Tuli 1995, Chen et al. 2002), (iv) or as an adjunct for providing lasting biological stability after decompression and debridement for active paravertebral vertebral disease.

Direct Operative Treatment with Antitubercular Drugs

This term indicates a direct surgical attack on the spinal lesion including evacuation of abscesses and curettage of the lesion. Wilkinson (1949), Hald (1954), Orell (1951), Kondo and Yamada (1957) were the first to report results of the treatment with antituberculosus drugs in conjunction with direct surgical attack on the spinal lesion.

A variety of opinions have been expressed by various workers in regard to the indications for the use of this combined method of treatment. Thus, Hald (1954) advocated that it should be employed more often than has been done so far. Fellander (1955), Boulvin (1960) and Debeyre (1964) performed the operation with little regard to factors such as the age of the patient and the stage or extent of the disease. Tuli et al. (1967–1975) operated only for failures and recurrences. In children, Wilkinson (1955) and Mukopadhaya (1956) found the indications to be wider than in adults. Further observations regarding radical operations for tuberculosis of the spine have been reported (1955–2003) by many workers (Serafinova and Malawski 1959, Hodgson et al. 1956, 1960, Fellander 1955, Kondo and Yamada 1957, Weinberg 1957, Roaf 1958, 1959, Shrivastava et al. 1961, Stock 1962, Cameron et al. 1962, Risko and Novosazel 1963, Masalawala 1963, Paus 1964, Donaldson and Marshall 1965, Lagenskiold and Riska 1967, Kohli 1967, Goel 1967, Guirguis 1967, Fang and Ong 1969, Baker et al. 1969, Jackson 1971, Bailey 1972, Kemp 1973, Chen et al. 1995, Govender 2002, Hassan 2003, Gokce et al. 2012, Garg et al. 2012, Khanna 2019).

Current Role of Direct Surgery in the Management of Spinal Tuberculosis

It is rather difficult to strictly compare the results of various series **(Table 23.1)** treated by conservative and operative treatment as the clinical material varies from center to center (Tuli 1973). Routine employment of newer and more effective antitubercular drugs (since 1970s) has also improved the outcome of nonoperative and operative treatment. Wilkinson (1949–1969) had an opportunity to compare the results of his series treated conservatively and those who underwent operation. Similarly, Paus (1964) compared the two series treated by himself. Somerville and Wilkinson (1965) treated 130 lesions by direct operation and achieved sound healing in 92% and reported relapse or recurrence in 12.5% of healed cases. They treated 105 patients with chemotherapy without operation (in cases "having relatively benign lesion") and achieved sound healing in 92% of such cases. Paus (1964) reported complete working capacity in 35% of 37 cases treated by ambulatory regime with antitubercular drugs. Of the healed cases there was a relapse in respect of back pain in one case and in respect of sinus in another. Out of 86 cases treated by him by radical operation and antitubercular drugs, 94% had complete working capacity. 11% of these cases underwent reoperation for relapse or failure.

Excisional therapy has been practised by many workers for all cases of tuberculosis of the spine with excellent results. The incidence of healing in cases treated by surgery combined with antitubercular drugs has been between 80 and 96%. Excisional surgery evidently evacuates tuberculous pus and debris, removes sequestra of disc and bone, opens up new vascular channels in ischemic areas, thus leading to reduction of general toxemia, reduction of total time of healing of the local lesion and probably improves the quality of healing especially in cases with extensive destruction and sequestration. On the other hand, there are certain cases of tuberculosis of the spine which do not have extensive destruction and sequestration which would heal without surgical intervention. The present day clinician is equipped with sophisticated investigations (CT scan/MRI) to diagnose tuberculous infection of the spine at a very early stage (predestructive or early destructive stage) and achieve excellent healing in nearly all such cases without the necessity of surgical intervention **(Fig. 23.1)**.

No "excisional surgery" obviates the necessity of continuation of antituberculosis drugs for the standard duration (18 months ±) for healing of the operated lesion and also the additional tuberculous lesions in other parts of body. Progressive bone destruction in spite of chemotherapeutic regime, failure to respond to conservative therapy and uncertainty in

Table 23.1: Comparison of results of different series of spinal tuberculosis treated by various regimes in post-antitubercular era (expressed as percentage).

Workers	*Mode of treatment*	*Clinical healing (%)*	*Neural recovery (%)*	*Death (%)*	*Relapse (%)*
Kondo, 1957	Streptomycin (SM) alone (nonoperative)	20.9	?	9.3	30.2
	Streptomycin with Albee's operation	35.5	?	0.0	35.5
	SM + focal debridement	52.0	?	2.1	2.1
Falk, 1958	Cases treated in 1946–1948 with SM alone and spinal arthrodesis in 69%	66.0	?	13.0	11.0
Stock, 1962 Hodgson, 1960	Surgical treatment by anterior approach	93.0	74.0	4.4	?
Konstam and Blesovsky, 1962	Antitubercular drugs, operation only for failure for paraplegia	96.0	89.0	1.5	2.0
Konstam, 1962	Antitubercular drugs primarily	86.0	99.0	?	?
Risko, 1963	Costovertebrotomy-spondylodesis = one rib resection (almost like costectomy) + post-spinal arthrodesis	82.0	95.0	1.0	7.0
Masalawala, 1963	Focal debridement with bone grafting	91.0	74.2	6.2	3.0
Kirkaldy-Willis, 1965	Surgical treatment by direct approach	86.0	79.0	3.4	?
Friedman, 1966	Antitubercular drugs primarily	97.0	?	4.1	18.8
Kohli, 1967	Radical surgery with antitubercular drugs	81.0	84.4	3.5	?
Arct, 1968 (patients >60 years)	Antitubercular drugs alone	26.0	0.0	18.0	31.0
	Anterolateral decompression + bone grafting	84.7	60.0	10.0	0.0
Wilkinson, 1969	Operative debridement (1940–1953)	80.0	?	2.0	20.0
	Operative debridement + chemotherapy (1954–1962)	95.0	–	2.0	5.0
Tuli, 1969, 1971	Antitubercular drugs; operation for failure only	95.0	80.0	8.0	?

? = difficult to calculate or not given clearly.

Note: The results are not strictly comparable because there are variations regarding clinical material, variety of antitubercular drugs used, criteria for clinical healing, and duration of follow-up during which death, "recurrence", or relapse are calculated. Only those series are tabulated where comparison was reasonably possible.

diagnosis are definite indications for surgery in active stage of the disease. A period of observation for about 2–3 months seems to be enough to judge these features. Another indication for evacuation of paravertebral abscess may be marked increase in its size in spite of rest and chemotherapeutic regime. Definite indications for late surgery are recrudescence of the local disease, development of neural complications or pain in the spine due to mechanical instability. Almost similar criteria are advised by many workers now (Somerville and Wilkinson 1995, Wimmer et al., 1997, Rajasekaran et al. 1998, Parathasarathy et al. 1999, Jain et al. 2003, Mukherjee et al. 2007, Dunn 2018, Andre's-Cano et al. 2018, Ahuja 2022).

Role of Surgery in Neural Complications

Opinion also varies regarding the role of surgery in tuberculous paraplegia (Capener 1967). A large group of surgeons performed debridement and decompression in all cases of tuberculosis of the spine irrespective of the status of neurological involvement (Ahn 1968, Donaldson 1965, Hodgson 1956–60, Kirkaldy-Willis 1965, Lagenskiold 1967, Masalawala 1963, Risko 1963). Others performed operative decompression only in those cases who did not respond to antitubercular drugs and rest (Griffiths 1952, 1956, Jones 1958, Roaf 1958,

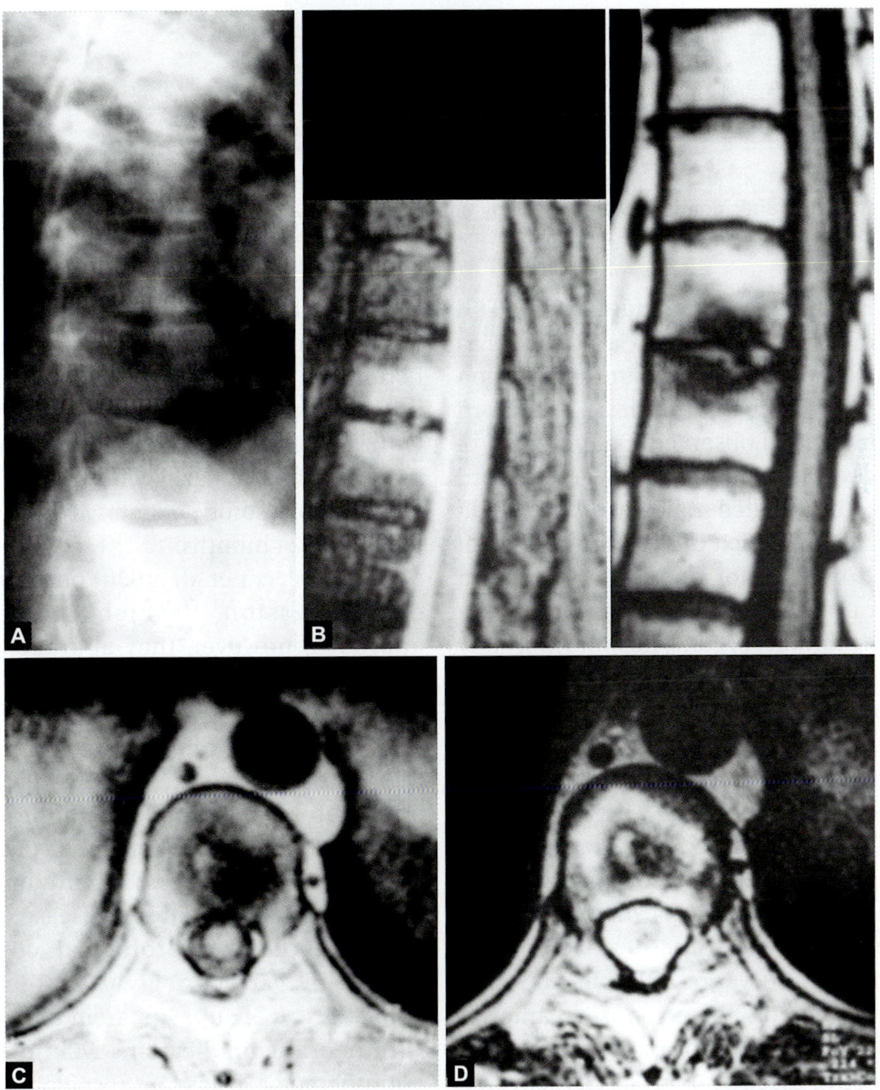

Figs. 23.1A to D: (A) Despite complaint of pain in the lower dorsal spine, systemic symptoms and persistent tenderness in the region of D9–D10, the plain X-rays did not reveal any gross abnormality except "straightening of dorsal kyphosis", (B to D) MRI however, clearly showed the lesion. The change in the signal intensity as observed in T1 and T2 signals suggested the collection of inflammatory exudates in the bodies of D9 and D10. Breach of the upper end plate of D10 is clearly visible in sagittal sections. The transverse sections show the destroyed area in the middle of vertebral bodies surrounded by the inflammatory exudates.

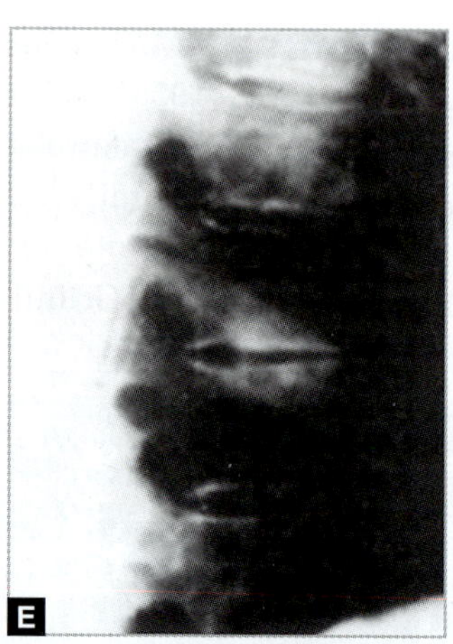

Fig. 23.1E: X-ray 1 year after domiciliary treatment by antitubercular drugs shows the healed status with diminished intervertebral disc space D9–D10, sclerosis of paradiscal margins, some restoration of dorsal curvature.

Konstam 1958, 1962, 1963, Seddon 1956, Tuli 1969). Bosworth (1952–63) and Campos (1955) felt that most reliable treatment is immobilization and early posterior spinal arthrodesis. Adendorff et al. (1987) in general observed that potential of neural recovery was related to the degree of cord compression. They treated majority of their adult patients with neural deficit or even those without neural deficit by anterior operation combined with bone grafting. They had rather significant postoperative mortality of 5.8%, hospital mortality was 2.1% for those without neural deficit, 6.3% for those with paraparesis and 10.9% for paraplegics. We feel such a high mortality is avoidable by more restricted indications for surgery and less extensive operations.

Hsu et al. (1988) reviewed 22 patients 7 years after treatment by anterior decompression and fusion in patients suffering from paraplegia of late onset. The mean time of development of paraplegia was 18 years after the onset of tuberculous spondylitis. The response to anterior decompression was better in patients who had evidence of active disease, 9 out of 12 recovered completely and 3 significantly. In patients with healed disease, the anterior decompression was technically more difficult and the recovery less satisfactory. Such 10 patients developed significant postoperative complications like neurological deterioration (2), cerebrospinal fistulae (3), and neuropraxia of cord (4). The period for most of the neural recovery in patients with active disease averaged 6–8 months. The recovery time in cases with healed disease was very variable, some patients who showed recovery took up to 24 months.

Though Hsu et al. (1988) performed anterior decompression through left thoractomy approach, however, they approached the cord from the lateral side through an intervertebral foramen by tracing the segmental nerve root, the bone (internal kyphos) in front of the cord was then carefully excised. We however, perform this operation by an extrapleural approach because the operation is directly at the site of the offending deformity, and it is a less hazarduous surgery for patients with long-standing disease.

Behavior of neurological complications treated by various regimes is summarized in **Table 23.1**. It is quite apparent that every patient with neural complications will not be cured by antitubercular drugs and rest alone, however, all patients do not need surgical decompression.

An absolutely conservative approach to Pott's paraplegia is considered unjustifiable as one might be losing very valuable time. Irreparable damage of the cord may take place if the deterioration progresses to complete loss of motor and sensory functions. However, universal radical extirpation seems to be unnecessary. The results obtained in the series, in which a middle path (Dickson 1967, Friedman 1966, Konstam 1962, Tuli 1969, 1970, 1975) was followed, were comparable with those reported in series treated by universal radical surgery (Paus 1964, Lagenskiold 1967, Ann 1968, Donaldson 1965, Griffiths 1979, Pun 1990, Louw 1990). In Konstam and Blesovsky's series out of 56 cases of paraplegia 28 (50%) recovered with antitubercular drugs and operative intervention was not needed in them. The other 28 (50%) were operated. In 26 cases of operated patients, simple operations like drainage of abscesses were done and only in two, anterolateral decompression was done. In these operated cases also 25 patients became well. In Friedman's (1966) series, spontaneous recovery from paraplegia was seen. In Roaf's (1958) series, 10 (43.4%) of 23 paraplegia cases recovered spontaneously and rest 13 (56.6%) needed operations, 3 (13.2%) costotransversectomy and 10 (43.4%) anterolateral decompression. Spontaneous recovery of neural complications was observed in 48% of cases on antitubercular drugs and bedrest in Tuli's (1969) series.

Apparently, the scenario of the patients with neurological complications presenting in specialized centers these days may not appear as favorable. In the Delhi University College of Medical Sciences GTB Hospital between 1987 and 1994, of the 360 cases of neural complications who presented in the department of orthopedics, 80% had absolute indications for operative decompression. This is because the first contact general physicians now put these patients on modern antitubercular drugs, and most of the neural complications produced by inflammatory causes resolve by the domiciliary treatment. Only those patients not responding to the above treatment seek opinion and admission in the specialized hospitals. Having performed an adequate mechanical decompression of the cord, most of the neural recovery takes place within one year, no significant neural recovery has been observed after 18 months of the operations.

Absolute Indications for Operative Decompression

One of the arguments offered by the advocates of universal extirpation in favor of exploration is that it enables the surgeon to rectify any errors in diagnosis based only upon clinical and radiological assessment. Since a noninflammatory lesion causing neurological complications is unlikely to respond to rest in bed and antituberculous drugs for a few weeks, such lesions would naturally be explored in the less radical programs as well. Whenever there is doubt about diagnosis surgical treatment is mandatory as it provides an opportunity to confirm the diagnosis. In general, workers who do not decompress every case (Jain 2020, Gan 2024), follow a middle path and they limit surgical decompression to the following situations: (1) Neurological complications which do not start showing signs of "progressive recovery" to a satisfactory level after a fair trial of conservative therapy (3–4 weeks), (2) patients with spinal caries in whom neurological complications develop during the conservative treatment, (3) patients with neurological complications which become worse while they are undergoing therapy with antituberculous drugs and bedrest, (4) patients who have a recurrence of neurological complication, (5) patients with prevertebral cervical abscesses, neurological signs and difficulty in deglutition and respiration, and (6) advanced cases of neurological involvement (Stage IV) such as marked sensory and sphincter disturbances, flaccid paralysis or severe flexor spasms. Older patients with neural complications require earlier operative decompression to avoid hazards of prolonged recumbency and immobilization.

Our Policy of Treatment (Middle Path Regime)

Because of a large number of patients of spinal tuberculosis, lack of adequate number of hospital beds, operating time and the trained medical staff, we have been treating our patients mostly on nonoperative lines with antituberculous chemotherapy, rest and spinal braces. Hospitalization has been restricted to the paraplegics who were unable to walk, or patients who required surgical evacuation of abscesses or debridement of vertebral lesion, or those who agreed for fusion of spine for extensive dorsal lesion in children or for an unstable and painful spinal lesion. Similar conditions also exist in other economically underdeveloped countries and one is forced to resort to such a line of treatment (Konstam et al. 1962, Kaplan 1959, Martini 1988, Kumar 1988) **(Table 23.1)**. Such a policy has stood the test of time and it is justified to call it the rational treatment (Wisneski 1991, Rajasekaran 2018, Khanna 2019, Jain 2020, Gan 2024).

a. *Rest* in hard bed or plaster of Paris bed: Plaster of Paris bed is not essential, however, it is rarely necessary for a few uncooperative patients or children who do not realize the value of rest. In the treatment of cervical (Tuli 1988, Chadha et al. 2007) and cervicodorsal lesions, traction (2–3 weeks) was used in the early stages to put the diseased part at rest.
b. *Drugs:* The policy of drug treatment is the same as outlined in Chapters 6 and 7. Our current general policy for an average adult is to start with "intensive phase" treatment comprising of daily dosage of isoniazid 300–400 mg, rifampicin 450–600 mg and ofloxacin 400–600 mg for 5–6 months. All replicating sensitive mycobacteria are likely to be killed by this bactericidal regime. The "continuation phase" treatment should last for 7–8 months where the aim is to attack the persisters, slow growing or intermittently growing or dormant or intracellular mycobacteria. It comprises of isoniazid and pyrazinamide (1500 mg per day) for 3–4 months, to be followed by isoniazid and rifampicin for another 4–5 months. The "prophylactic phase" consists of isoniazid and ethambutal (1200 mg) for 4–5 months. This is the time when the treated patient is back to his normal working environments. The aim is to offer prophylaxis to the patient during the time his body is developing adequate protective immunity. The doses and drugs were modified according to the weight of the patient, existing comorbidities and any adverse drug reactions. For patients who are hospitalized streptomycin replaces one of the drugs except isoniazid. Supportive therapy with multivitamins, hematinics if necessary and, high protein diet are advised. Valsalan et al. (2012) reported the efficacy of directly observed short-course (DOTS) chemotherapy of spinal tuberculosis. Our long-term observations of patients does not support short course chemotherapy for any patient of skeletal tuberculosis.
c. *Radiographs* and *ESR* are taken and patients are called for check-up at 3–6 months interval. Kyphosis was measured radiologically (Konstam and Blesovsky 1962, Tuli and Kumar 1971) as described by Dickson (1967) **(Fig. 23.2)**. For craniovertebral, cervicodorsal, lumbosacral regions and sacroiliac joints, MRI or CT scan may be advisable at 6–12 months interval for about 2 years.
d. *Gradual mobilization* of the patient is encouraged in the absence of neural deficit with the help of suitable spinal braces as soon as the comfort at the diseased site permits. After 3–9 weeks of starting of treatment, the patient is put on back extension exercises 5–10 minutes, 3–4 times a day as tolerated by the patient. Spinal brace is continued for about 18 months to 2 years when it is gradually discarded.
e. *Abscesses* are aspirated when near the surface, and 1 g of streptomycin with or without INH in solution is instilled at each

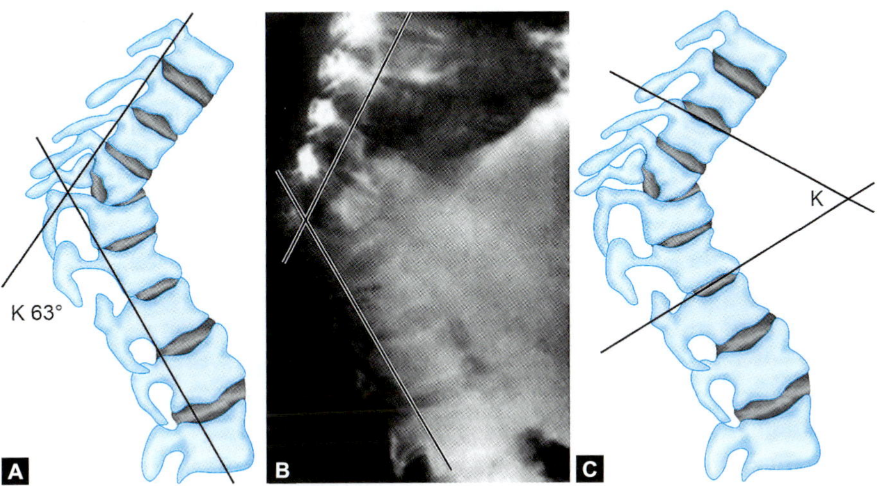

Figs. 23.2A to C: Method of measurement of angle of kyphosis (Dickson 1967). A line is drawn along the posterior margins of the bodies of the healthy vertebrae above and below the site of disease; angle "K" is the angle of kyphosis. Angle "K" increases with increase in the degree of kyphosis. Another method is by determining the angle between the upper end-plate of the normal vertebra proximal to the affected vertebrae and the lower end-plate of the normal vertebra distal to the affected vertebrae (C).

aspiration. Open drainage of the abscess is performed if aspiration fails to clear them. All radiologically visible paravertebral abscesses are not drained, drainage is incidental whenever a decompression is performed for Pott's paraplegia, or debridement is performed for an active tuberculous disease. Prevertebral abscesses in the cervical region can be aspirated or drained under local or general anesthesia when complicated by difficulty in deglutition and respiration. Drainage of a perispinal abscess *per se* may be considered when its radiological size increases markedly despite treatment.

f. *Sinuses* in a large majority of cases heal within 6–12 weeks from the onset of the treatment. A small number may require longer treatment and excision of the tract with or without debridement.

g. *Neural complications:* In the cases who started showing progressive recovery of neurological complications on triple drug therapy between 3 to 4 weeks and progressed to complete recovery, surgical decompression was considered unnecessary. Decompression of the cord for neurological complication should be performed for those cases who did not show progressive recovery after a fair trial of conservative therapy for a few weeks, or cases in which the patients developed the neurological complications during the conservative therapy, or in cases where the neurological status became worse while the patient was undergoing treatment with antitubercular drugs and bedrest, or cases who had a history of recurrence of neurological complication. In advanced cases with motor, sensory and sphincter involvement or those having severe flexor spasms, as well as in elderly patients, decompression was not delayed unduly. In other words, we performed decompression for absolute indications (Tuli 1969).

h. *Excisional surgery* is recommended for posterior spinal disease associated with abscess or sinus formation (with or without neural involvement) because of danger of secondary infection of the meninges if the disease does not come under control with drug therapy within 3–4 weeks.

i. *Operative debridement* is advised for cases who do not show arrest of the activity of spinal lesions after 3–6 months of the chemotherapeutic regime or cases with recurrence of disease.

j. *Posterior spinal arthrodesis* is recommended for symptomatic unstable spinal lesions in which the disease otherwise seems to be arrested. A lesion is considered mechanically unstable if inspite of the arrest of the vertebral disease the patient gets discomfort in the back on doing normal work. Radiologically, such lesions may show significant panvertebral destruction of more than two vertebrae and lack of regeneration of vertebral bodies during the process of healing. Main indications for surgical intervention on vertebral lesion are summarized in **Box 23.1**.

k. *Postoperative:* After decompression or debridement or arthrodesis the patients are nursed on a hard bed, when necessary (for children) a plaster of Paris bed has been used in initial 2–3 weeks. In cases with neural complications 3–5 months after the operation when the patient has made good recovery, the patient is gradually mobilized out of the bed with the help of spinal braces. In the absence of paraplegia, mobilization with spinal braces is started 2–3 months after the operation. The spinal brace is gradually discarded about 12–24 months after the operation.

BOX 1: Main indications for various operations for vertebral tuberculosis.

- Decompression (± fusion) for neurological complications which failed to respond to 3–6 weeks of conservative therapy/too advanced
- Debridement (± fusion) in failure of response after 3–6 months of nonoperative treatment
- Doubtful diagnosis
- Fusion for symptomatic mechanical instability after healing
- Debridement ± decompression ± fusion in recurrence of disease or of neural complication
- Prevention of severe kyphosis by posterior fusion ± debridement in young children with extensive dorsal lesions
- Anterior transposition of cord through extrapleural anterolateral approach for neural complications due to severe kyphosis

Note: Laminectomy has no place in tuberculosis of spine except for extradural granuloma/tuberculoma presenting as "spinal tumor syndrome", or a case of old healed disease (without much deformity) presenting with secondary "vertebral canal stenosis", or non-healing posterior spinal disease.

Operative Procedures Done by Us

For decompression and debridement, with or without bone grafting, cervical spine and cervicodorsal junction up to T1 have been approached through the anterior approach; dorsal spine and dorsolumbar junction has been approached through anterolateral approach or rarely through transpleural approach; lumbar spine and lumbosacral junction has been approached through extraperitoneal retro-psoas transverse vertebrotomy approach. Laminectomy has been performed by us for excising the diseased bones in some cases of posterior spinal disease and in cases of paraplegia due to extradural granuloma or tuberculoma. Anterior transposition of the cord through the anterolateral route was performed in cases with extreme degree (>60°) of kyphotic deformity and paraplegia.

Due to the efficacy of modern antitubercular drugs absolute indications for surgical intervention on the vertebral lesion are reduced to nearly 5% of uncomplicated cases, and to about 60% of cases with neurological deficit. All the patients who recover are able to return to their full activity within 6 to 12 months of the treatment. Active life is permitted first with suitable spinal braces which are gradually discarded within about 2 years.

Recrudescence of the Disease or Complications

Recurrence or relapse of a tuberculous lesion in the spine poses a special problem. Sometimes there may be a reactivation complicated by neurological involvement. Perhaps the commonest cause is a grumbling activity of infection caused by resistant strain of acid-fast bacilli in a patient with relatively poor general resistance. In such a situation, a thorough clinical and radiological examination may be helpful to localize the areas of activation. Special investigations like tomography or MRI, and/or myelography in cases of neural involvement may be of help to localize the disease.

Of the patients adequately treated with modern antitubercular drugs from 1965 to 1995, and followed for 20 years or more, the recurrence rate appears to be <5%. The cause of recurrence in those well-treated patients seems to be development of diabetes, prolonged use of steroids, use of immunosuppressive drugs (methotrexate) or nutritional debility associated with aging.

If the activity or complication cannot be controlled by new drugs, the diseased area is operated upon and thorough clearance is performed. Patient is treated by appropriate supportive therapy, new line antitubercular drugs in conjunction with isoniazid and a short post-operative course (3 weeks) of streptomycin. At the time of debridement, bone grafting may be performed if there is any evidence of instability; decompression of cord is performed when there is neural involvement, anterior transposition of the cord is mandatory if the kyphotic deformity is >60 degrees.

Results of Management by Following the Middle Path

All long-term results of any regime in the treatment of tuberculous spondylitis must be assessed in terms of achievement of **"favorable status"**. The universally accepted definition of a favorable status is: No residual neural impairment, no sinus or clinically evident cold abscess, no impairment of physical activity due to the spinal disease/lesion, and presence of radiologically quiescent disease.

The results presented here are based upon personal observations, upon nearly 900 cases, including 200 cases of tuberculous paraplegia. The number of cases which were available for various follow-up studies are mentioned in appropriate sections. Backache and tenderness was relieved in 96% cases at the end of 12 months treatment.

Sinuses: All the sinuses healed under the effect of antitubercular drugs within 1–7 months (average 3.3 months). Multiple sinuses healed almost simultaneously. There was no problem of persistent sinus formation even after extensive surgery. A small number of sinuses which failed to respond to drugs alone, healed by curettage or excision of the sinus tracks and change of drugs.

Sinus ramification is always greater than can be appreciated from the appearance of the openings or the quantity of the discharge. The sinus tracts lead into various directions and for great distances, therefore complete operative excision is difficult and indeed impracticable. Fortunately, with effective drug therapy, rarely is surgery necessary in the treatment of tubercular sinuses. Similar observations are reported by Kaplan (1959), Konstam and Blesovsky (1962), Paus (1964), Bosworth (1952, 1963), Hald (1954), Martini (1988), Jain et al. (2001), Moon (2014). Healing in multidrug resistant cases, or patients with HIV disease is extremely slow. The sinuses, ulcers, abscesses and operative wounds may not heal for many months despite multidrug therapy and attempted excisional surgery.

Palpable or Peripheral Cold Abscesses

In addition to systemic anti-TB drugs repeated aspiration and instillation of streptomycin (± isoniazid) was sufficient to heal 95% of abscesses, 5% healed by surgical evacuation. Majority of the abscesses were healed within 6 months. There were a few (<2%) abscesses which were not fully controlled in spite of surgical drainage and continuous treatment. These cases were probably having resistant strains. They presented with recurrence after a quiescent period varying between 6 and 12 months. Modern antitubercular drugs in conjunction with surgery were able to heal recurring cases. Percutaneous drainage has been suggested by Dave et al. (2014); surgical evacuation with postoperative suction—drainage (3–6 days) would be needed if the pus is too thick to be aspirated.

Deep-seated Radiological Perivertebral Abscesses

Observations regarding response to anti-TB drugs is based upon 72 cases who had deep-seated radiological abscess and in whom surgery was not done as the first procedure. 35% abscess shadows resolved spontaneously within 6–12 months **(Figs 23.3 to 23.5)**, in 45% the shadows regressed to a constant size and in 20% it appeared static.

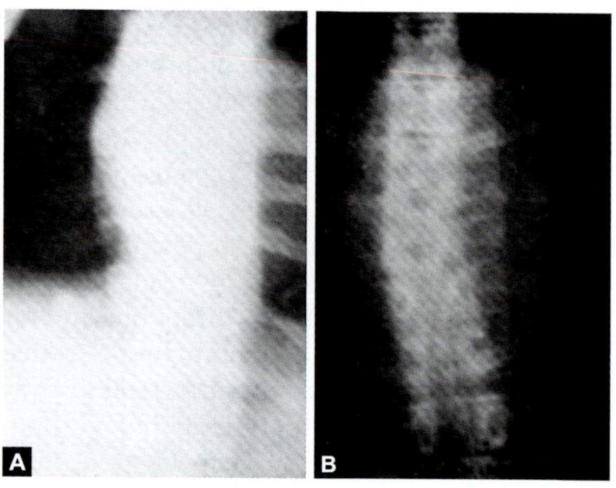

Figs. 23.3A and B: X-rays of an adult treated by antitubercular drugs alone. Note spontaneous resolution of the paravertebral abscess, (A) at the time of presentation, (B) after 8 months.

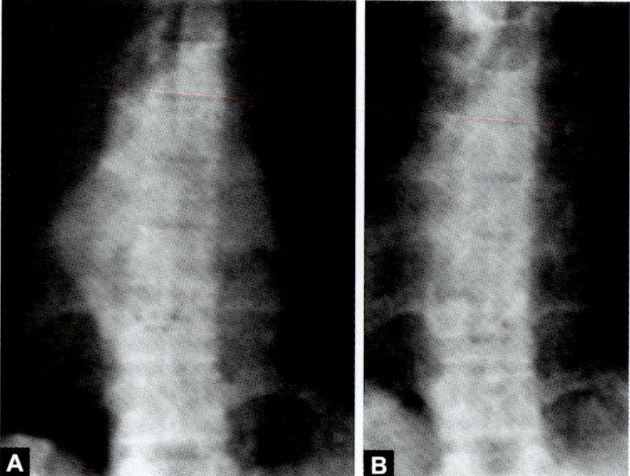

Figs. 23.4A and B: X-rays of an adult showing spontaneous resolution of a paravertebral abscess by antitubercular drugs without surgery, (A) at the time of presentation, (B) after 18 months.

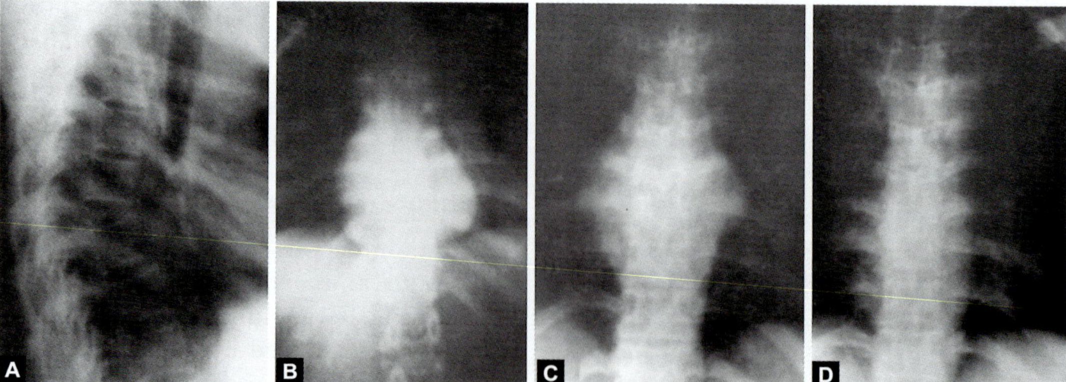

Figs. 23.5A to D: X-rays of dorsal spine (A, and B) at presentation show a large pear-shaped paravertebral shadow along with severe wedge-shaped collapse (almost vertebra plana) of dorsal 7 vertebral body and reduced intervertebral space between D7 and D8. Appearance of the paravertebral shadow 6 months after antitubercular drugs (C), and complete resolution of the shadow without surgery after one year (D).

In <1% of cases, the deep-seated paravertebral abscess required drainage because the size of the abscess increased markedly in successive X-rays in spite of treatment or it lead to difficulty in respiration and deglutition in the cervical region. Our observations compare favorably with those of Konstam and Konstam (1958), Kaplan (1959), Konstam and Blesovsky (1962), Konstam (1963), American Thoracic Society (1963), Friedman (1966, 1973) and Stevenson and Manning (1962). Presence of an abscess does not seem to deter the process of healing. Considering the results of present and other studies, it is suggested that a less aggressive attitude should be adopted towards radiologically demonstrable paravertebral abscess shadows. The drainage may be considered in cases with neurological complications and those having difficulty in deglutition and respiration, or abscesses which become much bigger in size despite adequate antitubercular therapy.

Neurological Complications

All the patients were given the standard treatment as previously outlined. The overall results for their response in 200 patients (during 1965–1974 in BHU Teaching Hospital) are summarized in **Table 22.2**. 38% recovered on conservative therapy alone and 6 patients died 3–4 weeks after admission and the beginning of treatment. The cause of death in these patients was moribund general condition and associated visceral tuberculous foci, tuberculous meningitis or both. Of the patients who recovered on conservative therapy in 9 cases, drainage of prevertebral abscess was performed in cervical or cervicodorsal lesions. In the remaining 118 patients who failed to respond to medicinal treatment or were too advanced to permit observation for a long time, operative decompression of the cord was performed. Of these 81 (69%) recovered fully, 13 (11%) had partial recovery sufficient to enable them to walk with moderate degree of support, 10 (8%) failed to respond appreciably though they had some improvement in sensations and in sphincter function; and 14 (12%) died. One death occurred 40 hours after operation due to hypostatic pneumonia; the other patients died between 4 and 52 weeks after decompression, the cause of death being tuberculous meningitis, uremia, an ascending urinary tract infection, renal failure and toxemia associated with decubitus ulcers.

The results of decompression in our series (during 1965–1974) viewed separately from those who responded to conservative regime may appear to be poorer than those in many other series in which surgical decompression was performed in all the patients. However, in the present series decompression was performed principally when the neurological signs failed to respond to conservative antituberculous treatment, while in the series in which decompression was performed in all patients, operation may have received credit for recoveries which would have occurred anyway on conservative therapy alone. The overall response in our series shows a success rate of 78.5% which compares favorably with the results of any other series.

The analysis of more recent (1987–2000) patients of tuberculous paraplegia or tetraplegia who were operated by us according to the criteria of middle-path-regime show much better neural recovery. Of >400 patients assessed up to 1 year after the operation, the outcome was complete recovery 85%, partial recovery enabling ambulation with some support 8% and negligible recovery (wheel chair bound) 7%. No mortality was observed within one year of the operations. This improvement in the clinical outcome is probably due to public awareness and reporting of patients at an early stage of disease, general availability of modern imaging modalities permitting early diagnosis and better understanding of offending pathology, and employment of more efficient antitubercular drugs.

In Konstam and Blesovsky's (1962) series out of 56 cases of paraplegia 28 (50%) became well only with antitubercular drugs and operative intervention was not needed in them. The other 28 (50%) were operated. In 26 of operated patients, simple operations like drainage of abscesses were done and only in 2, anterolateral decompression was done. In these operated cases also, 25 patients became well. In Friedman's (1966) series, 10 (43.4%) of 23 paraplegia cases recovered spontaneously, and rest 13 (56.6%) needed operations, 3 (13.2%) costotransversectomy and 10 (43.3%) anterolateral decompression. In Roaf's (1958) series as well spontaneous recovery from paraplegia was seen. This shows that a large number of cases of Pott's spine, with neurological complications, recover with an adequate course of modern anti-TB drugs alone. Operative decompression should be indicated in cases who fail to respond to drug therapy, advanced cases or cases who recur (Tuli 1969, 1985, Medical Research Council 1978–1998, Friedman 1973, Mehta 2001, Jain 2002, 2013, Dunn 2018, Khanna 2019).

Onset and Speed of Neural Recovery after Operation

The first objective evidence of neural recovery was observed 24 hours to 12 weeks after the decompression. No significant correlation between the onset and speed of recovery after decompression was found with other clinical data such as degree and duration of neural involvement. Most of the patients showed the first evidence of objective recovery within 3 weeks of the decompression, however, others took a longer time to recover. Four patients in the present series started showing recovery 10 and 12 weeks after decompression, 2 recovered completely and 2 had partial recovery. The time taken for near complete recovery varied between 3 and 6 months. No significant neural recovery occurred after 12–18 months of decompression. Clinical features which influence prognosis are shown in **Table 22.5**.

Plantar Response

Extensor plantar response, a sign of pyramidal tract involvement, lasted for a very long time. We had an opportunity to study this response 18 months after the onset of treatment in 65 patients who had achieved complete neurological recovery. In 36 cases (55.4%), the response was extensor on one or both sides, and in 29 cases (44.6%) it was flexor or equivocal. Early return of the flexor response was seen in cases of milder neurological involvement of a shorter duration.

Recurrence or Relapse of Neural Complications

One hundred patients of neural involvement who had completely recovered were followed-up for a period varying between 3 and 10 years. Two reported with recurrence of paraplegia after 3 years of complete recovery, one due to an extradural granuloma and one apparently due to severe kyphosis.

Of 144 patients without neural complication who had complete healing, 24 were followed up for >5 years. One hundred forty-one of these patients neither developed neurological complications nor relapse of the disease. One child who had a very severe kyphotic deformity reported back with neurological complications, 5 years after the first presentation. Two patients reported with recrudescence of the disease between 3 and 5 years.

Fate of Disc Space and Radiological Healing

Radiological Healing of Vertebral Tuberculosis without Operation

In the patients who at presentation showed intact intervertebral spaces due to central, anterior or appendiceal type of tubercular lesions, or patients diagnosed and treated at the "predestructive stage" the radiological appearance of the disc space remained unchanged and intact even at a long follow-up. Of the patients with classical paradiscal or metaphyseal variety of tubercular spondylitis followed for a period of 1–5 years after the start of treatment, 19% had fibrous replacement of the disc space **(Figs. 23.6 and 23.7)**, 12% had fibro-osseous and 69% had osseous replacement as judged by radiological examination **(Figs. 23.8 to 23.11)**. With longer follow-up there was shift from fibrous replacement towards osseous replacement of the intervertebral space. Moon (1987) observed that 36 months after the onset of antitubercular therapy intercorporeal bony fusion was observed in 36% of patients without surgery. Patients with retained disc space may exhibit lateral osteophytes on radiological examination, 5–10 years after the disease has healed.

It was further observed that in cases where the disc was completely destroyed and there was obliteration of the intervertebral spaces there were more chances for the lesion to heal by bony replacement of the disc space **(Figs. 23.11 to 23.14)**. Fate of the disc space on achieving the healed status depends more on its state when treatment was initiated rather than its location **(Table 23.2)**.

Radiological Healing of Vertebral Tuberculosis with Operation on the Diseased Vertebral Bodies without Bone Grafting

11% of cases had fibro-osseous and 89% had bony healing of the vertebral lesion **(Fig. 23.13)** when assessed between one and 5 years, after the operation. Over a period of observations from 1–10 years in our material, gradual increase in the incidence of bone block formation was recorded (Srivastava 1980–1981).

Radiological Healing of Vertebral Lesion

Following control of infection, the spine in most of the patients in the present series was capable of spontaneous stabilization without severe deformity. In a large percentage of lesions in which tubercular spondylitis was of the paradiscal or metaphysial variety, a spontaneous interbody bony or mixed fusion with clinical healing took place **(Table 23.2)**. In a much smaller group, clinical healing took place with fibrous replacement of the disc space between the involved vertebrae. Regeneration of involved vertebral bodies was observed in many cases

Figs. 23.6A and B: A young man diagnosed as tubercular spondylitis at the early destructive stage in 1986. The patient obtained a healed status by treatment with antitubercular drugs on domiciliary regime. The lesion achieved healing without increase in the kyphotic deformity, and with retention of the disc space (fibro-osseous healing—B).

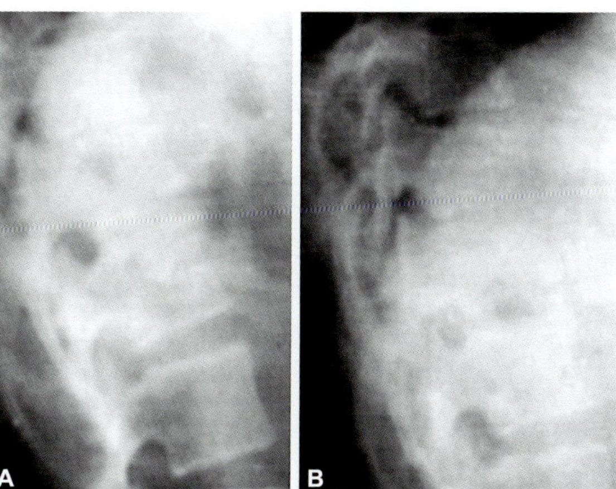

Figs. 23.7A and B: X-rays of a patient treated nonoperatively (A) at presentation, (B) after 2 years. Note regeneration of vertebral bodies and maintenance of the disc space (fibrous healing). The only evidence of old disease in X-ray seems to be a markedly diminished disc space.

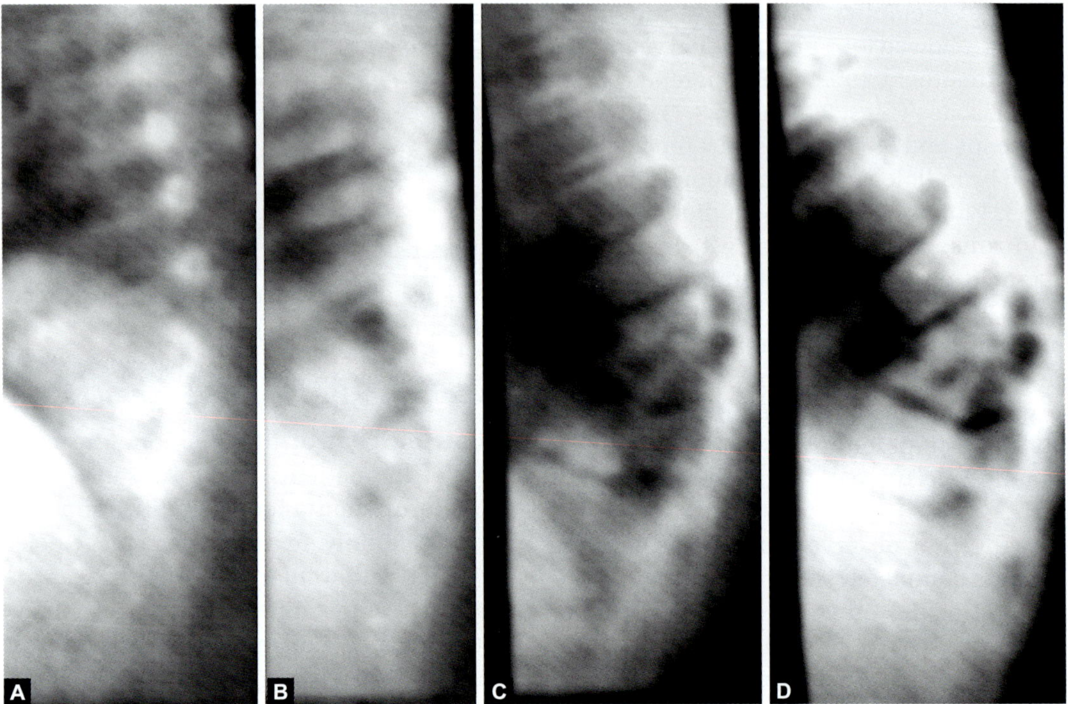

Figs. 23.8A to D: X-rays of a young patient showing a typical paradiscal lesion with marked diminution of the disc space and destruction of the adjacent vertebral bodies. Radiologically, the patient healed by osseous replacement of the disc space (osseous healing) and some regeneration of the involved vertebral bodies. There is formation of a "block vertebra"; (A) At presentation, (B) after 10 months, (C) after 22 months, (D) after 31 months at age 14 years (treated nonoperatively).

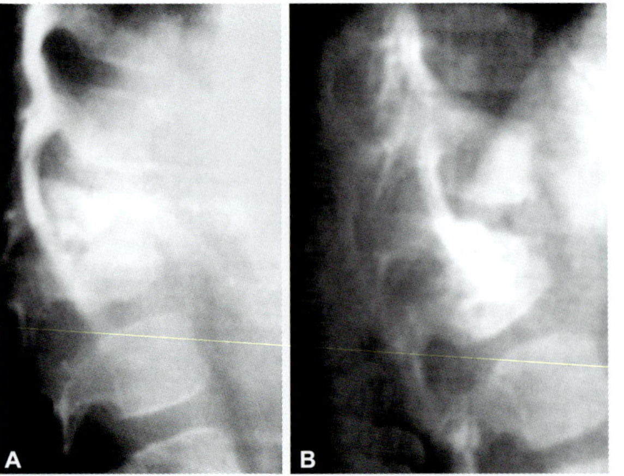

Figs. 23.9A and B: X-rays of a child showing a typical tuberculous lesion in the dorsolumbar region. Osseous healing was achieved by nonoperative treatment: (A) At presentation, (B) after 21 months.

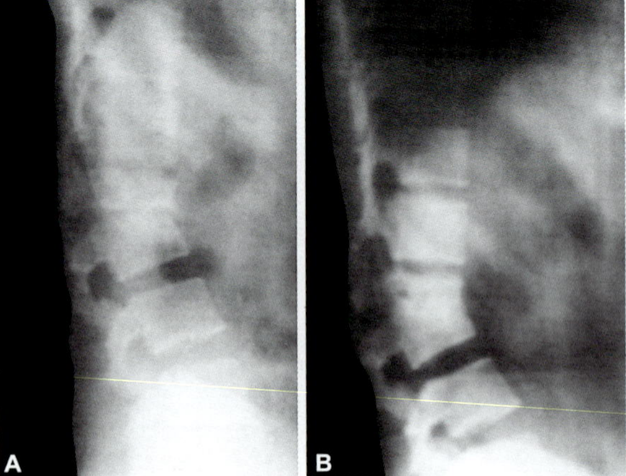

Figs. 23.10A and B: X-rays of an adult with a lumbar lesion treated nonoperatively. Note osseous healing, and no increase in the deformity; (A) At presentation, (B) 2 years after treatment.

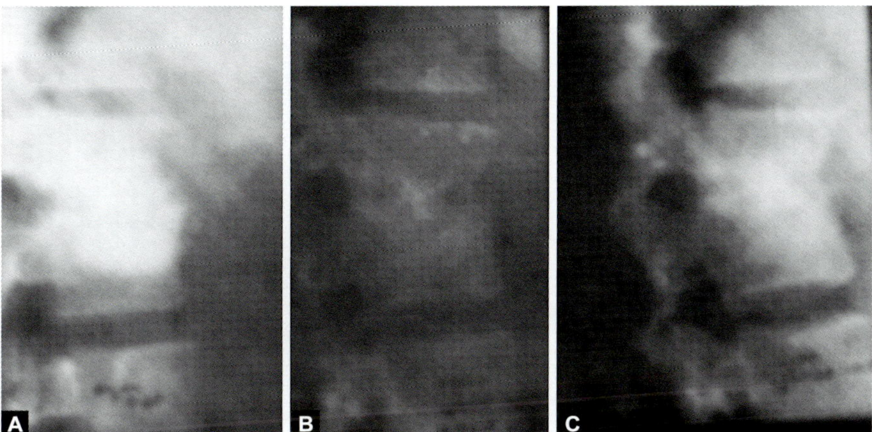

Figs. 23.11A to C: X-rays of an adult with a lumbar lesion treated nonoperatively. Note osseous healing and minimal increase in the kyphotic deformity, (A) At presentation, (B) after 11 months, (C) after 21 months (intercorporeal bone-block).

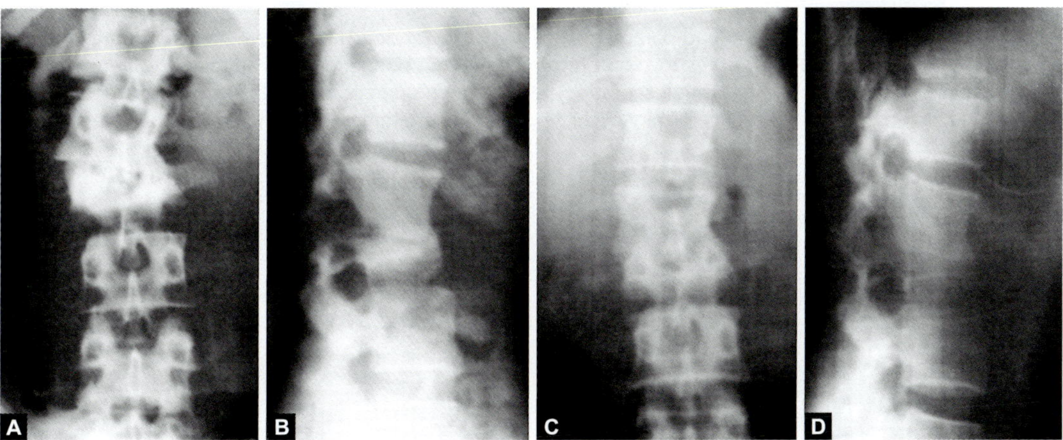

Figs. 23.12A to D: Tuberculosis of lumbar 1–2 vertebrae, (A and B) at presentation (C, and D) 1½ year after domiciliary treatment with antitubercular drugs, braces, and unrestricted activity. Note wedging of lumbar 2 vertebra in anteroposterior and lateral views and the resultant kyphoscoliotic deformity. Healing took place by spontaneous bone block formation by 18 months without increase in deformity.

under the influence of antitubercular drugs **(Figs. 23.14 to 23.16 and 23.19)**.

We observed many cases for 15 years, who under the influence of modern antitubercular chemotherapy achieved a healed status in which the intervertebral space remained intact **(Figs. 23.6, 23.15 and 23.16)** or was replaced by fibrous tissue. The incidence of local recrudescence in such cases does not seem to be more than those replaced by fibro-osseous or osseous tissue. Bony and mixed (fibro-osseous) replacement of the intervertebral space were not always synonymous with clinical healing. In four patients who had complete bony fusion the disease was still clinically active, another two had mixed fusion and active disease.

Course of Kyphosis of Spine in Patients not Operated Upon

Observations reported here are based upon long term follow-up of patients (Srivastava 1980-1981,

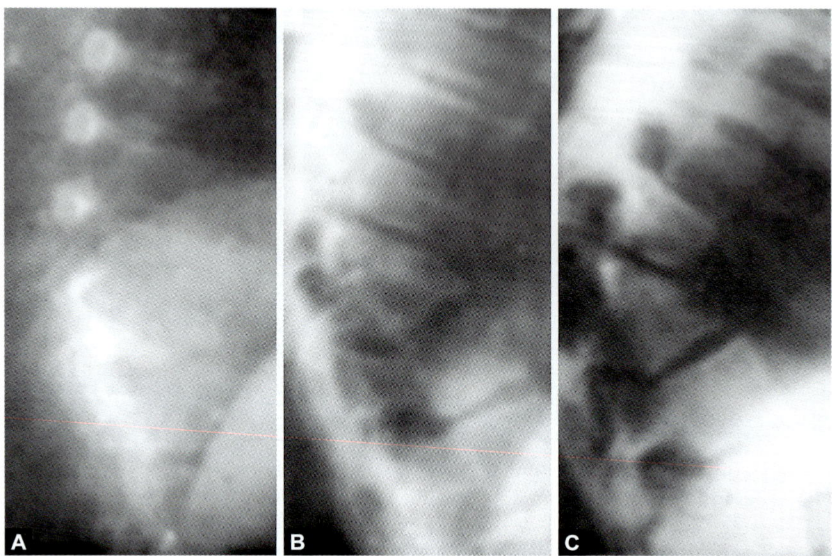

Figs. 23.13A to C: X-rays of a child who had paraplegia due to the lower dorsal lesion. As she failed to respond to drug therapy and rest, an anterolateral decompression was performed without bone grafting. Patient made complete and rapid neurological recovery. Successive x-rays (A) at presentation, (B) 1 year after operation, and (C) 2 years after operation revealed osseous healing and increase in kyphotic deformity by 20 degrees, concomitant posterior fusion might have minimized the deformity.

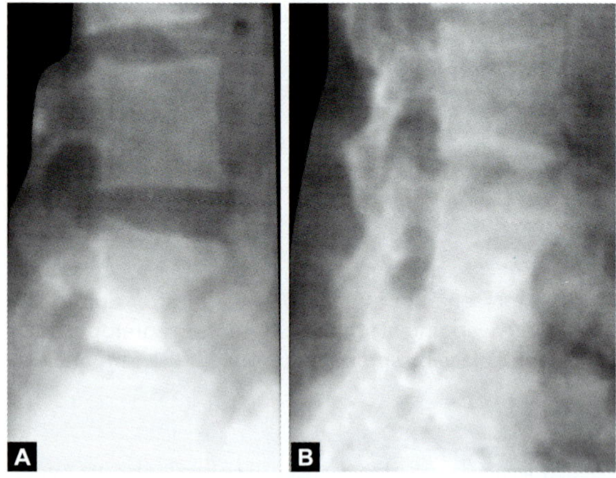

Figs. 23.14A and B: X-rays of an adult female with a lumbar lesion treated nonoperatively on domiciliary regime. Note marked regeneration of the destroyed vertebral bodies, spontaneous intercorporeal bone block formation, and no increase in the deformity, (A) at presentation, and (B) 31 months after treatment.

Table 23.2: Fate of disc space at various lesion sites 18 months after the onset of nonoperative treatment (1965–1974).

Level	*Number*	*Intact*	*Fibrous*	*Fibro-osseous*	*Osseous*
Cervical	2	0	0	2	0
Dorsal	38	2	6	22	8
Dorsolumbar	9	0	0	6	3
Lumbar	48	4	8	18	18
Lumbosacral	7	0	1	4	2
Total	104	6	15	52	31

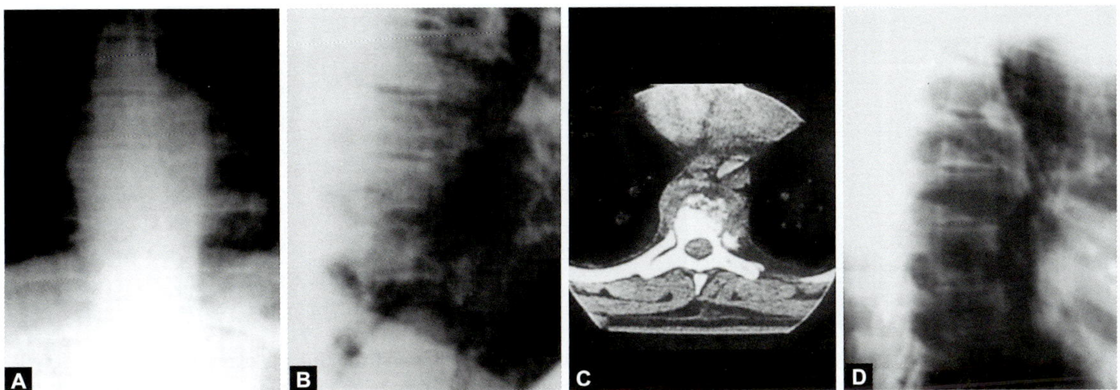

Figs. 23.15A to D: A young man with persistent mid-dorsal pain presented with X-rays of the dorsal spine (A and B). The anteroposterior view showed a paravertebral shadow, however, the lateral view suggested suspicious lesion D7 vertebral body. The CT scan (C) confirmed destructive lesion in the anterior half of D7, and presence of a paravertebral soft tissue abscess containing multiple small sequestrae. Diagnosis at an early destructive stage and prompt treatment by effective drugs healed the disease with negligible deformity. (D) X-ray 2 years after treatment showed reconstitution of the bony texture with slight diminution of the disc spaces D6–D7 and D7–D8.

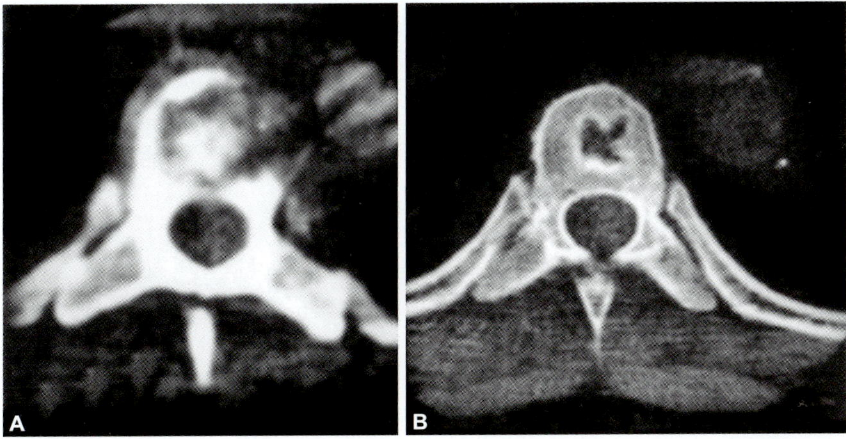

Figs. 23.16A and B: CT scan of the mid-dorsal spine of a doctor showing (A) the destructive lesion in the vertebral body (a cavity with sequestrum) and soft tissue shadow in the perivertebral region. The patient was treated by antitubercular drugs. The CT scan of the same area one year after the treatment; (B) Shows restitution of the destroyed vertebral body and resorption of soft tissue swelling and sequestrum.

Tuli 1975, 1985) from 5–13 years (mean 8 years). The angle of kyphosis increased by 10–30 degrees in 12%, >30 degrees in 3%, and in the remaining 85% the kyphosis either remained static, or decreased **(Fig. 23.19)**, or the increase was <10 degrees. Average increase in the kyphotic angle is about 15 degrees. All the cases with increase of kyphosis by >30 degrees, were in growing age at the onset of spinal disease, and all of them had involvement of three or more vertebral bodies. It seemed that multiple vertebral involvement, active growth and situation of the lesion in the thoracic spine were responsible for excessive increase in kyphosis **(Fig. 23.17)**. Increase of kyphosis was observed in 67% of thoracolumbar lesions, 55% of thoracic lesions and 33% of lumbar lesions.

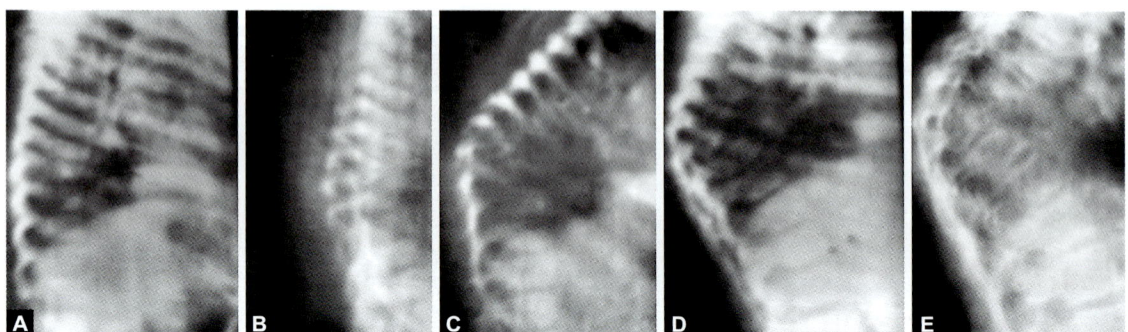

Figs. 23.17A to E: X-rays of a boy suffering from tuberculosis of D6–D9, followed from the age of 5–16 years: (A) in July 1977 only D8–D9 seem to be affected, (B) in November 1977 the disease is apparent from D6–D9 with mild kyphotic deformity, (C) in July 1978 the kyphosis has increased to 40 degrees, (D) in September 1981 though the disease remained healed the kyphotic deformity increased to 60 degrees, (E) in March 1989 at the age of 16 years the patient presented with a kyphotic deformity of 80 degrees and stage IV paraplegia. The patient had led an active life without neural deficit up to the age of 16 years. On operative decompression and anterior transposition of the cord no evidence of active disease was found. Debridement of the diseased part, and posterior spinal arthrodesis performed before the development of severe kyphosis (in 1977–1978) would have minimized the chances of severe deformity and late onset neural complications.

Table 23.3: Behavior of kyphosis in relation to age of patient, activity of disease, and number of vertebrae involved with a mean follow-up of 5 years (1965–1974) in 104 patients.

Increase in degrees	*No. of lesions*	*Age*		*Active*	*Non-active*	*Average no. vertebrae involved*
		*Children**	*Adults***			
Less than 6	72	18	51	1	68	2.5
6–10	12	5	6	0	11	2.4
11–15	9	4	5	2	7	2.8
16–20	4	1	3	0	4	3.0
21–25	1	0	1	0	1	2.0
26–30	0	0	0	0	0	0
31–35	2	1	1	0	2	3.5
36–40	0	0	0	0	0	0
41–50	0	0	0	0	0	0
51–100	3	2	1	1	2	6.6
More than 100	1	1	0	0	0	7

*Children: 14-years old and younger.
**Adults: 15-years old and older.

The relation of age, activity and the number of vertebral involvement to the increase in degree of kyphosis is summarized in **Table 23.3**. Four of the cases with severe kyphosis who had clinically and radiologically healed lesions at the end of treatment started showing neurological complications after 5-10 years of follow-up apparently due to the severe deformity. The conservative treatment in conjunction with triple or dual drug therapy does not prevent the progress of kyphosis (Friedman 1966, Konstam and Blesovsky 1962, Paus 1964, and Dickson 1967, Mechical Research Council 1978, Tuli 1995, Jain et al. 2014, Wong 2017). However, even spinal fusion operations (posterior type) have shown progress in kyphosis during the follow-up of patients. The observations regarding radiological kyphosis in the present series are compared with other reports in **Table 23.4**. In our series, an increase of 10 degrees or more of kyphosis was seen in only 20% of lesions during the period of their follow-up. In the rest (80%) of lesions, the curvature of spine either remained static or kyphosis increased by <10 degrees or kyphosis decreased. In our patients whose lesions had increase in kyphosis by >30 degrees, the disease was located in the dorsal spine. This is in agreement with Friedman (1966) and Puig Guri's (1947) observations. Puig Guri (1947) stated that the destruction of a thoracic vertebral body results in a posterior displacement of the center of motion, a subluxation at the level of the articular facets and increase in weight to be borne by the anterior part of the body. In the lumbar spine, the large bodies and vertical articular facets were more apt to telescope than to angulate. The cervical spine was prevented from telescoping by the interposition of transverse processes; and in this part of spine there was the least deformity. Incidence of kyphosis is more common in thoracic spine and this region is subjected to the greatest degree of angulation. All our cases who had increase of kyphosis by >30 degrees, had three or more vertebrae involved and all of these patients were <10 years of age at the onset of disease.

Younger age, multiple vertebral involvement and a dorsal lesion are responsible for most of those cases in which a severe degree of kyphosis takes place (Jain et al. 2004 and Rajasekaran 2012). Because of the pre-existing kyphotic curve in the dorsal spine the gravity perpetuates the deformity. Once the kyphotic deformity is <45 degrees probably the posterior spinal muscles are put to a mechanical disadvantage further adding to the deformity. Almost the whole of the deformity takes place during the phase of active spinal growth with or without active disease. Development of severe kyphotic deformity after clinical healing of disease and completion of growth of the vertebral column seems to be uncertain. The only nonoperative way to minimize the increase in kyphosis seems to be recumbency in early active stage and prolonged protection with suitable braces in the later stages.

In upper dorsal spine some degree of protection is provided by the rib cage against additional collapse and deformation. Patients with dorsal disease below the level of 9th rib have the worst prognosis regarding the development of kyphos. In addition to the osseous collapse of the anterior column, arrest of the growth potential of vertebral bodies, and tethering of anterior structures, horizontal orientation of posterior articular facets may lead to posterior subluxation of the diseased segment. In the lumbar spine, vertical orientation of the articular facets encourages telescoping (Rajasekaran 2002, Moon et al. 2002). Rajasekaran (1987, 1989, 2002) suggested that during growing age the deformity occurred in two phases: Phase I during active stage of disease caused by bone destruction and osseous collapse; in Phase II during the healed status of disease caused by arrest of growth potential of anterior column.

Unrestricted growth of the posterior elements of vertebrae in the presence of arrested growth of the vertebral bodies (during the growing phase of vertebral column) would lead to progressive kyphotic deformity. Because of pre-existing lordosis in cervical and lumbar spine the kyphotic deformity is less prominent. In the dorsal spine because of pre-existing kyphos the softened bones undergo collapse, telescopy, and significant kyphotic deformation. When the kyphotic angle at the disease site is >30 degrees, 80% of vertical forces are converted into translational forces (Rajasekaran 2007), thus creating kyphosis, translation and rotation (if destruction is asymmetrical). In the initial stages, the deformity is in a plastic state correctable to some extent by mechanical forces, in long-standing disease most of the deformity becomes fixed.

Table 23.4: Changes in radiologically demonstrated kyphosis in various series.

	Orthodox treatment				*Conservative treatment (ambulatory, dual drugs)*				*Radical operations*						*Middle path*			
	Hallock and Jones (1954)		*Bakalim (1960)*		*Konstam and Blesovsky (1962)*		*Paus (1964)*		*Cauchoix et al. (1961)*		*Paus (1964)*		**Prabhakar (1989)*		*Tuli and Kumar (1971)*		**Prabhakar (1989)*	
Changes	**No.**	**%**	**No.**	**%**	**No.**	**%**	**No.**	**%**	**No**	**%**	**No.**	**%**	**No.**	**%**	**No.**	**%**	**No.**	**%**
Increase of 10° or more	31	39.2	11	18.6	77	37.2	10	26.3	52	25	27	26.2	42	48	21	20	16	46
Decrease	3	3.8	0	0	8	3.8	1	2.6	0	0	1	1	2	2	2	2	0	0
No change or increase of >10°	45	57.0	48	81.4	122	59.0	27	71.1	159	75	75	72.8	45	50	81	78	19	54
Total number of lesions	79	100	59	100	207	100	38	100	211	100	103	100	89	100	104	100	35	100

*Thoracic or thoracolumbar only. Assessment is not reliable at cervicodorsal and lumbosacral regions.

Rajasekaran (2007, 2013) suggested radiographic signs to assess "spine-at-risk" for kyphotic deformity in children. These signs seen in lateral X-rays included: Separation of facet joints, posterior retropulsion of the diseased vertebral segments, toppling sign; and lateral translation of vertebral column as seen in anteroposterior views. We feel an active tuberculous disease in children <10 years of age showing destruction (not mere edema on MRI) of three or more vertebral bodies from C7 to L1 vertebrae must be kept under close observation, because these cases are at high risk for deterioration of kyphotic deformity. If deformity is progressive as seen in follow-up X-rays taken at 4–6-monthly intervals, posterior spinal fusion should be performed including one healthy vertebra proximal and distal to the destroyed vertebral bodies (Deshpande et al. 2012, Moon et al. 2012). Fusion of the anterior elements during the growing age should be avoided because that may negate any growth potential of the vertebral bodies.

Of the children operated according to above mentioned criteria and followed for 8–10 years (up to skeletal maturity), the angle of kyphotic deformity remained static or improved (by 5–10 degrees) or deteriorated by <10 degrees in approximately 95% of cases. In 5%, there was progress of kyphotic deformity by 11–15 degrees. In children with neural deficit, who underwent anterior debridement and decompression through extra pleural anterior operation (using the classical anterolateral approach) with concomitant posterior fusion, the behavior of the kyphotic angle as observed up to the skeletal maturity was practically similar. Earlier we were not doing posterior fusion for adult patients. However, since 1995 for any adult patient undergoing an anterior operation for non-recovering neural deficits, therapeutically refractory disease, uncertain diagnosis, panvertebral disease (with perceived instability), concomitant posterior spinal fusion was performed as a routine. Of these patients followed for 2 years or more, the average kyphotic angle at the diseased site increased by 10 degrees (range 0–30°). The author does not consider it justified to perform extensive operative procedures (Gokce et al. 2012) in children without clear signs of spine at risk for severe deformity. During growing years over zealous surgery on the vertebral bodies may jeopardize their growth potential, posterior spinal fusion is rational to minimize kyphotic deformity. Spinal "instability" in tuberculous infection is considered an important indication for operative stabilization, however there is no universally accepted definition for "instability" (Auja 2021).

Course of Kyphosis of Spine in Lesions Operated Upon without Bone Grafting

Adequate assessment of the progress of kyphotic deformity was performed on patients who were followed for periods from 2–6 years (average 3.2 years). Angle of kyphosis increased by 10–30 degrees in 19%, >30 degrees in 4% and in the remaining 77%, the kyphosis either remained static, or decreased, or the increase was <10 degrees. The deformity in the operated cases became stable by about 18 months in majority of the cases. In five cases, less than 8-year-old at the time of presentation with dorsal lesions, the kyphosis increased by 25 degrees even after 2 years of conventional anterior surgery, possibly because of unrestricted growth of posterior elements in the presence of restricted growth of anterior elements. Upadhyay et al. (1994) stated that there is no role of disproportionate unrestricted growth of posterior elements in the typical tubercular spondylitis responsible for severe kyphotic deformity. However, majority of their pediatric patients had the disease between D11 to L5 and they excluded the cases who had three or more vertebrae involved. Chen et al. (1995) obtained an average correction of kyphotic deformity by 10 degrees in adult patients treated by anterior debridement combined with anterior and posterior fusion.

The observations in various series are summarized in **Table 23.4**. There does not seem to be much difference regarding the behavior of kyphosis (in adults) whether the patients are treated by universal excisional surgery or by nonoperative medicinal therapy or by following a middle path regime (Paus 1964, Konstam and Blesovsky 1962, Tuli and Kumar 1971, Medical Research Council 1978, 1982, 1986, Martini 1988, Wong 2017).

Upadhyay et al. (1994), Moon et al. (2002) found no difference in the results of deformity in the lumbar spine between the group that had "anterior radical surgery" and the group that was treated by anterior curettage and debridement. Moon et al. (2002) in one of the recent analysis of lumbar spine disease treated by modern antitubercular drugs obtained spontaneous intercorporeal bone-block formation in nearly 70% of patients at 18 months and in 88% at 36 months. As observed by us, very early stage of disease healed without fusion with reconstitution of the vertebral bodies and diminution of the disc space. Absolute indications for surgery in lumbar spine disease appear to be non-resolving neurological complications, gross destruction of vertebral bodies with concomitant destruction of posterior elements (panvertebral destruction), and development of neurogenic claudication as a result of narrowing of lumbar canal secondary to healed status of tuberculous disease of long-standing.

The only operative procedure that has been claimed to prevent increase of kyphotic deformity is the radical excision and bone grafting performed in Hong Kong by pioneers of the radical operation themselves (Medical Research Council 1978–1982). At present, we feel that in young children having thoracic lesions with involvement of 3 or more vertebrae, recumbency in prone position in early active stage, and operative debridement (anteriorly if the disease is not healing or neural complications are not resolving by drugs), and bone grafting posteriorly for panvertebral stabilization **(Fig. 23.18)** may minimize the development of progressive kyphotic deformity (Tuli 1985, 1995).

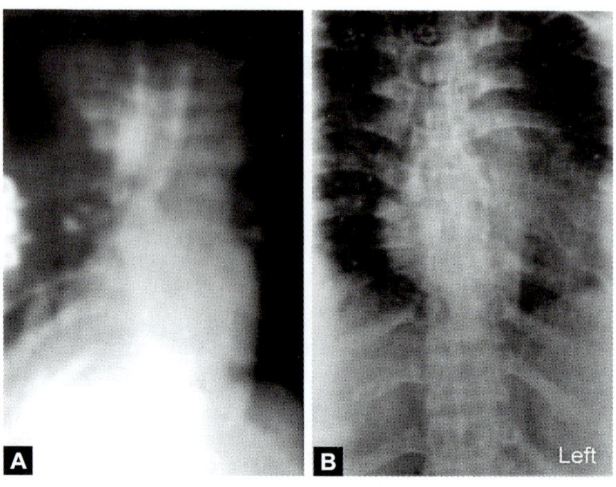

Figs. 23.18A and B: Pre-(A) and postoperative X-rays of a 12-year-old boy who was decompressed from D6 to D8, through anterolateral approach. At the same sitting posterior spinal fusion was performed (utilizing the excised ribs) with the hope to arrest the growth of posterior elements to minimize the increase in kyphotic deformity. In the postoperative X-ray (B) one can see the three ribs placed on the contralateral posterior elements.

The tuberculous granulations have the ability to erode and replace the involved bone. The cartilaginous growth plates, articular cartilage, and intervertebral disc are only indirectly affected because of lack of nutrition or due to erosion caused by granulomatous pannus. This accounts for the potential of preservation of the growth plates in children **(Fig. 23.19)**. Personal observations and studies in the literature (Schulitz et al. 1997) show that kyphotic deformity (during the growth period) behaved worst with "anterior debridement and anterior intercorporal fusion", the best behavior was with fusion of "posterior elements without anterior fusion". "Anterior and posterior combined fusion" showed intermediate behavior. A solid anterior interbody fusion during growth period appears to negate any growth potential of the vertebral bodies, thus leading to increase in kyphotic deformity **(Fig. 23.19)**.

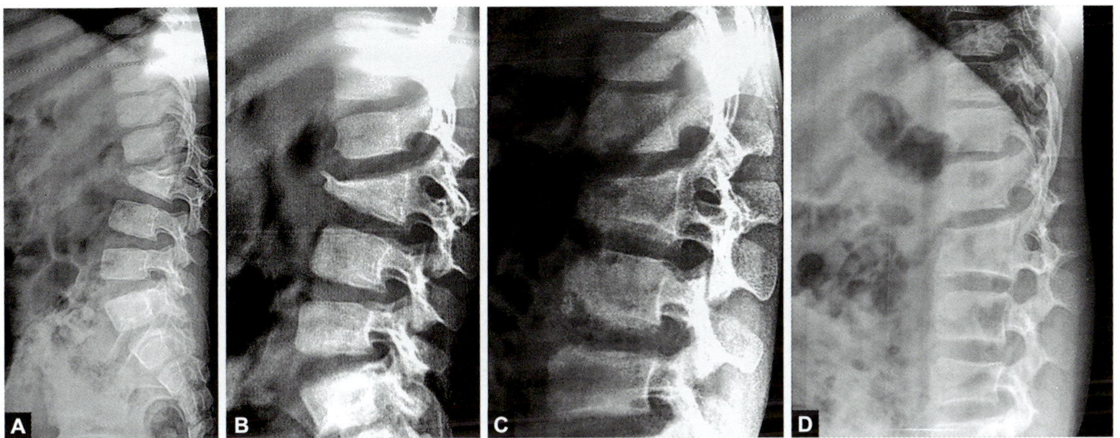

Figs. 23.19A to D: During growing age, despite tuberculous infection, the growth plates of vertebral bodies may retain some potential for growth of vertebral bodies: (A) Soon after the healing of disease, (B) 1 year, (C) 2 years (D) 3 years after the healed status of infection. One can appreciate the increase in the size of the destroyed vertebral bodies during the growing years due to the growth potential of apophysis on proximal and distal surface of the "bone block".

Clinical Healing Obtained by Anti-Tb Drugs in Cases without Neurological Complications

Almost all such cases were nonactive clinically and radiologically after 12 months of the drug therapy without surgery on the diseased vertebrae. All these cases were able to return to their work with full activity. Less than 5% of cases did not show a favorable response to drug therapy and adequate rest and these were subjected to direct surgical debridement in conjunction with newer drugs for a prolonged duration; all of them healed. Clinical healing of the patients was judged by local and general signs and symptoms, and radiological observations. After clinical healing patients engaged themselves in "normal activity" according to the criteria of Stevenson and Manning (1962) and had "complete working capacity" as described by Paus (1964). In our series, women patients were leading their normal family life and many were able to bear children without any signs of reactivation. Majority of the adult patients including farmers or daily wage earners were able to resume their pre-disease occupation and activities **(Figs. 23.20 to 23.22)**.

The overall incidence of healing by conservative antitubercular therapy in different series (Tuli 1973, Rajasekaran 2013, Khanna 2019) varies between 83% and 96.8%. In the series treated by excisional therapy, the incidence of healing has been between 80% and 96% (Hodgson 1960, Paus 1964, Wilkinson 1955, Yeager 1963, Chahal 1980) **(Tables 23.1, 23.5)**. The results of orthodox treatment obviously were poor because in those days antitubercular drugs were not available. The series treated by modern antitubercular drugs, conservatively or in conjunction with radical surgical extirpation, on the whole have good results (Girling et al. 1988). As the results of conservative therapy are satisfactory, we feel that the operative procedure should be reserved for complications of spinal tuberculosis, such as cases not responding favorably within 3–6 months, paraplegics not controlled by chemotherapy, abscesses not resolving by repeated aspirations, and painful and unstable spine. Many other workers have similar feelings (Chofnas 1964, Kaplan 1959, Medical Research Council 1982, 1993, Martini 1988, Prabhakar 1989, Khanna 2019, Shetty 2017, Rajasekaran 2018, Yadav 2020).

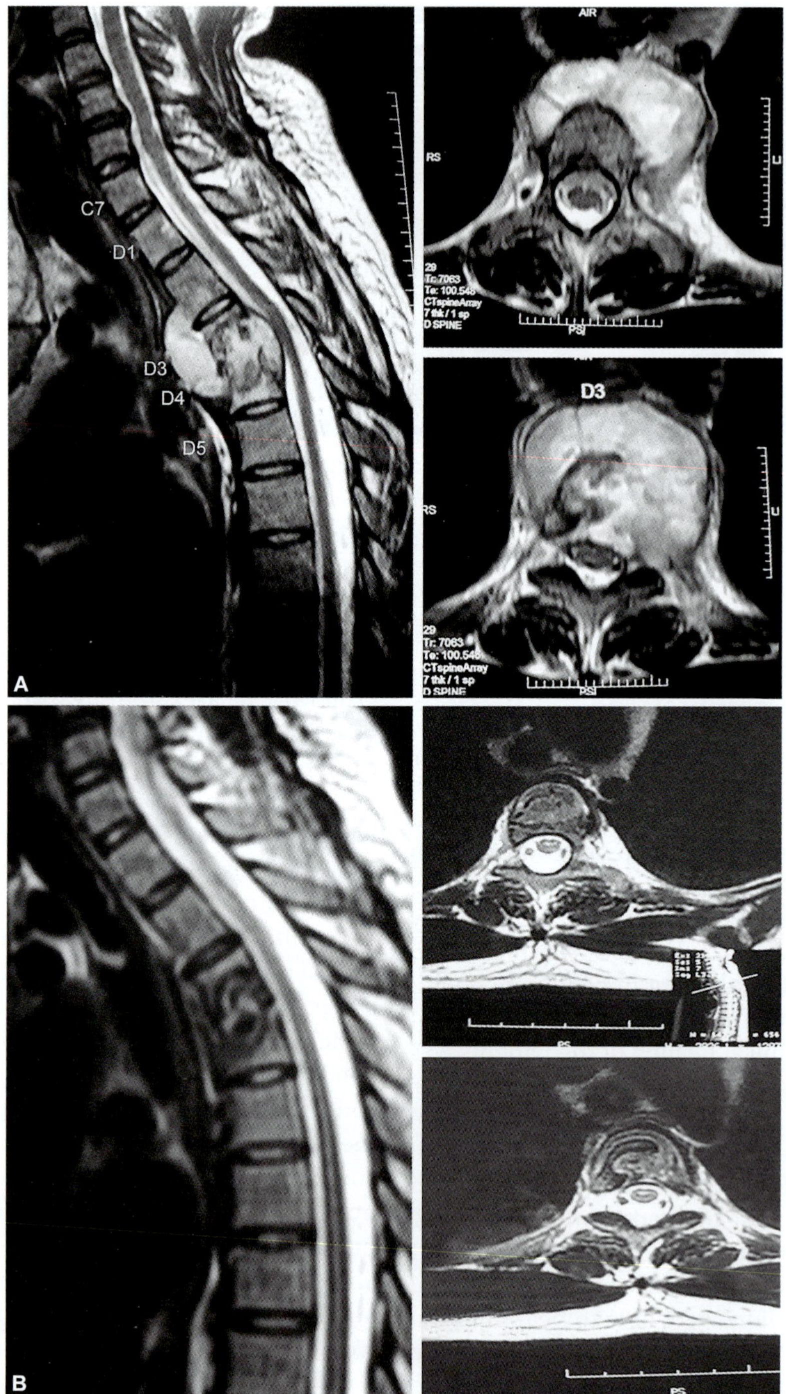

Figs. 23.20A and B: (A) MRIs showing a classical tuberculous lesion at presentation. Note the perivertebral abscess in the sagittal and axial views. (B) Shows complete healing of the osseous lesion and resolution of the paravetebral shadows after 12 months of antitubercular drugs without operation.

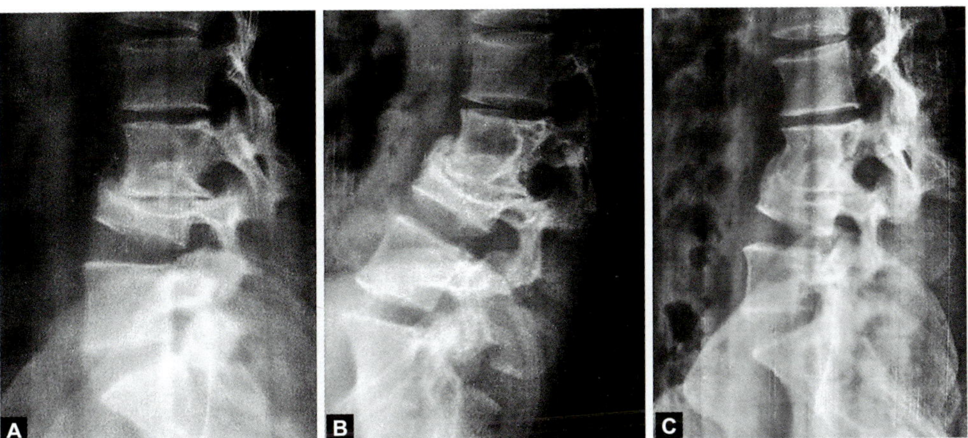

Figs. 23.21A to C: An adult was treated on domiciliary lines by autitubercular drugs and spinal brace. The disease at L3–L4 level healed by fibro-osseous tissue (A) which gradually converted into bony block during 3 years of follow up (B and C).

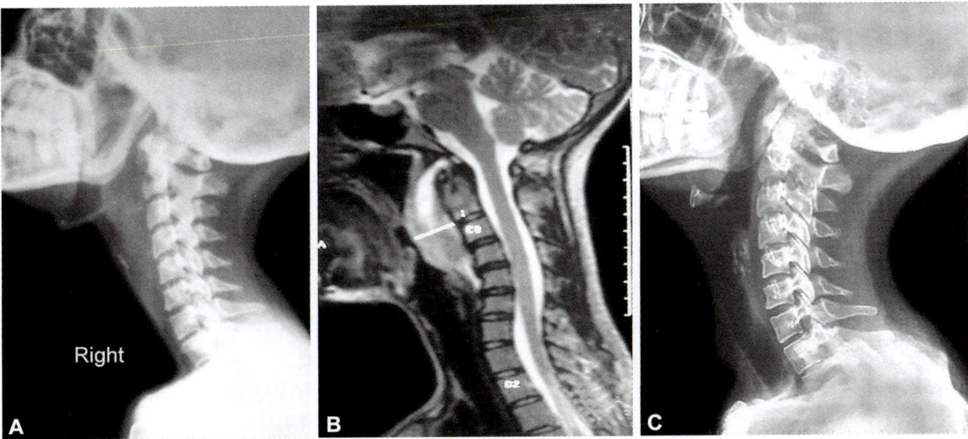

Figs. 23.22A to C: (A) X-rays of a young doctor showing destructive lesion of C1 and C2 with a prevertebral retopharyngeal soft tissue mass. (B) MRI of the same shows inflammatory changes in C1 and C2 with a soft tissue collection. The bright image in T2 sequence suggests fluid contents and the gray patchy shadows suggest fibrous and granulation tissue in the prevertebral mass. As the patient did not have any neural signs, or difficulty in deglutition and breathing, she was treated on domiciliary lines by SOMI bracing and multidrug therapy. Nine months after the therapy note complete resolution of the soft tissue mass and restitution of the destroyed bones. (C) No operation was performed.

Relapse or Recurrence or Complications

Assessment of exact statistics regarding the development of relapse/recurrence or complications of the disease is not possible in relation to a very long-term follow-up because these problems may occur at any period during the lifetime of a patient. Reactivation of the disease, recurrence of paraplegia or development of complications have been observed by us and many workers even during the era of antitubercular drugs as late as 20 years or more after healing (Martin 1970) irrespective of the primary treatment with or without operation.

One hundred eighty-one cases of tuberculosis of the spine, who had achieved clinical healing by following a middle path regime (between 1965 and 1974) could be followed-up by us for a period varying between 3 and 10 years. Two

Table 23.5: Comparison of clinical healing by various treatment modalities expressed as percentages.

Regime of treatment	***Mortality***	***Neural recovery***	***Clinical healing***
Orthodox pre-antimicrobial: Alvik (1949), Fellander (1955), Bakalim (1960), Kaplan (1959)	30–50	40–60	33–44
Conservative ambulatory (Dual Drug): Konstam and Blesovsky (1962) Dickson (1967) Prabhakar (1989)	5–15	60–70	83–90
Conservative nonambulatory (Triple drugs): Stevenson and Manning (1962) Friedman (1966)	0–10	60–80	93–96
Universal surgical extirpation: Hodgson and Wilkinson (1961) Stock (1962) Paus (1964) Prabhakar (1989)	0–10	75–80	80–96
Middle path: Roaf (1958) Tuli and Kumar (1971)	0–10	75–80	95

patients (treated earlier by surgery) reported with recurrence of paraplegia (one due to extradural granuloma and one due to severe kyphotic deformity); one child developed neurological complications apparently due to severe kyphotic deformity; 2 patients developed reactivation of the spinal lesion (one treated earlier by surgery and one had healed by drugs alone). One patient treated earlier by surgical debridement and bone grafting developed recrudescence of the vertebral lesion and died of generalized miliary tuberculosis probably because of resistant organisms. A higher incidence of relapse rate or development of other complications cannot be ruled out as some of such patients might not have reported to our institution for consultation. The cause of reactivation of the disease in spite of adequate treatment at the time of initial therapy appears to be lowered nutritional status, development of diabetes or compromised immune status, and/or resistant organisms.

The relapse rate reported by Somerville and Wilkinson (1965) and Paus (1964) was 12 and 11%, respectively of the healed cases. Kaplan (1959) reported 2% recurrence rate among 130 patients. In Konstam and Blesovsky's (1962) series, out of 207 patients only one had recurrence. The low rate of relapse is probably due to effective antitubercular drugs available these days. Yeager (1963) observed that prolonged use of "combined antimicrobial therapy has lowered the relapse rate to its lowest point in our history".

All recurrences and relapses with complications were treated by us by appropriate surgery (if needed) in conjunction with newer antitubercular drugs and supportive measures with very gratifying results.

Tuberculosis of the Cervical Spine

Between 1965 and 1982, 141 patients of cervical spine tuberculosis were treated in the orthopedic department of Banaras Hindu University. At the time of presentation half the patients showed a radiologically discernable increased prevertebral shadow. 34% (34 patients) had neural deficit.

A large majority (71%) was treated as outdoor patients. Only 43 patients were admitted because of neural deficit (34), or difficulty in deglutition (6), or for severe pain and deformity (3). Those admitted were put in cervical traction (3–8 weeks). Those treated in the outpatients were given rest to the neck using a four-post collar or Somi brace. All patients were given standard antitubercular drugs for about 18 months. Operations were performed for selective indications like: absence of spontaneous neural recovery (within 3–6 weeks), or failure of the control of activity of disease, or mechanical instability despite control of infection, or doubtful diagnosis. Of the 71 cases who had radiological prevertebral shadows, drainage was coincidental to decompression in 10 and to debridement in one; evacuation of abscess *per se* (for dysphagia) was required in 2. In the remaining 58, the "abscess shadows" gradually resolved within 6–12 months. Of the 34 patients with neural complications one died of moribund general condition (before surgery), and 22 recovered spontaneously (Tuli 1988). Surgical decompression through anterior approach, was done in 11 patients with neural complications, of which 9 recovered completely, one had partial recovery, one died of complications 4 days later. Amongst the classical paradiscal type of tuberculosis treated without surgery 70% healed by spontaneous bone block formation, and 30% healed by fibro-osseous replacement of the diseased area (as judged at 2 years of follow-up) without gross increase in the deformity **(Figs. 23.22 to 23.24)**. More recent studies report equally favorable outcome (Moon et al. 2007, Govender et al. 2007).

Despite the availability of MRI and CT scans a few patients of non-tuberculous pathologies may have images resembling tuberculous disease. In the period 1990–2000, we had one patient each where histological diagnosis turned out to be solitary metastasis, myeloma, lymphoma and chordoma **(Figs. 21.6 and 21.7)**.

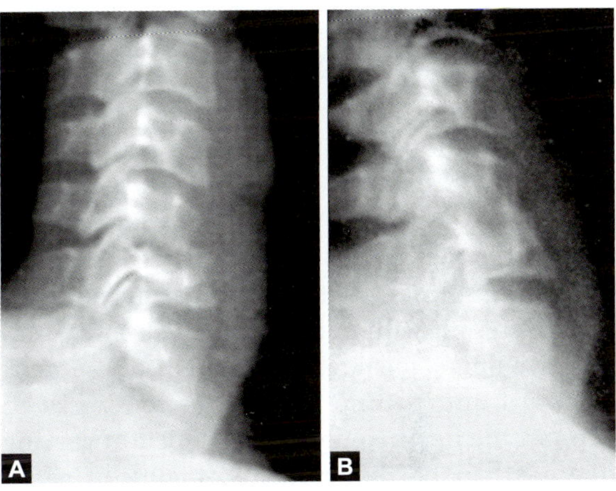

Figs. 23.23A and B: X-rays of a patient suffering from typical tuberculous disease of the cervical spine. Note marked diminution of the disc space, erosion of paradiscal margins, moderate degree of collapse of the vertebral bodies and localized prevertebral bulge of the soft tissues. The disease healed by a spontaneous bone block formation by domiciliary treatment using modern chemotherapy and four-post collar.

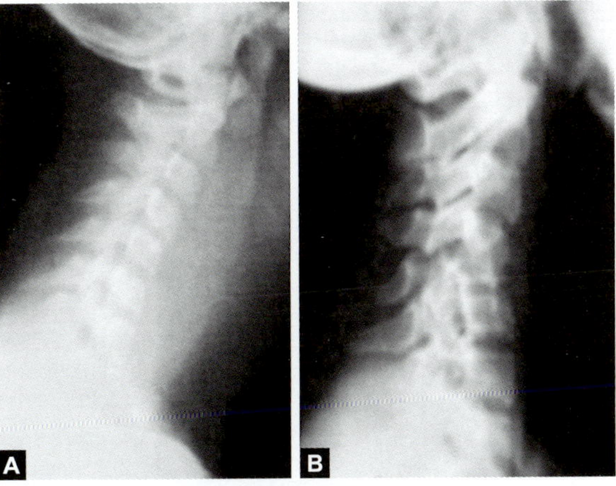

Figs. 23.24A and B: Tuberculosis of cervical spine C4–C6. At the time of presentation (A) there was a huge prevertebral soft tissue mass, diminution of the C4–C5 space, minimal changes in the texture of bone. The patient was treated on domiciliary lines by modern antitubercular chemotherapy and four-post collar. The result at the end of one year of treatment shows complete spontaneous resolution of the prevertebral shadow and healing by bone block formation between C4–C6 (B).

Tuberculosis of the Craniovertebral Region

Tuberculosis of the craniovertebral region is a rare localization **(Fig. 23.25)**. The incidence is probably < 1% of all cases of spinal tuberculosis (Tuli 1974). In general teaching hospitals in our country one can see 2–3 patients per year (Pandya 1971, Karapurkar 1988). Most of the patients would present with pain in the neck, limitation of movements, local tenderness, tilt of the neck (forward and to one side), and tendency to support the neck. Neurological deficit of varying degrees can be detected in 24–40% of cases at presentation (Tuli 1974, Karapurkar 1988, Lifeso 1987, Fang 1983). Radiologically, one can appreciate swelling in the retropharyngeal space, osteolytic erosions, and subluxation of atlantoaxial articulation. When osseous involvement occurs, earliest destruction takes place in the odontoid process. CT scan and MRI are the best modalities available now to observe the typical changes at the earliest stage of disease **(Figs. 20.25 to 20.29)**. In countries where tuberculous disease is common, it is rare for a nontuberculous pathology to produce the typical clinico-radiological picture (Lifeso 1987). At craniovertebral junction, the cervical cord is threatened by compression by tubercular abscess, granulation tissue or tubercular debris, atlantoaxial subluxation, upward translocation of odontoid, tubercular invasion of the cord or vascular ischemia due to local tuberculous pathology (Fang et al. 1983). Traction to the cervical spine (2–3 weeks) is one of the best methods to give rest to the part during the active stage of disease, when cord functions are threatened, and to reduce gross subluxation/dislocation (Tuli 1974, Chadha 2007). Under the cover of antitubercular drugs the disease gets healed, and a spontaneous stability is achieved within 3–6 months. About 2 months after treatment

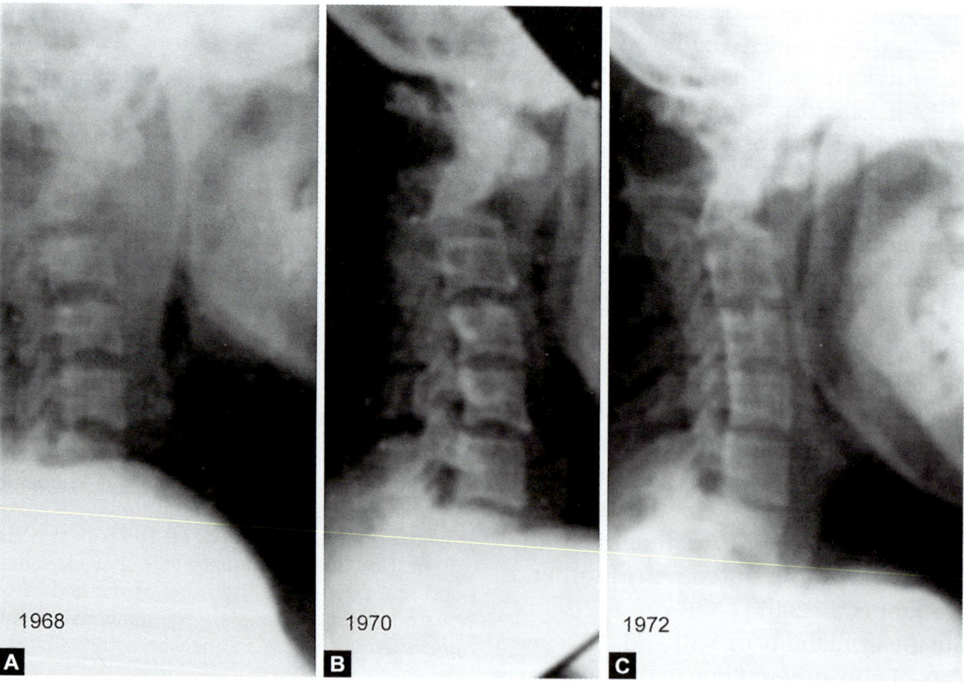

Figs. 23.25A to C: X-rays of a patient suffering from typical tuberculous disease of craniovertebral region. Note destruction of the anterior arches of C1 and C2, marked increase in the prevertebral soft tissue shadow and anterior subluxation of C1 over C2 (A-1968). The disease healed by treatment with skull traction, antitubercular drugs and four-post collar (B-1970, C-1972), note resolution of the prevertebral swelling, reconstitution of the destroyed bones and spontaneous stabilization of the subluxation.

in recumbent position, the patient should be encouraged mobilization with a four-post cervical collar or Somi brace. All normal activities, except head-loading, are permitted. In patients who do not recover the neural deficit, decompression is indicated. Those who do not undergo spontaneous stabilization of craniovertebral region as judged by lateral X-rays in flexion and extension done 3–6 months after the onset of treatment, require to be surgically fused. Whenever diagnosis is uncertain or the activity of the disease process or neural signs are not coming under control surgical exploration is warranted. Transoral approach is adequate for drainage of a prevertebral abscess or debridement of infected, soft and destroyed material (Wang 1981). Reposition of gross chronic displacement is not only impossible through this approach but may be even a dangerous exercise (Fang et al. 1983).

In case of doubt in diagnosis, and for assessment of extent of destruction in unstable cases CT scans and MRI studies are of significant help. If the craniovertebral region has been rendered mechanically unstable by the pathological process or by the anterior decompression, it is wise to achieve stability by posterior occipitocervical arthrodesis. The patient must be kept in skull traction or a halo device, or rest in recumbent position until posterior stabilization is sound. Depending upon the extent of anterior operation for cervical disease and the condition of patient, posterior arthrodesis may also be performed during the same operative session in one stage (from C1 to C7 level). To minimize the period of postoperative recumbency one may use metal implants to provide mechanical stability.

Tuberculosis of Sacrum and Coccyx

These are rare localization of tuberculous infection, probably < 1% of all spinal tuberculosis. Before general availability of MRI and CT scans for clinical use (prior to 1990), many such patients were suspected when abscesses, sinuses and ulcers had formed in the gluteal region or perianal area. Persistent pain in sacro-coccygeal region with local warmth and tenderness warrant investigations by modern imaging modalities.

When tuberculosis involves lower lumbar and sacral segments, tuberculous cold abscess may form anteriorly in the presacral space. Such abscesses were not demonstrable by conventional radiographs, however with the availability of CT scan and MRI images one can easily see varying sizes of abscesses from lumbosacral tuberculosis. When collection is large it may gravitate downwards in the presacral space **(Fig. 23.26)**. Occasionally, in neglected cases such large abscesses may point and drain spontaneously as chronic sinuses in the gluteal region or in perianal areas. If abscess is not subsiding by multidrug therapy or it is causing neural symptoms by pressure on the sacral nerves, it is prudent to establish dependent drainage.

As there is abundant loose areolar tissue in the presacral place, the cold abscess may gravitate towards the coccyx as a closed pyramidal pouch without attachment to the anterior surface of uninvolved sacral segments **(Fig. 23.26)**. Fourth and fifth sacral nerve roots may be sacrificed if needed during debridement of sacral disease, however, care must be taken not to damage the proximal three sacral nerves which contribute to form pudendal nerves.

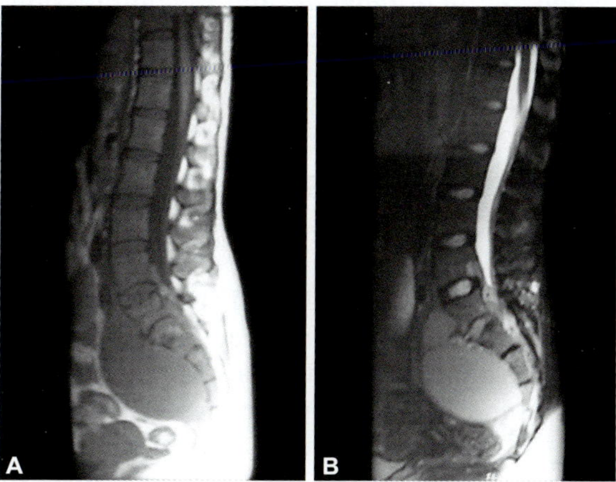

Figs. 23.26A and B: Presacral abscess as seen in the MRI, showing the fluid contents as (A) dark in T1, and (B) bright in T2 sequence. Osseous destruction is present at L5–S1.

CHAPTER 24

Operative Treatment

The effectiveness of currently available anti-TB drugs has obviated the need for surgical options in many cases. Following measures have been used successfully for treatment of spinal tuberculosis: Excision or debridement of diseased parts of the vertebrae, evacuation of a tuberculous abscess, arthrodesis of spine especially for mechanically unstable and painful spine and for prevention of severe kyphosis, and mechanical decompression of the cord for neural complications.

Any surgery on the vertebral column must ensure least disruption of the intact healthy columns. In the classical spondylodiscitis where the disease, destruction and compression is in the anterior columns, operation through anterior rout is the rational approach for debulking, debridement, and decompression; thus preserving the only biological stability the patient has, that is the posterior arch and ligament complex.

COLD ABSCESSES

Psoas Abscess

The palpable (peripheral) cold abscess if needed (failed aspiration) can be drained by standard surgical approaches. Iliopsoas abscess may be drained by anterior approach by making an 8–10 cm incision on the iliac crest one cm behind the anterior superior iliac spine. Cut external and internal obliquus abdominis muscles from the iliac crest and reach the inner surface of iliac bone. Palpate abscess and drain extraperitoneally. If the abscess (predominantly contained in psoas sheath) is pointing more posteriorly drain through the floor of the Petit's triangle. The floor is covered by obliquus internus abdominis muscle which requires to be incised (4–6 cm) between latissimus dorsi posteriorly, obliquus externus abdominis anteriorly and iliac crest inferiorly. Ludloff's approach is used for an abscess pointing on the medial side of thigh. Make a 2–3 cm incision distal to pubic tubercle longitudinally between gracilis and adductor longus muscle. Develop plane between adductor longus and brevis anteriorly, and the gracilis and adductor magnus posteriorly. Protect the posterior branch of obturator nerve and neurovascular bundle to gracilis. The abscess can be easily drained through the wound by developing a plane toward the lesser trochanter.

Cervical Spine Abscess

Cold abscess in the cervical spine is drained by making a transverse or longitudinal skin incision anterior or posterior to the sternocleidomastoid muscle depending upon the site of presentation of the abscess. It is wise to use suction drainage for nearly 72 hours after the surgery. If the size of the abscess is large (draining >300 mL in an adult), fluid must be replaced by intravenous route. Before making the incision it is wise to aspirate the swelling to exclude the possibility of an aneurysm or any other pathology.

SURGICAL APPROACHES

Treatment of tuberculous paraplegia is still controversial. Paraplegia of early onset associated with inflammatory causes is likely to recover in most of the cases, by antitubercular drugs alone. Paraplegia of late onset due to mechanical causes requires surgical decompression of the cord in majority. There are various approaches to different regions of the spine used by different workers **(Table 24.1)**.

Dorsal Spine

Anterolateral extrapleural approach as developed by Griffiths (1956), Seddon (1956) and Roaf (1959) has been used with some modifications by many workers (Arct 1968, Goel 1967, Kirkaldy-Willis 1965, Lagenskiold 1967, Paus 1964, Risko 1963, Tuli 1969, Wilkinson 1969, Korkusuz 1989, Jain et al. 2004, Wang 2016, Yang 2016, Gan 2024) for debridement of the diseased tissues, and for mechanical decompression of the cord, with or without bone grafting for achieving anterior spinal fusion. Most of the workers consider this approach as adequate for dorsal lesions. Transpleural anterior approach has been developed by Hodgson and Stock (1956, 1960) and used by many workers (Cauchoix 1957, Kirkaldy-Willis 1965, Kohli 1967, Masalawala 1963, Cook 1971, Jackson 1971) for tuberculous lesions of dorsal spine.

In treating active tuberculosis of the thoracic spine, Macrae (1957) (quoted by Cholmeley 1959) performed bilateral costectomy to evacuate any pus and then irrigated the area with streptomycin from each side through a catheter. Martin (1970, 1971) favored a "posterolateral approach" in which dura is exposed by hemilaminectomy first and then the operation is extended laterally to remove the posterior ends of 2–4 ribs, corresponding transverse processes and the pedicles. He considered the "anterolateral operation most difficult and tedious with risk of damage to the cord".

Indications for the choice of surgical approach to the dorsal spine are rather ambiguous. For example, Ahn (1968) recommended transpleural approach for long-standing cases and extrapleural anterolateral approach for early cases. On the other hand, Kirkaldy-Willis (1965) recommended transpleural approach for early cases and extrapleural anterolateral approach for chronic cases of long-standing. In fact, both these approaches provide adequate exposure for debridement or mechanical decompression and anterior bone grafting procedures. Both provide a good exposure of extradural space without further weakening of the vertebral column by removal of spinous processes and laminae as may happen in operations involving their removal. Transplural anterior spinal approach is, however, impracticable for operations on diseased vertebral bodies at the site of severe kyphotic deformities.

Cervical Spine

Cervical spine is best approached by anterior approach as developed by Smith and Robinson (1958, 1968). The involved region is explored by working between sternomastoid and carotid sheath laterally, and esophagus and trachea medially. The site may be localized under X-ray control. Similar approach has been successfully employed by Riley (1969) and others **(Table 24.1)**. Hodgson (1969) advocated an approach through the posterior triangle working by retracting sternomastoid, carotid sheath, trachea and esophagus anteriorly and to the opposite side.

Atlantoaxial Region

Fang and Ong (1962) developed transoral approach, and transthyrohyoid approach for such higher lesions. Operation is performed under anesthesia administered through tracheostomy tube. Hodgson et al. (1960, 1969) and Masalawala (1963, 1967) used similar approach successfully for this region. McAfee et al. (1987) developed a retropharyngeal extramucosal approach for cranio-atlantoaxial region.

Table 24.1: Main surgical approaches used by various workers in tuberculous lesions of different regions of vertebral column.

Workers	*C1–C2*	*Cervical*	*C7–D1*	*Dorsal*	*Dorsolumbar*	*Lumbar*	*L5–L1*
Cauchoix and Binet (1957)	—	Anterior	Trans-sternal anterior	Anterior transpleural decompression	—	—	—
Kirkaldy-Willis (1965)	—	Anterior	Transpleural through bed of 3rd rib	Anterolateral or transpleural	Anterolateral	Retroperitoneal sympathectomy or ureter approach	Transperitoneal, paramedian incision in Trendelenburg position
Hodgson et al. (1956,1960, 1969)	Transoral/ transthyroid like Fang and Ong (1962)	Through anterior triangle or through posterior triangle	Transpleural through bed of 3rd rib/split sternal for extensive lesion	Anterior transpleural decompression	Bed of 11th rib extrapleural extraperitoneal/left transpleural through bed of 9th rib	Renal approach	Transperitoneal in Trendelenburg position. Lower midline incision
Smith and Robinson, (1958), Riley (1969)	Anterior	Anterior	—	—	—	—	—
Lagenskiold and Riska (1967)	—	—	—	Anterolateral	Anterolateral	Anterolateral	—
Paus (1964)	—	Anterior	Anterior cervical	Anterolateral	Anterolateral	Retroperitoneal sympathectomy approach	Transperitoneal
Arct (1968)	—	—	—	Anterolateral	—	Retroperitoneal sympathectomy or ureter approach	Transperitoneal/ retroperitoneal of Harmon
Kemp et al. (1973)	—	Anterior	Anterior cervical	Trans-sternal for D3–D4. Anterior transpleural for D5–D12	Bed of 12th rib	Retroperitoneal approach	Retroperitoneal through oblique renal or "hemisection" incision
Tuli et al. (1969, 1975, 1979, 1988)	Transoral for drainage	Anterior	Low anterior cervical	Anterolateral or transpleural	Anterolateral	Transverse vertebrotomy retropsoas approach or retroperitoneal approach	Retropsoas transverse vertebrotomy or retroperitoneal

Cervicodorsal Region

Like atlantoaxial region cervicodorsal spine is also a difficult area to be exposed. Kirkaldy-Willis and Thomas (1965) used a transpleural thoracotomy approach through the bed of 3rd rib on left side. They also prescribed extrapleural anterolateral approach. Fang and Ong (1969) and Cauchoix and Binet (1957) described a technique for operation upon this region through an anterior, sternum splitting, extrapleural approach. Kemp et al. (1973) used trans-sternal approach for lesion at D3–D4. Robinson et al. (1962) and Paus (1964) approached this area through the anterior approach to the cervical spine. We have comfortably employed the anterior approach through a low cervical incision for lesions at C7–D1 (Tuli 1979). Lesions from C7–D2 have been debrided, debulked and decompressed by us through transverse low cervical approach with resection of upper border of manubrium sterni.

Thoracolumbar Region

It has been approached through extrapleural anterolateral exposure by Kirkaldy-Willis (1965), Paus (1964), Lagenskiold and Riska (1967). Hodgson et al. (1956–1969) described an extrapleural and extraperitoneal approach through the bed of 11th rib for this region.

Lumbar spine: It has been approached through a retroperitoneal approach (similar to kidney, ureter or sympathectomy exposure) by Arct (1968), and Hodgson et al. (1956, 1969), Kirkaldy-Willis (1965), Lagenskiold and Riska (1967), and Paus (1964).

Lumbosacral Region (L5–S1)

Kirkaldy-Willis (1965), Paus (1964), Arct (1968), Hodgson (1969) and Pun et al. (1990) described approaches through hypogastric paramedian transperitoneal approach. Trendelenburg position and extension of lumbosacral junction was found to be helpful in this exposure. Harmon (1963), Arct (1968) and Hodgson (1969) also described and used retroperitoneal approach. Lumbar and lumbosacral regions (L1–S1) have been approached by us through retroperitoneal sympathectomy approach, or through transperitoneal approach (for L5–S1 area). Since 1995 we prefer to use transverse vertebrotomy approach reflecting the psoas muscle anteriorly to reach the anterolateral surface of the lumbar vertebrae.

In general, junctional areas (craniovertebral, cervicodorsal, lumbosacral) are difficult for adequate exposures and no worker has an extensive experience of a particular approach. However, attention to the details of the technique described by various workers is helpful for satisfactory exposures. Opinion varies regarding the use of bone grafts after surgical debridement of the diseased vertebrae or after decompression of the spinal cord. Hodgson et al. (1956–1969) and Risko and Novosazel (1963) emphasized the use of bone graft after surgery. Many other surgeons consider it unnecessary in all cases. We feel that a common indication for use of bone grafts after excisional surgery of the diseased area are those cases where extensive excision leaves behind an unstable spine. The indications for bone grafting would become more selective if during debridement, debulking, and spinal cord decompression the surgeon does not remove the non-offending diseased or healthy bone. Whenever indicated we prefer posterior bone grafting for craniovertebral area, anterior grafting for cervical spine (C3–C6), posterior grafting for cervicodorsal junction (C6–D2) and anterior or posterior grafting for dorsal and lumbar spine. Main indications for surgery are summarized in **Table 23.2**.

OPERATIVE PROCEDURES

Excellent anesthesia, about 2–3 units of blood, surgical suction, cautery and experienced surgical team are essential prerequisites for these major procedures. Throughout the operative procedure the systolic blood pressure must never drop below 70 mm. During the preoperative period the patient, who has been lying paralyzed in bed for many weeks or months, is turned frequently and trained to lie on sides and in prone position in bed for 3–4 hours a day. He is taught deep breathing exercises and exercises for the limbs. Detailed description of certain common and useful procedures follows.

Approach to Atlanto-occipital and Atlantoaxial Region

It is difficult to approach the atlantoaxial joints from the side of the neck as numerous structures get in the way, such as the mandible, parotid salivary gland, internal carotid artery and vein and cranial nerves, while there is hardly any anatomy overlying these joints anteriorly, transoral of approach **(Fig. 24.1)** was adopted by Fang and Ong (1962).

The patient is positioned supine with head in 5–10 degrees hyperextension on a headrest. A preliminary tracheostomy is performed after induction of anesthesia, and a mouth gag of the Boyle-Davies type is inserted. The soft palate is folded back on itself and stitched so as to give adequate exposure. The uvula and soft palate may be bisected in the sagittal plane to improve the exposure or to permit visualization of the atlanto-occipital joint. The hypopharynx is packed and the posterior pharyngeal wall is palpated to locate the anterior tubercle of the atlas. An incision about 5 cm long is made along the median raphe with its center about 1 cm below the anterior tubercle. It should not extend too low down because subsequent closure will have to be carried out blindly. The incision is made down to bone and flaps are raised by blunt dissection to just short of the outer border of the lateral masses; to go beyond endangers the vertebral vessels. If these vessels are damaged, gelfoam (spongiostan) is used to control the bleeding. Dissection in this region is relatively avascular, though in children abundant lymphoid tissue may cause more oozing. In long-standing atlantoaxial subluxation or dislocation, dense scar tissue is encountered akin to that found in spondylolisthesis in the lumbosacral region.

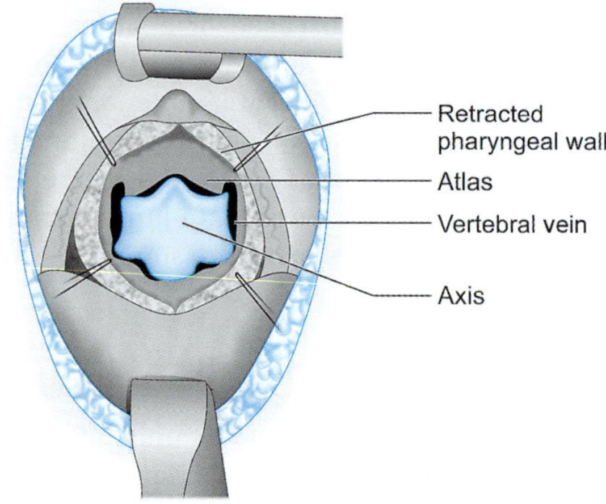

Fig. 24.1: Transoral anterior approach to atlantoaxial and atlanto-occipital regions.

Long stay sutures are used to retract the soft tissue flaps, thus exposing the underlying anterior arch of the atlas, the body of the axis and the atlantoaxial joints on each side **(Fig. 24.1)**. The diseased area is thus exposed and debrided. If a dislocation or subluxation is found the anterior part of the lateral masses of the atlas are gently levered back into place. If reduction is not possible with gentle force, as may happen in long-standing dislocations, fusion may be performed in the subluxated or dislocated position. To fuse the atlantoaxial joints, slots are made vertically across them, more medially than laterally to safeguard the vertebral vessels, and autogenous iliac grafts are inserted. The soft tissue flaps of the posterior pharyngeal wall are closed in layers successively as anterior longitudinal ligament, buccopharyngeal fascia, constrictor muscles and pharyngeal mucosa. Transoral debridement for reduction of pathological subluxation or dislocation is a major procedure and has a failure rate of 50% (Jain et al. 2000, 2002). Postoperative skull traction for 3–4 weeks would help stabilization of the fusion mass. If one is impelled for anterior bone grafting the patient should be managed by highly specialized surgeons. We have used the transoral approach to drain the prevertebral collection and debridement in a few patients.

Postoperative Management

The patient is given intravenous fluids for 1–2 days followed by a fluid diet until the pharyngeal wound is well-healed. The tracheostomy tube is left in place until bronchial secretions are reduced to normal amounts, usually for 7–10 days. It is a routine to keep patients on antibiotics to prevent wound infection. Patients are nursed in cervical traction (3–4 weeks) or on the plaster shell in children, and are kept in suitable cervical orthosis with limited activities until there is evidence of bony consolidation, which takes about 3 months. If the craniovertebral region does not become stable in about 3 months after anterior debridement with or without bone grafting, a posterior spinal fusion is indicated. Lateral view in flexion and extension would give a satisfactory assessment regarding mechanical stability. If the excursion between the dens and anterior arch of atlas is >3 mm, the craniovertebral region is considered unstable and warrants posterior spinal fusion (Tuli 1974, Jain 2000).

Anterior Retropharyngeal Approach to the Upper Part of the Cervical Spine (Clivus to Cervical-3, McAfee et al. 1987)

Upward extension of Smith-Robinson's anterior approach to the cervical spine has been developed at the Johns Hopkins Hospital, Baltimore (McAfee et al. 1987). This is in contrast to the commonly used transmucosal/transoral approaches to the atlas and axis *(vide supra)* where postoperative infection from the mucosal cavities is not uncommon.The extramucosal cranial extension is through the same fascial planes that are utilized in the standard anterior cervical approach. This approach is recommended only for an experienced surgeon who is thoroughly familiar with the anatomy and the fascial planes that are encountered/traversed during the standard anterior approach to the cervical spine. The maximum loss of blood in this approach has been calculated to be 1,200 mL. The approach to the upper part of cervical spine is recommended through the right side of the patient if the surgeon is right-handed. This is in contrast to the anterior approach to the cervical spine (cervical-3 to dorsal-1) which is as a rule performed from the left side of the patient as there is less chance of damage to the left recurrent laryngeal nerve.

The relevant fascial planes of the neck (which are continuous circumferentially) consist of: (1) The superficial fascia containing the platysma; (2) The superficial layer of the deep fascia surrounding both the sternomastoid muscles; (3) The middle layer of the deep fascia that encloses the omohyoid, sternohyoid, sternothyroid, and thyrohyoid muscles and the visceral fascia enclosing the trachea, esophagus, and recurrent nerves; and (4) The deep layer of the deep cervical fascia, which is divided into the alar fascia connecting the two carotid sheaths and fused midline to the visceral fascia, and the prevertebral fascia covering the longus colli and scalene muscles.

The operation must be performed (like other operations on cervical spine) with the skull traction on with 3–4 kg. With the patient awake, the neck is carefully extended by an active assisted movement as far as possible without precipitation or exaggeration of neurological symptoms. This position is designated as the maximum allowable position of extension of the neck, and it must not be exceeded at any time during the operative procedure.

A transverse submandibular incision is made from the symphysis menti to the tip of mastoid process. A vertical limb is extended from its middle only as far distally as is needed depending upon the requirement of the extent of the exposure.

The submandibular incision is made through the platysma muscle, and the superficial fascia and skin are mobilized in the subplatysmal plane of the superficial fascia. The marginal mandibular branch of the facial nerve is found with the aid of a nerve-stimulator after ligating and dissecting the retromandibular veins superiorly **(Fig. 24.2)**. The common facial vein is continuous with the retromandibular vein, and the branches of the mandibular nerve usually cross the latter vein superficially and superiorly. Ligate the retromandibular vein as it joins the internal jugular vein and keep the dissection deep and inferior to the vein. As the exposure is extended superiorly to the mandible, the superficial branches of the facial nerve are protected.

The anterior border of the sternocleidomastoid muscle is mobilized by longitudinally transecting the superficial layer of deep cervical fascia. This allows localization of the carotid sheath by palpation of the carotid arterial pulse. The submandibular salivary gland is resected, with care taken to suture its duct in order to prevent a salivary fistula. The jugular-digastric lymph nodes from the submandibular and carotid triangles can be resected and sent for histology. The posterior belly of the digastric muscle and the stylohyoid muscle are identified, and the digastric tendon is divided and tagged for later repair. Superior retraction at the base of the origin of the stylohyoid muscle can cause injury to the facial nerve as it exists from the skull. Division of the digastric and stylohyoid muscles allows mobilization of the hyoid bone and the hypopharynx to the opposite side. This maneuver helps to avoid exposure and opening of the nasopharynx, hypopharynx, and esophagus, which are considered to be contaminated with a high concentration of anaerobic bacteria.

The hypoglossal nerve, which is identified with a nerve-stimulator, is then completely mobilized from the base of the skull to the anterior border of the hypoglossal muscle; it is retracted superiorly throughout the remainder of the procedure **(Figs. 24.2 and 24.3)**.

The dissection then proceeds to the retropharyngeal space, between the contents of the carotid sheath laterally and the larynx and pharynx anteromedially. Superior exposure is facilitated by ligating the tethering branches of the carotid artery and internal jugular vein. Beginning inferiorly and progressing superiorly, ligation of the superior thyroid artery and vein, lingual artery and vein, ascending pharyngeal artery and vein, and facial artery and vein will help to mobilize the carotid sheath laterally. The superior laryngeal nerve, also identified with the help of a nerve-stimulator, is mobilized from its origin near the nodose ganglion to its entrance into the larynx **(Fig. 24.3)**.

The alar and prevertebral fasciae are transected longitudinally to expose the longus colli

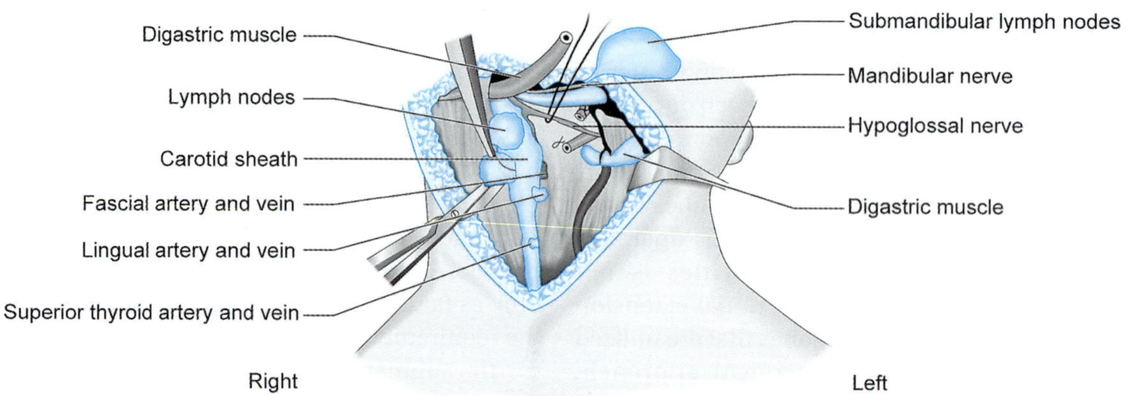

Fig. 24.2: Diagrammatic representation of retropharyngeal approach to the clivo-atlantoaxial region. Important structures after transecting the middle layer of deep fascia are exposed.

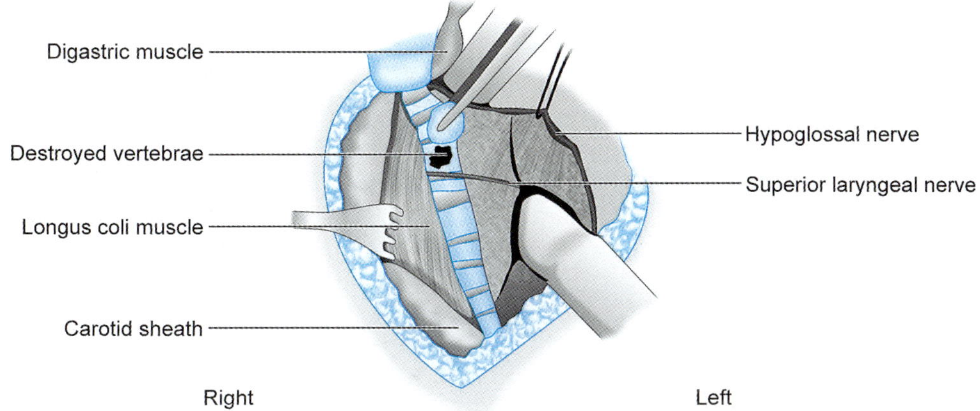

Fig. 24.3: Exposure of the important structures after cutting and retracting the prevertebral fascia and anterior longitudinal ligament.

muscles, which run longitudinally. It is very important at this point for the surgeon to gain orientation to the midline by noting the attachment of the left and right longus colli muscles as they converge toward the anterior tubercle of the atlas. The amount of rotation of the head away from the midline is gauged by palpating the mental protuberance of the mandible. Any rotation of the head is undesirable if the arthrodesis involves the anterior arch of the atlas, as it usually does. The surgeon's orientation regarding the midline of the cervical spine is maintained as the longus colli muscles are detached from the anterior surface of the atlas and axis. It is essential to maintain this orientation throughout the anterior decompression of the spinal cord so that the decompression may be carried far enough laterally to decompress the spinal cord but not so far laterally as to endanger the vertebral arteries. The anterior atlanto-occipital membrane is not disturbed but the anterior longitudinal ligament and part of vertebral bodies may be removed if necessary for visualization of the cord.

The anterior decompression is usually initiated by thoroughly removing the intervertebral disc between the second and third cervical vertebrae or the first normal disc at the caudad edge of the lesion **(Fig. 24.3)**. Visualization of the uncovertebral joints between these vertebrae helps to confirm the orientation of the midline, and the discectomy provides visualization of the posterior longitudinal ligament with minimum loss of blood. If a second cervical corpectomy is required, it is done with a high-speed burr.

In patients who do not have cranial settling due to basilar invagination of the odontoid process, the odontoid process can be retained to help to lock in the superior aspect of the strut graft. A fibular or tricortical iliac strut graft is fashioned into the shape of a clothespin. The two prongs of the clothespin are placed superiorly to straddle the anterior arch of the atlas. The inferior edge of the graft is tamped into the superior aspect of the body of the third cervical vertebra, which is undercut to receive the graft, thus helping to obtain stability. Closure is begun by reapproximation of the digastric tendon. Suction drains are placed in the retropharyngeal space and in the subcutaneous space. The platysma and skin are sutured in the standard fashion. We have no personal experience of using this technique.

Anterior Approach to the Cervical Spine

The C2–D1 **(Figs. 24.4 to 24.8)** cervical spine is best approached by anterior approach. If several vertebral bodies are to be exposed, a slightly oblique incision following the anterior/medial border of the sternocleidomastoid muscle may

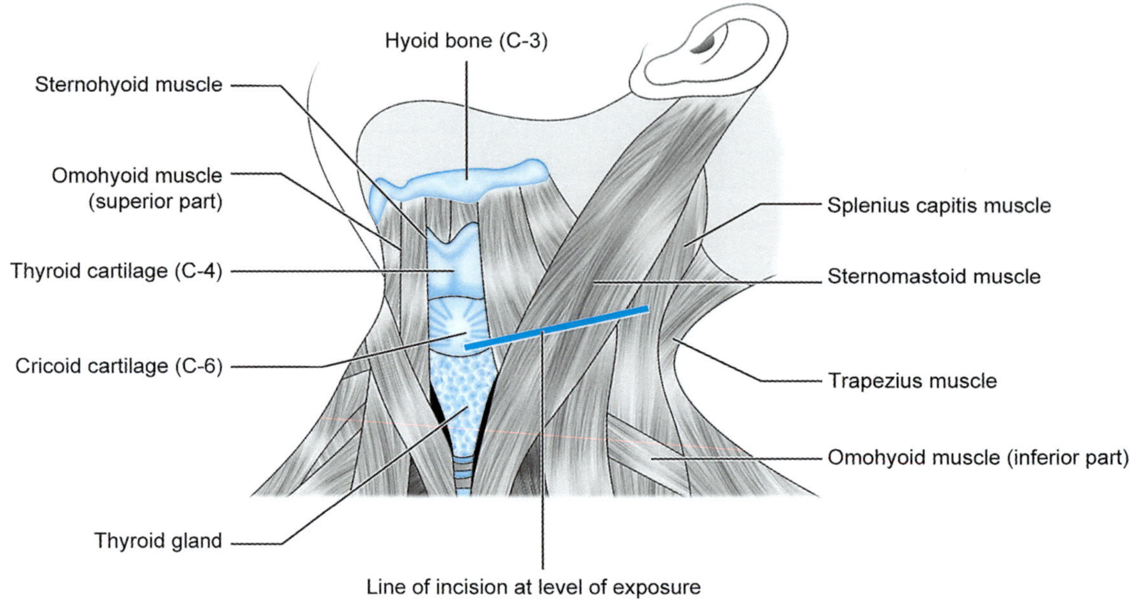

Fig. 24.4: Anterior approach to cervical spine.

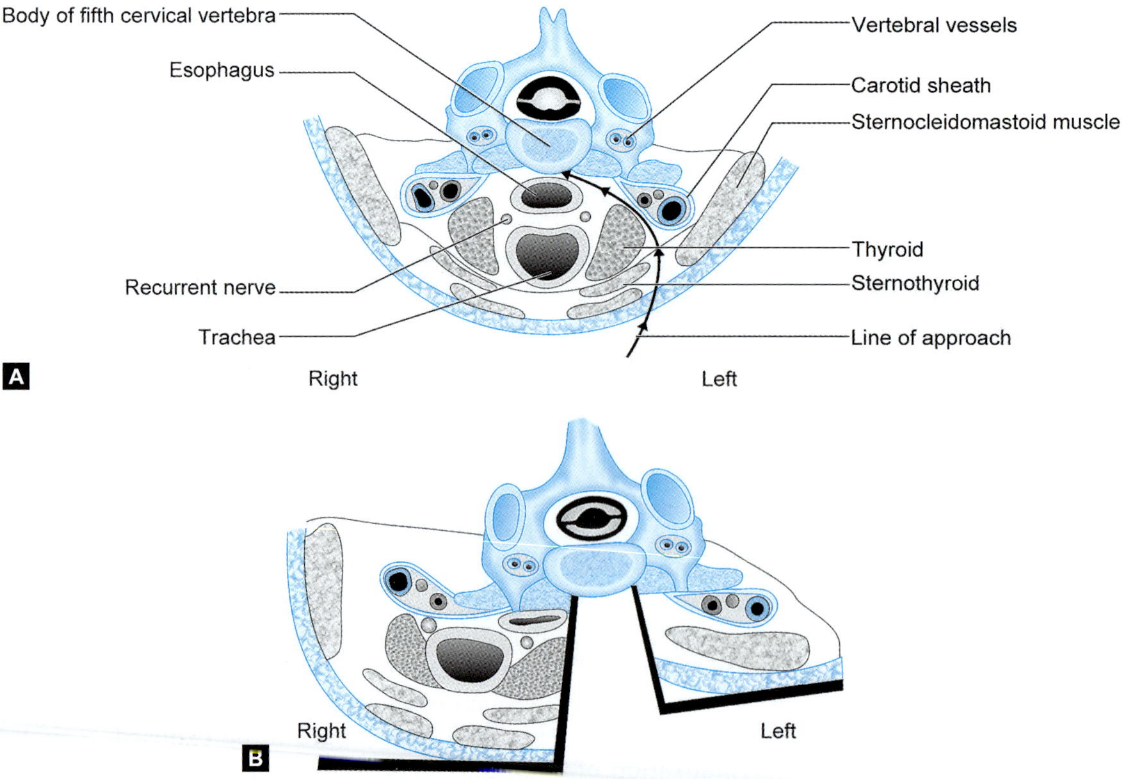

Figs. 24.5A and B: (A) Anterior approach to cervical spine, (B) Tissues retracted exposing fifth cervical vertebra.

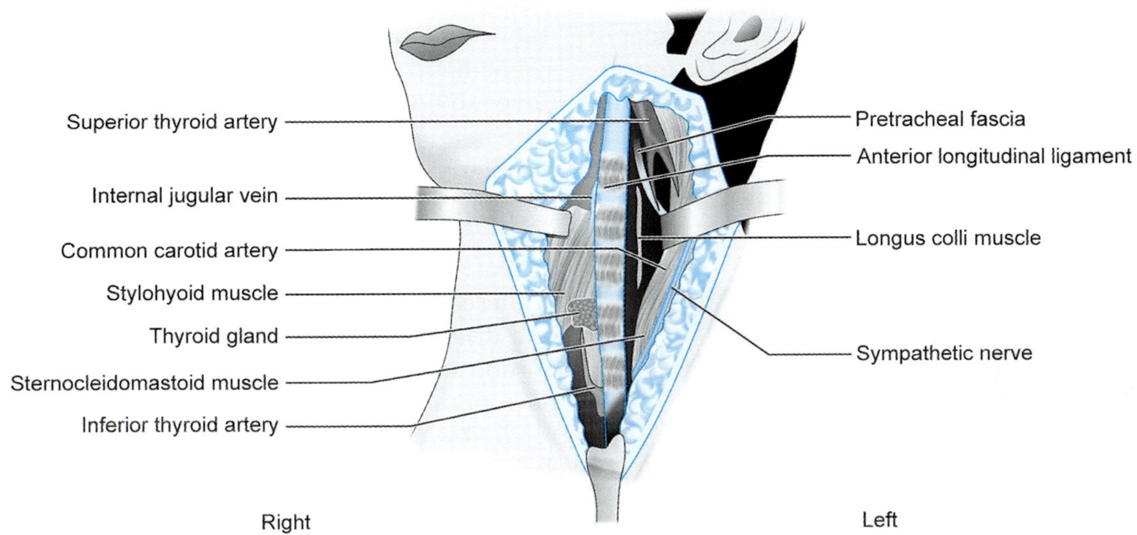

Fig. 24.6: Tissues retracted exposing cervical vertebrae.

be used. If only one or 2 vertebral bodies are to be exposed a short transverse incision at the appropriate level should be used. In cases with neurological involvement it is advocated to operate with about 3–6 kg of traction through skull tongs. Patient is kept supine with a low sand-bag in between the scapulae. It is preferable to work from the left side because there is less chance of injury to the recurrent laryngeal nerve. The recurrent nerve arises from the vagus at the level of the subclavian artery on the right and recurs below the subclavian artery and ascends between trachea and esophagus. The left recurrent nerve arises at the level of aortic arch and recurs around the arch to ascend in a like manner as on the right. Damage to the recurrent nerve may be caused by excessive retraction during anterior approach. This is less likely to happen with the left-sided approach as the left nerve, because of its longer vertical course, can tolerate retraction better.

A transverse skin incision is made at the level of the vertebrae to be operated, beginning the incision at the midline and extending it laterally for about 7–10 cm well over the belly of the sternocleidomastoid muscle. The skin and platysma are cut transversely in the same line. Then by blunt dissection or by gauze covered finger a gap is developed between the sternomastoid and carotid sheath laterally, and esophagus and trachea medially **(Figs. 24.4 to 24.8)**. Anterior surface of the cervical bodies are now visualized by retraction of esophagus, trachea/larynx, recurrent laryngeal nerve, thyroid gland, and the strap muscles toward the right side, and displacing the carotid sheath with its contents and sternomastoid muscle toward the left. The area to be operated must be confirmed by a lateral X-ray of the cervical spine with a shouldered drill point inserted into/near the suspected disc space. Thyroid arteries and veins, especially the middle vein, when present may need ligation if they come in the way. A longitudinal cut is made in the anterior longitudinal ligament in the midline of the exposed vertebral bodies. The longitudinal incision may open a perivertebral abscess, or the diseased vertebrae may be exposed by reflecting the anterior longitudinal ligament and the longus colli muscles. The sympathetic chain lies between the bodies and the transverse processes on the longus colli muscle fibers and should be protected. Tuberculous abscess and the diseased vertebrae are dealt with as required. Wound is closed over a suction drain after complete hemostasis. The most extensive decompression and arthrodesis for tuberculous quadriplegia which we performed were from lower border of C3 to upper border of C6 **(Fig. 24.8)**. Postoperatively, the patient is nursed with raised head end of the bed and maintenance of skull traction with 3–6 kg of weight for 2–3 weeks. Complications which may be associated with this operation are hematoma formation; injury to esophagus, trachea, dura, recurrent nerve, vagus nerve, sympathetic chain and vertebral artery. Careful dissection and attention to the details help to prevent them. Of the early 12 patients of cervical tuberculosis operated by us, one developed esophageal fistula which healed by the use of feeding tube and improvement in nutrition of the patient.

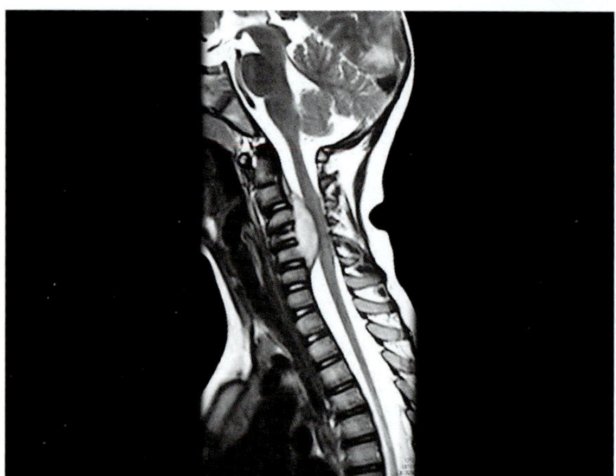

Fig. 24.7: While operating upon a case of tetraplegia it is mandatory to expose the posterior longitudinal ligament on the anterior surface of dura mater. The MRI picture shows the offending inflammatory tissues posterior to the destroyed and distorted segment of cervical spine.

Resection of one vertebral body or resection of a disc with paradiscal half of two vertebrae do not need any bone grafts or implants. The postoperative defect undergoes spontaneous repair by osseous or fibro-osseous tissue in 3–4 months. If the decompression entailed a segment longer than two vertebral bodies, it is wise to insert a strut bone graft fitted into the undercut proximal and distal bones. One may rarely supplement the graft with a buttress plate **(Fig. 24.8)**.

Transthoracic Transpleural Approach for Spine D1–L1

The chest is usually opened on the left side **(Fig. 24.9)** where it is easier to handle aorta. On the right side, the inferior vena cava being more

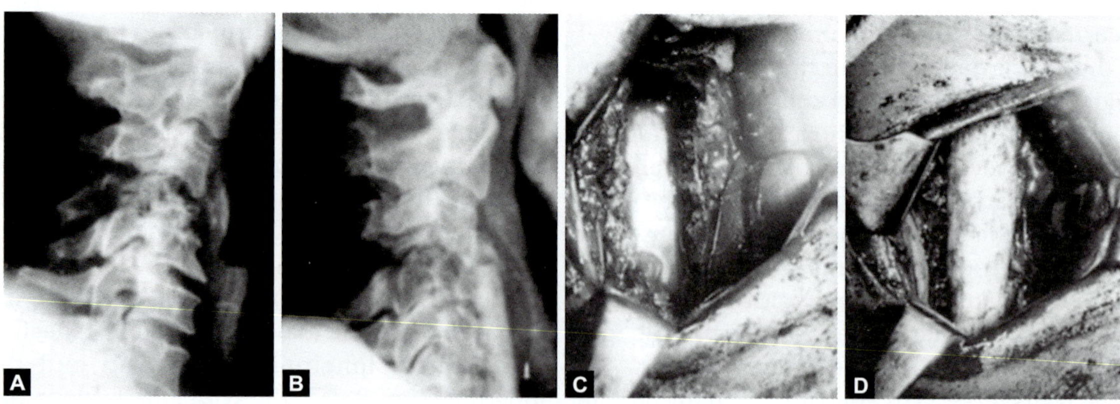

Figs. 24.8A to D: Lateral X-ray of cervical spine showing advanced tuberculous disease involving C3–C5 (A). There is gross destruction of C4 body and its disc spaces. Because the patient presented with quadriplegia of long-standing, decompression of the cord and bone grafting was performed through the anterior approach. Note the bone graft extending downwards from the distal border of C3 vertebral body (B). (C and D) Peroperative photograph of the same patient as shown in A and B. After removal of the diseased and offending vertebrae, discs, sequestra, inflammatory tissues and posterior longitudinal ligaments, one can see the cervical cord covered by dura (C-left). The gap created has been bridged by a snuggly fitting bone graft (D-right). Currently, we do not excise the posterior longitudinal ligament unless it is calcified or there is significant collection posterior to the posterior longitudinal ligament.

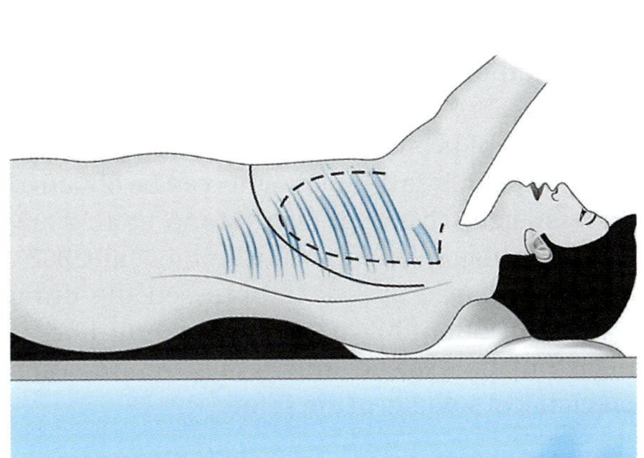

Fig. 24.9: Incision and position for transthoracic anterior approach: For left thoracotomy approach the patient is placed in right lateral position.

delicate is liable to be damaged while exposing the vertebral bodies. One may approach through the right thoracotomy where X-rays show an unusually large abscess on the right side with little or negligible bulge on the left side, or when left thoracotomy is difficult because of pulmonary complications, or prior operation.

For the left thoracotomy approach the patient is placed in the right lateral position and the surgeon stands on the dorsal side of the patient. An incision is made along the rib which in the mid-axillary line, lies opposite the center of the lesion. This is usually 2 ribs higher than the center of the vertebral lesion.

In patients with severe kyphosis, operative view is better if a rib is removed along the line of incision and a sand-bag or a bridge is used under the involved vertebrae to spread the ribs apart. When the lesion is situated at cervicodorsal region the highest rib that should be removed is the second rib. A J-shaped parascapular incision is required for lesions from C_7 to D_8 so that the scapula can be lifted off the chest wall and the appropriate rib can be selected for opening the chest. The muscles and the periosteum are cut over the selected rib from the costochondral junction to the posterior part of the rib. The selected rib is resected subperiosteally. In the bed of the rib, a small incision is made in the parietal pleura, in the absence of adhesions the lung falls away from the parieties. However, when adhesions are present, by gentle blunt dissection the parietal and visceral pleura are separated. Through the incision in the bed of the rib, index and middle fingers are introduced in the pleural cavity (which also help identifying the underlying adhesions), the opening is extended by cutting the parietal pleura with the help of scissors cutting over these fingers, and the wound edges are retracted by a self-retaining retractor. The lung is freed from the parieties as completely as possible. There may be adhesions between paravertebral abscess and the lung and/or aorta. Thick adhesions require cutting with cautery and careful hemostasis. Having freed the lung, it is retracted anteriorly displaying the aorta and any paravertebral bulge or the diseased area of the vertebral column **(Fig. 24.10)**. A plane is to be developed now between the descending aorta and the paravertebral abscess/diseased vertebral bodies. For this intercostal vessels and branches of hemiazygos veins opposite the site of disease have to be identified through the parietal pleura, dissected and cut between two ligatures. Now mobilize the aorta for displacement forward and to the right by making a longitudinal incision in the parietal pleura lateral to the aorta between the two ligatures. Use blunt dissection to retract the aorta and the contents of the mediastinum to the right and anteriorly. Opposite to D5–D10 vertebral bodies, the whole of (descending) aorta, (after cutting the intercostal arteries between two ligatures), cannot only be reflected to the right side with the help of spatulas but also lifted up on two loops. This permits extensive space to work on the front and left surface of vertebral bodies, and discs. In the presence of a severe kyphotic deformity, one is obliged to work in the depth of a depression—a very tedious job.

If a paravertebral abscess is present, it is opened by a T-shaped incision with the vertical limb of the T placed horizontally at the center of the diseased bodies and the horizontal limb of the T placed vertically medial to the lateral parts of the divided intercostal vessels. Two triangular flaps are then raised and retracted to expose the

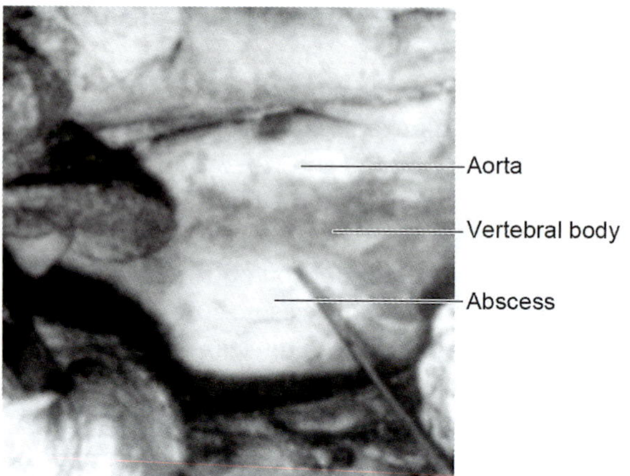

Fig. 24.10: Peroperative photograph while performing transthoracic transpleural anterior decompression at mid-dorsal level. Paravertebral abscess is clearly visible (shown by the black pointer), vertebral column and aorta are seen more anteriorly.

diseased vertebral bodies. The diseased area is then dealt as required by performing debridement or decompression with or without bone grafting. If one is operating for neurological complications, it is mandatory to expose the dural tube to the full extent of compressed area. An intercostal catheter is inserted through a small stab incision in the seventh or eighth intercostal space in the mid-axillary line and is connected to an underwater seal for 2 or 3 days. Chest is closed in layers. Govender (2001, 2002) reported the use of radical anterior debridement, and decompression for 41 patients with neurologic involvement. He stabilized the spine by allografts composited with autogenous rib (harvested during the operative procedure) and a single rod two screws construct. He felt that use of ribs alone did not give good results because of its unfavorable length-width ratio and a small surface area of contact with the adjacent recipient area of vertebral bodies. Earliest evidence of fusion and remodeling in adults was between 12 and 18 months, postoperatively.

Chen et al. (2002) reported their experience of treating 32 consecutive patients with a 2-stage surgical technique: Anterior debridement with anterior strut bone graft and in second stage (done around 11 days after the first) operation included posterior instrumentation with autogenous bone grafting. The overall results obtained by the authors were solid fusion in 97% (between 2 to 10 years), neurological recovery in 80% and correction of kyphotic angle by 17.3 degrees. We find that equally favorable results can be obtained by less aggressive approach (Moon et al. 2002, Jain 2002, Rajasekaran 2002, Bhojraj et al. 2002). Having exposed and decompressed the dural tube, non-offending parts of vertebral bodies need not be excised, this would retain some mechanical stability of the spine.

Anterolateral Decompression (D2–L1)

For the operation of anterolateral decompression the prone position has been described by Griffiths (1956), Seddon (1956) and Roaf (1959). We have been using the right lateral position (from 1964 to 2002 in >1,000 cases of tuberculous disease of the spine) and it has been found that lateral position avoids any venous congestion and excessive bleeding, and permits freer respiration; one can have a better look at the site of the lesion, and the lung and mediastinal contents easily fall anteriorly. We have been mostly approaching the spine from the left side.

Right-sided approach in the left lateral position was used in patients who required a reoperation because the first decompression from the left side was considered mechanically inadequate (26 patients), or having recovered from first decompression from the left side the patients reported back after a few years with recrudescence of the disease and neural deficit (four patients), or in patients (two cases) where the paravertebral shadow was exceptionally large on the right side, or in one patient who had situs inversus.

The site of decompression is as a rule satisfactorily localized from the standard anteroposterior and lateral X-rays. In patients who had more than one lesion and correlation of the neural deficit with a particular diseased area was not possible, descending and ascending myelograms were done to identify the offending

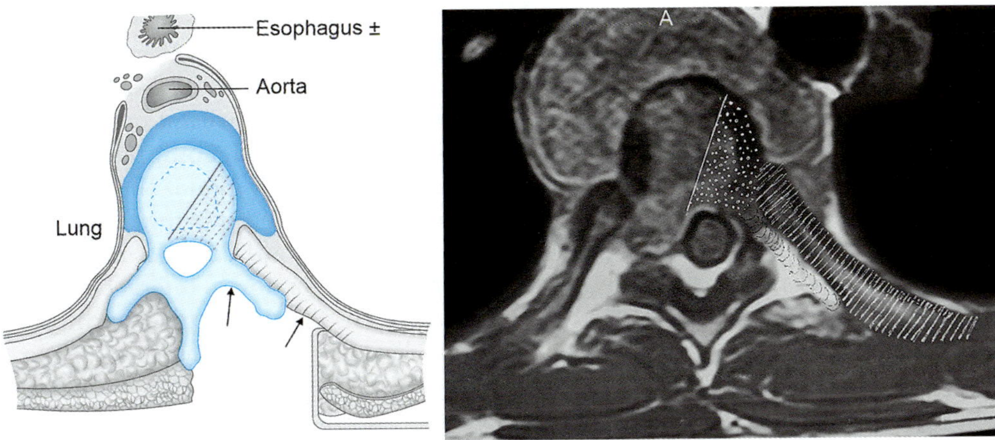

Fig. 24.11A: Diagram showing the classical anterolateral, extra plural approach to decompress the dural tube: Remove transverse process, underlying ribs and reach the diseased vertebral bodies.

site. Availability of MRIs and CT scans have eliminated the use of myelograms. The ribs articulating with the diseased vertebrae serve as the guide to the placement of the incision. Ribs are best identified by counting from below. For high dorsal lesions counting from first rib is more convenient. Resection of first rib is not advised.

A semicircular incision (convex laterally) is made starting from the midline about 6 cm proximal to the center of the diseased area, it is curved distally and laterally to a point about 9 cm from the midline and continues distally and medially to the midline about 6 cm distal to the center **(Fig. 24.11)**. The skin flap along with the deep fascia is elevated and retracted medially up to the midline; elevation of the flap along with the deep fascia minimizes the bleeding from the superficial fascia. The paraspinal muscles of the back are divided transversely starting from its lateral border coming up to the bases of the transverse processes of the diseased vertebrae. Medial parts of 2–4 ribs, which are articulating with the diseased vertebrae, and their transverse processes are exposed subperiosteally. Subperiosteal exposure of ribs is facilitated by separating the attachment of intercostal muscles and the periosteum by working from medial to lateral direction at the upper border of ribs, and lateral to medial direction at the lower border of ribs. This way one is working in the acute angle of attachment of the intercostal muscles.

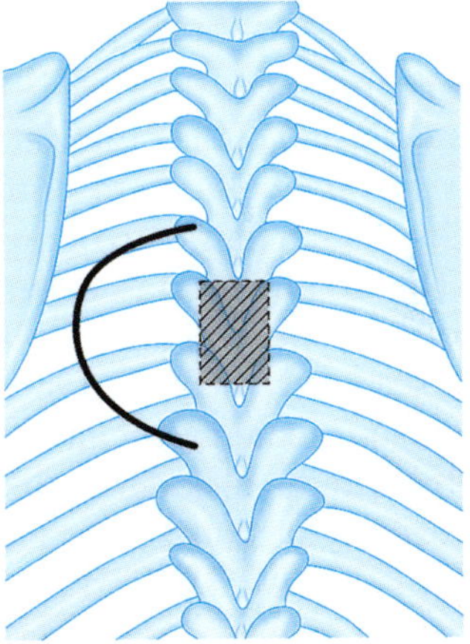

Fig. 24.11B: Incision for costotransversectomy and for anterolateral decompression.

A small curved gouge (Capner's type) is very useful for separating the transverse processes from the vertebral end of the ribs. The subperiosteally exposed transverse processes are resected from their base first. Two to four ribs, about 8 cm from the transverse processes are cut with a bone cutting forceps or a rib shear after completely freeing it subperiosteally. Curved gouge is gently pushed medially all around the rib up to its articulation with the vertebral column. The rib now is held from its lateral free end and is gently rotated and priced out subperiosteally till it is completely detached. Curved gouge, cutting cautery and sequestrum/bone holding forceps are very helpful in separating the medial end of the ribs from the vertebral column. Sometimes the rib breaks near its medial attachment when the remaining part may be removed with the help of a bone nibbler or a Cocker's forceps. If there is a paravertebral abscess it has already lifted up the periosteum and the anterior longitudinal ligament from the anterior and lateral surfaces of vertebral bodies and discs. A frank abscess (if present) would open out at this stage and suction facilities should be available to minimize contamination. This completes the operation of *costotransversectomy.*

If removal of the medial end of the rib does not drain out a suspected fluid abscess further exploration is done with the finger through the bed of the medial end of the removed rib skirting along the vertebral column to enter into the abscess cavity. Rough handling of the important structures (heart and aorta) anterior to the vertebral column should be carefully avoided. When the abscess cavity is found the liquid pus, semi-solid caseous material, small sequestra and necrotic debris can be dislodged with the finger and are removed by suction. Larger sequestra and necrotic debris can be dislodged by a curet and removed with the help of a sequestrum holding forceps, a Cocker's forceps or a curet itself. This completes the operation of *debridement.* In cases of tuberculous paraplegia, we as a routine, complete the operation of anterolateral decompression irrespective of the presence or absence of a cold abscess, as we feel that besides the paravertebral abscess, sequestra, tubercular debris and hard bony or osteocartilaginous salient may be responsible for the neural complication. Only on rare occasions when a tense abscess has been drained and the general condition of the patient is poor, have we completed the operation at this stage of costotrasversectomy.

In the normal course when anterolateral decompression is contemplated *one to three* additional transverse processes and ribs corresponding to the diseased area are resected. Excision of *3–4 ribs* provides a good exposure, especially when there is severe kyphosis and crowding of ribs, however, ordinarily one can perform adequate decompression even with excision of *two ribs* alone. Now the intercostal nerves are isolated starting from the lateral healthier area and traced medially to the intervertebral foramina. Intervertebral foramina can also be identified by inserting a curved blunt dissector into the foramina in between the pedicles. Cut the intercostal nerves *about 6 cm* lateral to the intervertebral foramina and let these hang or hold toward the opposite side away from the area for further operation. The lung covered with pleura, the periosteum of the excised ribs and the intervening costal muscles along with the intercostal vessels (arteries attached to the aorta and the veins attached to the vena cava) is gently retracted anteriorly. The connective tissue (anterior longitudinal ligament, periosteum and fibrous tissue) anterior to the position of intervertebral foramina and the resected transverse processes is carefully stripped off (using small periosteum elevator and chisel) from the lateral and anterior surfaces of the exposed vertebral bodies and the discs. Depending upon the extent of the vertebrae exposed insert subperiosteally one or two curved (2.5–5 cm broad) spatulae in front of the vertebral bodies and discs to be operated **(Figs. 24.12 to 24.15)**. The spatula safely holds the mediastinal contents and the lung anteriorly, away from the vertebrae. Self-retaining retractors are applied on the muscles proximal and distal to the excised ribs holding the lips of the wound apart. Avoid piercing the spikes of the retractors into the intercostal space lest it may perforate the pleura. Intercostal nerves serve as guide to the intervertebral foramina and the pedicles. The pedicles are palpated and seen; a curved blunt dissector inserted through the intervertebral foramina proximally and distally gives orientation of the exact position of the pedicles and the direction of the spinal canal which may be badly angulated; it also helps to separate any adhesions between the dura and the vertebral column, thus avoiding tear of dura while resecting the pedicles. A fine curved bone nibbler is useful to remove the pedicles bit by bit, removal of 2–4 pedicles exposes the dura laterally and one can see the position of the cord. Once the cord is visible further operation becomes easy.

With more experience and familiarity, after excision of the transverse processes and ribs,

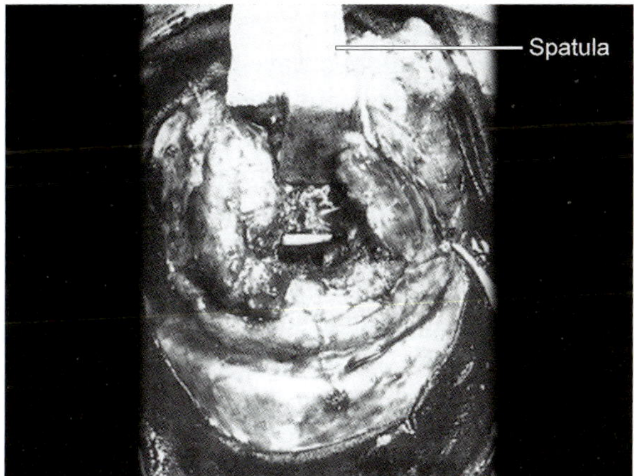

Fig. 24.12: Peroperative photograph at the completion of an anterolateral decompression. Note the semicircular flap of soft tissues raised for the retropleural approach. In this case, a strut bone graft was also inserted between the proximal and distal healthy vertebral bodies.

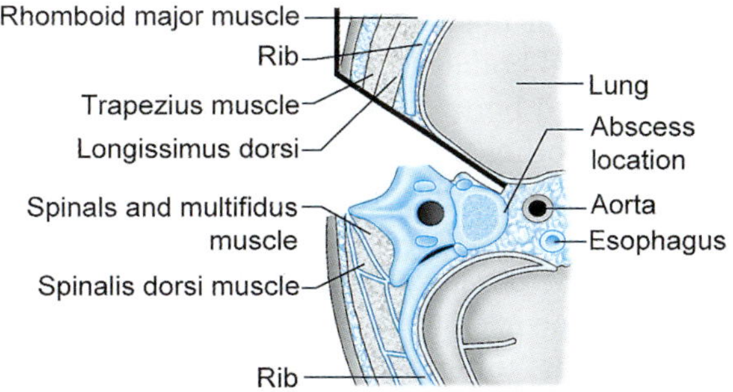

Fig. 24.13: Anterolateral approach to dorsal spine.

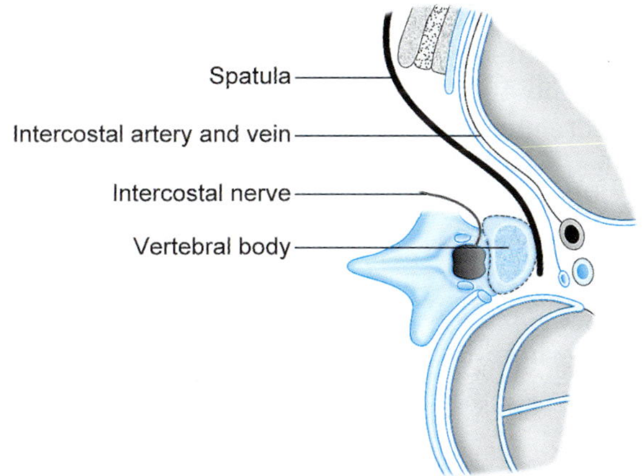

Fig. 24.14: Anterolateral approach to dorsal spine.

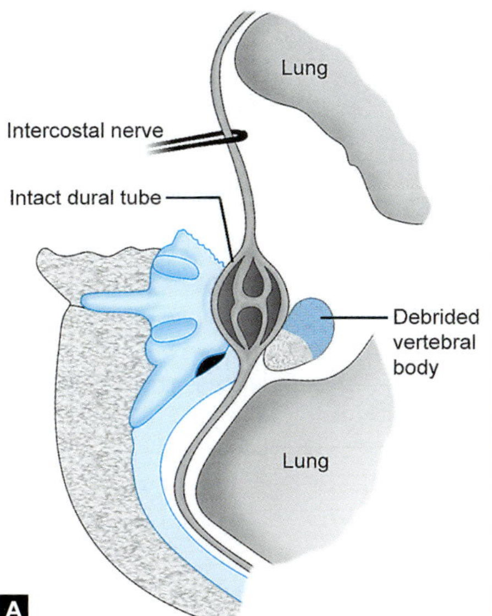

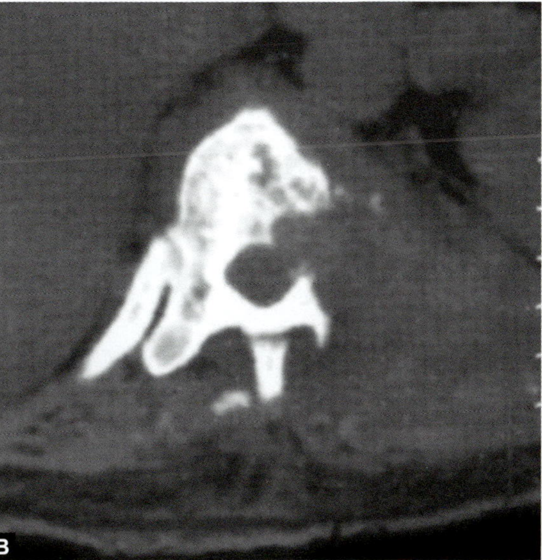

Figs. 24.15A and B: (A) Bones removed in anterolateral decompression, (B) CT scan of the operated patient showing the decompressed area, healing disease in the vertebral body and the intact posterior elements (postoperative follow-up).

one can clear the lateral and anterior aspects of the diseased bodies with the help of periosteum elevator and bone chisel. The diseased bodies, discs and other offending material anterior to the pedicles are resected and the cord is exposed anteriorly for about 4–8 cm depending upon the extent of the disease **(Figs. 24.14 and 24.15)**. In this way, one need not totally excise the pedicles. Bony ridges, tubercular sequestra and debris, caseous matter and any other offending tissue lying anterior to the cord are gently removed with the help of a small chisel, curet, rongeurs, and nibblers. The curved blunt dissector is again useful to separate the dura from the walls of the spinal canal. By this procedure one can (if required) resect almost the whole of the body of the vertebra **(Figs. 24.14 to 24.16)**. All offending diseased bodies and discs are removed and the cord ultimately comes to lie in a free place anteriorly. If required one can resect the (adjacent) diseased bodies and discs proximal and distal to the areas from where the ribs and transverse processes have been excised. This can be achieved easily by a curved goose-necked nibbler, curved rongeurs or curet without cutting the corresponding transverse process and the rib. We have never had any difficulty in performing a satisfactory decompression or working on the "other side" of the body of the vertebrae. If required, a strut bone graft may be inserted between the healthy bodies above and below **(Fig. 24.12)**. Before finally closing the wound, it is ensured that the exposed vertebrae left in the bed have bleeding surfaces. Any projecting ridges are removed, wound may be washed with saline and ultimately smeared with suitable antibiotics. The muscles and skin are sutured with/without any drainage.

During growing age in patients younger than 13 years, the vertebral bodies are predominantly made of cartilaginous tissue. Such a tissue does not offer a satisfactory bed for a strut bone graft. After completion of decompression in such patients, we have extended the dissection of the semicircular flap to the opposite side by extending

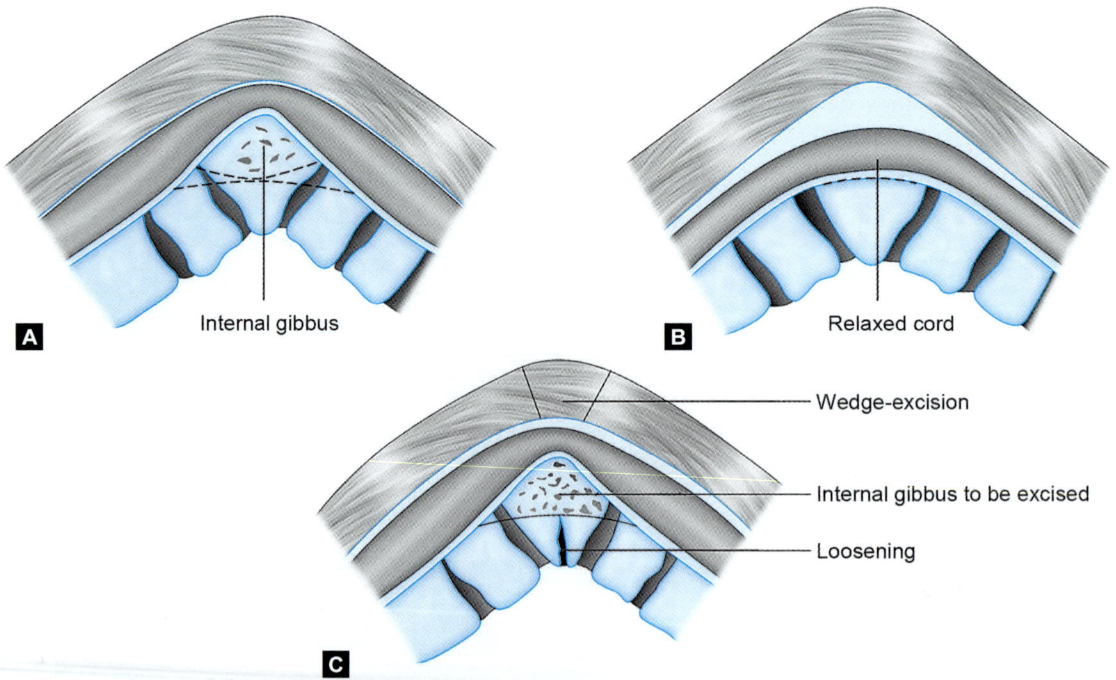

Figs. 24.16A to C: Diagrammatic representation of (A) excision of Internal gibbus, through anterolateral approach, (B) Anterior transposition of the cord, and (C) Suggested operation for fixed deformities: After anterior transposition of cord do osteotomy of anterior elements and wedge resection of posterior elements.

the proximal and distal ends of the incision by one cm across the midline. The paraspinal muscles are reflected laterally subperiosteally from the dorsum of spinous processes and laminae of the decompressed vertebrae (on the right side when decompressed through left approach). The exposed surfaces of spinous processes and laminae are decorticated and bridged with the ribs removed during the operation **(Figs. 23.20 and 24.17)**. The purpose of fusion is very well served at younger age by the posterior fusion rather than placement of grafts anteriorly. During growing age remove only the offending parts of vertebral bodies which are causing pressure on the dural tube. Avoid over-zealous "excisional surgery". The remaining part of vertebral bodies may still have some growth potential to negate the deterioration of kyphotic deformity. Since 1980s we have been performing this 360 degrees procedure for every case of anterolateral decompression. Such a combined operation has eliminated or minimized deterioration of kyphotic deformity. In patients followed for >2 years after the operation, average increase in the kyphotic angle was 10 degrees (0°–30°) **(Fig. 24.17)**.

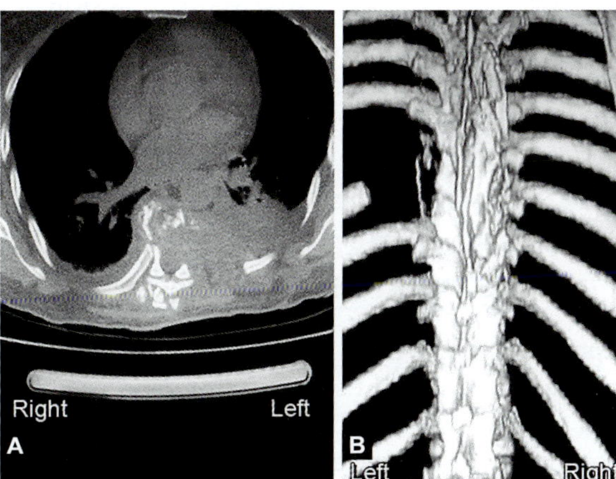

Figs. 24.17A and B: (A) Reconstructed CT-scan showing the quantity of decompression, and the extent of posterior graft in the right paraspinal gutter. (A) Cross-sectional CT-scan at mid-dorsal spine after anterolateral decompression, and posterior bone grafting. Note the adequacy of decompression of the dural tube, grossly destroyed vertebral body and (B) posteriorly placed bone grafts done in one sitting (360 degrees) procedure.

When expertise and facilities are not available for transthoracic or anterolateral approach one may use "posterior only approach" (Ukunda 2018). Basically, it comprises of laminectomy with pedicle fixation followed by costotransversectomy, unilateral or bilateral with bone grafting. The authors have used this approach for cervicodorsal, dorsal and dorso-lumbar regions. They re-emphasized that operative procedures for correction of deformity are more demanding when the disease is healed (rigid) as compared to the active disease (flexible).

OPERATIVE COMPLICATIONS AND IT'S PREVENTION

Excessive oozing from the paravertebral venous plexus and from the vertebral column is mostly due to pressure on abdomen or obstructed respiration. The avoidance of the abdominal pressure and maintenance of free air passages help a great deal to check this excessive oozing. Gravity helps to drain the blood away from the site of the operation if the foot (or head) end of the patient is lowered.

Bleeding from the paravertebral venous plexus and from the vessels in the dense fibrous tissues can rarely be troublesome. Selective coagulation using thin forceps, bipolar cautery and adequate local compression are of great help to stop such a bleeding. Avoid meticulously the use of electro-coagulation on the vessels entering into the intervertebral foramina. This area is considered a distribution center for blood supply to the spinal cord.

Excessive fall of blood pressure is noted in some patients even if the operative blood loss is replaced. This may be presumably due to the lag of activity of adrenal cortex; small quantities of corticosteroids may be required to control the same (Tyagi et al. 2007). Peroperative corticosteroids may also be given if the cord has been subjected to appreciable handling as may be required during anterior transposition of cord (in severe kyphotic deformity) or in cases of decompression for secondary canal stenosis, or paraplegia associated with healed disease.

Tear of the pleura is one of the complications especially in long-standing cases where pleura becomes adherent to the parieties. This usually happens when the ribs are being resected. This can be avoided by carefully resecting the ribs subperiosteally. It may be a time consuming process in most of the cases, however, this time is well worth spending. If a tear is made it should be carefully closed, and water seal drainage of the chest like transthoracic anterior approach is maintained. Repair the pleural tear (especially if the size is >1 cm) by nonabsorbable interrupted sutures. Prepare a No. 32 rubber catheter cut round at the tip with an additional hole on the side 2 cm away from the tip. Push the catheter mounted on an artery forceps through a stab in the seventh intercostal space in the mid-axillary line. One can see or feel through the operative field the catheter entering into the pleural cavity. Leave 4 cm of the catheter in the pleural cavity and attach it to an underwater seal for 48–72 hours. Expansion of the lungs assisted by the anesthesiologist at the time of last stitches helps in closing the pleural cavity. The drainage of the pleural cavity is effective so long as the water column is moving with the respiration. If the pleural tear occurred before the completion of decompression of the cord it may be worthwhile completing the operation as a transpleural procedure.

Tear of the dura is one of the rare complications which can be easily avoided by gently separating the dura from the vertebral column as stated earlier with the help of a curved blunt dissector before resecting the bone. If a tear is made it should be closed by continuous nonabsorbable sutures. If the tear is small and/or it is not possible to close it, a small piece of spongiostan or muscle helps to seal the leak. Close the wound meticulously in multi-layers and do not use postoperative suction drain. During the postoperative period, recumbent positive of patient for 48–72 hours would prevent leakage of cerebrospinal fluid and help sealing of the tear.

In our 700 operations performed between 1964 to 1987, seven patients had tear of pleura inadvertently. Four cases occurred during first 3 years of study, however, three tears occurred during the last 3 years. All these cases were treated by the insertion of underwater seal and repair of pleura. Five cases developed tear of dura while working close to the anterior aspect of the dural sheath. If the dural tear was larger than 1.5 cm it was repaired. Smaller tears sealed automatically by maintaining local pressure for a few minutes or by the use of a locally placed gelfoam/spongiostan or a piece of muscle.

Postoperative Care

The patient is nursed on a hard bed or rarely (small children) in a plaster of Paris posterior shell till about 3 months after the operation. Careful and assisted turning of the patient and possible exercises are permitted from first day of the operation. At the end of 3–4 months or when the patient has made good neural recovery whichsoever is later, the patient is mobilized out of the bed with the help of spinal brace. The spinal brace is gradually discarded after about 12–18 months of the operation.

ANTEROLATERAL APPROACH TO THE LUMBAR SPINE (LUMBOVERTEBROTOMY)

Approach **(Fig. 24.18)** is usually from the left side because on the right side inferior vena cava lies just anterior to the psoas major muscle. With the patient in right lateral position a semicircular incision (about 7 cm radius) convex laterally is given with the center of the incision opposite to the vertebral body(ies) to be exposed. Retract the skin flap medially and cut the paraspinal muscles (iliocostalis lumborum and longissimus dorsi muscles) transversely down to the transverse processes. Expose two transverse processes

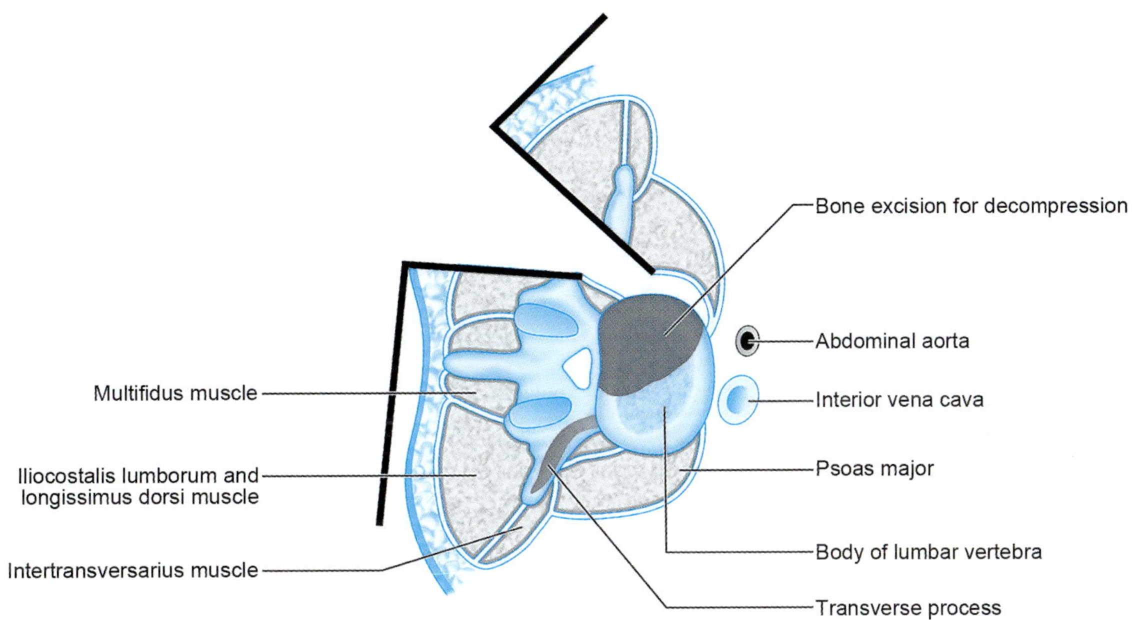

Fig. 24.18: Anterolateral approach to lumbar vertebrae from left side.

subperiosteally up to their bases. Remove the transverse processes of the vertebral bodies to be exposed, from their bases. Retract the cut paraspinal muscles proximally and distally with self-retaining retractors. At this stage, in the depth of the exposed area psoas major muscle will come into view. Retract the psoas muscle gently anteriorly and medially. Take care to protect the important vessels in front of the psoas, aorta on the left side and inferior vena cava on the right side, and the lumbar nerves which run from above downwards (anterior to the transverse processes) within the substance of the posterior part of the psoas, in the exposed area. Lumbar nerves must be protected and retracted (on suitable tapes) out of the way. Exiting lumbar nerves lie just in front of the transverse processes and must be protected by careful dissection. As an example, third lumbar nerve traverses in front of fourth transverse process. Retraction of nerves proximally and distally exposes an area of 5–9 cm. Starting from the anterior borders of the bases of resected transverse processes, using sharp osteotomes or periosteal elevators expose lateral and anterior surfaces of the vertebral bodies and discs subperiosteally. The periosteum, anterior longitudinal ligaments and the psoas are retracted gently anteriorly and medially. Insert two spatulae (subperiosteally) between the psoas and vertebral bodies. Anterolateral surface of the involved lumbar vertebrae is thus exposed for debridement, curettage, decompression, and bone grafting as needed.

Extraperitoneal Anterior Approach to the Lumbar Spine

Patient is placed **(Figs. 24.19 to 24.21)** in the 45 degrees right lateral position with a bridge centered over the area to be operated. The incision resembles that of nephroureterectomy or that of sympathectomy—extending from the renal angle posteriorly to the lower part of lateral margin of rectus abdominis anteriorly. The proximal and distal levels of the incision can be shifted cranially or caudally according to the vertebrae to be exposed. The layers of the abdominal muscles are split or incised in the line of the skin incision. The parietal peritoneum is gently stripped off (using your finger or a blunt dissector) the posterior

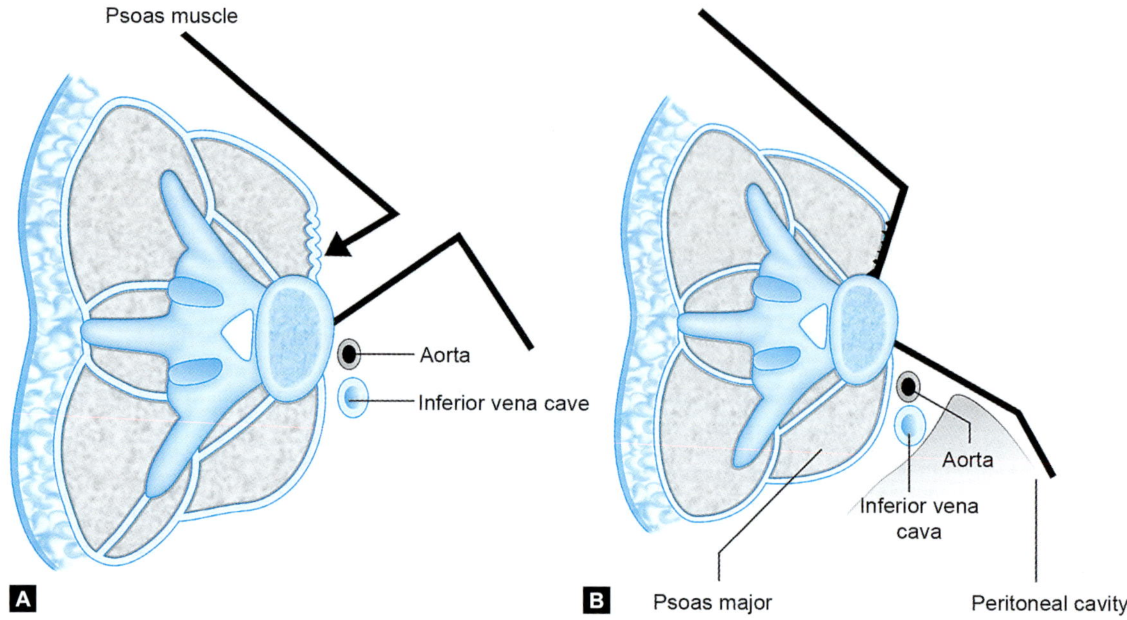

Figs. 24.19A and B: (A) Retroperitoneal anterior approach to lumbar vertebrae, from left side (B) Retroperitoneal anterior approach to lumbar vertebrae shifting left psoas laterally, aorta, vena cava and peritoneal contents to the right side.

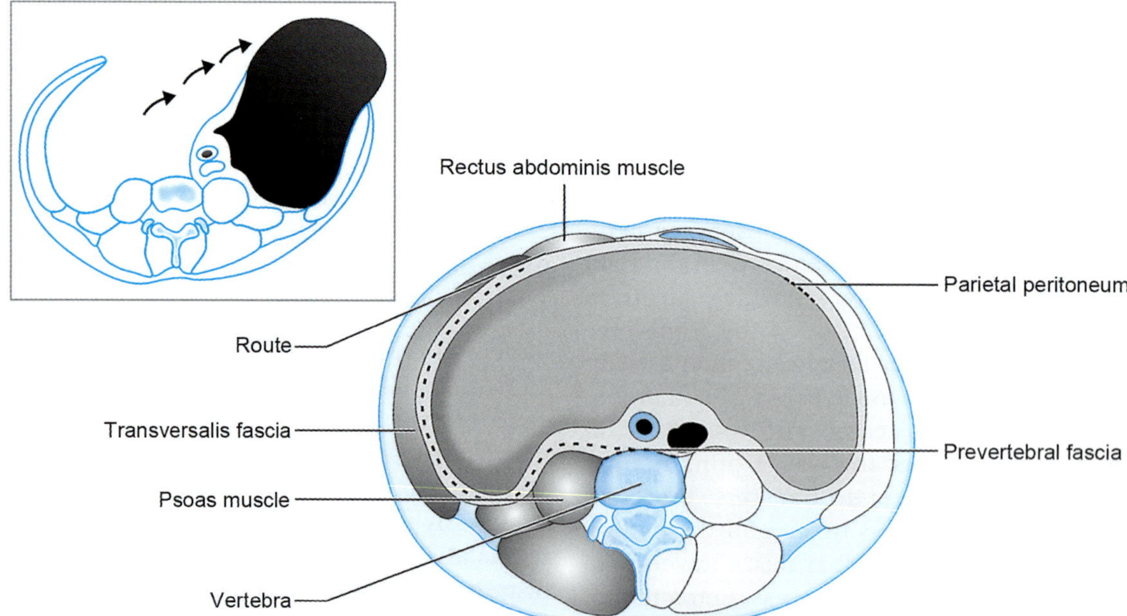

Fig. 24.20: Diagrammatic representation of the cross-section of abdomen demonstrating the plane (dotted line) of cleavage for the extraperitoneal approach to the lumbar vertebrae. One works lateral to the rectus abdominis sheath between the fascia transversalis and the peritoneum. Generally, one should start reflecting the peritoneum from the posterior part of the abdomen because maximum extraperitoneal fat is located there.

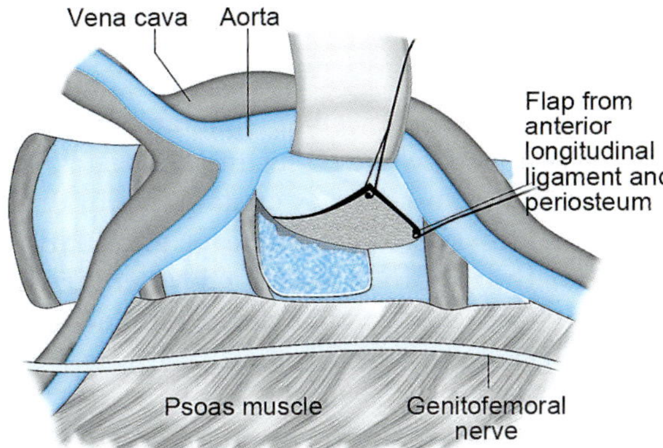

Fig. 24.21: Diagrammatic representation of the anterior retroperitoneal approach to the lower part of the lumbar vertebral bodies. The aorta and the inferior vena cava are mobilized and gently retracted to the right side. The diseased area is being exposed by lifting up a flap of anterior longitudinal ligament and the underlying periosteum.

abdominal wall and the kidney. The ureter must be visualized and protected as it may be reflected anteriorly along with the parietal peritoneum **(Fig. 24.21)**, it should be left resting on the psoas muscle. Use moist abdominal sponges to push the peritoneum and its contents to the right side. If a psoas abscess is present, the same is opened longitudinally in line with the psoas muscle fibers and after its evacuation the diseased bodies are exposed. In the contents of the psoas abscess, transversely running lumbar vessels may be seen which require ligation and division. Lumbar plexus of nerves is not encountered as it lies in the more posterior part of the psoas muscle. If no abscess is present the psoas muscle is stripped from its origins from the vertebral bodies and retracted laterally. The aorta and inferior vena cava are gently displaced to the right side after double ligation of the respective lumbar arteries and veins. The sympathetic chain may be reflected laterally with psoas major muscle. The diseased vertebral bodies are exposed and dealt with. Before closure the bridge under the trunk is lowered.

While operating upon the lumbar and lumbosacral regions the tips of the transverse processes of the lumbar vertebrae can be palpated in the lateral part of the operative field. This helps to identify the level for surgery.

Lumbosacral Region

Extraperitoneal Approach

Extraperitoneal approach from the left side is preferred because left common iliac vessels are longer than the right, and thus can be retracted toward the right side without undue tension. However, in cases with disease predominantly on the right side the approach from the right should be used. For the left sided approach, right lateral position as that for lumbar spine, a bridge in the lumbar region and lowered head of the table greatly facilitate the exposure. The skin incision starts in the midline midway between the symphysis pubis and the umbilicus and forms a lazy "S" to a point midway between the iliac crest and the lowest rib in the flank. The position of the incision may be shifted cranially or caudally according to the need. All the layers of subcutaneous tissue and fascia, external oblique, internal oblique, and transversalis muscles, are divided in the line of the skin incision. Abdominal muscles may be split if the direction of muscle fibers falls in the line of skin incision. Anteriorly, the anterior and posterior rectus sheaths are cut leaving the rectus abdominis intact. In the lateral part of the incision with the help of a wet sponge, define the extraperitoneal fat and work medially and posteriorly stripping the peritoneum to expose the psoas muscle, abdominal aorta and common iliac vessels. The ureter and spermatic vessels go forward toward the right side along with the parietal peritoneum **(Fig. 24.20)**. Lumbosacral region is cleared further by retracting psoas muscle laterally and pushing the extraperitoneal tissues with a piece of gauze. The left iliolumbar vein, lumbar vessels, and other occasional small vessels are ligated and divided, this permits displacement of common iliac vessels and aorta, and inferior vena cava to the right side. Lumbosacral region is thus exposed and dealt with as required. Special care and tedious dissection is required to expose lumbosacral region in cases with extensive destruction, spondylolisthesis or gross deformity.

Transperitoneal Hypogastric Anterior Approach

With the patient supine and Trendelenburg position of the table and a sand-bag at the back of lumbosacral junction to extend lumbosacral joint, midline incision is made from umbilicus to the pubis. Cut through skin, fascia, linea alba, and peritoneum. The intestines are retracted and retained upward with moist abdominal pads. The sacral promontory is exposed **(Fig. 24.22)**. The bifurcation of the aorta and left common iliac vein are identified proximal to the lumbosacral articulation. The parietal peritoneum over the lumbosacral region is incised in a longitudinal direction in the midline avoiding injury to the sacral nerve and sacral artery, and the ganglion of the sympathetic nerve. Any damage to the presacral nerves leads to retrograde ejaculation. Retraction of parietal peritoneum exposes the lumbosacral joint which can be dealt with as required.

After Exposing the Site of the Diseased Vertebrae

When a paravertebral swelling is palpable or visible it may be opened while dissecting and retracting structures. The abscess may contain thin or thick fluid pus, thick caseous tissue or granulation tissue or thick flbrotic tissue. On opening the abscess (if required by an incision parallel to the vertebral column) the contents are evacuated and cleared away. Next step is to remove the diseased bodies, sequestra from bones and discs and all unhealthy ligaments and diseased tissues. Use of chisels, curets, rongeurs, nibblers and suction would be required to clear the diseased tissues. If the aim is debridement and excision of the diseased tissue this much surgery is enough and one should proceed with closure. If one is dealing with a case of neurological involvement, decompression of the cord is mandatory. After clearing the diseased tissues posterior limit of the cleared area is judged and further tissues are removed to expose, the dural tube from the anterior aspect for the entire diseased area. Besides the vertebral bodies and intervertebral

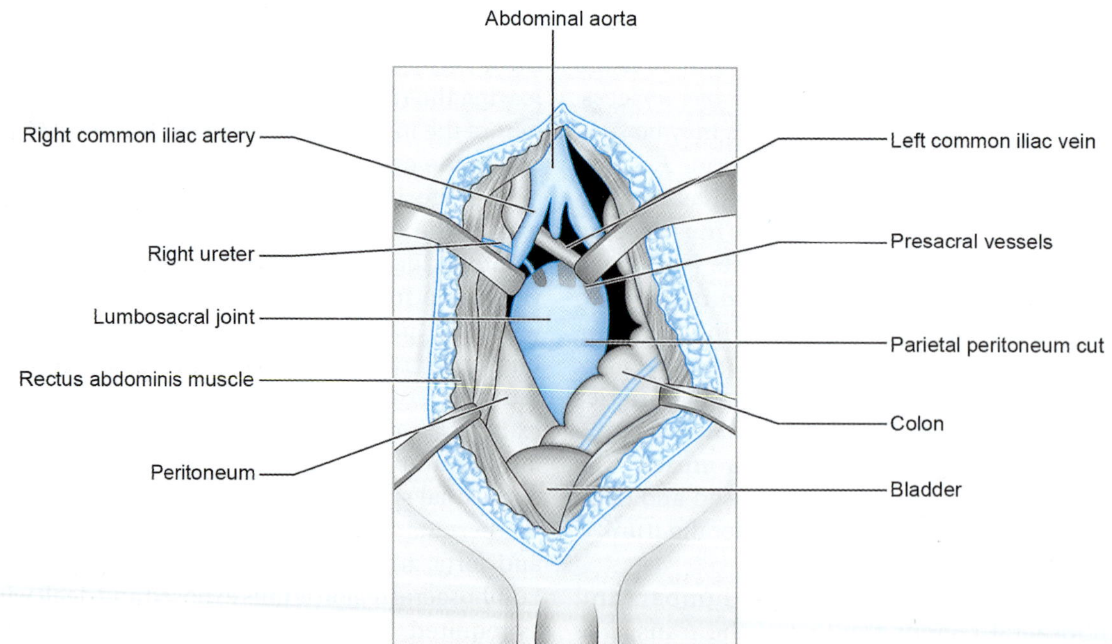

Fig. 24.22: Lumbosacral region exposed through suprapubic transperitoneal approach.

disc, the posterior longitudinal ligament and any tough or fibrotic or thick granulation is removed piecemeal, and the soft shiny dura is thus exposed. In case of severe kyphotic deformity, enough osseous tissues and the salient including the normal bone in front of the cord are removed till the cord lies anteriorly in a relaxed position **(Fig. 24.16)**. In an adult on an average 3–6 cm of cord is exposed anteriorly. Dura may or may not be pulsating at the end of the decompression. If the dura is not pulsatile, Hodgson (1969) suggested aspiration of cerebrospinal fluid through a small needle. If this failed, he did not hesitate opening the dura. We do not consider it justified to open the dura unless one suspects a concomitant intradural tuberculoma of the cord. In a case of neural involvement, decompression of the cord from the anterior aspect is essential, however, if the anterior most portions of the diseased vertebral bodies, well away from the dura are not particularly diseased this part can be left undisturbed without compromising the freedom to the cord. Care must be taken to leave behind healthy bleeding surfaces of the bones proximally and distally.

If an extensive gap is left behind after debridement and/or decompression and the vertebral column appears mechanically unstable, bone grafting is indicated. Slots are made, in the proximal and distal vertebral bodies, in the coronal plane. Rib (or any other available graft) is cut to the size as required. The operated area is sprung open by extending the spine by direct pressure on the spines of the operated area. Suitable length of one or two grafts from the ribs or iliac crest are inserted into the slots while the vertebrae are kept sprung apart. The release of the pressure at the back of the diseased spine would hold the grafts firmly. Streptomycin and nydrazide may be instilled locally and the wound is closed. In growing children, we advise against intercorporeal fusion, we as a rule perform concomitant posterior fusion. Thus, any growth potential of the vertebral bodies may negate the kyphotic deformity to some extent.

Exposure of Sacroiliac Joint

This operation is indicated for obtaining tissues from bones or soft tissues for confirmation of pathology, for debridement of the diseased joint in a therapeutically refractory case, or rarely for arthrodesis of a painful sacroiliac joint.

In lateral decubitus or prone position, make a semicircular incision through skin and subcutaneous tissues starting from 1–2 cm proximal to the level of posterosuperior iliac spine to 1–2 cm distal to the position of posteroinferior iliac spine. The incision is moderately convex laterally like a conventional incision for anterolateral decompression.

Lift and retract medially the skin flap along with the subcutaneous tissues. Strip the lumbosacral fascia and sacrospinous muscle along with periosteum from the posterior part of iliac bone and reflect it medially 1–2 cm. Similarly, strip the gluteus maximum origin with its thick aponeurosis and periosteum from the posterior part of iliac bone (from posterosuperior iliac spine to posteroinferior iliac spine) and reflect it laterally for 1.5–2.5 cm. Sacroiliac joint still covered by posterior part of iliac bone is thus exposed. To expose or enter the sacroiliac joint you have to remove the posterior part of iliac bone as needed. One to two cm of full thickness of iliac bone between the posterosuperior and posteroinferior iliac spines can be removed with an osteotome as a block to expose the sacroiliac joint and posterolateral part of sacrum. Avoid dissection or removal of bone distal to posteroinferior spine because that forms the superior border of greater sciatic notch. One can now perform curettage of cavities and debridement/excision of infected tissues. In a rare case if arthrodesis is desired, debride and decorticate the sacral side of joint and pack the sacroiliac joint with locally harvested bone grafts. If required one can remove 1–2 cm of lateral part of sacral ala along with the articular margin to reach the anterior surface of upper part of sacrum.

Drainage of Presacral Abscess

Place the patient in prone position and raise the buttocks on a sand-bag to position the hip in flexion. Make a midline longitudinal incision over the lower segments of sacrum and the coccyx. Remove the coccyx and carefully subperiosteally dissect the rectum anteriorly from the anterior surface of sacrum. Essentially, create a space going from below upwards in the midline of the anterior surface of the sacrum. Use packing gauze in the caudal part as you move upwards to minimize blood loss. Carry on the dissection upwards staying close to the midline of the anterior surface of sacrum till you reach the site of vertebral destruction and the isthmus of the cold abscess. The abscess may be attached to the bone only at the site of osseous lesions and that is the site where dissection will open the abscess cavity. Repair any perforation made in the rectal wall, secure hemostasis, insert a wide bore suction drain going up to the top of abscess cavity, close the wound in layers. The drainage tube is removed after 4–5 days.

With some experience one can do this operation in the lateral decubitus position of the patient with complete flexion of hips and knees. One may not excise the coccyx. Separate the soft tissue attachment on one side of the coccyx and lower three segments of sacrum. One may snip-cut lower half of sacrospinous ligament, this permits easy access to anterior surface of sacrum, you are now in front of the sacrum, the remaining dissection is the same as that after coccygectomy. Coccyx may exhibit varying degree of mobility after soft tissue release, it does not matter. It is wise not to open the sacral hiatus to avoid damage to S5 nerve root.

Posterior Spinal Arthrodesis

Since the introduction of anterior spinal clearance with the resultant sound healing and stability, the value of posterior spinal fusion (as a stand alone operation) has decreased. At present, its only practical use in tuberculosis of the spine is to control mechanical instability of the spine in otherwise healed disease, to stabilize the craniovertebral region in certain cases of tuberculosis or as a part of panvertebral operation **(Figs. 24.17, 24.24 and 24.28)**.

The posterior spinal arthrodesis operations are based upon the techniques of Albee and Hibbs. Albee (1911, 1930) aimed at fusion by uniting the spinous processes into one continuous bony ridge by a tibial graft inserted longitudinally into the split spinous processes across the diseased site. In the Hibbs (1912, 1918, 1928) operation, the fusion was induced by overlapping numerous small osseous flaps from contiguous laminae, spinous processes and articular facets. Most surgeons at present use a carefully performed Hibbs' type of arthrodesis with individual modifications (Neville 1971). The extent of the fusion currently is aimed to include the diseased area with one healthy vertebra each proximal and distal to it **(Figs. 24.23 and 24.24)**.

The operative procedure can be performed in lateral or prone position. The designated spinous processes and laminae are exposed through a midline longitudinal incision. With a curved hand-chisel, Capner's gouge, bone cutting forceps and nibblers the spinous processes are chipped off from their bases, thin shavings of bone are lifted along with the muscles exposing the rawed surfaces of laminae up to and including the posterior articulations.

As the bed for grafting is being prepared, assistants cut the spinous processes into chips, and harvest from tibia or posterior part of iliac bone, cancellous bone grafts. If needed, bone from a bank may be used, especially in children. The bone chips and slivers are distributed up and down the prepared bed in close contact with the raw areas and wound is closed in layers. Limited posterior fixation may be used to supplement the fusion area, or one may use a moulded brace, this may permit the patient with preserved neurology to be ambulatory 2–4 weeks, after the operation. In patients with neural deficit (which have a favorable chance of neural recovery), it is prudent

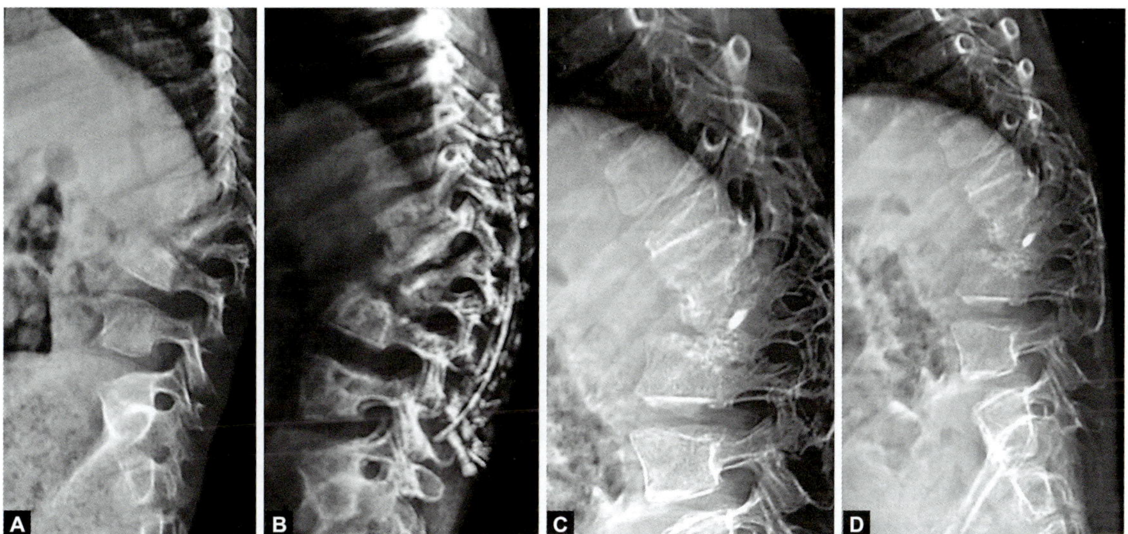

Figs. 24.23A to D: (A and B) Posterior fusion in a child with extensive disease >7 vertebrae; (C and D) Allogenic bone grafts succeeded in the arrest of deformation.

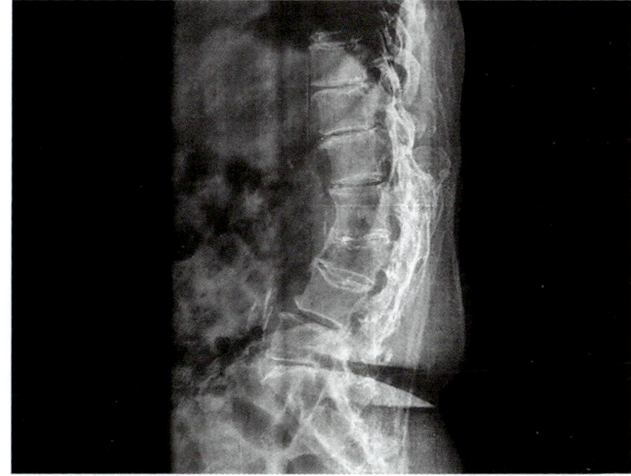

Fig. 24.24: A 20 years follow-up of posterior spinal fusion spanning L2–L4. Note the incorporated posterior bone mass and healed status of disease anteriorly.

to give rest to the operated spine for 8–12 weeks before encouraging the patient to sit and ambulate. Postoperatively, rest on a hard bed or in plaster of Paris bed is continued for about 8–12 weeks. The patient is encouraged back extension exercises after 6–8 weeks and ambulation in a suitable spinal brace after 8–12 weeks. The brace is continued for 6–9 months.

SURGERY IN SEVERE KYPHOSIS

The safest method of preventing severe kyphotic deformity is to identify the potential cases at high risk (active disease in patients younger than 10 years, dorsal lesion, involvement of three or more vertebrae (Tuli 1975, 1984) and subject them to a panvertebral operation including fusion of the posterior elements of the diseased vertebrae (Tuli 1995, Deshhande et al. 2012, Wong 2017).

It is unwise to rely solely on the anterior graft to prevent further collapse and increased kyphosis, in patients in whom the length of the graft or the extent of the disease exceeds two disc spaces. Additional measures such as an extended period of recumbency (about 6 months), prolonged use of brace (for 6–12 months), and concomitant or delayed (additional) posterior arthrodesis may improve the results (Tuli 1985, Rajasekaran 1989). Yau et al. (1974), Jain et al. (2014) pointed out that the kyphotic deformity may be unstable and progressive, particularly in childhood, and they believed that a severe deformity in the presence of active disease should be an absolute indication for debridement with or without decompression, correction and stabilization. Late reconstruction of a tuberculous kyphos was a difficult and dangerous procedure. Any significant correction of fixed kyphotic deformities involves many staged operations, the operative procedures required are, anteriorly at the site of disease, osteotomy of the posterior elements at the deformity and halopelvic or halofemoral traction postoperatively. The resultant correction rarely improves cosmesis, some loss of correction during follow-up is common, and the operation is frought with dangerous complications including permanent paralysis (Upadhyay et al. 1994).

Treatment of Paraplegia in Severe Kyphosis: (Anterior Transposition of the Cord)

Griffiths, Seddon and Roaf (1956) performed laminectomy first, then enough spinal nerve roots were divided on both sides to permit rotation and retraction of the theca so that enough bone from the front of the vertebral canal could be removed. Hyndman (1947) reported performance of this operation in 3 cases of paraplegia with severe kyphosis and bony fusion of the bodies in front. Two of his patients made rapid recoveries and one had a relapse. We, however, feel that excellent removal of internal kyphosis can be achieved through anterolateral approach **(Figs 24.16 and 24.25)** to permit the cord to lie in a relaxed anterior position. If required one may cut the intercostal nerves on the opposite side by making another paravertebral incision. Only intercostal nerves can be sacrificed to permit shifting of the cord, spinal nerve roots in other regions cannot be divided without significant loss of function **(Fig. 24.25)**. For treatment of kyphotic deformity Rajasekaran (2002) suggested stabilization of spine posteriorly followed by anterior debridement and bone grafting in active stage of disease. In healed stage with rigid deformity, he suggested anterior debridement first to be followed by posterior instrumentation and anterior fusion. Titanium cages filled with cancellous bone grafts and allografts have been used to bridge the defects of the anterior column by Govender and Prabhoo (1999). Yau et al. (1974) even with multistaged attempted correction of fixed kyphotic deformity reported mortality of 10% and average amount of correction obtained only 28%.

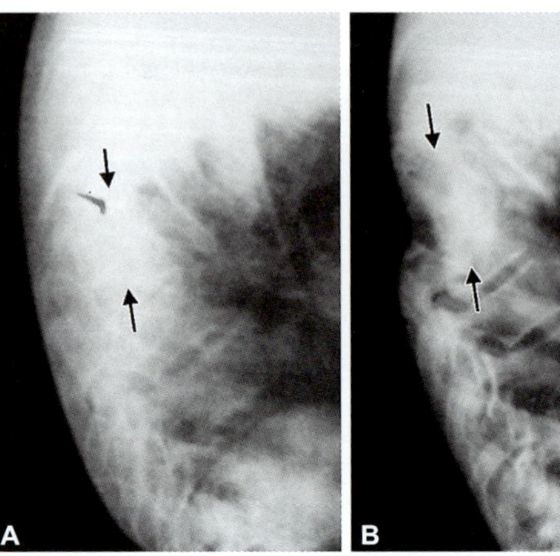

Figs. 24.25A and B: Radiographs of a patient with 90 degree kyphotic deformity in mid-dorsal region. The patient presented with late-onset paraplegia due to severe deformity for which anterior transposition of the cord was done, (A) before surgery, (B) after anterior transposition through anterolateral approach.

Anterior Transposition of the Spinal Cord and Possible Correction of Severe Kyphotic Deformity

This is an operation of some magnitude and should be undertaken by an experienced spine surgeon familiar with anatomy of the distorted spine. Following is the technique which we have used over the years in our institutions. Place the patient in lateral recumbent position. As for anterolateral decompression, the best approach is through the left side. However, if left side is badly scarred, one can go through the right side. After reflecting the soft tissues like standard anterolateral approach, identify three to four ribs which correspond to the kyphotic deformity. Remove 5-6 cm of three to four ribs subperiosteally, after having removed the corresponding transverse processes. Identify the intercostal nerves up to their exit from intervertebral foramina. The intercostals nerves or lumbar nerves in the lumbar spine give an orientation about the position of the dural tube. The intercostal or lumbar nerves and pedicles are anterior to the bases of resected transverse processes. No lumbar nerve should be sacrificed, however, two or three intercostal nerves can be sacrificed by sectioning the nerves 4–5 cm lateral to the intervertebral foramina. The medial segments of the intercostal nerves are held with small artery forceps and permitted to hang toward the floor with gravity (in the lateral decubitus position), these act as guide to the position of the dural tube. Using small sharp osteotomes, expose subperiosteally (starting just anterior to the pedicles) the lateral and anterior surface of the deformed vertebral bodies. Once you reach the anterior surface of the vertebral bodies, insert two or three flexible spatulae in front of the deformed vertebral bodies. In the dorsal spine, the spatulae are behind the contents of posterior mediastinum (aorta on the left side and vena cava on the right side). In the lumbar spine when you are reflecting the periosteum, the vertebral attachment of psoas muscle also gets reflected from the lateral and anterior surfaces of the lumbar vertebral bodies. Insertion of spatulae in front of lumbar vertebral bodies keeps the psoas muscle, sympathetic chain, ureter and the contents of peritoneal cavity anteriorly away from the next steps of surgery.

Exposure of the deformed vertebral bodies at the site of kyphos may require excision of tough fibrous tissue, sometimes containing calcified material. The site of kyphos may be osseous, chondro-osseous, fibro-osseous; rarely one may find a few beads of thick pus or caseous material. Using small sharp osteotomes or chisels or power burr or gooze necked nibblers, a gutter is created in the deformed mass of vertebral bodies **(Fig. 24.16)**. Anterior most 3–4 mm of the deformed kyphotic bones and posterior most 2–3 mm of bone anterior to the dural tube are not removed till the last stages of operation. The retention of thin bone anterior to the dural tube prevents anterior shift of the dural tube, while the gutter is being created for future anterior placement of the dural tube. The gutter in most cases should be 3–6 cm in length 1.5–2 cm in width and depth, still retaining the anterior border of the kyphos and a thin layer of contralateral surface of the vertebral bodies. Once an adequate space is created by the gutter, the thin layer of bone in front of the deformed dural tube is carefully removed permitting the dural tube shifting anteriorly in the gutter in more relaxed position. Do ensure that there are no sharp edges anterior to the dural tube proximally and distally. This completes the operation of anterior transposition of the spinal cord. Depending upon the clinical requirements and the surgical decision further supplementary procedures can be carried out: Bone grafting for mechanical instability, release of anterior most bone and shortening of posterior elements of the vertebral column for obtaining correction of deformity, adding posterior or anterior metal implants, etc. However, protection of the dural tube and its contents is of paramount importance during and after the operation. Though the outcomes of these procedures are not very gratifying, however, many surgeons use this approach with minor modifications (Upadhyay 1994, Wong et al. 2007, Jain et al. 2007).

Surgical Correction of Severe Kyphotic Deformity without Neural Complications

Most of the general orthopedic surgeons discourage the correction of such deformities because of the complications such a procedure is fraught with. Hodgson (1965, 1969) developed operative procedures to correct fixed spinal curves. Dommisse and Enslin (1970) reported on results of correction of fixed spinal deformities in 55 patients. Complications reported were permanent paraplegia in 4 patients, death in one, and average loss of operative correction was 50%. Having exposed the deformed area of spine (vide supra) the fundamentals of correcting a fixed spinal curve are first to perform an osteotomy on the concave side of the curve and wedge it open. The second step is to remove a boney wedge on the convex side and close this wedge. This operative correction is by no means an operation to be advocated for general use, however, there might be limited indications for extreme type of deformities in the hands of especially trained surgeons (Jain et al. 2007, Wong et al. 2007, Laheri et al. 2001, Wong 2017, Rajasekaran et al. 2018) **(Fig. 24.16)**.

The spine may be exposed through the transpleural anterior approach as described by Hodgson (1969) for thoracic spine, and through combined extrapleural and extraperitoneal approach for dorsolumbar regions. The anterior region to be wedged open is cleared of all unhealthy and soft tissues so that healthy bone is available proximally and distally for strength and insertion of autogenous bone grafts. While working backwards in the direction of the spinal canal, care must be exercised to avoid damage to the cord. Corresponding spinous processes, laminae, pedicles and transverse processes are exposed. Posterior elements are excised to remove the required size of wedge. During this process, theca is visualized throughout the extent of deformity. The next step is to open the wedge anteriorly and close the gap posteriorly. This is achieved by manual pressure posteriorly at the site of convexity and simultaneous use of vertebral spreaders anteriorly. The anterior wedge is held open temporarily by sterile wooden blocks till they are replaced by massive strong autogenous iliac grafts. The posterior wedge is closed and held securely by Harrington compression rods, their hooks being firmly fixed into the proximal and distal pedicles before completely opening the anterior wedge. As the posterior wedge is being closed and the hooks are approximated, strict watch is kept on the cord. If there is any pressure on the dural tube, the appropriate amount of the bone is nibbled off. Posterior parts of the ribs above and below the deformity may have to be excised for proper closure of the posterior wedge. Jain et al. (2008, 2007) suggested a combined single stage procedure of debridement and loosening of anterior elements, substraction osteotomy of pedicles, laminae and posterior elements, posterior bone grafting with posterior instrumentation (Hartshill loop). He obtained a mean correction of kyphotic deformity by 25° (6–42°) during a period of observation of 33 months after the procedure.

Postoperatively, patients are nursed on previously prepared anterior and posterior plaster shells or on a Stryker turning frame. After 8–12 weeks, the patient can be nursed on an ordinary bed and can be gradually mobilized wearing a suitable spinal support. Louis et al. (1970) advocated correction of spinal gibbosity in tuberculous lesions of the vertebral column by slow traction and corrective plaster casts before the operation. In cases that needed surgery, the anterior fusion was done in cervical spine. In dorsal and lumbar spine correction of deformity, bone grafting and plaster bed was used. In late cases, spinal osteotomy was performed.

We would not recommend the operative correction for fixed deformities proximal to the level of lumbar second vertebra. It is safest to prevent the development of severe deformity, if severe kyphosis is anticipated (guidelines *vide supra*) the diseased area should be fused by a panvertebral operation. The deformity that is not yet fixed may be corrected (to some extent) by halopelvic or halofemoral traction before being fused by operation. The maximum upper limit of traction is 13 kg through skull and 6.5 kg through each femur, the traction should be increased very gradually with close monitoring of the long tract functions. All the correction occurs within 3–4 weeks of traction. It is dangerous to add much correction on the operation table (Tuli 1995). In the absence of facilities for intraoperative monitoring of the cord function, we consider it inappropriate to add correction while doing surgery. Intraoperative cord function monitoring has been best done (during our operations) by Stagnara's wake-up test. Electrical monitoring of spinal cord function is another option, one should however be aware of false-positive and false-negative response as well. Any correction obtained should be before surgery for the "nonfixed" element of deformity, and in the postoperative period after the "loosening" effect of surgery, especially for severe kyphotic deformities proximal to lumbar one vertebra. We attempted correction of fixed kyphotic deformity in 2 children employing a panvertebral operation and a halopelvic apparatus. One child with the apex of deformity at D11 level had permanent deterioration of neural status. The other child with the apex of deformity at L2–L3 lost 50% of postoperative correction by 2 years after surgery.

For any fixed kyphotic deformity between dorsal one to lumbar one (>60 degrees) in an adult, do not rush in for operative corrections. Despite the availability of bone substraction osteotomies, multilevel vertebrectomies and spinal instrumentation, any clinically significant operative correction may lead to neural deterioration and complications (Rajasekaran et al. 2018). Let us not convert a walker to a non-walker. It may be wiser to keep these patients under close observation, and offer operative procedures when such a patient is likely to become a non-walker.

INSTRUMENTATION IN TUBERCULOUS SPINE

Halofixation (Pieron and Welply 1972) combined with pelvic traction (O'Brien et al. 1971) or with tibial traction (Schmidt 1971) or with sacral bars (Hardy 1971) had been safely employed in the treatment of severe spine deformities. Early results of the reported cases held some hope for possible application of this method in conjunction with surgery for correction of severe kyphotic deformities in tuberculosis of the spine. Louw (1990) used vascularized rib graft after decompression for neural deficit, preoperative kyphosis of 56 degrees was corrected to 27 degrees after surgery. There are a few reports (Govender 2002, Rajasekaran 2002, Govender and Prabhoo 1999, Hassan 2003, Yilmaz et al. 1999, Chen et al. 2002) of operative treatment for spinal tuberculosis where the authors have used instrumentation. We have used concomitant posterior instrumentation in 2 patients during the last 15 years for neurological complications due to panvertebral destruction. It is, however, difficult to eradicate the fear that infection will persist around the implant when placed in the area of tuberculous infection (Oga et al. 1993). Reactivation may occur any time during the life span of the patient. Re-operation to remove the anteriorly placed implants is complex and carries much higher risks than the original insertion (Yilmaz et al. 1999, Chen et al. 2002, Govender 2002).

There are reports and claims in a few publications (Benli et al. 2007, Jayaswal et al. 2007, Yilmaz et al. 1999) regarding the safety and efficacy of use of the anterior metallic implants in active tuberculosis of spine. The author, however, is not convinced regarding the advantages and safety of inserting a metallic implant in active disease of spine with softened bones. Since the introduction of these procedures in our metropolitan cities, the author happens to see at least one new patient every year with disturbing complications associated with anterior implants. The complications that have been seen are deterioration of neural deficit, discharging sinuses or ulcers traceable to the implants, loosening and displacements of implants, and pathological subluxation/displacement at the diseased area **(Figs. 24.26, 24.27, 24.30, 24.31)**. Even the primary operating surgeons are hesitant to venture the removal. If one is impelled to use a metallic implant after anterior debridement and decompression, it is safest to use posterior implants; the implants get purchase in healthy bones and removal if warranted is simpler and safer (Jain et al. 2007, 2011, Moon et al. 1995, Garg et al. 2012).

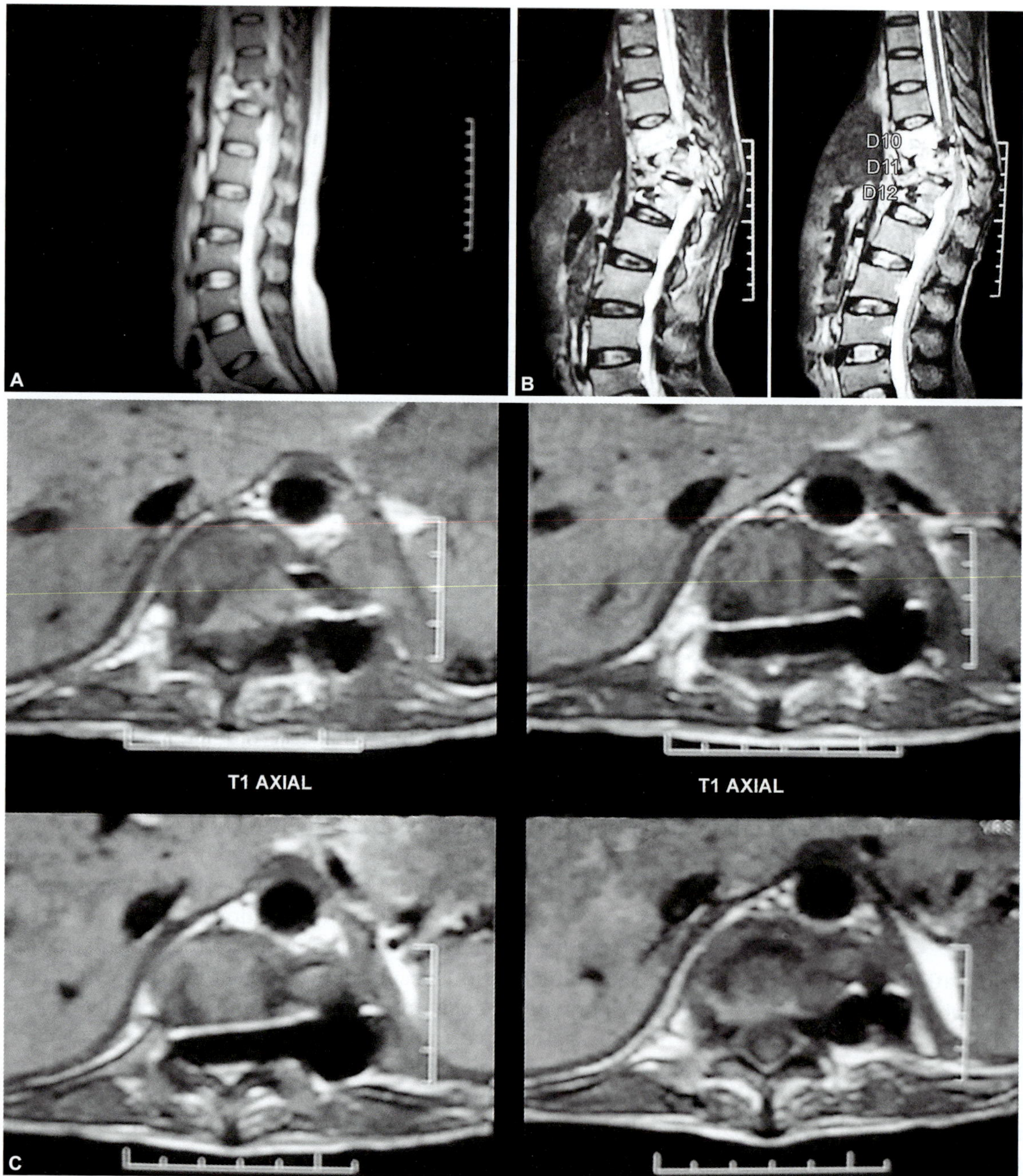

Figs. 24.26A to C: (A) Tuberculosis of D11 (predominately central type) with a paravertebral abscess presented with stage I neural signs in a 27-year-old female. Note no gross displacement of the vertebral column. (B) Anterior fixation resulted in gross anteroposterior instability and displacement. Postoperative MRI of the same patient, 2 years after operation shows the vertebral displacement, encroachment of the vertebral canal and persistence of active infection. (C) Axial cuts of MRI T1, 2 years after operation show abscesses around the implants and encroachment of the vertebral canal by the screws.

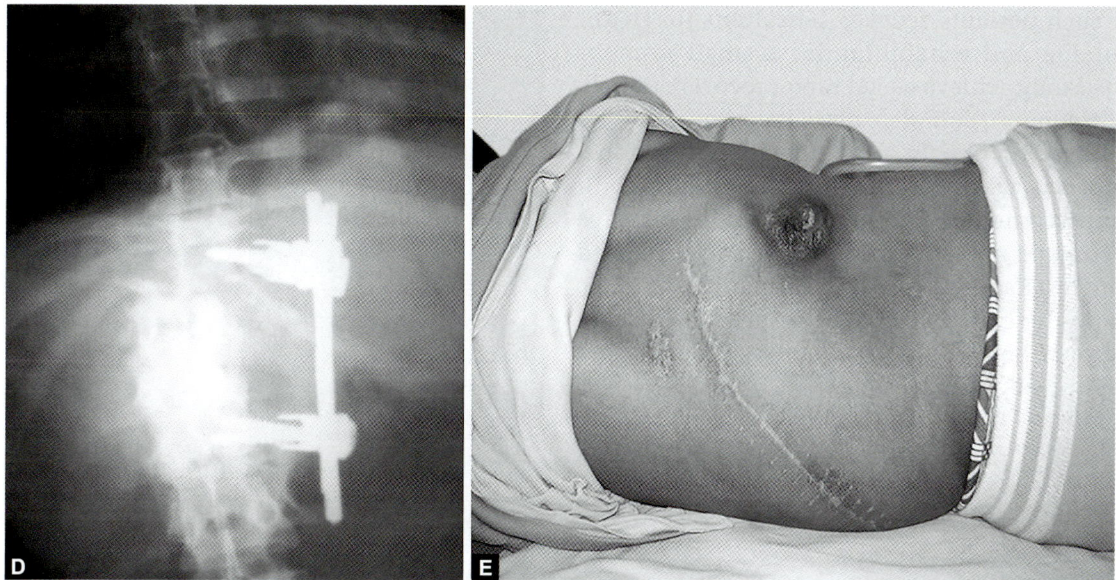

Figs. 24.26D and E: (D) The implant has disengaged. (E) The young lady remained permanently paralyzed with an indwelling catheter and discharging sinus after the ill-advised anterior implant fixation.

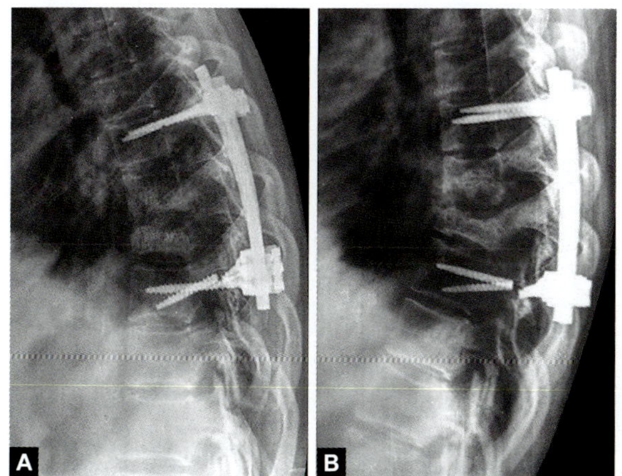

Figs. 24.27A and B: Tuberculosis of mid-dorsal spine in an adult has been fixed with posterior instrumentation for "possible stabilization". The destroyed paradiscal vertebral bodies in an adult would heal by bone formation and telescopy to some extent. The implant prevented telescoping and the metal underwent fatigue and fracture, (A) 9 months after fixation, and (B) 12 months after fixation.

RE-OPERATION FOR DECOMPRESSION

One is impelled for a repeat surgery if the earlier operation, (i) did not improve the neural status and the postoperative myelogram/MRI reveal persistent mechanical compression, or (ii) the operation was at incorrect level, or (iii) the earlier operation was an ill-advised laminectomy for the classical spondylodiscitis. As the tissue planes are lost, the reoperations are time consuming and there is more blood loss. Special care is required to minimize iatrogenic instability of the vertebral column. We as a rule perform the anterolateral decompression from the unoperated side and concomitantly do the spinal fusion placing the bone grafts on the decorticated laminae, or corresponding transverse processes where the earlier operation was laminectomy **(Figs. 24.28 and 24.29)**. Many of such patients recover sensations for better nursing and rehabilitation, a small number pleasantly achieve useful motor recovery to walk with support, complete neural recovery however seldom occurs. In very unstable situations, one may add posterior instrumentation with multisegmental fixation. Minimally invasive technique are being tried in highly specialized centers (Kandwal et al. 2012, Huang et al. 2000, Kapoor et al. 2005). These procedures are however highly complex requiring expertise and sophisticated infrastructure.

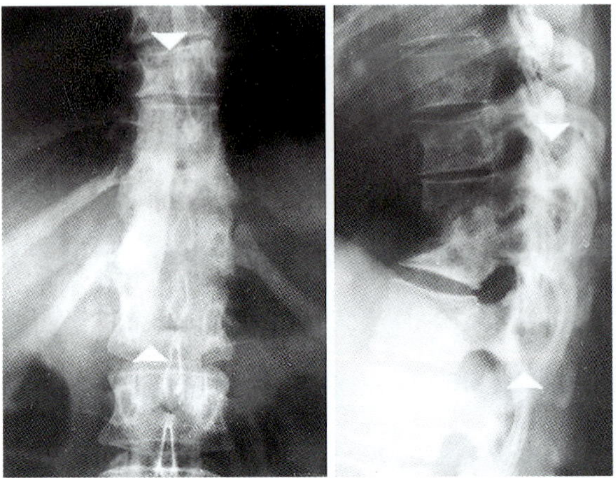

Fig. 24.28: A wrong level operation performed at D8–D9 for tuberculous paraplegia caused by D10–D11 lesion. These are follow-up X-rays 6 months after the second operation. Note the healed disease anteriorly and incorporated graft (arrow heads) on the right-sided laminae and no significant increase in deformity

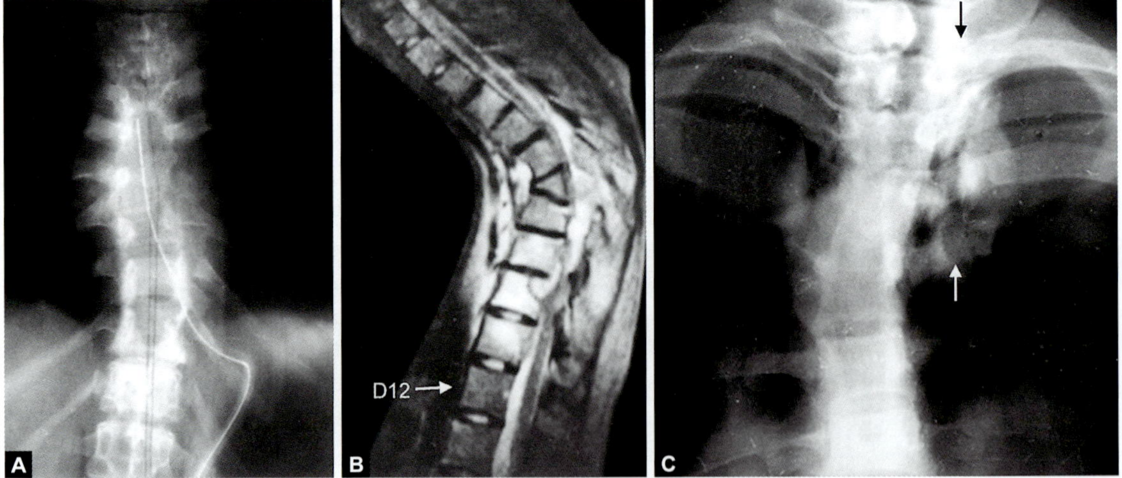

Figs. 24.29A to C: (A) Ill-advised laminectomy for classical spondylodiscitis resulted in (B) gross postoperative instability, kyphotic deformity and no neural recovery. (C) Anterolateral decompression for a similar situation was combined with inter-transverse fusion at re-operation on left side (arrow heads).

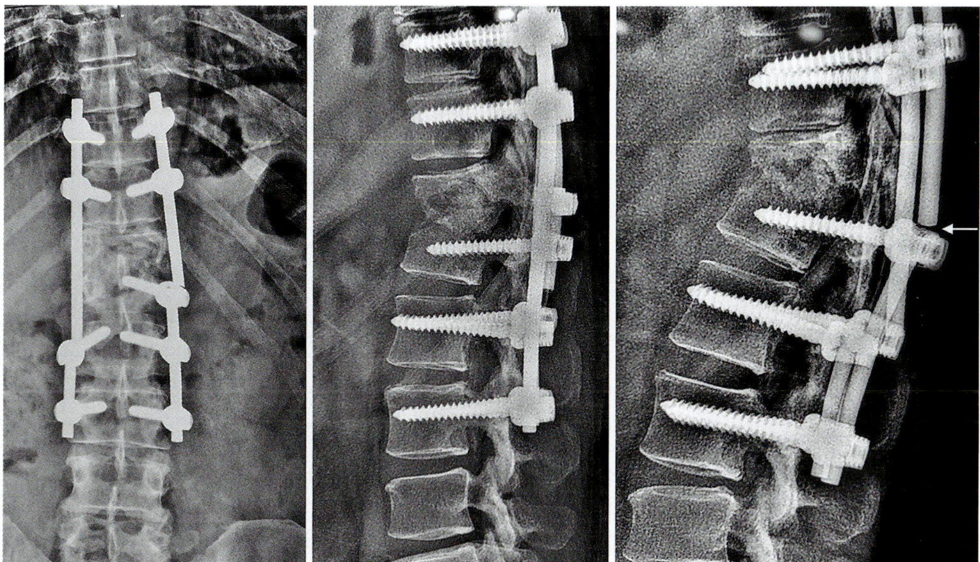

Figs. 24.30: Attempted posterior implants fixation for stabilization of active tuberculosis of D12–L1 vertebrae. Part of the implant is inserted at the site of active disease. Despite the use of anti-TB drugs and implant the activity of infection persisted and implant broke because of metal fatigue (arrow).

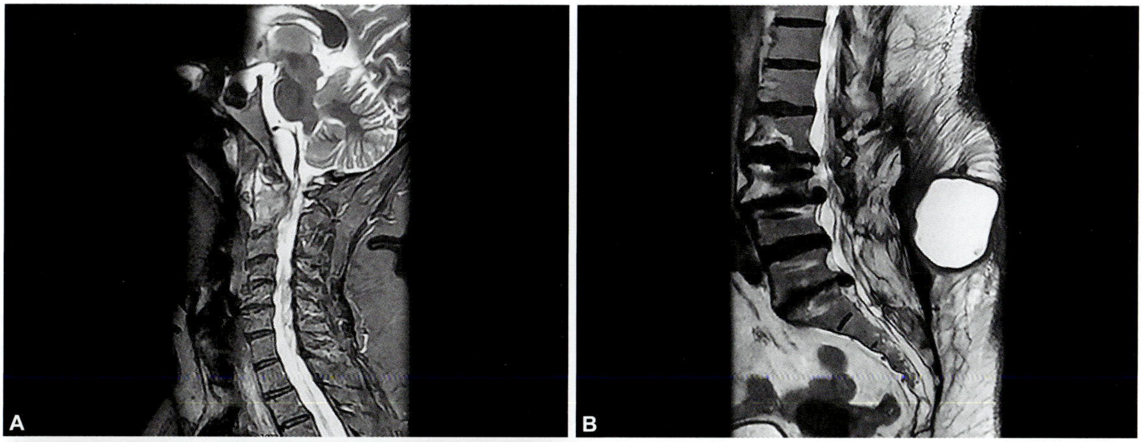

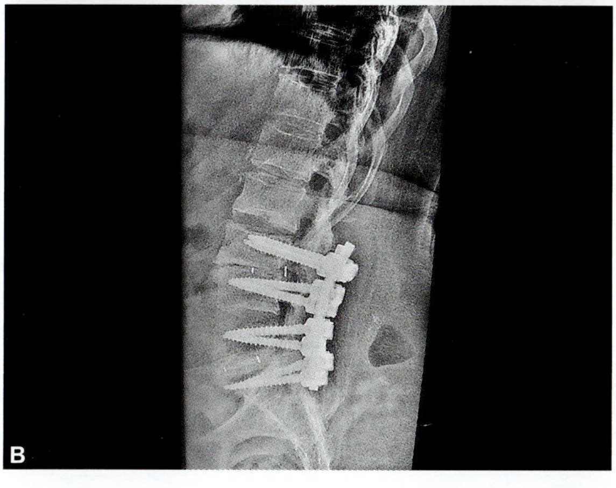

Figs. 24.31A to C: Implants in the diseased bones perpetuates the activity of infection: Observe collection of pus at the operative site. Tuberculosis at craniovertebral junction: (A) Showing involvement of C1, C2 and base of skull. (B and C) Collection of pus around the implants in lumbar spine disease.

Spinal Braces

In economically advanced countries, one is impressed with the high degree of sophistication and beauty of the orthopedic appliances. However, such appliances require the availability of material and parts which add to the cost and require especially trained technical personnel to manufacture and repair them. Plastic materials are now available in India; for preparing sophisticated braces in all metropolitan cities. The principle for making, measuring and the extent of the braces, however, remain the same. Metal and leather spinal braces are practical braces which also can be made and used effectively, especially in those countries where tuberculous disease is endemic. Such braces can be easily repaired by local artisans. Prominent bony points and ridges are protected by suitable padding with sponge rubber and felt pads. Spinal braces are mostly used for ambulation of cases of spinal tuberculosis. The nature of the brace depends on the level of the lesion **(Figs. 25.1 and 25.2)**.

For disease from *fourth dorsal to second lumbar vertebrae* the traditional spinal brace extends from the seventh cervical spine to the lower end of the sacrum. It is held closely fitting into the lumbar and dorsal region by a waist band, a band passing round between the iliac crest and the great trochanters, groin straps and shoulder straps. This **Taylor brace** may control a simple kyphotic deformity but has little control on a scoliotic deformity. The upper end of the brace, in standing posture, remains away from the spine by two fingers. The brace is bent and moulded over a kyphotic deformity. Use of a **Milwaukee brace** or a **Jewett brace** is recommended for tuberculous lesions in the dorsal spine throughout the growing age, especially if the number of vertebrae involved is more than 2, or there is panvertebral disease, or radiologically there is wedging in anteroposterior as well as in lateral views, or after performance of a panvertebral operation. Anterior spinal hyperextension **(ASH) brace** has been found to be more acceptable by young girls and ladies as it gets accommodated in the contours of the body and clothings. The rigid metal upright extends anteriorly from the symphysis pubis to manubrium sterni, a band passing around the trunk holds the upright in front and a pad over the vertebral column. In our current practice, ASH brace has replaced the Taylor brace for adults.

For disease of the upper dorsal spine involving *dorsal one to dorsal third* vertebrae, there is no simple brace to control the spine effectively. The only satisfactory method of bracing is to extend the usual spinal brace upwards with the attachment of cervical collar **(Figs. 25.3 and 25.4)**. Extended **SOMI** (Sternal Occipital Mandibular Immobilizer) brace is another option.

For disease of the cervical spine from *cervical first to cervical seventh* vertebrae, adequate splintage can be provided by a four post-collar having two vertical rods with turn-buckles in

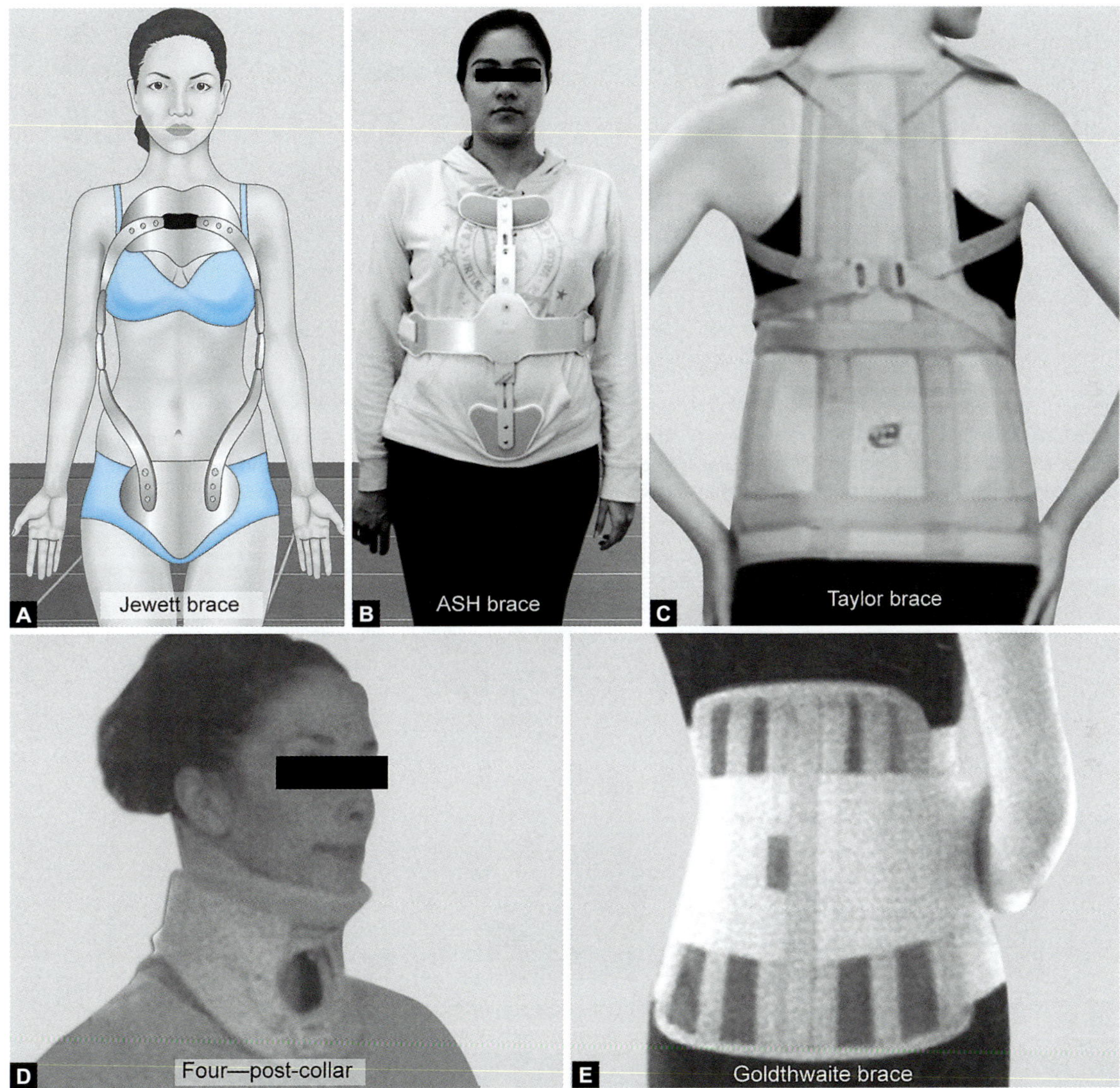

Figs. 25.1A to E: Commonly used spinal braces (A to C) for lesions from fourth dorsal to second lumbar, (D) for lesions from first to seventh cervical vertebrae, (E) for lesions from third lumbar to lumbosacral region.

front and two at the back. When the degree of destruction and the stage of healing of the disease in cervical spine requires less support, a block leather collar reinforced with aluminum strips or made of thermoplastic material is adequate (like **Philadelphia collar**). SOMI brace has been more acceptable to many patients because it eliminates the two uprights at the back of the neck, it leaves the back particularly free except the occipital pad.

When the disease involves the lower lumbar *(third lumbar and below)* and lumbosacral region a **Goldthwaite brace** or a lumbar corset of block leather or thermoplastic material provides adequate form of immobilization. This brace should be well-moulded on the back of sacrum and around the iliac crests, anteriorly the corset should be cut away in the region of the groin so that full flexion of the hip joints is possible and the patient is able to sit and squat.

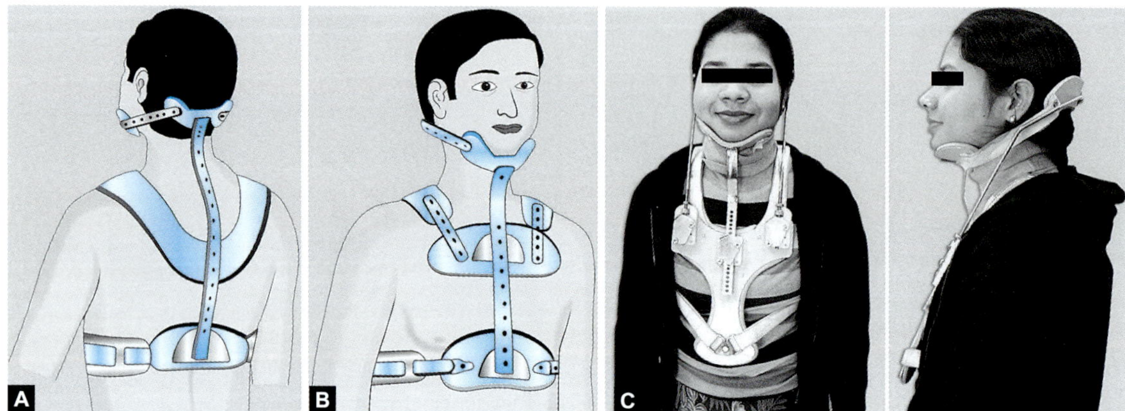

Figs. 25.2A to C: Cervicodorsal junction is a very difficult area for satisfactory bracing. A Taylor brace extended to four-post collar, or a SOMI (Sternal Occipital Mandibular Immobilizer) brace with cauded extensions shown in the figure, provides some protection. (C) A clinical photograph of an extended SOMI brace.

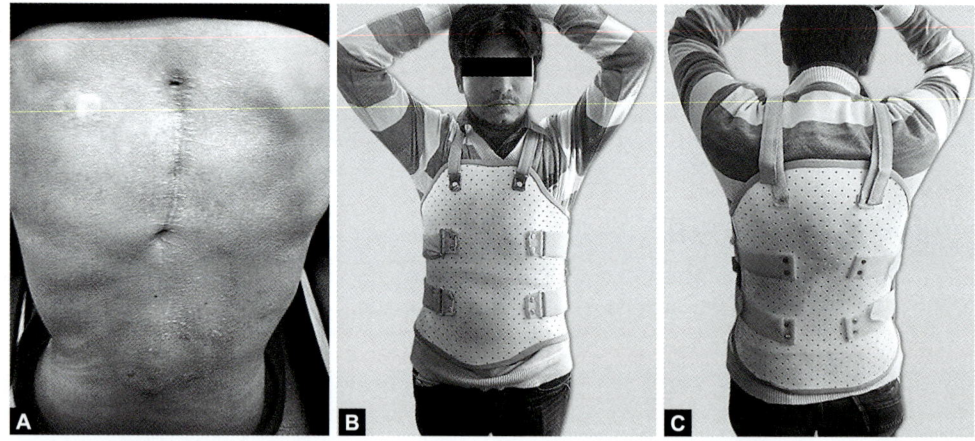

Figs. 25.3A to C: Whole spine brace for a patient of disseminated tuberculosis of spine.

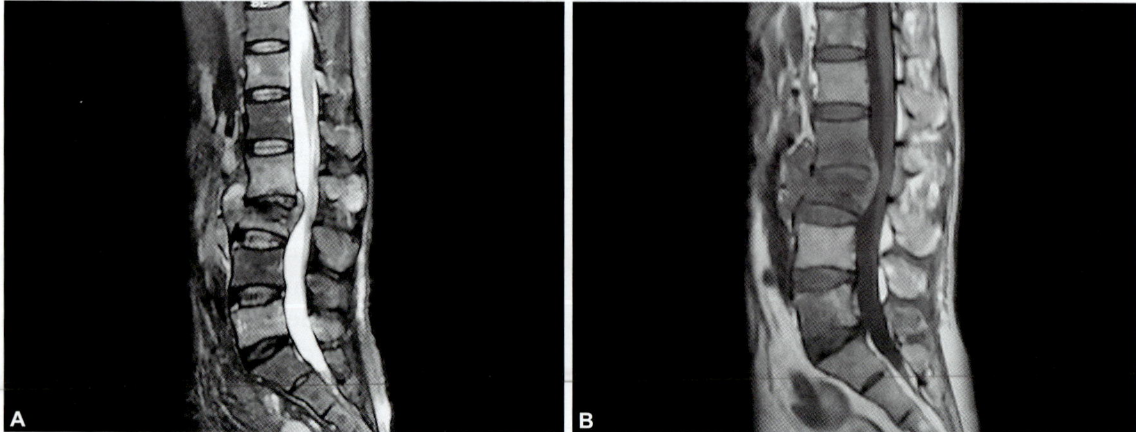

Figs. 25.4A and B: On healing of infection, the diseased bone generally gets repaired by normal bone textures, rarely however, the repaired bone may be replaced by fat: (A) At presentation (B) 2 years after healed status.

CHAPTER 26

Relevant Surgical Anatomy

VERTEBRAL BODIES

A vertebral body may be compared **(Fig. 26.1)** to a compressed long bone, with an intervertebral disc interposed between the bodies. A thin layer of hyaline cartilage intervenes between the disc and the vertebral body, sometimes regarded as part of the body and sometimes as that of intervertebral disc. The hyaline cartilage (growth plate) fits accurately over the body of the vertebra as an epiphysis which determines the growth of the vertebral bodies. The growth of the vertebral bodies occurs, as in the long bones, at these epiphyseal plates by the process of endochondral ossification. At about the age of 6 years, a ring or annular epiphysis appears as a narrow cartilaginous rim lying on the periphery of the cephalic and caudal surfaces of the respective vertebral bodies **(Fig. 26.1)**. These represent the traction epiphysis and take no part in the longitudinal growth of the vertebral column. Calcification in these ring epiphyses starts at about 8 years and they fuse with the vertebral bodies at about the age of 18 years. Thus, between 8 and 18 years of age, the ring epiphysis is visible radiologically as a separate center from the vertebral body. Such an appearance following a back injury may be misinterpreted as a chip fracture.

The interior of a vertebra is made up of cancellous bone, containing red marrow and

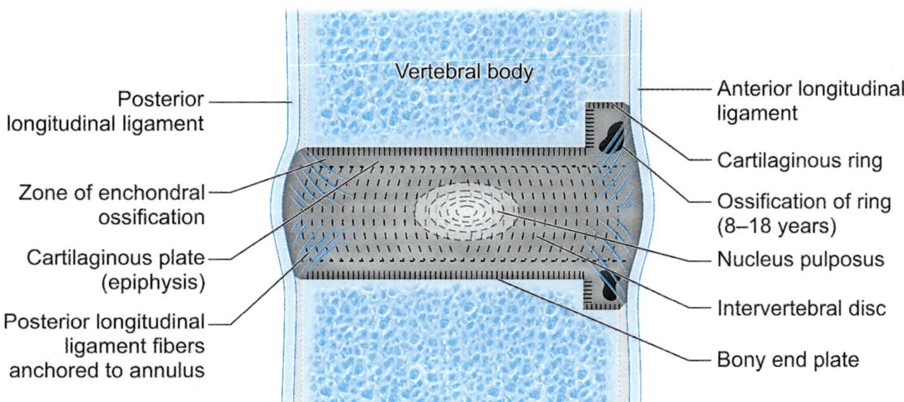

Fig. 26.1: Diagrammatic representation of sagittal section of the intervertebral disc and the adjacent vertebral bodies.
Courtesy: Turek SL. Orthopedics: Principles and their Application, 2nd edition. Lippincott, Philadelphia.

reticuloendothelial depots. The cancellous bone in each vertebral body is covered superiorly and inferiorly by a thin end plate of bone which is perforated by numerous tiny holes. The bacillemic tuberculous infection may start anywhere in the vertebral body but it is more often close to the epiphyseal plates. This area corresponds to metaphyseal region of a growing long bone which has the main lymphoreticular elements and has very rich blood supply distributed by tortuous vascular loops and arcades. The heights of the vertebral bodies are affected by the normal stresses of weight bearing during the growth period. In the absence of normal stresses, an increase in the height of the healthy vertebral bodies ("tall vertebrae") becomes manifest, as observed in patients who develop severe kyphotic deformity **(Fig. 26.2)** during their growing age. This phenomenon does not occur after discontinuance of longitudinal growth of the vertebrae.

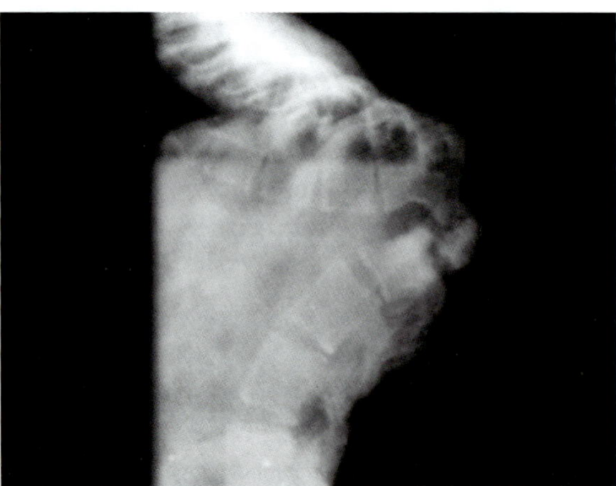

Fig. 26.2: X-ray of a patient with severe kyphotic deformity of long-standing (Walker at presentation). The disease and deformity occurred during the growing period, therefore, due to the absence of normal stresses on the vertebral column the part of the spine distal to the deformity has developed "tall vertebrae". The development of the diseased vertebral bodies is markedly restricted due to damage to their growth cartilage plates, however, unrestricted growth of their posterior elements has resulted in a kyphotic deformity of 145 degrees.

INTERVERTEBRAL JOINT

The vertebrae from the second cervical to the first sacral articulate by (i) a series of fibrocartilaginous joints formed by the intervertebral discs between the vertebral bodies, and (ii) a series of paired synovial joints between the posterior articular processes. The latter are sometimes designated as apophyseal joints. The capsule of these synovial joints is loose to permit sliding movements between the contiguous facets. A true **tubercular synovitis** may occur in these apophyseal joints, in suboccipital or in the atlantoaxial joints. A typical vertebra articulates at six articulating surfaces, two discs, two proximal facet joints, two distal facet joints. Any fusion of the vertebral column (especially long segment) leads to disturbed kinematics and results in premature adjacent level degenerative changes.

INTERVERTEBRAL DISC

The fibrocartilaginous interverterbal discs lie between the bodies of the vertebrae **(Fig. 26.1)**. They function chiefly as fluctuant shock absorbers and are liable to be affected by trauma, degenerative changes, infections and other diseases. The vertical height and circumference of the intervertebral discs correspond to the size of the intervening vertebrae, being small in the cervical region and correspondingly large in the lumbar spine. The configuration of the discs contributes to the curvature of the vertebral column, being thicker on the convex side of the curves of the vertebral column.

Each disc is composed of a semigelatinous central portion, the **nucleus pulposus**, and a thick peripheral ring of lamellated fibrous tissue, the **annulus fibrosus**, both separated from the bodies of the adjacent vertebrae by a thin cartilaginous plate. The fibers of the annulus are attached to the cartilage plates, anterior and posterior longitudinal ligaments and to the edges of the vertebral bodies. The nucleus pulposus develops from notochord and is composed of a white glistening mucoid material. It has been estimated that in the lumbar spine, in an average healthy young adult the gelatinous material is under a pressure of 10–15 kg to a square centimeter, while loaded in the standing position, the intradiscal pressure is 50% less in recumbent position. In case of an area of deficiency in the hyaline cartilage and bone end plate, the nucleus pulposus sometimes herniates into the cancellous bone of the vertebral bodies, where it may get encircled by reactive bone to become a Schmorl's node. In osteoporosis, and generalized demineralizing state the nucleus may bulge the bony end plate inwards, causing characteristic biconcave vertebral bodies and biconvex intervertebral disc spaces. The intervertebral discs (white in T2 MRI) present maximal elasticity up to 30th year of life. As age advances, the water content of the nucleus falls (black in MRI), its elasticity diminishes, the nucleus becomes granular and friable; the annulus becomes progressively thinner and weaker, and the discs show gradual attrition. With degeneration or attrition of the disc, transmission of forces of weight has to be borne more by the vertebral bodies, posterior elements and the facet joints. In old age, when the discs are dehydrated, osteoporosis initially would show as depression of the proximal end-plates (due to body weight) of vertebral bodies.

In fetal life, small blood vessels penetrate the annulus from the vertebrae, but these regress soon after birth. By the age of about 18 years, the disc is practically avascular. The nutrition of the intervertebral disc is apparently dependent on the diffusion of fluid from the adjacent vertebral bodies.

BLOOD SUPPLY OF THE VERTEBRAL COLUMN

Blood supply of the vertebrae follows the embryological pattern, branches from each segmental intercostal artery or lumbar artery supplying adjacent halves of two vertebrae, the lower half of the one above and the upper half of the one below and the intervening disc region. This occurs because the adjacent part of any two vertebrae and the intervertebral disc develop from the same somites. One vertebral body has developed from four somites, two of the left and two of the right side, thus each vertebral body gets blood supply from four arterial systems. Inside the vertebral bodies the arterioles terminate as tortuous loops under the epiphyseal end plates, where it is suggested that they lack anastomosis with each other and behave functionally as endarteries (Somerville and Wilkinson 1965). If these end-arteries are blocked an infarct may result. It has been shown by injection techniques in fresh cadavers, that each vertebral body may have 15–18 nutrient arteries with a free central anastomosis (Schmorl and Junghanns 1959). Spread of infection through the arterial route, offers an explanation for the most frequent early localization of spinal tuberculous lesions in the very vascular juxta epiphyseal (metaphyseal), paradiscal areas of the vertebral bodies. In addition to the spread of infection through the arterial flow, it is possible that the epidural and peridural plexus of veins, described by Batson (1940), also plays a part in the localization of lesions in some cases of spinal tuberculosis. The veins from the vertebral column drain into Batson's perivertebral plexus of veins, the largest veins from the vertebrae emerge from the posterior aspect of bodies to join the postcentral anastomosis. The plexus has ramifications into the base of brain and chest wall and has free anastomosis with the intercostal, lumbar and pelvic veins. The blood in the Batson's plexus probably flows in all the directions depending upon the movements of chest, coughing and straining. Retrograde flow of blood from infected viscera to the spine may be responsible for spread of infection from the diseased organs to the vertebral column. However, as yet it is uncertain whether the spread of infection is by paravertebral plexus of veins or by the lymphatics in the walls of the veins (Hodgson et al. 1969). The spread along Batson's perivertebral plexus may account for the frequent observation of involvement of multiple adjacent vertebrae, the presence of multiple skipped lesions in the spinal column, the association of tuberculous abscesses on the chest wall with vertebral tuberculosis and the special association of tuberculous meningitis with spinal tuberculosis particularly in children.

THE BONY VERTEBRAL CANAL

It is relatively larger (than the corresponding spinal cord) and is of triangular outline in the cervical and lumbar regions where free movements also occur. However, its size is smaller in the thoracic region where it is of circular outline and has limited motion. Thus, even minor space occupying lesions at the thoracic level lead to early interference of the cord functions. In fact, this region was designated as the "paraplegic level" by Butler and Seddon (1935) who stated that 85% paraplegic complications occur in the thoracic region.

BLOOD SUPPLY TO THE SPINAL CORD

Blood reaches the spinal cord by way of an anterior and two posterior spinal arteries **(Figs. 26.3 and 26.4)**. The anterior spinal artery is formed by the union of branches from the terminal portion of the vertebral arteries at the level of foramen magnum. This artery descends as a single trunk on the anterior surface of the spinal cord and terminates along the filum terminale. Posterior arteries which may be duplicated in parts, also begin as branches of the vertebral artery near the lateral margin of medulla oblongata and descend on the dorsolateral surface of the spinal cord (posterior to the spinal roots) to the cauda equina. During their course downwards these arteries receive a succession of small segmental arterial branches, as anterior and posterior radicular arteries, which enter the spinal canal **(Fig. 26.4)** through the intervertebral foramina. Electrocoagulation at intervertebral foramina or medial to it must be avoided.

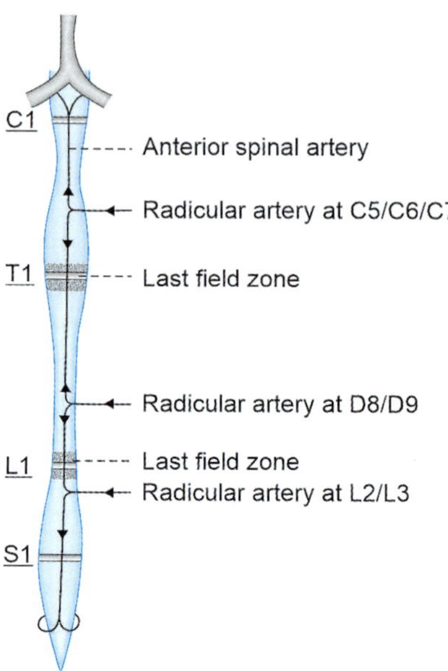

Fig. 26.3: Anterior spinal artery showing the probable direction of blood flow and major anterior radicular arteries. The shaded areas indicate the "last field" zones.

The radicular arteries originate at respective levels from vertebral arteries, the intercostal arteries, the iliolumbar and the sacral arteries. Of particular importance are six to eight large anterior radicular arteries (Epstein 1965, Chakravorty 1969), the largest of which is the **arteria radicularis magna** or the great spinal artery of Adamkiewicz which originates from a left intercostal or lumbar artery between the 10th thoracic and second lumbar segments and passes on a lumbar ventral nerve root to the cord. Next in size are those in the cervical and lower thoracic regions as shown in the diagram **(Fig. 26.3)**. The areas of the cord best supplied with blood are those in proximity to these large anterior radicular arteries. The caudad and cephalad ends of the respective vessels usually provide less blood to the corresponding spinal segments. These "last field" zones are most likely to suffer from an insufficiency of blood. In general, these areas are situated at about the junction of cervicodorsal segments and the dorsolumbar segments **(Fig. 26.3)**. The anterior

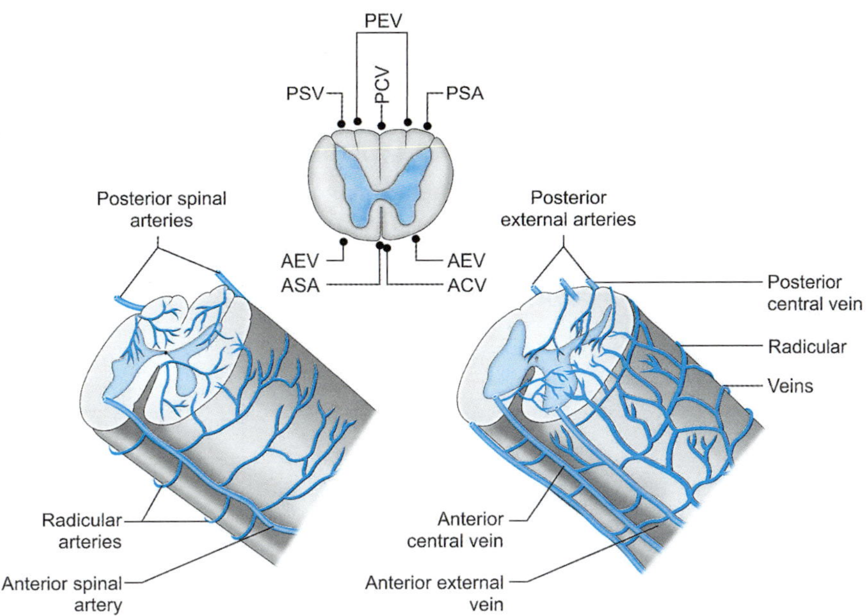

Fig. 26.4: Arteries and veins of spinal cord shown in horizontal section.
(ACV: anterior central vein; AEV: anterior external vein; ASA: anterior spinal artery; PCV: posterior central vein; PEV: posterior external vein; PSA: posterior spinal artery)

spinal artery supplies approximately the anterior two-thirds of the transverse area of the spinal cord. The remaining posterior part is supplied by the 2 posterior spinal arteries. These anastomose freely, and send communicating vessels to those of the anterior spinal artery. Minor variations even in the main supplying arteries are not at all uncommon.

Interference with the blood supply of the spinal cord may be a rare complication of inflammatory endarteritis or thrombosis. Ischemia of the cord may also result from extensive or repeated surgical intervention on the vertebral column. Isolated anterior spinal artery thrombosis may lead to symptoms primarily involving the motor tracts. More extensive involvement may result in complete and permanent loss of cord function.

CROSS-SECTIONAL TOPOGRAPHY OF THE SPINAL CORD

Gross configuration of cross-sections of the cord is clearly delineated on axial T2 MRI scans or CT myelogram sections. One can see the central gray matter having a characteristic **butterfly or H-shaped** configuration formed by the dorsal and ventral horns. The white matter is composed of 3 funiculi on right and left halves each, divided into anterior, lateral, and posterior funiculi by the dorsal and ventral horns. The middle of the gray matter is traversed by the central canal, lined by the ependymal cells, and containg cerebrospinal fluid (CSF). The dialatation of the ependymal canal is called hydromyelia, whereas **syringomyelia** is defined as CSF dissection through the ependymal lining to form a paracentral cavity. Often both these conditions coexist and intercommunicate, and are grouped as **hydrosyrinomyelia**. With the availability of MRI and CT scans such cavitations have been observed by us in a few cases of long-standing tuberculous paraplegics.

The spinal cord ends as conus medullaris, at about the level of lumbar one vertebral body. The lumbosacral nerve roots, however, continue distally contained in the dural sac as cauda equina. The segmental nerve roots leave the dural sac at appropriate levels, each nerve distal to the vertebra of the same member, from D1 to S5.

Normally, the odontoid tip is <5 mm above the McGregor's line (posterior edge of hard palate to the lower point on the occiput). Any destructive lesion at atlanto-occipital joint may lead to proximal (basilar) migration of odontoid process with neural complications. Basilar invagination, >5 mm upward migration of odontoid process is generally associated with complications. In the lateral images of cervical spine usually hyoid bone is seen at the level of cervical 3rd vertebral body, thyroid cartilage is at the level of C4–C5 vertebral bodies and cricoid cartilage is at the level of C6 vertebral body. The dural sac continues up to the level of sacral two vertebra.

Take Home Key Points

Apurv Mehra

Chapter 1: Epidemiology and Prevalence

It is estimated that India alone has got one-fifth of the total world population of tuberculous patients. Of all the patients suffering from tuberculosis, nearly 1–3% have involvement of the skeletal system.

Regional Distribution in TB-endemic Countries

- The most common chronic vertebral infection, however, is tuberculosis.
- Vertebral tuberculosis is the most common form of skeletal tuberculosis.
- Mandible and temporomandibular joint appear to be the least common location.
- The most common cause of chronic osteomyelitis of rib is tuberculosis.

Prophylaxis against Tuberculosis and BCG Vaccination

The protection afforded by BCG in the control of tuberculosis is estimated to be in the region of 80%. For prophylaxis isoniazid is usually used in a dose of 5 mg/kg body weight daily continued for at least 6 months. We prefer a combination of isoniazid and rifampicin for 4–6 months.

Chapter 2: Pathology and Pathogenesis

Hematogenous dissemination from a primarily infected visceral focus. Based upon radiologist observations nearly 7% of cases of spinal tuberculosis had "skipped lesions" in the vertebral column and 12% had involvement of other bones and joints in addition to spine.

Osteoarticular Disease

- Articular cartilage destruction begins peripherally.
- Initial focus starts in the metaphysis in the growing age, and at the end of the bone in adults.
- Cartilaginous tissue is resistant to tuberculous destruction.
- In patients who have optimum or competent immunity, the disease generally starts as tuberculous synovitis and the course is usually slow.
- Flakes or loose sheets of necrosed articular cartilage, and accumulations of fibrinous material in the synovial fluid may produce "rice bodies" in synovial joints.
- Necrosis of subchondral bone by the ingrowth of tuberculous granulation tissue (pannus) on each side of the joint line may develop "kissing lesion" and/or "kissing sequestra".

Spinal Disease: Typical paradiscal lesion and tubercular foci in the extremities are considered due to spread by way of arteries.

The Tubercle: Epithelioid cells are the characteristic feature of the tuberculous reaction. Langhans giant cells are probably formed by fusion of a number of epithelioid cells, these are formed only if caseation necrosis has occurred, and often they contain tubercle bacilli.

Cold Abscess: A cold abscess is formed by a collection of products of liquefaction and the reactive exudation.

Tubercular Sequestra: Following the infection, marked hyperemia and severe osteoporosis takes place. As a result of ischemic changes sometimes sequestration takes place usually appearing as "coarse sand" and rarely forming a definite radiologically visible sequestrum. The intervertebral disc is not involved by disease; the size diminishes because of lack of its nutrition (blood supply). Pressure on neural structures is more likely in the thoracic spine where the caliber of the vertebral canal is relatively small, but it also contains the cord and not cauda equina.

Types of the Disease: Caseous exudative type.

Granular Type: The lesion in children is generally "caseous exudative type" while in adults it is more likely to be of "granular type" with minimal destruction.

Immunopathology of Skeletal Tuberculosis

Mycobacterium tuberculosis and *Homo sapiens* have lived in symbiosis since the ascent of man on earth. The helper subset of T-lymphocytes are central to cell-mediated immunity against tuberculous infection.

Immunodeficient Stage and Looming Tuberculosis Epidemic

The most alarming features are that people with AIDS virus are getting infected with atypical tuberculous bacilli (which were earlier considered generally non-pathogenic), and many of these strains already show resistance to a large number of antitubercular drugs. The incidence of tuberculosis in patients with AIDS is almost 500 times the incidence in the general population (Barnes et al. 1991).

Immunomodulation

The following outline is suggested: 150 mg of levamisol is given at night for 3 consecutive days at weekly intervals for a total of 45 tablets. Four injections are administered once a month. The first and second are 0.1 mL intradermal BCG injections, and the third and fourth are intramuscular DPT (diphtheria + pertussis + tetanus vaccine) injections.

Chapter 3: The Organism and its Sensitivity

Mycobacterium Tuberculosis

- Most of the skeletal tuberculosis is now caused by bacilli of human type.
- Ideally speaking the diagnosis of tuberculous infection should be confirmed by the demonstration of tubercle bacilli in the skeletal tuberculous lesion.

Mycobacterium Cultures

In our efforts at Banaras Hindu University, positive results were obtained in 60% of cases of osteoarticular tuberculosis. Osteoarticular disease is a paucibacillary infection.

Disease Caused by Atypical Mycobacteria

Typical mycobacteria are as a rule not resistant to more than one main drug, whereas most of the atypical mycobacteria are found resistant to many commonly used drugs.

Chapter 4: Evolution of Treatment of Skeletal Tuberculosis

Natural Course of Skeletal Tuberculosis without Chemotherapy: The diseases passed through three stages spanned over a period of 3–5 years. The stage of onset (synovial disease). In the second stage of destruction. The survivors entered the third stage of repair and ankylosis, occurring after 2–3 years of onset of the disease. In prechemotherapy era by the end of 5 years after diagnosis: 50% were dead, 25% were living with grumbling disease and 25% had healed status.

Post-antitubercular Era

Most of the workers at present continue the chemotherapeutic regime for 12–18 months. For optimal results, the drugs must be used in combination, for a long time and uninterruptedly. Remarkable healing of osteoarticular tuberculosis with drugs alone occurs especially in patients treated at predestructive and early destructive stage of disease. Osseous tubercular lesions are relatively more resistant than synovial lesions.

Sinuses and Ulcers

Under the influence of antitubercular drugs most of the sinuses heal within 3–4 months without surgical intervention.

Relapse of the Disease or Recurrence

Modern antitubercular drugs are the most important therapeutic measures in skeletal tuberculosis. Anti-tubercular drugs must be continued for about 18 months and must include isoniazid.

Chapter 5: Diagnosis and Investigations

General Clinical Picture: Skeletal tuberculosis mostly occurs during first three decades of life; no age, however, is immune. During sleep, the muscle spasm relaxes and permits movement between the inflamed surfaces resulting in pain causing the typical night cries (especially in children).

Diagnosis: In the affluent societies, corticosteroids, alcoholism, prolonged illness, diabetic state, anticancer chemotherapy, immunosuppressive drug therapy (in organ transplants), and old age are the probable predisposing factors.

Roentgenogram

- Localized osteoporosis is the first radiological sign of active disease.
- The synovial fluid, thickened synovium, capsule and pericapsular tissues may cause a soft tissue swelling. With the involvement of articular cartilage, the joint space (articular cartilage space shows diminution in the X-rays).
- In the center of a tuberculous cavity, there may be a sequestrum of cancellous bone or calcification of the caseous tissue, which gives an appearance of an irregular soft, feathery, coke-like sequestrum.
- The subperiosteal reaction occurs much earlier in pyogenic arthritis. Plaques of irregular calcification (dystrophic calcification) if present in the wall of a chronic abscess or sinus, is almost diagnostic of tuberculous infection of long-standing.

Blood: Raised ESR, however, is not necessarily a proof of activity of the infection. Repeated estimation at 3–6 months intervals gives a valuable index to the activity of the disease.

Mantoux (Heaf) Test: A negative test, in general, rules out the disease. A positive test suggests exposed to infection. Positive test converting to negative may suggest immunocompromise.

Biopsy: Epitheliod cells surrounded by lymphocytes in the configuration of a tubercle (even without central necrosis or peripheral foreign-body giant cells) is an adequate histological evidence of tuberculous pathology in a patient who has been diagnosed so clinicoradiologically.

Examination of Synovial Fluid: The glucose content is markedly reduced, protein levels are elevated with a poor mucin clot. Synovial joint aspirate is an excellent material for polymerase chain reaction (PCR) for tuberculosis.

Modern Imaging Techniques: Show the predestructive lesions like edema or inflammation of the bone in active disease.

Chapters 6 and 7: Principles of Management of Osteoarticular Tuberculosis Anti-TB Drugs

Stage I: Synovitis
Range of movements present is >75%.

Stage II: Early arthritis
There is preservation of movements between 50 and 75%.

Stage III: Advanced arthritis
There is nearly 75% loss of movements and the restriction is in all directions.

Stage IV: Advanced arthritis with subluxation or dislocation
Wandering/migrating acetabulum

Surgery in Tuberculosis of Bones and Joints: No surgical resection is a substitute for a prolonged course of antitubercular drugs and supportive therapy.

Extent and Type of Surgery: Fusion of a major joint is now rarely indicated as a primary mode of treatment. "Functional treatment" for articular tuberculosis is helpful in majority.

Chapter 8: Tuberculosis of the Hip Joint

- Next only to spinal tuberculosis. Starts from acetabular roof.
- Rarely, the disease may start in the synovial membrane.
- When the initial focus starts in the acetabular roof, the joint involvement is late.
- *Cold abscess*: Femoral triangle, medial, lateral or posterior aspects of thigh, ischiorectal fossa, or pelvis.
- Along the neighboring vessels and nerves to reach the surface.

Clinical Features

- First three decades
- The limp is the earliest and commonest symptom
- Muscle spasm in lower abdominal muscles, and in the adductors of the thigh on attempting sudden abduction-external rotation at the hip joint.

Stage I: Tubercular synovitis

- Irritable hip
- Only extremes of movements are limited and painful.

Stage II: Early arthritis
Spasm of adductors and flexors the hip assumes a deformity of flexion, adduction (presenting as apparent shortening) and internal rotation. True/real shortening of not >1 cm.

Stage III: Advanced arthritis
Nearly 75% loss of movements and the restriction is in all directions. True shortening of >1 cm.

Stage IV: Advanced arthritis with subluxation or dislocation

- Upper end of femur may displace upwards and dorsally in the wandering or migrating acetabulum, may have protrusio acetabuli, mortar and pestle appearance.
- Flexion, abduction and external rotation with the lateral aspect of thigh of the diseased hip resting on the bed. This may be due to continuous adoption of the latter posture for relief of pain, or due to the destruction of iliofemoral Y ligament by the tuberculous process.
- *Coxa magna*: Resembling acetabular "dysplasia". Coxa vara may also occur rarely.

Classification of Radiological Appearance

Normal appearance, travelling acetabulum, dislocated hip, Perthes type, protrusion acetabuli, atrophic type, mortar and pestle type, coxa breva. If the joint space was reduced to 3 mm or less, the outcome could be predicted as poor for motion.

Prognosis

- Early disease may heal leaving a normal or nearly normal hip joint.
- Healing in the state of advanced arthritis generally results in fibrous ankylosis.

Management

- All patients during active stage are treated by multidrug therapy, and traction to correct the deformity (if present) and to give rest to the part.
- Traction relieves the muscle spasm, prevents or corrects deformity and subluxation, maintains the joint space, minimizes the chances of development of migrating acetabulum and permits close observation of the hip. Palpable cold abscess may be aspirated.
- Usually after 4–6 months of treatment the patient may be permitted ambulation with suitable orthosis and crutches.
- The ideal position for ankylosis of hip joint in adults is neutral between abduction and adduction, 5–10 degrees of external rotation, and flexion depending upon age (between 10 degrees in children and 30 degrees in adults).

Management in Children: Traction

Osteotomy

- Sound ankylosis in bad position require upper femoral corrective osteotomy.
- The ideal site for corrective osteotomy is as near the deformed joint as possible.

Arthrodesis

- Direct intracapsular fusion is favored.
- Healed or active disease after the completion of growth potential of bones of the hip joint. This procedure provides a painless hip joint. At present rarely indicated.
- Some degree of shortening (3.5–5 cm) is unavoidable.

Stage of Disease and Operative Procedure

- Arthrotomy and synovectomy
- Some cases maintain good functional range of movements. Other options are osteotomy, sound arthrodesis, Girdlestone's type excisional arthroplasty or by total joint replacement in selected cases in adults.
- One may try total joint arthroplasty about 1–3 years after complete healing of infection.

Surgical Approaches to the Hip Joint

- The anterior iliofemoral approach or anterolateral approach.
- In the proximal part of the plane, about 5 cm distal to the hip joint, one may find a leash of blood vessels (from lateral femoral circumflex artery) entering into the medial surface of tensor fasciae lata muscle.
- This incision of the capsule divides the reflected head of the rectus femoris that blends with the capsule at the superior margin or the capsule.

Alternative Approaches

- Southern approach of Moore, because he came from southern part of USA.
- Relatively little bleeding occurs because the split is through the water-shed or superior gluteal artery (supplying the proximal half of gluteus maximus) and inferior gluteal artery (supplying the distal half).

Joint Debridement or Joint Clearance

- The synovectomy at the best is a subtotal one but nevertheless is adequate.
- Possible complications of synovectomy and debridement include avascular necrosis of femoral head, slippage of the proximal femoral epiphysis in children, and fracture of the femoral neck or acetabulum.

Arthrodesis

- Almost eliminated the absolute indications.
- Effect of arthrodesis of the hip joint on early development of degenerative osteoarthrosis in the lumbosacral spine, ipsilateral knee, and contralateral hip.
- More than 18 years of age the best position for fusion of the hip joint is 10–30 degrees of flexion (depending upon age), no abduction or adduction (in adults), and 5–10 degrees of external rotation.

Excision Arthroplasty of Hip Joint

- Divide the femoral head and acetabular rim flush with the outer surface of the ileum, divide the femoral neck at its base a little proximal and parallel to the intertrochanteric line. One can err to make the bone section a little more horizontal, but it is unwise to err to make it more vertical. Postoperatively traction in 30–50 degrees of abduction maintained for 2–4 months, along with exercises.
- After 3 months of operation, the patients were encouraged to walk using a walker or crutches. The crutches were usually discarded 5–9 months after the operation and the patient was advised to use a walking stick generally in the contralateral hand. Shortening can be minimized.

Instability in Excision Arthroplasty: Supplementary operations are suggested, especially for the young patients; pelvic support osteotomy.

Replacement Arthroplasty: Over-zealous replacement in active disease did not result in impressive improvement in hip function. Mobility in general was considerably improved if operated after healed status.

Relevant Surgical Anatomy of the Hip Joint

- The opening of the acetabulum faces laterally, downwards (about 30 degrees), and forwards (about 30 degrees).
- The forward inclination or the angle of anteversion in an adult is 10–30 degrees.

- Neck-shaft angle is 125 degrees. A neck-shaft angle of <125 degrees is referred to as coxa vara and the angle >125 degrees (i.e., more vertical neck) is called coxa valga.
- The weakest (thinnest) part of the hip joint capsule is situated posteriorly, and the femoral head is most vulnerable to posterior dislocation in flexion-adduction position of the hip joint.

Chapter 9: Tuberculosis of the Knee Joint

The knee joint is the largest joint in the body.

Pathology

As a rule, osseous erosion by the pannus starts at the site of synovial reflections, i.e., at the margins of the articular cartilage, and the capsular attachments. In advanced stage—triple dislocation (triple deformity), i.e., flexion of joint, posterior subluxation of tibia, lateral subluxation and lateral rotation, and abduction of tibia.

Clinical Features

- Appreciated earliest in medial parapatellar fossa.
- Thickened synovium gives a boggy (doughy or semielastic) feel and can be rolled between the fingers and the underlying femur. It is best palpated on the medial side of knee because vastus medialis remains muscular up to its insertion to patella and wasting is appreciated early.
- In the synovial disease only terminal restriction of movements, quadriceps muscles show gross wasting and there is regional lymphadenopathy.
- Currently articular tuberculosis is best managed by "functional treatment".

Differential Diagnosis

- In doubtful cases, biopsy for histological and microbiological investigations is mandatory.
- However, a negative PCR does not exclude tuberculosis.
- PCR positive can be false positive in TB endemic countries.

Treatment

Nonoperative treatment with antitubercular drugs is employed in tubercular synovitis and in children.

Operative Treatment

Arthroplasty operations are now considered more rational for healed status of advanced disease in adults. Arthrodesis may be considered as a rare indication for post-arthroplasty uncontrolled infection.

Surgical Techniques

Synovectomy of Knee Joint

- Most of the synovectomies are subtotal.
- The surgeon before closure should test if one can achieve at least 90 degrees of flexion of the knee joint easily. Any obstructing intra-articular lesion or extra-articular adhesions should be cut carefully, capsulectomy or capsulotomy performed, to obtain the desired flexion on the operation table.

Synovectomy with Debridement (Joint Clearance)

The pannus when present is stripped off the underlying articular surfaces. Smaller areas of destruction are curetted. Larger areas of destruction on articular surfaces and margins are curetted and filled up with cancellous bone grafts obtained from nearby healthy bone. If >50% of articular cartilage is destroyed the outcome is likely to be less than half of the normal range of joint motion. Synovectomy and joint debridement can also be done by arthroscopic procedure.

Postoperative Regimen for Synovectomy with or without Debridement

- Knee joint kept in about 5–10 degrees of flexion with the help of a rolled towel or a small pillow behind the knee. Exercises at ankle and static quadriceps exercises are started the same evening. Within a day or two of the operation, knee bending exercises active (or +/– assisted) are done within the range of tolerable pain at hourly basis. In the presence of deformity postoperative traction may be needed.
- *Ambulation*: Started about one month after the operation when the patient can perform knee flexion to 90 degrees and is able to lift the limb with extended knee against gravity. Crutches are gradually discarded between 3 and 6 months, and orthosis is gradually discarded between 18 and 24 months.

Arthrodesis of the Knee Joint

- This operation may be now rarely indicated in advanced tubercular arthritis stage IV with triple dislocation or especially after failed or uncontrolled infection after joint replacement.
- A patient with gross ankylosis (with or without deformity) has nothing to lose except "pain" after arthrodesis. Whenever in doubt, the "acceptability test" of this operation is advisable by simulating the functional restrictions imposed by arthrodesis of the knee joint.
- No more than a few degrees (5–15 degrees) of flexed position of arthrodesis is desirable. There should be no lateral angulation. The neutral position in the long axis of leg is achieved by the screw-home movement of the tibia, placing the tibial tubercle a little lateral to the midline of thigh (giving 5–7 degrees of external rotation).
- Charnley's compression apparatus was used as a routine for arthrodesis.

- Appropriate antibiotic and chemotherapy is continued for 12–18 months.
- In patients with severe flexion deformity (>90 degrees), care must be taken to prevent damage to the neurovascular bundles by sudden correction of deformity.
- About 8 cm of upper end of fibula is excised to relieve any tension on the lateral popliteal nerve on straightening the knee.

Arthroplasty for Tuberculous Arthritis

- After completing 18 months course of ATT at least 1–3 years disease-free period must be there.
  Note: Disease-free refers to the entire body should be disease free.
- Arthrodesis may be the only practical option for uncontrolled infection after joint replacement.

Relevant Surgical Anatomy of the Knee Joint

Any disease involving the synovium would easily extend to the communicating synovial prolongations and present as popliteal cysts/swellings. The cruciate ligaments are intracapsular and extrasynovial.

Chapter 10: Tuberculosis of the Ankle and Foot

Tuberculosis of Ankle: Synovium, especially in children.

Clinical Features: The ankle joint is usually held in plantar flexion.

Management: Nonoperative functional treatment in most of the patients.

Operative Treatment

Surgery is indicated for cases that are not responding to antitubercular drugs, or when the diagnosis is in doubt. Arthrodesis of ankle or pantalar arthrodesis should be restricted to cases with persistent pain or deformity and never solely for the radiological evidence of joint damage.

Surgical Technique

Exposure of Ankle Joint

- Anterolateral approach
- If there is concomitant involvement of subtalar joint, its fusion, in addition to the ankle is indicated in the same sitting pantalar arthrodesis.
- Every sensate foot can heal with good function.

Tuberculosis of Foot

- Commoner sites of involvement are calcaneum, subtalar, and mid-tarsal joints.
- Endarteritis of the nutrient artery of tarsal bone in such lesions is common and many would show a cavity with or without typical coke-like sequestrum on the X-rays. Comparative X-rays of both feet are of great help.

Relevant Surgical Anatomy of the Ankle and Foot

A synovial-lined cavity exists between each pair of tarsal bone, and these joints frequently communicate with one another. This explains the ease with which an infective lesion spreads to many tarsal joints.

Chapter 11: Tuberculosis of the Shoulder

- Incidence of concomitant pulmonary tuberculosis is high. Infection starts from head of the humerus or synovium. Painful limitations of abduction and external rotation occur early.
- Dry atrophic form (caries sicca) exclusively in adults.

Management

- Immobilized on abduction frame orthosis.
- If diagnosed at an early stage, one may obviate the use of abduction frame.
- Response to chemotherapy and splintage is as a rule favorable.
- In an advanced case abduction frame is desirable to permit healing of shoulder infection in glass holding position or saluting position.

Operative Technique

- Arthrodesis for tuberculosis of shoulder is currently seldom indicated.
- The position of the shoulder for arthrodesis should be such as to allow the hand to reach the midline of the body in front, to reach the face and ipsilateral trouser pocket (with the elbow flexed).

Relevant Surgical Anatomy of the Shoulder Joint

- 4 to 1 disproportion between the large spherical humeral head and the shallow glenoid fossa.
- It is wise to appreciate that the medial epicondyle of humerus faces in the same direction (and a little backwards) as the articular surface of the humeral head.
- Humeral head is retroverted by 30 degrees.
- Functional movement of shoulder: For first 90 degrees of abduction:

For every 3 degrees of movement at glenohumeral articulation one degree of movement is occurring at scapulothoracic articulation. This ratio is almost reversed for the movements beyond 90 degrees; for every one degree of scapulohumeral movement there is 3 degrees of scapulothoracic movement.

Chapter 12: Tuberculosis of the Elbow Joint

Infection starts from synovium or olecranon or the lower end of humerus. Supratrochlear and/or axillary lymph nodes are enlarged in nearly one-third of the patients.

Management: In a unilateral case, 90 degrees of flexion and midprone position of the forearm is advisable. With a range of flexion from 30 to 130 degrees one can perform all activities of daily life.

Arthrodesis: Rare indication for unilateral disease a position of 90 degrees flexion is described. For a rare bilateral case, one elbow should be placed at 110 degrees flexion to reach the mouth and face and the other at 65 degrees to attend to personal body hygiene.

Chapter 13: Tuberculosis of the Wrist

Clinical Features

- Enlargement of supratrochlear and/or axillary lymph nodes is highly suggestive of an infective pathology. A case of monoarticular rheumatoid arthritis may strongly resemble tuberculosis. Rheumatoid disease may sometimes have regional reactive lymphadenopathy.
- Posteroanterior (PA-view) X-ray of both wrists with ulnar deviation provides maximum information especially in early stages of any disease/disorder. Capitate is the most common bone to be infected.

Management

Splintage of the wrist in 10–15 degrees of dorsiflexion ad forearm in midprone position.

Operative Treatment

Surgical intervention is rarely indicated.

Relevant Surgical Anatomy of the Wrist

It is worth recalling that the most useful movement of the wrist is one of dorsiflexion combined with radial deviation, and palmar flexion combined with ulnar deviation.

Chapter 14: Tuberculosis of Short Tubular Bones

Tuberculous dactylitis; the hand is more frequently involved than the foot; spindle-shaped expansion; spina ventosa.

Tuberculosis of the Joints of Fingers and Toes

In countries where typical mycobacterial disease is disappearing atypical (non-typical) mycobacterial infections due to *Mycobacterium kansasii* or *marinum* have been reported.

Chapter 15: Tuberculosis of the Sacroiliac Joints and Sacrum

- Sacroiliac joint is a true synovial joint.
- Disease is relatively more common in women of child-bearing age.

Clinical Features

Goldthwait's sign and Faber test are positive in active stage of disease.

Management

Conservative treatment as for lower lumbar disease gives satisfactory outcome.

Operative Debridement and Arthrodesis of Sacroiliac Joint

Operative treatment is only indicated in refractory cases.

Chapter 16: Tuberculosis of Rare Sites, Girdle and Flat Bones

See Figure 1.2.

Chapter 17: Tuberculous Osteomyelitis

Tuberculous Osteomyelitis without Joint Involvement

- Tuberculous osteomyelitis (without involvement of joints), especially of long tubular bones, is so infrequent that it often fails to attract the attention of the clinician.
- BCG osteomyelitis of long bones may resemble the clinical features of tuberculous osteomyelitis.

Tuberculosis of Long Tubular Bones

- Disseminated skeletal tuberculosis was considered to be very rare.
- When imaging modalities (MRIs or isotope bone scans) are employed to scan the body, additional active, subclinical tuberculous foci can be detected in about 40% of patients.

Chapter 18: Tuberculous of Tendon Sheaths and Bursae

The most common site of involvement is the flexor tendons of the hand (compound palmar ganglion).

Tuberculous Bursitis

It can occur in any bursal sheath.

Chapter 19: Spine Tuberculosis—Clinical Features

Age and Sex

It is most common during first three decades. The disease is equally distributed among both sexes. During the last two decades, we have been observing another peak of such cases above the age of 60 years probably because of increase in the population of senior citizens and those with compromised immune status.

Symptoms and Signs

Active stage

Insidious; during sleep, the muscle spasm relaxes permitting movement between the inflammed surfaces resulting in the typical night cries.

Unusual Clinical Features

Tuberculosis as a cause of persistent backache must be remembered. Vertebral tuberculosis may present as "spinal tumor syndrome" with neural deficit. Case having a pulmonary lesion with pain in the spine may be case of ankylosing spondylitis and requires to be differentiated from tubercular spondylitis.

Abscesses and Sinuses

Far away from the vertebral column along the fascial planes or course of neurovascular bundles; psoas sheath; ıliac fossa; lumbar triangle; upper part of the thigh below the inguinal ligament or even track downwards up to the knee; iliopsoas abscesses can lead to pitfalls in diagnosis; they can give rise to hip flexion deformity—"pseudo-hip flexion" deformity. Iliopsoas abscess source: dorsal 10th vertebra to the sacrum; sacroiliac joint, pelvic bones and hip joint; what is generally expressed as clinically palpable "psoas abscess" in reality is an iliopsoas abscess.

Analysis of Clinical Material

95% of patients reporting in the BHU hospital between 1965 and 1974, had varying degrees of kyphosis at presentation.

Regional Distribution of Tuberculous Lesions in the Vertebral Column (in the pre-MRI Era—Observed by Conventional X-rays)

Lower thoracic and thoracolumbar region. In Cleveland's (1942) series, the peak incidence was at the 11th thoracic vertebra, the incidence curve falling away more or less smoothly in each direction along the vertebral column. Cervical spine tuberculous being more common in children.

Vertebral Lesion

The majority of patients there are the typical paradiscal lesions. Tuberculosis of vertebral arches is very rare.

Associated Extra-spinal Tubercular Lesions

Spinal tuberculosis is always the result of a hematogenous dissemination from a primary focus. A pulmonary and/or visceral and/or glandular tubercular lesions could be detected in 12% of patients. Employing modern imaging techniques (MRI/isotope scan) would demonstrate an additional subclinical skeletal or visceral tuberculous lesion in approximately 40% patients clinically presenting as spinal tuberculosis.

Chapter 20: X-ray Appearance and Findings on Modern Imaging

Number of Vertebrae Involved

Average number of vertebrae involved at each site was 3 for children and 2.5 for adults.

Paradiscal Type of Lesion is the most common type and narrowing of the disc is often the earliest radiological finding. Foci of <1.5 cm in diameter are not demonstrable in a conventional radiograph. The narrowing of the disc may represent either atrophy of the disc due to lack of nutrition or prolapse of the nucleus pulposus into the soft necrotic vertebral bodies now often observed in MRI studies.

Paravertebral Shadows

The normal space between the pharynx and cervical spine above the level of cricoid cartilage is 0.5 cm and below this level it is 1.5 cm. Seventh cervical to fourth dorsal vertebrae require good quality X-rays or MRIs to be diagnosed at an early stage. In the lateral view, normally the tracheal shadow is concave anteriorly. Between C7 to D4 vertebrae the distance between the tracheal shadow (air shadow) and the vertebral column if >8 mm indicates the disease. Abscesses below the level of fourth dorsal vertebrae produce typical fusiform shape. If the abscess is too large it may take the shape of generalized broadening of the mediastinum. A psoas abscess can be aspirated through the iliac fossa or Petit's triangle. Thoracic spine tense paravertebral abscess of long standing may show a scalloping effect (aneurysmal phenomenon), saw tooth appearance radiologically.

Kyphotic Deformity (Angulation of Spine with Convexity Posteriorly)

Forward wedging of one or two vertebral bodies would produce a small kyphos (knuckle kyphosis), wedge collapse of 3 or more vertebral bodies would produce an angular kyphosis, and moderate wedging of a large number of vertebrae would create a round kyphosis not unlike osteoporotic kyphos. "Tall vertebrae" can develop only when the disease occurred during the growth period. They are seen distal to the kyphotic deformity.

Central Type of Lesion (Tuberculosis of the Centrum): May result in vertebra plana.

Skipped Lesions: Defined if one or more of healthy vertebrae present between the two lesions.

Anterior Type of Lesion: Common in thoracic spine in children. "Scalloping effect" or "aneurysmal phenomenon" or "saw-tooth appearance" in tuberculosis of the spine.

Lateral Shift and Scoliosis: Almost all such cases occurred in the lower dorsal and lumbar spine, it is an indicator of involvement of posterior spinal segment in addition to anterior damage.

Natural Course of the Disease: When a paradiscal lesion is diagnosed early (predestructive stage) and treated adequately, healing may take place leaving behind no radiological deformity or defect except a moderately diminished disc space. Remarkable regeneration of the destroyed vertebrae may be observed in children.

Modern Imaging Techniques

MRI is an excellent modality to judge the disease at a predestructive stage and to assess the health of the cord; additional involvement; detected in >40% of cases. In countries where tuberculosis is endemic, a typical clinical and radiological appearance of tuberculosis may be sufficient reason to begin treatment without biopsy.

Clinico-radiological Classification of Typical Tubercular Spondylitis

Stage I, if diagnosed in time and treated effectively would heal without leaving any deficit.

Biological Healing and Imaging

MRI done up to 5 months after the start of multidrug therapy may show abnormal signal in more extended area, this is not due to destruction but is because of hyperemic reparative reaction.

Chapter 21: Differential Diagnosis

In clinical practice, there are some cases (about 5% in Indian-subcontinent) whose final diagnosis is revealed only by examination of diseased tissue obtained by operation. Conditions to be considered are:

Pyogenic infections, typhoid spine, brucella spondylitis, mycotic spondylitis, histiocytosis-X, local developmental abnormalities of the spine, spinal osteochondrosis, traumatic conditions, osteoporotic conditions, spondylolisthesis, hydatid disease

Tumorous Conditions

- Hemangioma
  - Most common benign tumor of the vertebral column,
  - Incidence of 10.7% of MRI of spine (cervical to sacral),
- Corduroy appearance in X-rays and MRIs.

Secondary Neoplastic Deposits are the commonest malignant neoplasms of the vertebral column.

- Most common primary malignancy is multiple myeloma
- Discs on either side remain unaffected for a long time in tumorous conditions.

CT-guided core biopsy or fine needle aspiration biopsy in expert hands may give a tissue diagnosis in early 80% of cases. Failing semi-invasive techniques, operation is justified.

Chapter 22: Neurological Complications

Incidence

- The overall incidence has been reported between 10 and 30%.
- More common during first three decades of life.
- Highest incidence of paraplegia associated with disease of the lower thoracic region.
- Most common pathology for nontraumatic paraplegia in developing countries still remains tuberculosis.

Group A: Early Onset Paraplegia

Inflammatory edema, tuberculosis granulation tissue, tuberculous abscess, tuberculous caseous tissue or rarely ischemic lesion of the cord. Recovery favorable in non ischemic lesions.

Group B: Late Onset Paraplegia

More than 2 years after the healing of tuberculosis, tuberculous caseous tissue, tubercular debris, sequestra from vertebral body, angular deformity, narrowing vertebral canal. Prognosis is less favorable.

Gross Neural Signs

- Ankle clonus
- Extensor plantar response with or without brisk tendon reflexes
- Clumsiness (incoordination) or spasticity or jumpiness
- Sensory deficit
- Spontaneous flexor spasm
- Sphincter disturbances

Pathology of Tuberculous Paraplegia

- Inflammatory edema
- Cause of early cases of neurological deficits

Extradural Mass

Tuberculous osteitis of the vertebral bodies.

Bony Disorders

Up to 60% of vertebral canal encroachment may be compatible with intact neural status.

Changes in Spinal Cord

MRI studies have revealed myelomalacic and syringomyelic changes. Up to 60% of vertebral canal encroachment may be compatible with intact neurology.

Signs and Symptoms of Pott's Paraplegia Associated with Disease Proximal to Lumbar First Vertebra

The first signs of interference: twitching of muscles in the lower limbs and clumsiness while walking.

- Diseased area in the spine lies anterior to the cord
- The motor tracts are more sensitive to compression of the cord
- Position and vibration are the last to disappear

Prolonged Stretching of the Cord over a Severe Deformity:

- Stretched cord may be more vulnerable to other causes, then decompression, release of cord, and anterior transposition may lead to recovery
- Rarely stretching leads to interstitial gliosis or atrophy of cord (may be visualized by myelo-CT and/or by MRI) which does not recover completely.
- Diffuse extradural granuloma or tuberculoma or peridural fibrosis: Present as spinal tumor syndrome, laminectomy may help.

Classification of TB Paraplegia

Stage I: The patient is not aware of the deficit. On examination, reflexes may be brisk, with plantars being extensor.

Stage II: Patient is aware of the deficit. The patient is ambulatory. Signs of spastic paraparesis are present.

Stage III: Nonambulatory. Paraplegia in extension. Sensory deficit <50%. Bladder bowel not involved.

Stage IV: Nonambulatory. Paraplegia in flexion. Flexor spasms or flaccid. Sensory deficit >50%. Bladder bowel involvement, loss of vibration and joint sensation.

Prognosis for Recovery of Cord Function

Cord involvement	Better prognosis	Relatively poor prognosis
Duration	Shorter	Longer (>12 months)
Type	Early onset	Late onset
Speed onset	Slow	Rapid
Age	Younger	Older
General condition	Good	Poor

Treatment of Pott's Paraplegia

Not to rush in for surgery so long as the patient is able to walk.

Chapter 23: Management and Results

Results of Operations on the Diseased Vertebrae in the Preantitubercular Era

General outlook regarding surgery, therefore, was aptly summarized by Calot (1930) as, "the surgeon who, so far as tuberculosis is concerned, swears to remove the evil from the very root, will only find one result waiting him-the death of his patient".

Role of Direct Surgery in the Management of Spinal Tuberculosis

- Chemotherapy with braces achieved sound healing in 92% of such cases.
- Progressive bone destruction in spite of chemotherapeutic regime, failure to respond to conservative therapy and uncertainty in diagnosis are definite indication for surgery in active stage of the disease. Observation for about 2–3 months seems to be enough to judge these features.

Absolute Indications for Operative Decompression

Whenever there is doubt about diagnosis surgical treatment is mandatory as it provides an opportunity to confirm the diagnosis.

- Neurological complications which do not start showing signs of progressive recovery to a satisfactory level after a fair trial of conservative therapy (3–4 weeks).
- Neurological complications develop during the conservative treatment:
  - Which become worse
  - Recurrence of neurological complication
  - Difficulty in deglutition and respiration in cervical spine disease
  - Marked sensory and sphincter disturbances

Main indications for various operations for vertebral tuberculosis

- Decompression (± fusion) for neurological complications which failed to respond to 3–6 weeks of conservative therapy/too advanced
- Debridement (± fusion) in failure of response after 3–6 months of nonoperative treatment
- Doubtful diagnosis
- Fusion for symptomatic mechanical instability after healing
- Debridement ± decompression ± fusion in recurrence of disease or of neural complication
- Prevention of severe kyphosis by posterior fusion ± debridement in young children with extensive dorsal lesions
- Anterior transposition of cord through extrapleural anterolateral approach for neural complications due to severe kyphosis

Note: Laminectomy has no place in tuberculosis of spine except for extradural granuloma/tuberculoma presenting as spinal tumor syndrome or a case of old healed disease (without much deformity) presenting with secondary "vertebral canal stenosis", or non-healing posterior spinal disease.

Results of Management by following the Middle Path

- Favorable status is no residual neural impairment, no sinus or clinically evident cold abscess, no impairment of physical activity due to the spinal disease/lesion, and presence of radiologically quiescent disease.

- All the sinus healed under the effect of antitubercular drugs within 1–7 months (average 3.3 months).

Deep-seated Radiological Paravertebral Abscesses

The drainage may be considered in cases with neurological complications and those having difficulty in deglutition and respiration, or abscesses which become much bigger in size despite adequate antitubercular therapy.

Neurological Complications

The overall success rate is about 80% which compares favorably with the results of any other series.

Onset and Speed of Neural Recovery after Operation

The first objective evidence of neural recovery was variable: 24 hours to 12 weeks after the decompression. Despite decompression about 8% do not recover because of intrinsic damage of cord.

Plantar Response: Extensor plantar response, a sign of pyramidal tract involvement, lasted for a very long time even after decompression-operation (first to appear and last to resolve).

Radiological Healing of Vertebral Tuberculosis with Operation on the Diseased Vertebral Bodies without Bone Grafting: 11% of cases had fibro-osseous and 89% had bony healing of the vertebral lesion when assessed 2 years after operation.

Radiological Healing of Vertebral Lesion: Bony and mixed (fibro-osseous) replacement of the intervertebral space were not always synonymous with clinical healing.

Course of Kyphosis of Spine in Patients not Operated Upon

All the cases with increase of kyphosis by >30 degrees, were in growing age at the onset of disease, and had involvement of three or more dorsal vertebral bodies.

Thoracic spine

Destruction of a thoracic vertebral body results in a posterior displacement of the center of motion, a subluxation at the level of the articular facets and increase in weight to be borne by the anterior part of body. In the lumbar spine, the large bodies and vertical articular facets were more apt to telescope than to angulate.

- Only nonoperative way to minimize the increase in kyphosis seems to be recumbency in active stage and prolonged protection with suitable braces in the later stages.
- Dorsal disease below the level of 9th rib has the worst prognosis regarding kyphos.

Course of Kyphosis of Spine in Lesions Operated Upon without Bone Grafting

There does not seem to be much difference regarding the behavior of kyphosis whether the patients are treated by universal excisional surgery or by nonoperative medicinal therapy or by following a middle path regime.

The best behavior was with fusion "posterior elements without anterior fusion".

Fusion of the anterior elements during the growing age should be avoided because that may negate any growth potential of the vertebral bodies.

Clinical Healing in Cases without Neurological Complications

Almost all such cases were nonactive clinically and radiologically after 12 months of the drug therapy without surgery on the diseased.

Tuberculosis of the Cervical Spine

Those admitted were put in cervical traction (3–8 weeks). Those treated in the outpatients were given rest to the neck using a four-post collar or SOMI brace, along with routine anti-TB drugs.

Chapter 24: Operative Treatment

The effectiveness of chemotherapy has obviated the need for surgical therapy in many cases. Any surgery on the vertebral column must ensure least disruption of the intact healthy columns.

Surgical Approach

Dorsal Spine

Anterior transthoracic or extrapleural anterolateral (ALD) approaches provide adequate exposure for debridement, mechanical decompression and anterior or posterior bone grafting procedure.

Anterior spinal approach is, however, impracticable for operations on severe kyphotic deformities, ALD or lumbar-transverse vertebrotomy are practicable.

Cervical Spine: Anterior approach.

Atlantoaxial Region: Transoral approach or posterior approach.

Cervicodorsal Region: Anterior approach through a low cervical incision for lesion at C7-D1, lesion from C7 to D2 have been debrided, debulked and decompressed by us through transverse low cervical approach with resection of upper border of manubrium sterni.

Lumbosacral Region (L5–S1)

Transverse vertebrotomy approach reflecting the psoas muscle anterior to reach the anterolateral surface of the lumbar vertebrae.

Bone grafts help stability and negate deformation.

Anterolateral Decompression (D2–L1)

- Right lateral position
- Approaching the spine from the left side
- The ribs articulating with the diseased
- Severe as the guide to the placement of the incision
- Ribs are best identified by counting from below
- Semicircular incision (convex laterally)
- 6 cm proximal to the center of the diseased area
- Laterally to a point about 9 cm from the midline
- About 6 cm distal to the center
- Elevation of the flap along with the deep fascia
- Medial parts of 2–4 ribs, which are articulating with the diseased vertebrae, and their transverse processes are exposed subperiosteally.
- 2–4 ribs, about 8 cm from the transverse process are cut with a bone cutting forceps: this completes costotransversectomy. Expose anterolateral surface of verterbal bodies.
- Debride the diseased bone and decompress dural tube. In cases of paraplegia
- Complete the operation of anterolateral decompression
- Excision of 3–4 ribs provides a good exposure

Intercostal nerves serve as guide to the intervertebral foramina and the pedicles. Only intercostal nerves can be sacrificed while doing anterolateral decompression but no nerve to be sacrificed in cervical or lumbar region.

Operative Complication and their Prevention

Tear of the pleura, tear of the dura, if the dural tear was larger than 1.5 cm it was repaired.

Postoperative Care

- At the end of 2–3 months or when the patient has made good neural recovery.
- Patient is mobilized out of the bed with the help of spinal brace.
- The spinal brace is gradually discarded after about 12–18 months of the operation.

Anterolateral Approach to the Lumbar Spine (Lumbovertebrotomy)

Approach is usually from the left side.

Surgery in Severe Kyphosis

- Identify the potential cases at high risk, perform posterior spinal fusion.
- Extended period of recumbency and prolonged use of brace would minimize deterioration.

Treatment of Paraplegia in Severe Kyphosis (Anterior Transposition of the Cord)

Excellent removal of internal kyphosis can be achieved through anterolateral approach.

Instrumentation in Tuberculous Spine

Author, however, is not convinced regarding the advantages and safety of inserting a metallic implant in active disease of spine with softened bones.

If one is impelled to use a metallic implant after anterior debridement and decompression, it is safest to use posterior implant; the implants get purchase is healthy bone and removal if warranted is simpler.

Re-operation for Decompression

- Did not improve the neural status and the postoperative myelogram/MRI reveal persistent mechanical compression.
- The operation was at incorrect level
- The earlier operation was an ill-advised laminectomy
- Symptomatic canal stenosis after a healed disease
- Nonresponder to reactivated infection
- Persistent infection related to implant

Chapter 25: Spinal Braces

- Fourth dorsal to second lumbar vertebrae, spinal brace extends from the seventh cervical spine to the lower end of the sacrum.
- Taylor brace may control a simple kyphotic deformity but has little control on a scoliotic deformity. Milwaukee brace or a Jewett brace is recommended for tuberculous lesions in the dorsal spine throughout the growing age, anterior spinal hyperextension brace has been found to be more acceptable by ladies.
- Dorsal one to dorsal third vertebra, there is no simple brace to control the spine effectively, hybrids are available.
- Cervical first to cervical seventh; Philadelphia collar or four post-collar.
- For lower lumbar (third lumbar and below) and lumbosacral region; a Goldthwaite brace or a lumbar corset.

Bibliography

SECTION I AND II

General Considerations and Extra-spinal Regional Tuberculosis

A

Abbott LC, Lucas DB. Arthrodesis of the hip in wide abduction. J Bone Joint Surg. 1954;36A:1129.

Adjard A, Martini M. Tuberculosis of the hip in adults. Int Orthop. 1987;11:227-33.

Agarwal A, Suri T, Verma I, Kumar SK, Gupta N, Shaharyar A. Tuberculosis of the hip in children—a retrospective analysis of 27 patients. Indian J Orthop. 2014;48:463-9.

Aggarwal VK, Nair D, Khanna G, Verma J, Sharma VK, Batra S. Use of amplified *Mycobacterium tuberculosis* direct test (Gen-probe Inc., San Diego, CA, USA) in the diagnosis of tubercular synovitis and early arthritis of knee joint. Indian J Orthop. 2012;46:531-5.

Agoramoorthy G. India needs to refine a strategy to tackle the tuberculosis epidemic. Lancet Infect Dis.. 2017;17:23-4.

Albrook D, Kirkaldy-Willis WH. The restoration of articular surfaces after joint excision. J Bone Joint Surg. 1958;40B:742-6.

Allen BW, Mitchison DA, Darbyshire J, Chew WWK, Gabriel M. Examination of operation specimens from patients with spinal tuberculosis for tubercle bacilli. J Clin Pathol. 1983;36:662-6.

Allen SC. A case in favour of Poncet's disease. Br Med J. 1981;283:952.

Ambekar AP, Joshipura JCN. Classification and treatment of tuberculosis of hip joint: analysis of 104 cases. Ind J Surg. 1973;35:309-15.

American Thoracic Society. Sub-committee on surgery and the committee on therapy. The present status of skeletal tuberculosis. Am Rev Respir Dis. 1963;88:272.

Andre T. Studies on the distribution of tritium-labelled dihydrostreptomycin and tetracycline in the body. Acta Radiol Suppl. 1956;142.

Antti-Poika I, Vankka E, Santavirta S, Vastamaki M. Two cases of shoulder joint tuberculosis. Acta Orthop Scand. 1991;62:81-3.

Arora A. Basic Science of host immunity in osteoarticular tuberculosis—a clinical study. Ind J Orthop. 2006;40:1-15.

Arora A, Nadkarni B, Dev G, Chattopadhya D, Jain AK, Tuli SM, et al. Use of immunomodulators as an adjunct to autitubercular chemotherapy in clinically non-responsive patients of osteoarticular tuberculosis. J Bone joint Surg. 2006;88-B:264-9.

Arora S, Sethi S. Isolated tubercular tenosynovitis in children: report of seven cases. JR Ped Orthop. 1994;14:752-4.

Autzen B, Elberg JJ. Bone and joint tuberculosis in Denmark. Acta Orthop Scand. 1988; 59:50-2.

Azouz EM. Computed tomography in bone and joint infections. J Canad Assoc Radiol. 1981;32:102.

B

Babhulkar S, Pande S. Tuberculosis of the hip. Clin Orthop. 2002;398:93-9.

Babhulkar SS, Pande SK. Unusual manifestation of osteoarticular tuberculosis. Clin Orthop. 2000;398:114-20.

Bailey TB, Akhtar M, Ali MA. FNA biopsy in the diagnosis of tuberculosis. Acta Cyto. 1985;29: 732-6.

Barclay WR, Elbert RH, Le Roy GV, Manthei RW, Roth LJ. Distribution and excretion of radioactive isoniazid in tuberculous patients. J Am Med Assoc. 1953;151:1384-8.

Barnes PF, Barrows SA. Tuberculosis in the 1990's. Ann Intn Med. 1993;119:400-10.

Barnes PF, Block AB, Davidson PT, Snider DE. Tuberculosis in patient with human immunodeficiency virus infection. New Engl J Med. 1991;324(23):1644-50.

Bastian I, Colebunders R. Treatment and prevention of multidrug-resistant tuberculosis. Drugs. 1999;58:633-66.

Bavadekar AV. Osteoarticular tuberculosis in children. Progress in Ped Surg. 1982;15:131-51.

Bayrakci K, Daglar B, Tasbas BA, Agar M, Gunel U. Tuberculosis osteomyelitis of symphysis pubis. Orthopedics. 2006;29:948-50.

Bell WJ, Brown PP. Bacterial resistance in cases of pulmonary tuberculosis in Accra, West Af Med J. 1961;10:140-7.

Benjamin B, Khan MRH. Hip involvement in childhood brucellosis. J Bone Joint Surg. 1994;76B:544-7.

Benkeddache Y, Gottesman H. Skeletal tuberculosis of the wrist and hand: A study of 27 cases. J Hand Surg. 1982;7:593-600.

Besser MI. Total knee replacement in unsuspected tuberculosis of the joint. Br Med J. 1980;280:1434.

Beveridge M. Burden of orthopaedic disease in developing countries. J Bone Joint Surg. 2004;86(8):1819-22.

Bick EM. Classics of Orthopaedics. JB Lippincot Co, Philadelphia, 1976.

Bickel WH, Kimbrough RF, Dahlin DC. Tuberculous tenosynovitis. J Am Med Assn. 1953;151:31-5.

Bickel WH, Young H, Pfuetze KH, Falls G, Norley T. Streptomycin in tuberculosis of bones and joints. J Am Med Assoc. 1948;137: 682-7.

Bickel WH. Streptomycin in skeletal tuberculosis. Surg Gynecol Obstet. 1948;89: 244-5.

Bittar EA, Petty W. Girdlestone arthroplasty for infected total hip arthroplasty. Clin Orthop Relat Res. 1982;170:83-7.

Bosworth DM, Wright HA. Streptomycin in bone and joint tuberculosis. J Bone Joint Surg. 1952;34A: 255-66.

Bosworth DM. Modern concepts of treatment of tuberculosis of bones and joints. Ann N Y Acad Sci. 1963;106:98-105.

Boutin RD, Brossman J, Sartoris Dj, Reilly D, Resnick D. Update on imaging of orthopaedic infections. Ortho Clin N Am. 1998;29:41-65.

Brittain HA. Architectural Principles in Arthrodesis, 2nd Edition, Livingstone, Edinburgh, 1952.

Broderick C, Hopkins S, Mack DJF, Aston W, Pollock R, Skinner JA, Warren S. Delays in the diagnosis and treatment of bone and joint tuberculosis in the United Kingdom. Bone Joint J. 2018;100-B:119-24.

Buchman J, Koval RP. Surgical treatment of tuberculosis of bones and joints under an umbrella of antituberculosis and antibiotic drugs. NYJ Med. 1961;61:3657-72.

Buck P, Morrey BF, Chao EYS. The optimum position of arthrodesis of the ankle. J Bone Joint Surg. 1987;69A:1052-62.

Bush DC, Schneider LH. Tuberculosis of the hand and wrist. J Hand Surg. 1984;9A:391-8.

C

Calandruccio RA, Gilmer WS, Jr. Proliferation, regeneration, and repairs of articular cartilage of immature animals. J Bone Joint Surg. 1962;44A;431-55.

Calot T. Sur Le meilleur traitment localdes tuberculoses doses, articulations et ganglions lymphatiques. Acta Chir Scand. 1930;67:206-26.

Campbell JAB, Hoffman EB. Tuberculosis of the hip in children. J Bone Joint Surg. 1995;77B: 319-26.

Campbell's Operative Orthopaedics, Ed Crenshaw, AH Edi. VII, CV Mosby Company, St Louis, Missouri, USA, 1987.

Campos. Bone and joint tuberculosis and its treatment. J Bone Joint Surg. 1955;37A:937-66.

Canetti G. The Tubercle Bacillus in the Pulmonary Lesion of Man. New York, Springer, 1955.

Caparros AB, Sousa M, Ribera Zabalbeascoa J, Uceda Carrascosa P, Mkoya Corral F. Total hip arthroplasty for tuberculous coxitis. Int Orthop. 1999;23:348-50.

Chadha M, Agarwal A, Kumar S. Spinal tuberculosis with concomitant spondylolisthesis, coexisting entities or 'cause and effect'? Spinal Cord. 2006;44:399-404.

Chalmers BP, Weston JT, Osmon DR, Hanssen AD, Berry DJ, Abdel MP. Prior hip or knee prosthetic joint infection in another joint increases risk three-fold of prosthetic joint infection after primary total knee arthroplasty: a matched control study. Bone Joint J. 2019;101B:91-7.

Chapman JS. The atypical mycobacteria. Am Rev Resp Dis. 1982;125:119-24.

Charnley J, Houston JK. Compression arthrodesis of the shoulder. J Bone Joint Surg. 1964;46B:614-20.

Charnley J. Compression arthrodesis. E&S Livingstone lid., London, 1953.

Chow SP, Ip FK, Lau JHK, Collins RJ, Luk KDK, So YC, et al. *Mycobacterium marinum* infection of the hand and wrist. J Bone Joint Surg. 1987;69A:1161-8.

Chow SP, Yau A. Tuberculosis of the knee: a long term follow-up. Int Orthop. 1980;4:87-92.

Citron KM. Tuberculosis-chemotherapy. Br Med J. 1972;1:426-8.

Cleveland M. Surgical treatment of joint tuberculosis. Surg Gynecol Obstet. 1935;61: 503-20.

Collins DH, Dodge OG. Tuberculosis in Pathology of Bone. Butterworth and Co, London, 1966; 216-19.

Compere EL, Kleinberg S, Kleiger B, Moore PH, Stewart MJ, Wright PB. Evaluation of streptomycin therapy in controlled series of 90 cases of skeletal tuberculosis. J Bone Joint Surg. 1952;34A:288-97.

Coventry MB. The first use of streptomycin for bone tuberculosis: A 47-year follow-up. J Bone Joint Surg. 1994;76B:673-5.

Crofton J. Drug treatment of tuberculosis. Br Med J. 1960;2:370.

Currie MA. Profile of spine and joint tuberculosis of Pakistan's Afghan frontier. Ann R ColL Surg Eng. 1984;66:105-07.

D

Dahl HK. Examination of pH in tuberculous pus. Acta Orthop Scand. 1951;20:176.

Davidson PT, Horowitz I. Skeletal tuberculosis: A review with patient presentations and discussion. Am J Med. 1970;48:77-84.

Davidson PT, Le HA. Drug treatment of tuberculosis. Drugs. 1992;43:651-73.

Davies PDO, Humphries MJ, Byefield SP, et al. Bone and joint tuberculosis. A survey of notifications in England and Wales. J Bone Joint Surg. 1984;66B:326-30.

Debeyre J. Present treatment of bone and joint tuberculosis (in French) 27: 702-10; Rev

Tuberc. (Paris) abstracted in Am Rev Respir Dis. 1964;90:823-84.

Deroy MS, Fisher H. Treatment of tuberculous bone disease by surgical drainage combined with streptomycin. J Bone Joint Surg. 1952;34A: 299-329.

Dewan R, Gangal SV, Chandrashekar S, Suryanarayana Murthy P. Turnover of Phospholipids in whole cell and membranes of *M. tuberculosis* H37RV. Indian J Biochem Biophys. 1987;24:278-81.

Dhillon MS, Aggarwal S, Prabhakar S, Bachhal V. Tuberculosis of the foot: An osteolytic variety. Indian J orthop. 2012;46:206-11.

Dhillon MS, Goel A, Prabhakar S, Aggarwal S, Bachhal V. Tuberculosis of the elbow: A clinicoradiological analysis. Indian J Orthop. 2012;46:200-5.

Dhillon MS, Nagi ON. Tuberculosis of the foot and ankle. Clin Orthop. 2002;398:107-13.

Dhillon MS, Singh P, Sharma R, Gill SS, Nagi ON. Tuberculous osteomyelitis of the cuboid: a report of four cases. J Foot Ankle Surg. 2000;39:329-35.

Dhillon MS, Tuli SM. Osteoarticular tuberculosis of foot and ankle. Foot Ankle Int. 2001;22:679-86.

Dixon JH. Non-tuberculous mycobacterial infection of the tendon sheaths in the hand. J Bone Joint Surg. 1981;63B:544-7.

Duraiswami PK, Tuli SM. Five thousand years of orthopaedics in India. Clin Orthop. 1971;75: 269-80.

Dutt AK, Moers D, Stead WW. Short course chemotherapy for extra pulmonary tuberculosis: nine years' experience. Ann Intern Med. 1986;104:7-12.

E

East African/British Medical Research Councils. Isoniazid with thioacetazone in the treatment of pulmonary tuberculosis in East Africa-Second thioacetazone investigation. Tubercle, Lond. 1963;44:301-33.

Edeiken J, Depalma AF, Moskowitz H, Vernan S. Cystic tuberculosis of bone. Clin Orthop. 1963;28:163-8.

Editorial. Tuberculosis retrospect and prospect. Clinician. 1968;32:1-2.

Eskola A. Cementless total replacement for old tuberculosis of the hip. J Bone Joint Surg. 1988;70B:603-6.

Eskola A, Santavirta St, Konttinen YT, Tallroth K, Lindhom ST. Arthroplasty for old tuberculosis of the knee. J Bone Joint Surg. 1988;70B:767-9.

Evans TE. Tuberculosis of bones and joints: with special reference to influence of streptomycin and application of radical surgical technics to certain effects and complications of tuberculous lesions. J Bone Joint Surg. 1952;34A:267-78.

F

Falk A. A follow-up study of the initial group of cases of skeletal tuberculosis treated with streptomycin, 1946-48. The United States Veterans Administration and Armed Forces Cooperative studies of tuberculosis. J Bone Joint Surg. 1958;40A:1161-8.

Fehring TK, Keith AF, Angela H, et al. What's new in musculoskeletal infection. J Bone Joint Surg. 2019;101(14):1237-44.

Fellander M, Hiertonn TV, Wallmark G. Studies on the concentration of streptomycin in the treatment of bone and joint tuberculosis. Acta Tuber Scand. 1952;27:176-89.

Fellande berculosis osteitis following BCG vaccination. Acta Orthop Scand. 1963;2:116-26.

Formicola V, Milanesi Q, Scarsini C. Evidence of spinal tuberculosis at the beginning of fourth millennium BC from Arena Candide cave (Liguria, Itlay). Int Orthop. 1987;11:315-22.

Fox W. Realistic chemotherapeutic policies for tuberculosis in the developing countries. Br Med J. 1964;1:135-42.

Fox W. The chemotherapy and epidemiology of tuberculosis. Lancet. 1962;473:413-7.

Franceschi F, Longo UG, Ruzzini L, Denaro V. Isolated tuberculosis of patellar tendon. J Bone Joint Surg. 2007;89-B:1525-26.

Friedman B, Kapur VN. Newer knowledge of chemotherapy in the treatment of tuberculosis of bones and joints Clin. Orthop. 1973;97:5-15.

Friedman B, Kapur VN. The management of tuberculosis of the knee joint. Am Rev Resp Dis. 1970;101:265-9.

G

Gale DW, Harding ML. Total knee arthroplasty in the presence of active tuberculosis. J Bone Joint Surg. 1991;73B:1006-07.

Gangadharan PRJ. Drug resistance in tubercle bacilli and its importance in the chemotherapy and epidemiology of the tuberculosis. Ind J Tuberc. 1967;14:65-70.

Gangadharan PRJ. Drug resistance. Ind J Tuberc. 1967;14:63-4.

Ganguli S, Bardwan PM. Drug sensitivity of strains of *Mycobacterium tuberculosis* isolated at Poona. Ind Med Res. 1960;48:394-9.

Garcla-Porrua C, Gonzalez-Gay MA, Sanchez-Andrade A, Vaquez-Caruncho MB. Arthritis in the right great toe as the clinical presentation of tuberculosis. Arthritis Rheumat. 1998;41:374-5.

Girdlestone GR. Tuberculosis of Bone and Joint 3rd Edn. Revised by EW Somerville and MC Wilkinson. London. Oxford University Press. 1965.

Girdlestone GR. Tuberculosis of bones and joints. Modern Trends in Orthopaedics, series, I, pp. 35, Butterworth and Co., London, 1950.

Girling DJ, Darbyshire JH, Humphries MJ, O'Mahoney SG. Extrapulmonary tuberculosis. Brll Med. Bulletin. 1988;44:738-56.

Goldschmidt RB. The challenge of tuberculosis. Current Orthop. 2000;14:18-25.

Gollwitzer H, Langer R, Diehl P, Mittelmeier W. Chronic Osteomyelitis due to *Mycobacterium chelonae* diagnosed by polymerase chain reaction homology matching J Bone Joint Surg. 2004;86:1296-301.

Goris ML. Bone scintigraphy in osteomyelitis. J Nuc Med. 1986;27:566.

Goyal RK, Sen PC. Laboratory diagnosis of tuberculosis in the present antibiotic era. Curr Med Practice. 1962;5:239-45.

Grange JM. The rapid diagnosis of paucibacillary tuberculosis. Tubercle. 1989;70:1-4.

Griffiths DL. Tuberculosis of bones and joints. Modern Practice in Tuberculosis. Vol. II, Butterworth and Co., London, 1952;302-35.

Griffiths JF, Kumta SM, Leung PC, Cheng JCY, Chow LTC, Metreweli C. Imaging of musculoskeletal tuberculosis: A new look at an old disease. Clin Orthop. 2002;398:32-9.

Gupta R, Dhillon MS, Bahadur R, Nagi ON. Multifocal involvement of the foot in tuberculosis. Ind J Foot Surg. 2000;15:55-9.

Gupta SK. The treatment of synovial tuberculosis of the knee by a method with unrestricted activity. Ind J Orthop. 1982;16:14-8.

Gupta SP. Resistance of tubercle bacilli to drugs. Ind J Tuberc. 1962;10:146-9.

H

Hald J. The value of histological and bacteriological examination of tuberculosis of bones and joints. Acta Orthop Scand. 1964;35:91-9.

Hald J. Treatment of bone and joint tuberculosis with streptomycin and PAS. Acta Tuberc Scancd. 1954;30:82-104.

Hall WH, Falk A, Lyon RH. Growth and drug resistance of tubercle bacilli from pulmonary tuberculous lesions after prolonged combined chemotherapy. In Transaction of the 15th

Conference on the Chemotherapy of Tuberculosis, Washington DC, Veterans Administration. 1956;176-80.

Halsey JP, Reeback JS, Barnes CG. A decade of skeletal tuberculosis. Ann Rheum Dis. 1982;41: 7-10.

Hanngren A, Andre T. Distribution of a 3 H-dihydro-streptomycin in tuberculous guinea pigs. Acta Tuberculosea et Pneumologica Scandinavica. 1964;45:14-20.

Hanngren A. Studies on the distribution and fate of C 14 and T-labelled p- aminosalicyclic acid (PAS) in the body. Acta Radiol, Supplement. 1959;175.

Hardinge K, Williams Etienne A, McKenzie D, Charnley J. Conversion of fused hips to low friction arthroplasty. J Bone Joint Surg. 1977;59B:385-92.

Harikrishna J, Sukaveni V, Kumar DP, Mohan A. Cancer and tuberculosis. J Ind Acad Cli Med. 2012;13:142-4.

Harris HW. Current concepts of the metabolism of antituberculous agents. Ann. NY Acad Set. 1963;106:43-7.

Harris RI, Coullhard HS, Dewar FP. Streptomycin in treatment of bone and joint tuberculosis. J Bone Joint Surg. 1952;34A:279-87.

Hecht RH, Meyers M, Thornhill-Joynes M, Montgomerie JZ. Reactivation of tuberculous infection following total joint replacement. J Bone Joint Surg. 1983;66A:1015-6.

Held M, Laubscher M, Zar HJ, Dunn RN. Gene Xpert polymerase chain reaction for spinal tuberculosis. Bone joint J. 2014;96-B:1366-9.

Hever E, Risko T. Studies on streptomycin levels of blood and abscess. Acta Tuber Scand. 1960;38:40-50.

Hillerdal O, Hint V, Siogreu I. Tuberculosis therapy and drug resistance. Nord. Med Bull Hyg. 1961;65:902-05.

Hobby GL, Johnson PM, Baytar-Pepimyik V. Primary drug resistance: A continuing study of drug resistance in tuberculosis in a veteran population within the United States; Amer Rev Resp Dis. 1974;110:96-8.

Hodgson AR, Fang D. Tuberculosis of the hip in children, Hip Disorders in Infants and Children. In: Chung SMK (Ed), Lea and Febiger, Philadelphia (USA). 1981;221-33.

Hodgson AR, Smith TK. Tuberculosis of the wrist. Clin Orthop. 1972;83:72-83.

Hoffman EB, Allin J, Campbell JAB, Leisegang FM. Tuberculosis of the knee Clin Orthop. 2002;398:100-6.

Holmdahl HCS. Tuberculosis of knee: A review of 170 cases. Acta Orthop Scand. 1951;20:19-49.

Hunt DD. Problems in diagnosing osteoarticular tuberculosis, J Am Med Assoc. 1964;190:95-8.

Hutchins PM. Skeletal tuberculosis in the Lothian region of Scotland. A ten year survey. J Roy Coll Surg, Edin. 1984;29:167-71.

J

Jain AK, Dhammi IK, Modi P, Kumar J, Sreenivasan, Saini NS. Tuberculosis spine: Therapeutically refractory diseae. Indian J Orthop. 2012;46:171-8.

Jain AK, Kumar S, Shiv V, Singh H, Tuli SM. Retrofascial pyogenic iliac fossa abscess. Acta Orthop Scand. 1992;63:53-6.

Jain AK, Jain P, Jaggi K, et al. Drug-resistant bone, joint and spine tuberculosis: Evolution of diagnosis and treatment. Ind J Orthop. 2024;58(6):661-8.

Jambhekar NA, Kulkarni SP, Madur BP, Agarwal S, Rajan MGR. Application of the polymerase chain reactin on formalin-fixed, paraffin-embedded tissue in recognition of tuberculous osteomyelitis J Bone Joint Surg. 2006;88-B: 1097-101.

Jellis JE. Human immunodeficiency virus and osteoarticular tuberculosis. Clin Orthop. 2002;398:27-31.

Johnson E, Lidgren L, Rydholm U. Position of shoulder arthrodesis measured with Moire' photography. Clin Orthop. 1989;238:117-21.

Johnson R, Barnes KL, Owen R. Reactivation of tuberculosis after total hip replacement. J Bone Joint Surg. 1979;61B:148-50.

Jungling D. Osteitis tuberculosa cystica. Fortsch Roentgenstr. 1936;27:375.

Jupiter JB, Karchner AW, Lowel JD, Harris WH. Total hip replacement in the treatment of adult hips with current or quiescent sepsis. J Bone Joint Surg. 1981;63A:194-200.

Jutte PC, Van Loenhout-Rooyackers JH, Borgdorff MW, Van Horn JR, Increase of bone and joint tuberculosis in the Netherlands. Jr Bone Jt Surg. 2004;86:901-4.

K

Kaplan CJ. Conservative therapy in skeletal tuberculosis: an appraisal based on experience in South Africa. Tubercle (London). 1959;40:335-68.

Karlson AG. Mycobacteria of surgical interest. Surg Clin North Am. 1973;53:905-12.

Katayama R, Hami Y, Oyak K, Tanaka J, Maruno E. The chemotherapy of bone and joint tuberculosis. Observations on clinical disease. Ann Tuberc. 1954;5:59-94.

Katayama R, Itami Y, Maruno E. Treatment of the hip and knee-joint tuberculosis: an attempt to retain motion. J Bone, Joint Surg Am. 1962;44A:897-917.

Keegan GM, Learmonth ID, Case CP. Orthopaedic metals and their potential toxicity in the arthroplasty patient. J Bone Joint Surgery. 2007;89B:657-73.

Kerri O, Martini M. Tuberculosis of the knee, Int Orthop (SICOT). 1985;4:153-57.

Khan SA, Varshney MK, Hasan AS, Kumar A, Trikha V. Tuberculosis of the sternum. A clinical study J. Bone Joint Surg. 207;89B:817-20.

Kim SJ, Postigo R, Koo S, Kim JH. Total hip replacement for patients with active tuberculosis of the hip: A systematic review and pooled analysis. Bone Joint. 2013;95B: 578-82.

Kim YH. Total knee arthroplasty for tuberculous arthritis. J Bone Joint Surg. 1988;70A:1322-30.

Kim YY, Amn BIH, Bae KD, Ko CO, Jung DL, Byung MK, et al. Arthroplasty using the Charnley prosthesis in old tuberculosis of the hip. Clin Orthop. 1986;211:116-21.

Kim YY, Han DY, Park BM. Total hip arthroplasty for tuberculous coxarthrosis. J Bone Joint Surg. 1987;69A:718-27.

Kim YY, Ko CU, Ann JY, Yoon YS, Kwak BM. Charnley low friction arthroplasty in tuberculosis of the hip. J Bone Joint Surg. 1988;70B:756-60.

Kim YY, Ko CU, Lee SW, Kwak BM. Replacement arthroplasty using the Charnley prosthesis in old tuberculosis of the hip. Int. Orthop. 1979;3:81-8.

Koga Y, Kono S, Mabuchi K. A long term follow-up of the resection interposition arthroplasty of the knee using chromicised fascia lata. Int Orthop (SICOT). 1988;12:9-15.

Kondo E, Yamada K. End result of focal debridement in bone and joint tuberculosis and its indications. J Bone Joint Surg. 1957;39A:27-31.

Krantz JJC, Carr CJ. The Phormocologic Principles of Medical practice. William and Wilkins Co. Baltimore. 1958;4:204-19.

Kumar K, Saxena MBL. Multifocal Osteoarticular Tuberculosis. Int Orthop. (SICOT) 1988;12:135-8.

Kumar S, Agarwal A, Arora A. Skeletal tuberculosis following fracture fixiation. A report of five cases. J Bone Joint Surg. 2006;88-A:1101-06.

L

Lacy NJ, Viegas SF, Calhoun J, Mader JT. *Mycobacterium marinum* flexor tenosynovitis. Cl Orthop. 1989;238:288-93.

LaFond EM. An analysis of adult skeletal tuberculosis. J Bone Joint Surg. 1958;40A:346-64.

Lakhanpal VP, Singh H, Sen PC, Tuli SM. Bacteriological study in osteoarticular tuberculosis. Ind J Orthop. 1976;10:13-7.

Lakhanpal VP, Singh H, Tuli SM, Sen PC. *Mycobacterium kansasii* and osteoarticular lesions. Acta Orthop Scand. 1980;51:471-3.

Lakhanpal VP, Tuli SM, Singh H, Sen PC. The value of histology, culture and guinea pig inoculation in osteoarticular tuberculosis. Acta Orthop Scand. 1974;45:36-42.

Lal H, Jain UK, Kannan S. Tuberculosis of pubic symphysis: four unusual cases and literature review. Clin Orthop. 2013;471:3372-80.

Lattimer JK, Rosenberg S, Chowdhury BK, Apperson J, Wechsler H. Genitourinary tuberculosis. Results of therapy. In Transaction of the twenty-first research conference in Pulmonary Disease, Washington DC, Veterans Administration. 1962;78-86.

Lauckner JR. The treatment of tuberculosis in the tropics. J Trop Med Hyg, 1959;62:1-9.

Lauckner JR. Tuberculosis in developing countries. Br Med J. 1964;1:766.

Lee AS, Campbell JAB, Hoffman EB. Tuberculosis of the knee in children, J Bone Joint Surg. 1995;77B:313-18.

Leff A, Lester TW, Addington WW. Tuberculosis. A chemotherapeutic triumph but a persistent socio-economic problem. Arch Ind Med. 1979;139:1375-7.

Leibe H, Koehler H, Kessler P. Osteo-artikulare Tuberculosis: Ruckblick-gegenwartiger Stand von Diagnostik and Therapie. Zentralbl Chir. 1982;107:322-42.

Leibert E, Schluger NW, Bonk S, Rom WH. Spinal tuberculosis in patients with human immunodeficiency virus infection. Clinical presentation, therapy and outcome. Tuber Lung Dis. 1996;77:329-34.

Lettin AWF, Neil MJ, Citron ND, August A. Excision arthroplasty for infected constrained total knee replacements. J Bone joint Surg. 1990;72B:220-4.

Leung PC. Tuberculosis of the hand. Hand. 1978;10:285-91.

Lindberg L. Experimental skeletal tuberculosis in the guinea pig. A method for producing local lesions and autoradiographic study of their accessibility to tritium-labelled dihydrostreptomycin. Acta Orthop Scand, Supplement. 1967;98.

Luck JV. A transverse anterior approach to the hip. J Bone Joint Surg. 1955;37A:534-9.

Lynder AF. Tuberculosis of the greater trochanter: a report of eight cases. J Bone joint Surg. 1982;64B:185-8.

M

Mackaness GB, Smith N. Am Rev Tuberc. 1952;66:125-33.

Madras Tuberculosis Chemotherapy Center. Bull. WHO. 1960;23:535-85.

Mallolas JI, Gatell JM, Rovira M, Conget JI, Trilla A, Soriano E. Vertebral arch tuberculosis in two human immunodeficiency virus seropositive heroin addicts. Arch Intern Med. 1988;148:1125-7.

Manjul KK, Dhammi IK, Jain AK. Unusual skeletal tuberculosis lesion in ribs and ischium. Ind J Orthop. 2000;34:304-5.

Martin T, Cheke D, Natyshak I. Broth culture the modern 'guinea pig' for isolation of mycobacteria. Tubercle. 1989;70:53-6.

Martini M, Benkeddache Y, Medjani Y, Gottesman H. Tuberculosis of upper limb joints. Int Orthop. 1986;10:17-23.

Martini M, Boudjema A, Hannachi MR. Tuberculosis of bone tuberculous osteomyelitis. Acta Orthop Belg. 1981;47:95-103.

Martini M, Boudjeman A, Hannachi MR, Tuberculous osteomyelitis: A review of 125 cases. Int Orthop 1986;10:202-87.

Martini M, Gottesman H. Results of conservative treatment in tuberculosis of the elbow. Int Orthop. 1980;4:83-6.

Martini M, Gottesman H. Tuberculosis of the elbow in tuberculosis of the bones and joints. In: Martini M, Springer-Verlag (Eds), New York, Berlin, Heidelberg. 1988;87-96.

Martini M. Ed. Tuberculosis of the Bones and Joints. Springer-Verlog, Heidelberg. 1988;87-96.

Masood S. Diagnosis of tuberculosis of bone and soft tissue by fine-needle aspiration biopsy. Diagnostic Cytopathology, 8, 1992.

May VR Jr. Shoulder fusion. A review of fourteen cases. J Bone Joint Surg. 1962;44A:65-76.

McCullough CJ. Tuberculosis as a late complication of total hip replacement. Acta Orthop Scand. 1977;48:508-10.

McCullough CJ. Tuberculosis as a late complication of total hip replacement. Acta Orthop Scand. 1978;48:171-4.

Medlar EM, Bernstein S, Reeves F. The demonstration of streptomycin resistant tubercle bacilli in necropsy specimens. Am Rev Tuberc. 1951;63:449-58.

Meltzer RM, Deehl LK, Karlin JM, Silvan SH, Scurran BL. Tuberculous arthritis: A case study and review of the literature J Foot Surg. 1985;24: 30-9.

Menard V. (1894). Cited by Griffith, et al., 1956.

Meng CM. Tuberculosis of the mandible J Bone Joint Surg. 1940;22:17-27.

Menon NK. Intermittent chemotherapy of pulmonary tuberculosis. XVIII International Tuberculosis Conference, Munich, October 5-9, 1965.

Menon NK. Scientific Contributions of the Tuberculosis Chemotherapy Centre, Madras. J Ind Med Assoc. 1966;47:82-8.

Mercer W. Then and Now. The history of skeletal tuberculosis. JR Coll Surg Edinb. 1964;9:243-54.

Millet J, Moreno A, Fina L, Bano L, Orca P, Cayla J. Factors that influence current tuberculosis epidemiology. Eur Spine J. 213;(22 suppl);539-48.

Misgar MS, Nazir AM, Tsering N. Partial synovectomy in the treatment of tuberculosis of the knee. Int Surg. 1982;67:53-5.

Mitchison DA, Chalmer J. Musculoskeletal tuberculosis in Musculo-skeletal Infections Eds. Hughes, SPE and Fitzgerold, R Blackwell Publishers. 1986;186-215.

Mitchison DA. The action of antituberculosis drugs in short course chemotherapy. Tubercle. 1985;66:219-25.

Mittal R, Gupta V, Rastogi S. Tuberculosis of the foot, J Bone Joint Surg. 1999;81B:997-1000.

Mohan V, Danielsson L, Hosni G, Gupta RP. A case of tuberculosis of the scapula. Acta Orthop Scand. 1991;62:79-80.

Moon MS, Kim SS, Lee SR, Moon YW, Moon JL, Moon SI. Tuberculosis of hip in children: A retrospective analysis. Indian J Orthop. 2012;46:191-9.

Moon MS, Kim S, H Moon, Dong K. *Mycobacterium Tuberculosis* in spinal tuberculosis. Asian Spine J. 2017;138-49.

Mousa AR, Muhtaseb SA, Almudallal DS, Khodeir SM, Marafie AA. Osteoarticular complications of brucellosis: A study of 169 cases. Rev Infect Dis. 1987;9:531-43.

Mukopadhya B. Role of excisional surgery in bone and joint tuberculosis Hunterian Lecture. Ann Roy Coll Surg (Eng.). 1956;18:288-313.

N

Neogi DS, Yadav CS, Kumar A, Khan SA, Rastogi S. Total hip arthroplasty in patients with active tuberculosis of the hip with advanced arthritis. Cl Orthop Relat Res. 2010;468:605-12.

Newton P, Sharp J, Barnes KL. Tuberculosis of peripheral joints an often missed diagnosis. J Rheumatology. 1986;13:187-9.

Nocera RM, Sayle B, Rogers C. 99mTc-MDP and Indium-111 chloride scintigraphy in skeletal tuberculosis Clin. Nucl Med. 1983;8:418-20.

Norden CW. Experimental osteomyelitis. I. A description of model. J Inf Dis. 1970;122:410-8.

O

O'Connor BT, Steel WM, Sanders R. Disseminated bone tuberculosis. J Bone Joint Surg. 1970;52A:537-42.

Ohtera K, Kura H, Yamashita T, Ohyama N. Long term follow-up of tuberculosis of the proximal part of the tibia involving the growth plate. J Bone Joint Surg. 2007;89-A:399-403.

Orell S. Chemotherapy and surgical treatment in bone and joint tuberculosis. Acta Orthop Scand. 21:109-203.

Orell S. Streptomycin in the surgical treatment of bone and joint tuberculosis. Acta Orthop Scand. 1951;2;1951;21:113-20.

Ormerod LP, Grundy M, Rahman MA. Multiple tuberculous bone lesions simulating metastatic disease. Tubercle. 1989:70:305-7.

Ostman P. Combined surgical and chemotherapy of abscesses in bone and joint tuberculosis. Acta. Orthop. Scand. 1951;21:204-10.

P

Park JW, Jeon IH, Kim Ys, Yoon JO, Kim JS, Chang JS, et al. Non-tuberculous mycobacterial infection of the musculoskeletal system. Bone Joint J. 2014,96-B,1561-5.

Prasad R, Saxena H, Gupta N, Tanzeem M, Naorem R. Treatment of Drug-Resistant Tuberculosis: Current Status. Ann Natl Acad Med Sci (India). 2021;57:68-73.

Prasad R, Singh A, Gupta N. Adverse Drug Reactions with First-Line and Second-Line Drugs in Treatment of Tuberculosis. Ann Natl Acad Med Sci (India). 2021;57:16-35.

Pablos-Mendez A, Raviglione MC, Laszlo A, et al. Global surveillance for antituberculosis-drug resistance, 1994-1997. New Engl J Med. 1998;338:1641-9.

Pamra SP. Symposium on Chemotherapy of tuberculosis in developing countries. Ind J Tuberc. 1967;15:30-2.

Pandey S. Modified anterior approach to the hip joint. Personal Comm-unication-Ranchi 1985.

Papavasiliou VA, Petropoulos AV. Bone and Joint tuberculosis in childhood. Acta Orthop Scand. 1981;52:1-4.

Parkinson RW, Hodgson SP, Noble J. Tuberculosis of the elbow: A report of five cases. J Bone Joint Surg. 1990;72B:523-4.

Pascon EG, Leung JP. TB arthritis. Current Orthop. 2000;14:197-204.

Patel MR. Mycobacterial infections in Operative Hand Surgery Ed. David Green Churchill Livingstone expected 1997.

Patel PR, Patel DA, Thakker T, Shah K, Shah VD. Tuberculosis of shoulder joint, Ind J Orthop. 2003;37:109-12.

Patel S, Collins DA, Bourke BE. Don't forget tuberculosis. Ann Rheum Dis. 1995;54:174-5.

Panico CT, Oliveira PR, Carvalho VC, Anjos AM, Melo VF, Lima AL. Clinical–epidemiological profile of confirmed cases of osteoarticular tuberculosis. J Bone Joint Infect. 2023;8:11-7.

Pigrau-Serralach, Rodrignez-Pardo. Bone and Joint tuberculosis. Eur Spine J. 2013;22(Suppl):556-66.

Pouchot J, Vinveneux P, Barge J, Boussougant Y, Grossin M, Pierre J, et al. Tuberculosis of the sacroiliac joint: clinical features, outcome, and evaluation of closed needle biopsy in 11 conservative cases. Am J Med. 1988;84:622-8.

Q

Qi-qiu W, Xi-kuan N, Wu-chang T. The concentrations of four antituberculous drugs in cold abscesses of patients with bone and joint tuberculosis. Chinese Med Jr. 1987;100:819-22.

R

Ramakrishnan T, Gopinathan KP, Suryanarayana-Murthy P, Intermediary metabolism of mycobacteria. Bact Rev. 1972;36:65-108.

Ramlakan RJS, Govender S. Sacroiliac Joint tuberculosis. Int orthop. 2007;31:121-4.

Rasool MN, Govender ST, Naidoo KS. Cystic tuberculosis of bone in Children. J Bone Joint Surg. 1994;76B:113-7.

Raunio P. The role of non-prosthetic surgery in the treatment of rheumatoid arthritis by fusions and auto-arthroplasties. Ann Chir Gynaecol. 1985;74(Suppl. 198):96-102.

Reichman LB. Tuberculosis elimination; what's to stop us? Int J Tuberc Lung Dis. 1997;1:3-11.

Reigstad O, Siewers P. A total hip replacement infected with *Mycobacterium bovis* after intravesicular treatment with Bacille-Calmette-Guerin for bladder cancer. J Bone Joint Surg. 2008;90B:225-7.

Rickert J. On Patient Safety: Latent tuberculosis—How we can help address this problem. Clin Orthop Relat Res. 2023;481:1682-3.

Roaf R, Kirkaldy-Willis WH, Cathro AJM. Surgical treatment of bone and joints tuberculosis. Edinburg E & S. Livingstone Ltd. 1959.

Robins RHC. Tuberculosis of wrist and hand. Br J Surg. 1967;54:211-8.

Rook GA, Hernandez—Pando R. T-cells helper types and endocrines in the regulation of tissue-damaging mechanisms in tuberculosis. Immunobiology. 1994;191:478-92.

Rowe CR. Arthrodesis of the shoulder used for treating painful conditions. Clin Orthop. 1983;173:92-6.

Rowe CR. Ed. Shoulder. Churchill Livingstone, New York, 1988.

Runnyon EH. Anonymous mycobacteria in pulmonary disease. Med, Clin North Amer. 1959;43:273-90.

S

Sanchis-Olmos V. Skeletal tuberculosis. The Williams & Wilkins Co, Baltimore, 1948.

Sandher DS, Al-Jibury M, Paton RW, Ormerod LP. Bone and joint tuberculosis: cases in Blackburn between 1988 and 2005. J Bone Joint Surg. 2007;89-B:817-820.

Sandhu HS, Kalhan BM, Dogra S. Management of tuberculosis of the hip joint. current concepts in bone and joint tuberculosis. In: Shanmughasundaram TK (Ed), 147-Periyar EVR Road, Madras 600 010, India 1983.

Sankaran B. Tuberculosis of bones and joints. Ind J Tuberculosis. 1993;40:109-19.

Santavirta S, Eskola A, Kontten YT, Tallroth K, Lindholm ST. Total hip replacement in old tuberculosis: A report of 14 cases. Acta Orthop Scand. 1988;59: 391-5.

Saraf SK, Tuli SM. Tuberculosis of hip: a current concept review. Ind J Orthop. 2015;49:1-9.

Saxena PS, Sharma RK. Value of histopathology, culture and guinea pig inoculation in osteoarticular tuberculosis. Int Surg. 1982;67: 540-7.

Scott JE, Taor WS. The changing pattern of bone and joint tuberculosis. J Bone Joint Surg. 1982;64B:250.

Seber S, Göktürk E, Günal I. Giant tuberculous abscess without primary focus. Acta Orthop Scand. 1993;64:109.

Sepheriadou-Mavropoulou T, Yannoulopoulos A. Tuberculosis of the Jaws J Oral Maxillofac Surg. 1986;44:158-62.

Serafinova R, Malawski S. Principles of treatment of active bone and joint tuberculosis by direct intervention on the lesion. Chir Narzadow Ruchu. 1959;24:437-54.

Sevastikoglou J, Wernerheim B. Some views on skeletal tuberculosis. A statistical report. Acta Orthop Scand. 1953;23:67-84.

Sevastikglou RD, Vauer JH, Murray HL, Kalamarides JJ. Result of treatment of skeletal tuberculosis in Central New York, NYJ Med. 1951;51:2731-6.

Severance RD, Bauer JH, Murray HL, Kalamarides JJ. Results of treatment of skeletal tuberculosis in Central New York, NYJ Med. 1951;51:2731-6.

Shanmugasundaram TK. A clinicoradiological classification of tuberculosis of hip in current concepts in bone and joint tuberculosis. Ed. 147-Periyar EVR Road, Madras 600 010, India, 1983.

Shanmugasundaram TK. Bone and joint tuberculosis, Indian J. Orthop. 2005;39:1958.

Shannon FB, Moore M, Houkom JA, Waecker NJ JR. Multifocal cystic tuberculosis of bone. Report of a case. J Bone Joint Surg. 1990;72A:1089-92.

Sharma SV. Cystic skeletal tuberculosis, Ind J Orthop. 1978;12:65-70.

Sharma SV, Varma BP, Khanna S. Dystrophic calcification in tubercular lesions of bursae Acta Orthop Scand. 1978;49:445-7.

Shembekar A, Babhulkar S. Chemotherapy for osteoarticular tuberculosis. Clin Orthop. 2002;398:20-6.

Sherwani R, Tilak V, Alam S, Sherwani MKA. Carpal tunnel syndrome as the rare initial manifestation of tuberculosis. Ind J Orthop. 2000;34:282-3.

Sidhu AS, Singh AP, Singh AP. Total hip replacement in active advanced tuberculous arthritis. J Bone Joint Surg. 2009; 91B:1301-4.

Silber JS, Whitfield SB, Anbari K, et al. Insidious destruction of the hip by *Mycobacterium tuberculosis* and why early diagnosis is critical. J Arthoplasty. 2000;15:392-7.

Silva JF. A review of patients with skeletal tuberculosis treated at the University Hospital, Kuala Lumpur. Int Ortho. 1980;4:79-81.

Singh B. Tech Rept, to ICMR, 1956;140.

Sinha BN. Osteoarticular tuberculosis. Ind J Tuberc. 1958;5:134-48.

Skoura E, Zumla A, Bomanji J. Imaging in tuberculosis. Int J Infect Dis. 2015;32:87-93.

Smith AD, Yu HI. Streptomycin combined with surgery in treatment of bone and joint tuberculosis. J Am Med Assoc. 1950;142:1-7.

Solheim LF, Kjelsberg F. Recurrent mycobacterial osteomyelitis. Report of a case due to *Mycobacterium avium* intracellulare scrofulaceum complex and BCG innoculation. Arch Orthop Traum Surg. 1982;192:277-80.

Somerville EW, Wilkinson MC. Girdlestone's tuberculosis of bone and joints. 3rd Ed. Oxford University Press, London, 1965.

Southwood TR, Hancock EJ, Petty RE, Malleson PN. Tuberculous rheumatism (Poncets' disease) in a child. Arthritis Rheum. 1988;31:1311-3.

Srivastava KK, Garg LD, Kochar VL. Tuberculous osteomyelitis of the clavicle Acta Orthop Scand. 1974;45:668-71.

Srivastava TP, Anand R. Results of treatment of tuberculosis of elbow joint by chemotherapy and early mobilisation. Unpublished data Banaras Hindu University, 1984.

Srivastava TP, Singh S. Osteoarticular tuberculosis in children. Thesis Banaras Hindu University, Unpublished data, 1987.

Srivastava TP. Tuberculosis of the Elbow Joint_ Proceedings of the Combined Congress of the International Bone and Joint tuberculosis Club and Indian Orthopaedic Association, Madras, India. 1983;12:26-9.

Standford JL, Standford CA. Immunotherapy of tuberculosis with *Mycobacterium vaccae*-NCTC 11659. Immunobiology. 1994;191:555-63.

Stanford JL, Gange JM. The promise of immunotherapy for tuberculosis. Respiratory Med. 1994;88:7.

Steiner P, et al. Primary drug resistance in children; Amer Rev Resp Dis. 1974;110:98-100.

Stevenson FH. The chemotherapy of orthopaedic tuberculosis. J Bone Joint Surg. 1954;36B:5-22.

Stroebel AM, Daniel TM, Lara JHK. Serologic diagnosis of bone and joint tuberculosis by an enzyme-linked immunoabsorbent assay. J Infect Dis. 1982;146:280-3.

Su JY, Lin SY, Liao JS. Tuberculous arthritis of the knee. J West Pacific Orthop Assoc. 1985;22:11-6.

Sunderam G, McDonald RJ, Maniatis JO, Kapila R, Reichman LB. Tuberculosis as a manifestation of the acquired immunodeficiency syndrome (AIDS). JAMA. 1986;256:362-6.

Suryanarayana-Murthy P, Brodie AF. Phosphorylation coupled to the soluble malate vitamin K reductase of *Mycobacterium phlei* Bacteriol. Proceedings. 1966;70.

Sural S, Soni A, Kashyap A, Ahmad V, Hanif M, Khanna A. Spectrum of drug resistance in musculoskeletal tuberculosis. Indian J Orthop. 2021;55(4):907-11.

Sutker WL, Lankford LL, Tompsett R. Granulomatous synovitis. The role of atypical mycobacteria. Rev Infect Dis. 1979;1:729-34.

Sweany HC, Levingston SA. Standnichenko AMS. Tuberculous infection in people dying of causes other than tuberculosis. Am Rev Tuberc. 1943;48:131-73.

T

Tang SC, Chow SP. Tuberculosis of the shoulder: Report of 5 cases treated conservatively. J Roy Coll Surg Edin. 1983;283:188-90.

Tanka M, Matsui H, Tsuji H. Atypical *Mycobacterium osteomyelitis* of the fibula. Int Orthop. 1993;17:48-50.

Thomas O. (1875). Disease of the hip, knee and ankle. Cited by Paus, 1964.

Thornhill TS, Rodney MD, Dalziel W, Sledge CB. Alternatives to arthrodesis for the failed total knee arthroplasty. Clin Orthop. 1982;170:131-40.

Tian Q, Na L, Cao S, Tian Z, Guo Z. Clinical features and surgical management of tuberculous arthritis of the sacroiliac joint: a retrospective analysis of 33 patients. BMC Surg. 2022;22: 322-31.

Tuberculosis Chemotherapy Centre, Madras. Isoniazid plus thioacetazone compared with two regimens of isoniazid plus PAS in the domiciliary treatment of pulmonary tuberculosis in South Indian patients. Bull WHO. 1966;34:483.

Tuberculosis Research Centre, Madras. Ethambutol and Isoniazid for the treatment of Pulmonary Tuberculosis: A controlled trial of four regimens; Tubercle, 1981;61:13-29.

Tuli SM. Preliminary observations of the affect of immunomodulation in multidrug resistant cases of osteoarticular tuberculosis Ind J Orthop. 1999;33:83-5.

Tuli SM, Brighton CT, Morton HE, Clark LW. Experimental induction of localised skeletal tuberculous lesions and accessibility of such lesions to antituberculous drugs. J Bone Joint Surg. 1974;56B:551-9.

Tuli SM, Mishra S. Penetration of antitubercular drugs in cold abscesses of skeletal tuberculosis and in tuberculous joint aspirates. Ind J Orthop. 1983;17: 14-8.

Tuli SM, Mukherjee SK. Excision arthroplasty for tuberculous and pyogenic arthritis of the hip. J Bone Joint Surg. 1981;63B:29-32.

Tuli SM, Sinha GP. Skeletal tuberculosis_"Unusual" lesions, Ind J Orthop. 1969;3:5-18.

Tuli SM. Challenge of therapeutically refractory and multidrug resistant tuberculosis in orthopedic practice. Ind J Orthop. 2002;36:211-3.

Tuli SM. Mutidrug resistant tuberculosis: a challenge in clinical orthopaedics. Ind J Orthop. 2014;48:235-7.

Tuli SM. General principles of osteoarticular tuberculosis. Clin Orthop. 2002;398:11-9.

Tuli SM. Judicious management of tuberculosis of bones, joints and spine. Ind J Orthop. 1984;19: 147-66.

U

Ueng W-N, Shih C-H, Hseuh S. Pulmonary tuberculosis as a source of infection after total hip arthroplasty: a report of two cases. Int Ortho. 1995;19:55-9.

V

Varma BP, Krishnamurthy T. Serological tests for brucellosis in clinico-radiologically diagnosed cases of osteoarticular tuberculosis (unreported). 1973.

Versfeld GA, Solomon A. A diagnostic approach of tuberculosis of bones and joints. J Bone Joint Surg. 1982;64E:446-9.

Vielgut I, Putzl L, Thomüller I, et al. Musculoskeletal tuberculosis revisited: bone and joint tuberculosis in Austria. Arch Orthop Trauma Surg. 2023;143(7):3845-55.

Vishwakarma GK, Khare AK. Amniotic arthroplasty for tuberculosis of the hip, a preliminary clinical study. J Bone Joint Surg. 1986;68B:68-74.

Vohra R, Kang HS. Tuberculosis of the elbow, a report of 10 cases. Acta Orthop. Scand, 1995;66: 57-8.

Vos AM, Meim A, Verver S, et al. High incidence of pulmonary tuberculosis persists a decade after immigration. The Netherlands, Emerg. Infect Dis. 2004;4:736-739.

W

Watson JM. Tuberculosis in Britain today (Editorial). BMJ. 1993;306:221-2.

Wang Y, Wang J, Xu Z, Li Y, Wang H. Total hip arthroplasty for active tuberculosis of the hip. Int Orthop. 2010;34:1111-4.

Watts H, Lifeso RM. Current concepts review: Tuberculosis of bones and joints. J Bone Joint Surg. 1996;78A:288-98.

WHO/HTM/TB/2012.6.2012. Global tuberculosis report.

Wier JA. The present status of ambulatory therapy of tuberculosis. Ann NY Acad Sci. 1963;106: 148-50.

Wild AN, Brems JJ, Boumphrey FRS. Arthrodesis of shoulder: Current indications and operative technique. Orthop Cl North America. 1987;18: 463-72.

Wilkins EG, Hnizdo E, Cope A. Addisonian crisis induced by treatment with rifampicin. Tubercle. 1989;70:69-73.

Wilkinson AG, Roy S. Two cases of Poncet's disease. Tubercle. 1984;65:301-3.

Wilkinson MC, Notley B. Synovectomy and curettage in tuberculosis of joints. J Bone Joint. Surg 1953;35B:209-23.

Wilkinson MC. Observations on the pathogenesis and treatment of skeletal tuberculosis. Ann R Coll Surg Engl. 1949;4:168-92.

Wilkinson MC. Tuberculosis of the hip and knee treated by chemotherapy, synovectomy and debridement: A follow-up study, J Bone Joint Surg. 1959;51A:1343-59.

Williams GT, Williams WJ. Granulomatous inflammation: A review. J Clin Potho. 1983;36: 723-33.

Wilson JN. Tuberculosis of the elbow: A study of 31 cases. J Bone Joint Surg. 1953;35B:551-60.

Winder F. The antibacterial action of streptomycin isoniazid and PAS in Chemotherapy of Tuberculosis. Butterworth and Co., London 1964;111-49.

Wolfgang GL. Tuberculous joint infection. Clin Orthop. 1978;136:257-63.

Wray CC, Roy S. Arthroplasty in tuberculosis of the knee, two cases of missed diagnosis. Acta Orthop Scand. 1987;58:296-8.

Y

Yeager RL. Opening remarks. Ann of NY Acad Sci. 1963;106:3-4.

SECTION III

Tuberculosis of the Spine

A

Adendorff JJ, Boeke EJ, Lazarus C. Tuberculosis of the spine, Results of management of 300 patients, JR Coll Surg Edin. 1987;32:152-5.

Ahn BH. Treatment for Pott's paraplegia. Acta Orthop Scand 1968;39:145-60.

Ahuja K, Kandwal P, Ifthekar S, et al. Development of Tuberculosis Spine Instability Score (TSIS): An Evidence-Based and Expert Consensus-Based Content Validation Study Among Spine Surgeons. Spine (Phila Pa 1976). 2022;47:242-51.

Albee FH. The bone-graft operation for tuberculosis of the spine. J Am Med Assoc. 1930;94:1467-71.

Albee FH. Transplantation of a portion of the tibia into the spine for Pott's disease: A preliminary report. J Am Med Assoc. 1911;57:885-6.

Andrés-Cano P, Cerván A, Rodríguez-Solera M, et al. Surgical infection after posterolateral lumbar spine arthrodesis: CT analysis of spinal fusion. Orthop Surg. 2018;10(2):89-97.

Anley CM, Brandt AD, Dunn R. Magnetic resonance imaging findings in spinal tuberculosis: Comparison of HIV positive and negative patients. Indian J Orthop. 2012;46:186-90.

Alvik I. Tuberculosis of the spine. I. An analysis and follow-up study of 507 patients; II. The mobility of the lumbar spine after tuberculous spondylitis. Acta Chir Scand (Suppl). 1949;141.

Arct MW. Operative treatment of TB of the spine in old people. J Bone Joint Surg. 1968;50A:255-67.

Arizono T, Oga M, Shiota E, Honda K, Sugioka Y. Differentiation of vertebral osteomyelitis and tuberculous spondylitis by magnetic resonance imaging. Int Orthop. 1995;19:319-22.

Arora S, Sabat D, Maini L, et al. Isolated involvement of the posterior elements in spinal tuberculosis: a review of twenty-four cases. J Bone Joint Surg. 2012;94-A:151.

B

Babhulkar SS, Tayado WB, Babhulkar SK. Atypical spinal tuberculosis. J Bone Joint Surg. 1984;66B:239-42.

Bailay HL, Gabriel M, Hodgson AR, Shin JS. Tuberculosis of the spine in children, operative findings and results in one hundred consecutive patients treated by removal of the lesion and anterior grafting. J Bone Joint Surg. 1972;54A:1633-57.

Bakalim G. Tuberculous spondylitis: A clinical study with special reference to the significance of spinal fusion and chemotherapy. Acta Orthop Scand (Suppl). 1960;47.

Baker W de C, Thomas TG, Kirkaldy-Wills WH. Changes in the cartilage of the posterior intervertebral joints after anterior fusion. J Bone and Joint Surg. 1969;51B:736-46.

Batson DV. The function of the vertebral veins and their role in the spread of metastasis. Ann Surg. 1940;112:138.

Bell GR, Stearns KL, Bountti PM, Boumphrey FR. MRI diagnosis of tuberculous vertebral osteomyelitis. Spine. 1990;15:462-5.

Benli IT, Kaya A, Aearoglu E. Anterior instrumentation in tuberculous spondylitis**:** Is it effective and safe? C1 Orthop. 2007;460:108-16.

Berges O, Sassoon C, Roche A, Vanel D Psoas. Abscess of tuberculous origin without visible vertebral lesions. J Radiol (Paris). 1981;62:467-70.

Bhatnagar A, Chakraborty KL, Jain CM, Mishra P, Gupta A, Chopra MK. Diagnosis and assessment of treatment response of Pott's spine using Technetium-99m citrate. A new methodology. Ind J Orthop. 2000;34:245-7.

Bhojraj S, Nene A. Lumbar and lumbosacral tuberculous spondylodiscitis in adults. J Bone Joint Surg. 2002;84-B:530-34.

Boachie-Adjei O, Squillants RG. Tuberculosis of the spine. Orthop Cl, North America. 1996;27: 95-103.

Booysen JT, Vlok GJ, Newton DA, Debeer JF. Magnetic resonance imaging in tuberculous spondylitis. J Bone Joint Surg. 1989;7IB:716 (proceedings).

Bosworth DM, Della Pictra A, Rahilly G. Paraplegia resulting from tuberculosis of the spine. J Bone Joint Surg. 1953;35A:740-57.

Bosworth DM, Wright HA, Fielding JW, Goodrich ER. A study in the use of bank bone for spine fusion in tuberculosis. J Bone Joint Surg. 1953;35A:329-32.

Bosworth DM. Circumduction fusion of the spine. J Bone Joint Surg. 1956;38A: 263-9.

Boulvin R. (1960). Quoted by Paus, in treatment for tuberculosis of the spine. Acta Orthop Scand. (Suppl) 1964;72.

Boxer DI, Pratt C, Hine AL, McNicol M. Radiological feature during and following treatment of spinal tuberculosis. Br J Radiol. 1992;65:476-9.

Buchelt M, Lack W, Kutschera HR, Katterschafka T, Kiss H, Schneider B, et al. Comparison of tuberculous and pyogenic spondylitis: An analysis of 122 cases. Cl Orthop. 1993;296:192-9.

Buchelt. Comparison of tuberculous and pyogenic spondylitis, an analysis of 122 cases. Cl. Orthop. 1993;296:192-9.

Buchowski JM, Adogwa O. What's new in spine surgery. J Bone Joint Surg Am. 2019;101(12): 1043-49.

Butler RW. Paraplegia in Pott's disease, with special reference to the pathology and etiology. Br J Surg. 1935;22:738-68.

C

Cameron JAP, Robinson CLN, Robertson DE. Radical treatment of Pott's disease and Pott's paraplegia by extirpation of diseased area and anterior spinal fusion. Am. Rev. Respir. Dis 1962;86:76-80.

Capener N. (1933). Quoted by Seddon, HJ, Pott's paraplegia prognosis and treatment. Br J Surg. 1935;22:769-99.

Capener N. Vertebral tuberculosis and paraplegia. J Bone Joint Surg. 1967;49B:605-06.

Cauchoix J, Binet JP. Anterior surgical approaches to the spine. Ann R Coll Surg Engl. 1957;21:237-43.

Cauchoix J, Mechelany EF, Tersen G, Morel G, Cotrel Y. (1961) Quoted by Paus, 1964.

Chadha M, Agarwal A, Singh AP. Craniovertebral tuberculosis: a retrospective review of 13 cases managed conservatively. Spine. 2007;32:1629-34.

Chahal AS, Jyoti SP. The radical treatment of tuberculosis of spine. Int Orthop. 1980;4:93-9.

Chakravorty BG. Arterial supply of the cervical spinal cord and its relation to the cervical myelopathy in spondylosis. Ann R Coll Surg Engl. 1969;45:232-51.

Chandler FA, Page MA. Tuberculosis of the spine. End result series studied at the Children's Memorial Hospital, Chicago. J Bone Joint Surg. 1940;22:851-9.

Chatterjee ND, Hira M, Ghosh T, Goswami A. Unsusual presentation of tubercular osteomyelitis of femur. In Jr Orthop. 2003;37:205-6.

Chen WJ, Chen CH, Shich CH. Surgical treatment of tuberculous spondylitis. 50 patients followed for 2-8 years. Acta Orthop Scand. 1995;66:137-42.

Chen WJ, Wu CC, Jung CH, Chen LM, Niu CC, Lai PL. Combined anterior and posterior surgeries in the treatment of spinal tuberculous spondylitis. Clin Orthop. 2002;398:50-9.

Chofnas I, Surrett NE, Severn HD. Pott's disease treated without spinal fusion. Ann Rev Respir Dis. 1964;90:888-98.

Choksey MS, Powell M, Gibb WR, Casey AT, Geddes JS. A conus tuberculoma mimicking an intramedullary tumour: A case report and review of literature. Br J Neurosurg. 1989;31:117-21.

Cholmeley JA. Tuberculous disease of the spine. In Modern Trends in Diseases of the Vertebral Column. In: Nassim R, Burrows HJ (Eds). Butterworth and Co London. 1959;137-41.

Cleveland M, Bosworth DM, Fielding JW, Smyrnis P. Fusion of the spine for tuberculosis in children. J Bone Joint Surg. 1958;40A:91-106.

Cleveland M, Bosworth DM. Pathology of tuberculosis of spine. J Bone Joint Surg. 1942;24:527-46.

Cloward RB. Complications of anterior cervical disc disease. Cl Surg. 1971;69:175-82.

Cook WA. Transthoracic vertebral surgery. Ann Thoracic Surg. 1971;12:54-68.

Cordero M, Sanchez I. Brucellar and tuberculous spondylitis. J Bone Joint Surg. 1991;73B:100-03.

D

Danaviah S, Govender S, Gordon ML, Cassol S. Atypical mycobacterial sypondylitis in HIV-negative patients identified by genotyping. JBone Joint Surg. 2007;89B:146-8.

Dave BR, Kurupati RB, Shah D, Degulamadi D, Borgohain N, Krishnan A. Outcome of percutaneous continuous drainage of psoas abscess: A clinically guided technique. Indian J Orthop. 2014;48:67-73.

de Roos A, van Persijn van Meerten EL, Bloem JL, Bluemm RG. MRI of tuberculous spondylitis. Am J Roentgenol. 1986;147:1979-82.

de Roos A, van Persijn van Meerten EL, Bloem JL. MRI of tuberculous spondylitis. Am J Rad. 1986;147:79-82.

Desai SS. Early diagnosis of spinal tuberculosis by MRI. J Bone Joint Surg. 1994;76B:863-9.

Deshpande SS, Mehta R, Yagnik MG. Short term analysis of healed post-tubercular kyphosis in younger children based on principles of congenital kyphosis. Ind J Orthop. 2012;46:179-85.

Dickson JAS. Spinal tuberculosis in Nigerian children: A review of ambulant treatment. J Bone Joint Surg. 1967;49B:682-94.

Dobson J. Tuberculosis of spine. J Bone Joint Surg. 1951;33B:517-31.

Dommisse GF, Enslin TB. Hodgson's circumferential osteotomy in the correction of spinal deformity (Proceedings). J Bone Joint Surg. 1970;52B:778.

Donaldson JR, Marshall CE. Pott's disease. Ind J Surg. 1965;27:765-73.

Dott NM. Skeletal traction and anterior decompression in the management of Pott's paraplegia. Med J. 1947:54:620-27.

Dunn RN, Husien MB. Spinal tuberculosis. Review of current treatment. Bone Joint J. 2018;100-B:425-31.

E

Editorial Pott's paraplegia. Br Med J. 1968;2:638-9.

Eismont EJ, Bohlman HH, Soni PL, et al. Pyogenic and fungal vertebral osteomyelitis with paralysis. J Bone Joint Surg. 1993;65A:19-29.

Epstein BS. The Spine: A Radiological Text and Atlas. Lea and Febiger, Philadelphia, 1965.

F

Fang D, Leong JCY, Fang HSY. Tuberculosis of the upper cervical spine. J Bone Joint Surg. 1983;65B:47-50.

Fang HSY, Ong GB. Direct anterior approach to the upper cervical spine. J Bone Joint Surg. 1962;44A:1588-604.

Fang HSY, Ong GB. Radical treatment of cervicodorsal spinal tuberculosis. Jr Coll Surg Edinb. 1969;14:20-30.

Fellander M. Radical operation in tuberculosis of the spine. Acta Orthop. Scand (Suppl) 1955;19.

Ferrand J, Chitour S, Sporn Z, Mehdi M. Direct approach to Pott's disease by bony replacement and correction of kyphosis. J Chir (Paris) 1967;93:43-58. Abstracted in Surg Gynecol Obstet.1967;125:933.

Fountain SS, Hsu LCS, Yau ACMC, Hodgson AP. Progressive kyphosis following solid anterior spine fusion in children with tuberculosis of the spine. J Bone Joint Surg. 1975;57A:1104-07.

Francis IM, Das DK, Luthra UK, et al. Value of radiologically guided fine needle aspiration cytology (FNAC) in the diagnosis of spinal tuberculosis: A study of 29 cases. Cytopathology. 1999;10:390-401.

Friedman B. Chemotherapy of tuberculosis of the spine. J Bone Joint Surg. 1966;48A:451-74.

G

Garg B, Kandwal P, Upendra BN, Goswami A, Jayaswal A. Anterior versus posterior procedure for surgical treatment of thoracolumbar tuberculosis: A retrospective analysis. Ind J Orthop. 2012;46:165-70.

Garceu GJ, Bardy TA. Pott's paraplegia. J Bone Joint Surg. 1950;32A:87-96.

Gan J, Zhang C, Tang D, Du X. Surgical treatment of spinal tuberculosis: an updated review. Eur J Med Res. 2024;29(1):588-99.

Goel MK. Pott's paraplegia. Ind J Surg. 1964;26: 825-32.

Goel MK. Treatment of Pott's paraplegia by operation. J Bone Joint Surg. 1967;49B:674-81.

Gokce A, Ozturmen Y, Mutlu S, Gokay NS, Tonbul M, Caniklioglu M. The role of debridement and reconstructin of sagittal balance in tuberculosis spondylitis. Ind J Orthop. 2012;46:145-9.

Govender S, Parbhoo AH. Support of the anterior column with allograft in tuberculosis of the spine. J Bone Joint Surg. 1999;81B:106-09.

Govender S, Parbhoo AH, Kumar KPS, Annamalai K. Anterior spinal decompression in HIV-positive patients with tuberculosis. J Bone Joint Surg. 2001;83B:864-7.

Govender S, Ramnarain A, Danaviah S. Cervical spine tuberculosis in children. Cl Orthop. 2007;460:78-85.

Govender S. The outcome of allografts and anterior instrumentation in spinal tuberculosis. Clin Orthop. 2002;398:60-6.

Green PWB. Anterior cervical fusion. A review of thirty-three patients with cervical disc degeneration. J Bone Joint Surg. 1977;59B:236-40.

Grewal KS, Singh M. Tuberculosis of spine. Ind J Surg. 1956;18:394-405.

Griffiths DL, Seddon HL, Roaf R. Pott's Paraplegia. Oxford University Press, London, 1956.

Griffiths DL. The treatment of spinal tuberculosis. In Mc Kibbin, B Ed. Recent Advances in Orthopaedics. 1979;3:1-17.

Griffiths DLL. Short course chemotherapy in the treatment of spinal tuberculosis: A report from the Medical Research Council's Working Party. Proceedings of the spring meeting of the British Orthopaedic Association, Llandune, UK, 17-19 April, 1985. J Bone Joint Surg. 1986;68B:158.

Gropper GR, Acker JD, Robertson JH. Computed tomography in Pott's disease. Neurosurgery. 1982;10:506-08.

Guirguis AR. Pott's paraplegia. J Bone Joint Surg. 1967;49B:658-67.

Gupta AK, Kumar C, Kumar P, Verma AK, Nath R, Kulkarni CD. Correlatin between neurological recovery and magnetic resonance imaging in Pott's paraplegia. Ind J Orthop. 2014;48:366-73.

Gupta SK, Ganguly SK, Tuli SM, Kumar S. Lateral vertebral shift in tuberculosis of spine, Ind J Radiology. 1973;27:254-7.

H

Hahn MS. Clinical study of spinal tuberculosis. New Medicine Jr. 1977;20:1-6.

Hallock H, Jones B. Tuberculosis of spine. J Bone Joint Surg. 1954;36A:219-40.

Hardy JH, Grossling HR. Combined Halo and Sacral Bar fixation: A method for immobilization and early ambulation following extensive spine fusion. Clin Orthop. 1971;75:205-8.

Harmon PH. Anterior excision and vertebral body fusion operation for intervertebral disc syndromes of the lower lumbar spine. Clin Orthop. 1963;26:107-27.

Harrington KD Metastatic disease of the spine J Bone Joint surg. 1986;68A:1110-5.

Hassan MG. Anterior plating for lower cervical spine tuberculosis. Int Orthop. 2003;27:73-7.

Hayes AJ, et al. Spinal tuberculosis in developed countries: Difficulties in diagnosis. JR Coll Surg Edinb. 1996;41:192-69.

Hibbs RA, Risser JC. Treatment of vertebral tuberculosis by the spine fusion operation. J Bone Joint Surg. 1928;10:805-14.

Hibbs RA. An operation for Pott's disease of the spine. J Am Med Assoc. 1912;59:433 6.

Hibbs RA. Treatment of vertebral tuberculosis by fusion operation. J Am Med Assoc. 1918;71:1372.

Hodgson AR, Skinsnes OK, Leong CY. The pathogenesis of Pott's paraplegia. J Bone Joint Surg. 1967;49A:1147-56.

Hodgson AR, Stock FE, Fang HSY, Ong GB. Anterior spinal fusion: The operative approach and pathological findings in 412 patients with Pott's disease of the spine. Br J Surg. 1960;48:172-8.

Hodgson AR, Stock FE. Anterior spinal fusion for the treatment of tuberculosis of the spine. J Bone Joint Surg. 1960;42A:295-310.

Hodgson AR, Stock FE. Anterior spine fusion. A preliminary communication on the radical treatment of Pott's disease and Pott's paraplegia. Br J Surg. 1956;44: 266-75.

Hodgson AR, Wong W, Yau ACMC. X-ray Appearance of Tuberculosis of the Spine. Charles C. Thomas, Illinois, 1969.

Hodgson AR, Yau ACMC. Anterior surgical approaches to the spinal column, in Recent Advances in Orthopaedics. In: Apley AG (Ed). J and A Churchill, London. 1969;289-323.

Hodgson AR, Yau ACMC. Penetration of lung by the paravertebral abscess in tuberculosis of the spine. J Bone Joint Surg. 1968;50B:243-54.

Hodgson AR. Correction of fixed spinal curves (A preliminary communication). J Bone Joint Surg. 1965;47A:1221-7.

Hodgson AR. Report on the findings and results in 300 cases of Pott's disease treated by anterior fusion of the spine. J West Pacific Orthop Assn. 1964;1:3-7.

Hoffman EB, Crosier JH, Cremin BJ. Imaging in children with spinal tuberculosis: A comparison of radiography, computed tomography and magnetic resonance imaging. J Bone Joint Surg. 1993;75B:233-9.

Hsu LCS, Cheng CC, Leong JCY. Pott's paraplegia of late onset; the causes of compression and results after anterior decompression, J Bone Joint Surg. 1988;70B:534-8.

Huang JJ, Hsu RW, Chen SH, Liu HP Video-assisted theracoscopic surgery in managing tuberculous spondylitis. Clin Orthop. 2000;379:143-53.

Hughes JT. Pathology of the spinal Cord. Lloyd-Luke, London, 1966.

Humphries MJ, Gabriel M Lee YK. Spinal tuberculosis presenting with abdominal symptoms: A report of two cases. Tubercle. 1986;67:303-07.

Hussan K, Elmorshidy E. Anterior versus posterior approach in the surgical treatment of tuberculous spondylodiscitis of thoracic and lumbar spine. Eur Spine J. 2016;25:1056-63.

Hyndman OK. Transplantation of the spinal cord. Surg Gynecol Obstet. 1947:84:460-4.

I

Ito H, Tsuchiya J, Asami G. A new radical operation for Pott's disease. J Bone Joint Surg. 1934:16:499-515.

J

Jackson JW. Spinal tuberculosis. Postgrad Med J. 1971;47:723-4.

Jackson JW. Surgical approaches to the anterior aspect of the spinal column. Ann, R Coll Surg Engl. 1971;48:83-98.

Jain AK. Tuberculosis of the spine: a fresh look at an old disease. J Bone Joint Surg Br. 2010;92(7): 905-13.

Jain AK, Aggarwal A, Dhammi IK, Aggarwal PK, Singh S. Extrapleural anterolateral decompression in tuberculosis of the dorsal spine. Jr. Bone Joint Surg. 2004;86-B:1027-31.

Jain AK, Aggarwal A. Mehrotra G. Correlation of canal encroachment with neurological deficit in tuberculosis of spine. Int Orthop (SICOT). 1999;23:85-6.

Jain AK, Aggarwal PK, Arora A, Singh S. Behavior of the kyphotic angle in spinal tuberculosis. Int Orthop. 2004;28:110-4.

Jain AK, Arora A, Kumar S, Sethi A, Avtar R. Measurement of prevertebral soft tissue space in cervical spine in an Indian population. Ind J Orthop. 1994;28:27-31.

Jain AK, Dhami IK, Sinha S, Kumar V. Management of tuberculosis of spine. Ind J Orthop. 2003;35:194-9.

Jain AK, Dhammi IK. Tuberculosis of the spine: A review. Cl Orthop. 2007;460:39-49.

Jain AK, Dhammi IK, Prasad B, Sinha S, Mishra P. Simultaneous anterior decompression and posterior instrumentation of the tuberculous spine using an anterolateral extrapleural approach. J Bone Joint Surg. 2008;90-B:1477-81.

Jain AK, Jaggi KR, Bhayana H, Saha R. Drug-resistant spinal tuberculosis. Indian J Orthop. 2018;52(2):100-7.

Jain AK, Jain P, Jaggi K, Suresh A, Yadav M, Gain A, Gupta H. Drug-resistant bone, joint and spine tuberculosis: Evolution of diagnosis and treatment. Indian J Orthop. 2024;58(6):661-8.

Jain AK, Jain S. Instrumented stabilization in spinal tuberculosis. Int Orthop. 2012;36:285-92.

Jain AK, Jena A, Tuli SM. Correlation of clinical course with magnetic resonance imaging in tuberculous myelopathy. Neurol India. 2000;48:132-9.

Jain AK, Kumar J. Tuberculosis of spine: neurological deficit. Eur Spine J. 2013:22(Suppl 4):624-33.

Jain AK, Kumar S, Tuli SM. Tuberculosis of spine (C_1-D_4). Spinal Cord. 2000;37:362-9.

Jain AK, Mahishwari AV, Jena S. Kyphus correction in spinal tuberculosis. Cl Orthop. 2007;460:117-23.

Jain AK, Rajasekaran S, Jaggi KR, Myneedu VP. Tuberculosis of the Spine. J Bone Joint Surg Am. 2020;102(7):617-28.

Jain AK, Singh S, Sinha S, Dhammi IK, Kumar S. Intraspinal tubercular granuloma—An analysis of 17 cases. Ind Jr Orthop. 2003;37:182-5.

Jain AK, Sreenivasan R, Mukunth R, Dhammi IK. Tubercular spondylitis in children. Ind J Orthop. 2014;48:136-44.

Jain AK. Treatment of tuberculosis of the spine with neurologic complications. Clin. Orthop. 2002;398:75-85.

Johns D. Syphilitic disorders of the spine. J Bone Joint Surg. 1970;52B:724-31.

Jones BS. Pott's paraplegia in Nigerian. J Bone Joint Surg. 1958;40B:16-25.

Jones R, Lovett RW. Orthopaedic Surgery. London, 1923.

K

Kafle G, Garg B, Mehta N, Sharma R, Singh U, Kandasamy D, et al. Diagnostic yield of image-guided biopsy in patients with suspected infectious spondylodiscitis: a prospective study from a tuberculosis-endemic country. Bone Joint J. 2022;104-B(1):120-6.

Kamara E, Mehta S, James C M Brust, Jain AK. Effect of delayed diagnosis on severity of Pott's disease. Int Orthop. 2012;36(2):245-54.

Kandwal P, Garg B, Upendra BN, Chowdhury B, Jayaswal A. Outcome of minimally invasive surgery in the management of tuberculous spondylitis. Ind J Orthop. 2012;46:159-64.

Kapoor SK, Agarwal PN, Jain BK Jr, Kumar R. Video-assisted thoracoscopic decompression of tubercular spondylitis. Clinical evaluation. Spine (Phila PA 1976). 2005:30E:605-10.

Karapurkar AP. Tuberculous atlantoaxial disease including dislocations. Nimhans Journal. 1988;6suppl.:89-98.

Kastert J. (1951). Quoted by Paus B. in Treatment for tuberculosis of the spine. Acta Orthop. Scand. (Suppl) 1964;72.

Kemp HBS, Jackson JW, Jeremiah JD, Cook J. Anterior fusion of the spine for infective lesion in adults. J Bone Joint Surg. 1973;55B:715-34.

Khanna K, Sabharwal S. Spinal tuberculosis: a comprehensive review for the modern spine surgeon. The Spine Journal. 2019;19:1958-70.

Kirkaldy-Willis WH, Glyn Thomas T. Anterior approaches in the diagnosis and treatment of infections of the vertebral bodies. J Bone Joint Surg. 1965;47A:87-110.

Kohli SB. Radical surgical approach to spinal tuberculosis. J Bone Joint Surg. 1967;49B:668-73.

Konstam PG, Blesovsky A. The ambulant treatment of spinal tuberculosis. Br J Surg. 1962;50:26-38.

Konstam PG, Konstam ST. Spinal tuberculosis in Southern Nigeria with special reference to ambulant treatment of thoracolumbar disease. J Bone Joint Surg. 1958;40B:26-32.

Konstam PG. Spinal tuberculosis in Nigeria. Ann R Coll Surg Engl. 1963;32:99-114.

Korkusuz Z, Binnet, MS, Isiklar ZU. Pott's disease and extrapleural anterior decompression. Results of 108 consecutive cases. Arch Orthop Trauma Surg. 1989;108:349-52.

Kumar K. Tuberculosis of spine: Natural history of disease and its judicious management, J West Pac Orthop Ass. 1988;25:1-18.

Kumar KA. Clinical study classification of posterior spinal tuberculosis. Int Orthop. 1985;9:147-52.

Kumar M, Kumar R, Srivastva AK, Nag VL, Krishnani N, Maurya AK, et al. The efficacy of diagnostic battery in Pott's disease: A prospective study. Ind J Orthop. 2014;48:60-6.

Kumar S, Jain AK, Dhammi IK, Aggarwal AN: Treatment of intraspinal tuberculoma. Cl Orthop. 2007;460:62-6.

L

Lagenskiold A, Riska EB. Pott's paraplegia treated by anterolateral decompression in the thoracic and lumbar spine. Acta Orthop Scand. 1967; 38:181-92.

Laheri VJ, Badhe NP, Dewanany GT. Single stage decompression, anterior interbody fusion and posterior instrumentation for tuberculous kyphosis of the dorsolumbar spine. Spinal Cord. 2001;39:429-36.

Lichtenstein L. Histiocytosisa X: Integration of eosinophilic granuloma of bone, 'Letterer

Siwe disease' and 'Schuller-Christian disease' as related manifestations of a single nosolgic entity. Arch Pathol. 1953;56:84-102.

Lichtor J, Lichtor A. Paleo-pathological evidences suggesting precolumbian tuberculosis of spine. J Bone Joint Surg. 1957;39A:1938-9.

Lifeso R. Atlantoaxial tuberculosis in adults. J Bone Joint Surg. 1987;69B:183-7.

Lifeso RM, Weaver P, Harder EH. Tuberculous spondylitis in adults. J Bone Joint Surg. 1985;64A:1405-13.

Louis R, Conty CR, Pouye I. Operation of Pott's disease with correction of gibbosity (Chirugie du mal de Pott avec correction des gibbosites). J Chin. 1970;99:401-16.

Louw JA. Spinal tuberculosis with neurological deficit. J Bone Joint Surg. 1990;72B, 686-93.

M

Madras Experiment. Lancet. 1961;2:532-3.

Madras Tuberculosis Chemotherapy Centre. A concurrent comparison of home and sanatorium treatment of pulmonary tuberculosis in South India. Bull WHO. 1959;21:51-144.

Madras Tuberculosis Chemotherapy Centre. Bull. WHO. 1960;23:535-85.

Mann JS, Cole RB. Tuberculous spondylitis in the elderly: Potential diagnostic pitfall. Br Med J. 1987;294:1149-50.

Martin AN. Anterior cervical discectomy with or without interbody bone graft. J Neurosurg. 1976;44:290-95.

Martin NS. Pott's paraplegia (A report on 120 cases). J Bone Joint Surg. 1971;53B:596-608.

Martin NS. Tuberculosis of the spine (A study of the results of treatment during the last twenty-five years). J Bone Joint Surg. 1970;52B:613-28.

Masalawala KS. Operative treatment in tuberculosis of the spine. Ind J Surg. 1963;25:311-5.

Masalawala KS. Tuberculosis of vertebral column. A review of evolution of therapy. Ind J Surg. 1967;29:219-26.

Me Afee PC, Bohlman HH, Riley LE, Robinson RA, Southwick WO, Nachlas NE. The anterior retropharyngeal approach to the upper part of the cervical spine. J Bone Joint Surg. 1987;69A: 1371-83.

Medical Research Council. 5-year assessments of controlled trials of ambulatory treatment, debridement and anterior spinal fusion in the management of tuberculosis of the spine. Studies in Bulawayo (Rhodesia) and in Hong Kong: VI Report. J Bone Joint Surg. 1978;60B:163-77.

Medical Research Council. A 10-year assessment of controlled trials of inpatient and outpatient treatment and of Plaster of Paris jackets for tuberculosis of the spine in children on standard chemotherapy. J Bone Joint Surg. 1985;67B:103-10.

Medical Research Council. A 10-year assessment of a controlled trial comparing debridement and anterior spinal fusion in the management of tuberculosis of the spine in patients on standard chemotherapy in Hong Kong: VIII report. J Bone Joint Surg. 1982;64B:393-8.

Medical Research Council. A 15-year assessment of controlled trials of the management of tuberculosis of the spine in Korea and Hong Kong. J Bone Joint Surg. 1998;80B:456-62.

Medical Research Council. A 5-year assessment of controlled trials of in-patient and out-patient treatment and of plaster-of-paris jackets for tuberculosis of the spine in children on standard chemotherapy. J Bone Joint Surg. 1976;58B: 399-411.

Medical Research Council. A controlled trial of ambulant outpatient treatment and inpatient rest in bed in the management of tuberculosis of the spine in young Korean patients on standard chemotherapy. J Bone Joint Surg. 1973;55B: 678-97.

Medical Research Council. A controlled trial of six-month and nine-month regimens of chemotherapy in patients undergoing radical surgery for tuberculosis of the spine in Hong Kong: Tenth report. Tubercle. 1986;67:243-59.

Medical Research Council. Controlled trial of short-course regimens of chemotherapy in the ambulatory treatment of spinal tuberculosis: results at three years of a study in Korea. J Bone Joint Surg. 1993;75B:240-8.

Mehta JS, Bhojraj SY. Tuberculosis of the thoracic spine. A classification based on the selection of surgical strategies. J Bone Joint Surg. 2001;83B: 859-63.

Misra UK, Kalita J. Somatosensory and motor evoked potential changes in patients with pott's paraplegia. Spinal Cord. 1996;34:272-6.

Mittal VA. Anterior spinal artery angiography in Pott's paraplegia. Ind J Orthop. 1990;24:57-9.

Mohanty J, Kurain SP, Somesth KT. Computed tomography in tuberculous Spondylitis: Appearances and staging. Ind J of Orthop. 2000:34:240-4.

Mondal A. Cytological diagnosis of vertebral tuberculosis with fine-needle aspiration biopsy. J Bone Joint Surg. 1994;76A:181-4.

Moon MS. Tuberculosis of spine: current views in diagnosis and management. Asian Spine J. 2014;8(1):97-111.

Moon MS. Development in the management of tuberculosis of the spine. Curr Orthop. 2006;20:132-40.

Moon MS, Ha KY, Sun DH, et al. Pott's paraplegia. Clin Orthop. 1996;323:122-8.

Moon MS, Kim I, Woo YK, Park YO. Conservative treatmentoftuberculosisofthethoracicandlumbar spine in adults and children. Int Orthop. 1987;11: 315-22.

Moon MS, Kim SS, Lee BJ, Moon JL. Spinal tuberculosis in children: Retrospective analysis of 124 patients. Ind J Orthop 2012;46:150-8.

Moon MS, Moon JL, KIM SS, Moon YW. Treatment of tuberculosis of the cervical spine. Cl Orthop. 2007;460:67-77.

Moon MS, Moon YW, Moon JL, Kim SS, Sun DH. Conservative treatment of tuberculosis of the lumbar and lumbosacral spine. Clin Orthop. 2002;398:40-9.

Moon MS, Woo YK, Lee KS, Ha KY, Kim SS, Sun DH. Posterior instrumentation and anterior interbody fusion for tuberculous kyphosis of dorsal and lumbar spines. Spine. 1995;20:1910-16.

Moutla T, Fowles JV, Kassab MT. Pott's paraplegia: A clinical review of operative and conservative treatment in 63 adults and children. Int Orthop. 1981;5:23-9.

Mukherjee SK, Dau AS. Anterior lumbar fusion in Pott's disease. Cl Orthop. 2007;460: 93-9.

Mukopadhaya B, Mishra NK. Tuberculosis of the spine. Ind J Surg. 1957;19:59-81.

N

Nand S. Pott's spine. Acta Orthop Beig. 1972;38:209-16.

Nene AB, Patil S, Kathare AP, et al. Six versus 12 Months of Anti Tubercular Therapy in Patients With Biopsy Proven Spinal Tuberculosis: A Single Center, Open Labeled, Prospective Randomized Clinical Trial-A Pilot study. Spine (Phila Pa 1976). 2019;44(1):E1-E6.

Neville GH Jr, Davis WL. Is surgical fusion still desirable in spinal tuberculosis. Cl Orthop. 1971;75:179-87.

O

O'Brien JP, Yau ACMC, Smith TR, Hodgson AR. Halo pelvic traction. J Bone Joint Surg. 1971;53B:217-29.

Oga M, Arizono T, Takasita M, Sugioka Y. Evaluation of the risk of instrumentaion as a foreign body in spinal tuberculosis. Clinical and biologic study. Spine. 1993;18:1890-4.

Olmarker K, Holm S, Rosenqvist AL, Rydevck B. Experimental nerve root compression. Presentation of a model for acute, graded compression of the porcine cauda equina, with analyses of neural and vascular anatomy. Spine. 1991;16:61-9.

P

Pande KC, Babhulkar SS. Atypical spinal tuberculosis. Clin Orthop. 2002;398:67-74.

Pande KC, Pande SK, Babhulkar SS. An atypical presentation of tuberculosis of the spine. Spinal Cord. 1996;34:716-9.

Pandya SK. Tuberculous atlantoaxial dislocation (with remarks on the mechanism of dislocation). Neurology Inida. 1971;19:116-21.

Parathasarathy R, Sriram K, Satha T, et al. Short course chemotherapy for tuberculosis of the spine: A comparison between ambulant treatment and radical surgery: Ten-year report. J Bone Joint Surg. 1999;81B:464-71.

Parmar H, Shah J, Patkar D, Varma R. Intramedullary tuberculomas: MR findings in seven patients. Acta Radiol. 2000;41:572-7.

Patel J, Upadhyay M, Kundnani V, et al. Diagnostic efficacy, sensitivity, and specificity of Xpert MTB/RIF assay for spinal tuberculosis and rifampicin resistance. Spine (Phila Pa 1976). 2020;45(3):163-9.

Patel P, Patel D, Shah K, Agarwal D. Tuberculosis of the lumbosacral junction. Ind J Orthop. 2000;34:252-5.

Pattisson PRM. Pott's paraplegia: An account of the treatment of 89 consecutive patients. Paraplegia. 1986;24:77-91.

Paus B. Treatment for tuberculosis of the spine. Acta Orthop Scand (Suppl). 1964;72.

Pawar UM, Kundnani V, Agashe V, et al. Multidrug-resistant tuberculosis of the spine--is it the beginning of the end? A study of twenty-five culture proven multidrug-resistant tuberculosis spine patients. Spine (Phila Pa 1976). 2009;34(22):E806-10.

Perros P, Sim DW, Maclntyre D. Psoas abscess due to retroperitoneal tuberculous lymphadenopathy. Tubercle. 1988;69:290-301.

Pieron AP, Welply WR. Halo traction. Acta Orthop Beig. 1972;38:147-56.

Pott P. Remarks on that kind of palsy of the lower limbs which is frequently found to accompany a curvature of the spine and is supposed to be caused by it. London, 1779.

Prabhakar R. A controlled trial of short-course regimens of chemotherapy in patients receiving ambulatory treatment or undergoing radical surgery for tuberculosis of the spine. Ind J Tub. Supp 1989;36.

Puig Guri J. The formation and significance of vertebral ankylosis in tuberculous spines. J Bone Joint Surg. 1947;29:136-48.

Pun WK, Chow SP, Luk KDK, Cheng CL, Hsu LCS, Leong JCY. Tuberculosis of the lumbosacral junction. J Bone Joint Surg. 1990;72B:675-8.

R

Rahman NU. Atypical forms of spinal tuberculosis. J Bone Joint Surg. 1980;62B:162-5.

Rajasekaran S, Rajoli SR, Aiyer SN, et al. A Classification for Kyphosis Based on Column Deficiency, Curve Magnitude, and Osteotomy Requirement. J Bone Joint Surg Am. 2018;100-A:1147-56.

Rajasekaran S, Shanmugasundaram TK, Dheenadharyalan J, Shetty DK. Tuberculous lesions of the lumbosacral region: A 15 year follow up of patients treated by ambulant chemotherapy. Spine. 1998;23:1163-7.

Rajasekaran S, Shanmugasundaram TK. Prediction of the angle of gibbus deformity in tuberculosis of the spine. J Bone Joint Surg. 1987;69A:503-08.

Rajasekaran S, Soundararajan DCR, Shetty AP, et al. Spinal tuberculosis: current concepts. Global Spine J. 2018;8:96S-108S.

Rajasekaran S, Soundarapandian S. Progression of kyphosis in tuberculosis of the spine treated by anterior arthrodesis. J Bone Joint Surg. 1989;71A:1314-23.

Rajasekaran S. Buckling collapse of the spine in childhood spinal tuberculosis. Cl Orthop. 2007;460:86-92.

Rajasekaran S. The natural history of post-tubercular kyphosis in children: Radiological signs which predict late increase in deformity. J Bone Joint Surg. 2001;83B:954-62.

Rajasekaran S. Natural history of Pott's kyphosis. Eur Spine J. 2013:22(suppl 4);634-40.

Rajasekaran S, Khandelwal G. Drug therapy in spinal tuberculosis. Eur Epine J. 2013;22(Suppl):587-93.

Rand C, Smith MA. Anterior spinal tuberculosis: Paraplegia following laminectomy. Ann R Coll Surg Engl. 1989;71:105-09.

Riley LH, Robinson RS, Johnson KA, Walker AE. The results of anterior interbody fusion of the cervical spine. Review of ninety-three consecutive cases. J Neuro Surg. 1969;30:127-33.

Risko T, Novasazel T. Experience with radical operations in tuberculosis of the spine. J Bone Joint Surg. 1963;45A:53-68.

Roaf R. Tuberculosis of the spine. J Bone Joint Surg. 1958;40B:3-5.

Robinson RA, Walker AE, Ferlic DC, Wiecking DK. The results of anterior interbody fusion of the cervical spine. J Bone Joint Surg. 1962;44A: 1569-87.

Rychlicki F, Messori A, Recchioni MA, et al. Tuberculosis spondylitis: A retrospective study on a series of 12 patients operated on in a 25-year period. J Neurosurg Sci. 1998;42:213-9.

S

Safran O, Rand N, Kaplan L, Sagiv S, Floman Y. Sequential or simultaneous, same-day anterior decompression and posterior stabilization in the management of vertebral osteomyelitis of the lumbar spine. Spine. 1998;23:1885-90.

Schmidt AC. Halo-Tibial traction combined with Milwaukee brace. Clin Orthop. 1971;77:73-83.

Schmieden V. Die operative chirurgie der Wirbelsaule Langenbecks. Arch Klin Chir. 1930;162:388-477; Cited by Paus 1964.

Schmorl G, Junghanns H. The Human Spine in Health, and Disease. New York, Grune, 1959.

Schulitz KP, Koth R, Leong JC, Wehling P. Growth changes of solidly fused kyphotic bloc after surgery for tuberculosis. Spine. 1997;22: 1150-5.

Seddon HJ. Pott's Paraplegia in Modern Trends in Orthopaedics. II Series Ed Sir Harry Platt. 1956;230-4.

Seddon HJ. Pott's Paraplegia, prognosis and treatment. Br J Surg. 1935;22:769-99.

Shanmugasundaram TK. Tuberculosis of spine. Ind J Tuberculosis. 1982;29:213-21.

Shaw NE, Thomas TG. Surgical treatment of chronic infective lesions of the spine. Br Med J. 1963;1:162-4.

Shetty AP, Viswanathan VK, Kanna RM,et al. Tubercular spondylodiscitis in elderly is a more severe disease: a report of 66 consecutive patients. Eur Spine J. 2017;26:3178-86.

Shrivastava PK, Singhal SL. Anterior spinal fusion: Preliminary report on direct radical intervention in Pott's spine and Pott's paraplegia. Ind J Surg. 1961;23:452-66.

Shufflebarger HL, Grimm JO, Buiv. Anterior and posterior spinal fusion. Staged versus same day surgery. Spine. 1991;16(8):930-3.

Silverman JF, Larkin EW, Carney M, Weaver MD, Norris HT. Fine needle aspiration cytology of tuberculosis of the lumbar vertebrae (Pott's disease). Acta Cytol. 1986;30:538-42.

Simmons EH, Bhalla SK. Anterior cervical discectomy and fusion. J Bone Joint Surg. 1969;51B:225-37.

Singh V, Kumar A, Patond KR. Extraosseus extradural spinal tuberculosis–A case report. In Jr Orthop. 2005;10:62-3.

Smith AD. Tuberculosis of the spine. Clin Orthop. 1968;58:171-6.

Smith AS, Weinstein MA, Mizushima A, Coughlin B, Hayden SP, Lakin MM, et al. MR imaging characteristics of tuberculous spondylitis versus vertebral osteomyelitis. Am J Roentgenol. 1989;153:399-405.

Smith GW, Robinson RA. The treatment of certain cervical spine disorders by anterior removal of the intervertebral disc and interbody fusion. J Bone Joint Surg. 1958;40A:607-24.

Srivastava TP, Tuli SM. Hydatidosis of the spine and femur: A report of two cases. Ind J Orthop. 1974;5-7:86-9.

Stevenson FH, Manning CW. Tuberculosis of the spine treated conservatively with chemotherapy, series of 72 patients collected 1949-54 and followed to 1961. Tubercle (Edin). 1962;43:406-11.

Stock FE, Hodgson AR. Anterior spinal fusion. Review of 5 years' work. Aust NZJ Surg. 1962;31:161-70.

T

Tian, et al. 2022.

Travlos J, Toit G Du. Spinal tuberculosis: beware the posterior elements. J Bone Joint Surg. 1990;72B:722-3.

Tuli SM, Kumar K, Sen PC. Penetration of antitubercular drugs in clinical osteoarticular tubercular lesions. Acta Orthop Scand. 1977;48:362-8.

Tuli SM, Kumar S. Early results of treatment of spinal tuberculosis by triple drug therapy. Clin Orthop. 1971;81:56-70.

Tuli SM, Srivastava TP, Verma BP, Sinha GP. Tuberculosis of spine. Acta Orthop Scand. 1967;38:445-58.

Tuli SM. Anterior approach to the cervical spine. Ind J Orthop. 1979;13:23-33.

Tuli SM. Historical Aspects of Pott's disease (Spinal Tuberculosis). Eur Spine J. 2013;22(suppl): 529-38.

Tuli SM. Judicious management of tuberculosis of bones, joints and spine. Ind J Orthop. 1985;19:147-66.

Tuli SM. Results of treatment of spinal tuberculosis by "middle-path" regime. J Bone Joint Surg. 1975;57B:13-23.

Tuli SM. Severe kyphotic deformity in tuberculosis of the spine: Current concepts. Int Orthop. 1995;19:327-31.

Tuli SM. Treatment of neurological complications in tuberculosis of the spine. J Bone Joint Surg. 1969;51A:680-92.

Tuli SM. Treatment of tuberculosis of the spine. Ind J Surg. 1973;35: 195-213.

Tuli SM. Tuberculosis of cervical spine. Nimhans Jr. 1988;6Suppl:79-83.

Tuli SM. Tuberculosis of the craniovertebral region, Clin Orthop. 1974;104:209-12.

Tuli SM. Tuberculosis of the spine: A historical review. Cl Orthop. 2007;460:29-38.

Tuli SM. Tuberculosis of the spine; Amerind Publishing Co, New Delhi, 1975.

Tyagi A, Girotra G, Mohta M, Bhardwaj R, Sethi AK. Autonomic dysfunction and adrenal insufficiency in thoracic spine tuberculosis. Cl Orthop. 2007;460:56-61.

U

Ukunda UNF, Lukhele MM. Posterior-only surgical approach in the treatment of tuberculosis of the spine. Bone Joint J. 2018:100-B:1208-13.

Upadhyay SS, Saji MJ, Sell P, Sell B, Hsu LCS. Spinal deformity after childhood surgery for tuberculosis of the spine (A comparison of radical surgery and debridement). J Bone Joint Surg. 1994;76B:91-8.

Upadhyay SS, Saji MJ, Sell P, Yau AIMC. The effect of age on the change in deformity after radical resection and anterior arthrodesis for tuberculosis of the spine. J Bone Joint Surg. 1994;76A:701-8.

V

Valsalan R, Purushothaman R, Raveendran MK, Zacharia B, Surendran S. Efficacy of directly observed treatment short-course intermittent regimen in spinal tuberculosis. Indian J orthop. 2012;46:138-44.

Vyaghreswarudu C, Reddy Y. Evaluation of treatment in tuberculosis of spine. Ind J Surg. 1964;26:911-24.

W

Walmsley R. Anatomy and development. In Modern Trends in Diseases of the Vertebral Column. In: Nassim R, Burrows HJ (Eds). Butterworth and Co, London, 1959;1-28.

Wang LX. Peroral focal debridement for treatment of tuberculosis of the atlas and axis. Chinese J Orthop. 1981;1:207-9.

Wang ST, Ma HL, Lin CP, et al. Anterior debridement may not be necessary in the treatment of tuberculous spondylitis of the thoracic and lumbar spine in adults; a retrospective study. Bone Joint J. 2016;98-B:834-39.

Watts HG, Lifeso RM, Tuberculosis of bones and joints. Current Concepts Review. J Bone and Joint Surg. 1996;78A:288-98.

Weinberg JA. The surgical excision of psoas abscesses resulting from spinal tuberculosis. J Bone Joint Surg. 1957;39A:17-27.

Weinstein JN, McLain RF. Primary tumors of the spine. Spine. 1987;12:84-851.

Wilkinson MC. Curettage of tuberculous vertebral disease in the treatment of spinal caries. Proc R Soc Med. 1950;43:114-6.

Wilkinson MC. The treatment of tuberculosis of spine. J Bone Joint Surg. 1955;37B:382-91.

Wilkinson MC. Tuberculosis of the spine treated by chemotherapy and operative debridement. A long term follow-up study. J Bone Joint Surg. 1969;51A:1331-42.

Wimmer C, Ogon M, Sterzinger W, Landauer F, Stockl B. Conservative treatment of tuberculous spondylitis: A long-term follow-up study. J Spinal Disord. 1997;10:417-9.

Wisneski RJ. Infectious disease of the spine. Orthop Cl North America. 1991;22:491-501.

Wong YW, Leong JCY, Luk Kok. Direct internal kyphectomy for severe angular tuberculous kyphosis. Cl Orthop. 2007;460:124-9.

Wong YW, Samartzis D, Cheung KMC, Luk K. Tuberculosis of the spine with severe angular kyphosis. Bone Joint J. 2017;99-B:1381-8.

Y

Yadav G, Kandwal P, Arora SS. Short-term outcome of lamina-sparing decompression in thoracolumbar spinal tuberculosis. J Neurosurg Spine. 2020;33(5):627-34.

Yang P, Zang Q, Kang J, Li H, He X. Comparison of clinical efficacy and safety among three surgical approaches for the treatment of spinal tuberculosis: a meta-analysis. Eur Spine J. 2016;25:3862-74.

Yau ACMC, Hsu LCS, O'Brien JP, Hodgson AR. Tuberculous kyphosis: correction with spinal osteotomy, halopelvic distraction, an anterior and posterior fusion. J. Bone Joint Surg. 1974;56A:1419-34.

Yilmaz C, Selek HY, Gurkan I, Erdemli B, Korkusuz Z. Anterior instrumentation for the treatment of spinal tuberculosis. J Bone Joint Surg. 1999;81A:1261-7.

Yin XH, Liu SH, Li JS, et al. The role of costotransverse radical debridement, fusion and postural drainage in the surgical treatment of multisegmental thoracic spinal tuberculosis: a minimum 5 year follow up. Eur Spine J. 2016:25:1047-55.

Index

Page numbers followed by *f* refer to figure, *fc* refer to flowchart, and *t* refer to table.

A

F

G

H

Q

R

S

T